PHARMACOCHEMISTRY LIBRARY – VOLUME 7

THEORETICAL DRUG DESIGN METHODS

PHARMACOCHEMISTRY LIBRARY, edited by W. Th. Nauta and R. F. Rekker

Volume 1 The Hydrophobic Fragmental Constant. Its Derivation and Application. A Means of Characterizing Membrane Systems
by R. F. Rekker

Volume 2 Biological Activity and Chemical Structure. Proceedings of the IUPAC-IUPHAR Symposium held in Noordwijkerhout (The Netherlands), August 30—September 2, 1977
edited by J. A. Keverling Buisman

Volume 3 Pharmacochemistry of 1,3-Indandiones
edited by W. Th. Nauta and R. F. Rekker

Volume 4 Strategy in Drug Research. Proceeding of the second IUPAC-IUPHAR Symposium held in Noordwijkerhout (The Netherlands), August 25—28, 1981
edited by J. A. Keverling Buisman

Volume 5 The Chemistry and Biology of Antibiotics
by V. Betina

Volume 6 Quantitative Approaches to Drug Design. Proceedings of the Fourth European Symposium on Chemical Structure — Biological Activity: Quantitative Approaches, Bath (U.K.), September 6—9, 1982
edited by J. C. Dearden

Volume 7 Theoretical Drug Design Methods
by R. Franke

PHARMACOCHEMISTRY LIBRARY
Editors: W. Th. Nauta and R. F. Rekker

Volume 7

THEORETICAL DRUG DESIGN METHODS

by

RAINER FRANKE

Institute of Drug Research,
Research Centre of Molecular Biology and Medicine,
Academy of Science of the GDR,
Berlin, GDR

ELSEVIER

Amsterdam — Oxford — New York — Tokyo 1984

This book is a largely revised and extended English translation of "Optimierungsmethoden in der Wirkstofforschung — Quantitative Struktur-Wirkungs-Analyse", published in 1980 as "Sonderband 2" in the series "Beiträge zur Forschungstechnologie", by Akademie-Verlag, Berlin. It has been translated by J. C. van Gerven in co-operation with the author.

Published in coedition with Akademie-Verlag, Berlin, DDR

This book is exclusively distributed in all non socialist countries by

Elsevier Science Publishers
Molenwerf 1
P. O. Box 211, 1000 AE Amsterdam, The Netherlands

Distributors for the U.S.A. and Canada

Elsevier Science Publishing Company, Inc.
52 Vanderbilt Avenue
New York, NY 10017

Library of Congress Cataloging in Publication Data

Franke, Rainer.
Theoretical drug design methods.
(Pharmacochemistry library ; v. 7)

Translation of: Optimierungsmethoden in der Wirkstoff-forschung.
"Published in coedition with Akademie-Verlag, Berlin, DDR"—T.p. verso.
Includes bibliographical references and index.
1. Structure-activity relationship (Pharmacology)—Mathematical models. I. Title. II. Series. [DNLM: 1. Structure—Activity relationship. 2. Chemistry, Pharmaceutical—Methods. 3. Models, Chemical. W1 PH272L v.7 / QV 744 F8290]

RM301.42F7313 1984 615'.7 83-20781
ISBN 0-444-99634-6 (Vol. 7)
ISBN 0-444-41564-5 (Series)

ISBN 0-444-99634-6 (Vol. 7)
ISBN 0-444-41564-5 (Series)

With 44 Figures and 88 Tables

Printed in the German Democratic Republic

Foreword

In the Introduction to this series in the first volume of the Pharmacochemistry Library we announced that one of the aims of the new series would be to publish basic text-books for the teaching of Quantitative Structure — Activity Relationships (QSAR).

In compliance with this intention, the Editors are fortunate to be able to present as Volume 7 the English version of Professor Rainer Franke's book "Optimierungsmethoden in der Wirkstofforschung", originally published by Akademie Verlag, Berlin, German Democratic Republic, in 1980.

The English text is not merely a translation but rather an updated version with rewritten and new passages, including some that review the literature that has become available since the publication of the original German version.

In our opinion, this publication will be useful to all workers interested in the QSAR field and should enable them to keep abreast of developments in QSAR research.

We also feel that the volume not only satisfies the prerequisites of a basic text-book for teaching purposes but goes beyond this objective, and with this in mind we would like to recommend it to all colleagues engaged in the theory and practice of QSAR.

The book is divided into 15 chapters and includes an Appendix on some principles of linear regression analysis.

An extensive treatise on the extra-thermodynamic approach to the relations between physico-chemical properties on the one hand, and chemical and biological features of compounds on the other, is supplemented by a comprehensive review of more modern methods which came into use during the last years. A wide variety of well documented examples derived from nearly all research areas where QSAR methods demonstrates the power but also limitations of QSAR based approaches to drug design.

May 1983

W. Th. Nauta
R. F. Rekker

Contents

I. Introduction and Formulation of Problems

The design of new compounds for particular purposes is a problem with various aspects. Nearly always it implies that from a wide range of structures those must be selected which meet the requirements most closely. At one time the procedure was to synthesize compounds more or less at random and to see whether they showed the properties desired. In view of the ever increasing number of chemical compounds and in particular the heavier demands to be met by new chemicals, this method is no longer effective; it is too time-consuming, guarantees too little success and is too expensive. As a consequence it was necessary to seek other ways for finding novel compounds. There are, of course, differences in the approach to the search for, e.g., a new dyestuff, a better photosensitizer or a new drug, for each of these has its own specific features, but the basic question — what lines are to be pursued to find the desired compound at minimal cost in the briefest time and with maximal safety — always remains the same. The current situation is characterized by an extremely unfavourable relation between research costs and relevant information obtained. What matters most is to derive clear rules so that access to the information hidden in the individual facts becomes possible. This will require a set of special theoretical methods essentially comprising *quantitative relations between chemical structure and the properties of interest.* In practice, this approach permits rational decisions on further syntheses to be made so that the probability of designing compounds with the desired properties is materially increased.

In the present treatise the application of this approach is illustrated with respect to drug research, an area of special significance which in recent years has witnessed the development of novel technologies. While the specific features of drug research serve as a starting point in this treatise, the results may, in principle, be extended to other problems and research areas as well.

Drugs[1]) are of major importance to human health and nutrition on account of their action on biological and pathological processes. Thus, ca. 70% of clinical results are obtained through medication, and the annual benefit of the world-wide application of pesticides in agriculture runs into thousands of millions of dollars. The use of drugs has shown considerable world-wide increase in recent years, and this tendency will continue until at least the year 2000. This applies not only to already available compounds but especially to new agents with improved or novel properties and ranges of application. Extremely high demands are made on the quality of the new agents. They must be more effective and specific than existing compounds, produce no undesirable side effects in the case of therapeutic application, and aid prophylaxis. In agricultural chemistry more and more emphasis is placed on highly selective, low-residue and en-

---

[1]) By drugs are meant all biologically active compounds, which evoke a desired biologic effect. This definition includes not only human therapeutics but also compounds applied in the veterinary field, and agrochemicals.

vironmentally safe chemicals. These requirements can no longer be satisfied by the classical and essentially empirical mode of research alone. The chance of discovering a new agent has diminished to 1 in 10000 and will decrease even further, whereas development costs have risen to more than 40 million dollars per new drug (cf., the development costs of some 4 million dollars at the start of the 1960's). The range of chemical compounds is virtually boundless, and it will never be possible to explore it fully. This is particularly true in the search for new therapeutics, because the multitude of biological systems and the tests they require have added a new dimension. A random selection from a group of compounds is extremely unlikely to be successful. Thus SPINKS [1] concluded from a retrospective analysis of corresponding test data that for such a procedure to yield one suitable anticonvulsant 400000 compounds would have to be screened. The situation is even more unfavourable with anticancer and antiviral agents, SPINKS claiming that in a purely randomized search some $4 \cdot 10^8$ compounds would have to be investigated before a therapeutically applicable drug would be discovered.

Therefore, any procedure is unavoidably bound to consist of the selection of *sub-systems* from a large group of compounds. A sub-system is in general understood to represent a number of chemical compounds formed by substantial variations in a given parent structure, referred to as the *lead compound*. Needless to say, such a sub-system represents no more than a relatively small segment of the chemical universe. The underlying assumption is that the chance of discovering compounds with the biological properties desired is greater in that segment than in any other. Unfortunately, there are as yet almost no sound criteria by which sub-systems can be selected on the basis of this rationale, so that even the first step in the search for new drugs, which is usually called "*lead generation*", involves a high degree of uncertainty. The most important approaches currently employed to obtain sub-systems or promising lead compounds are as follows (see, e.g. [2, 3]):

1. Mass Screening

As already pointed out, mass screening is, at best, not very effective in finding novel drugs. It must not be forgotten, however, that many of the drugs which came into use in the past were found by just this procedure. The experience and intuition of medicinal chemists have helped to reduce the stochastic nature of mass screening techniques. Mass screening will continue to be applied especially in such areas where rationales for more selective search procedures are difficult to find.

2. Haphazard Discoveries

The discoveries of antifebrin and phenacetin [4] are striking examples. Naphthalene was initially tested as a vermicide. However, it did not show this property but instead a strongly antipyretic action. On subsequent investigation it was found that the test compound was not naphthalene but acetanilide(!) which then became commercially available as antifebrin.

At about the same time, tons of p-aminophenol were available as a by-product in the Bayer factories, and following the discovery of antifebrin, it was converted into p-ethoxyacetanilide to yield phenacetin, which is still in use. It was found later that phenacetin is converted *in vivo* to p-hydroxyacetanilide, and this compound is now also in clinical use (paracetamol).

3. Modification of natural compounds

Accidental findings have frequently played a major role here and continue to do so. A well known example is FLEMINGS discovery of penicillin [5]. The bleeding so often noted in cattle fed on improperly stored hay (sweet clover disease) let to the discovery of dicumarol, a compound that by inhibiting prothrombin synthesis acts as an anticoagulant. A whole family of other anticoagulants have since been derived from dicumarol. 6-Methoxybenzoxazolinone, a pesticide naturally occurring in some maize varieties, was discovered as a result of the resistance to destruction of these plants by weevil larvae. A list of drugs and pesticides accidentally found in this way could be made, and especially in the last few years efforts have been made to further explore this area.

4. Discovery and exploration of side effects

Experience acquired in clinical medicine and pharmacology often plays a decisive role, as illustrated clearly by the case of the sulfonamides. Originally developed as chemotherapeutic agents, sulfonamides produced many side effects, which were subsequently cultivated by appropriate modification of their structure. Among drugs obtained in this way are oral antidiabetics (tolbutamide, chlorpropamide), saluretics (chlorathiazide, furosemide) and antihypertensives (diazoxide).

5. Investigation of drug metabolites

It is by no means uncommon for a drug to be the precursor (pro-drug) of an active ingredient generated metabolically *in vivo*. A classical example of this is sulfanilamide which is a cleavage product of bacteriostatically inactive prontosil rubrum. Its discovery has led to a wide variety of chemotherapeutically active sulfonamides.

6. Chemical modification of natural, endogenous substances

In principle, there are two approaches. Through introduction of so-called bioisosteric groups it is possible to develop drugs similar in action to the model substance itself (mimetics). The object is to obtain compounds exhibiting biologically more favourable properties (e.g., in pharmacokinetic terms) or which are cheaper, that is easier to synthesize.

Another possibility is to alter the structure in such a manner (e.g., by introducing so-called deceptor groups) that antimetabolites, antagonists, antivitamins or antihormones are formed. For this procedure to be meaningful, however, there should be no uncertainty as to the site of action of the drug and the biochemical and physiological consequences of its attack. To a greater or lesser extent there is always the danger that the resulting compounds will exhibit a relatively wide range of side effects and, in extreme instances, even highly toxic compounds are obtained. The latter is, for example, the case with certain cytostatics designed on the basis of the antimetabolite principle. A striking — although in its current form rare — example of the biochemical application of the antimetabolite principle is to be found in the development of the anti-gout agent allopurinol [4]. Allopurinol was prepared by structural modification of xanthine, the substrate of xanthinoxidase, and is an active inhibitor of this enzyme, thereby blocking the degradation of xanthine to the gout-inducing factor uric acid and producing the therapeutic effect. Fortunately, xanthine is rapidly excreted and allopurinol interferes with neither the regulation of nucleotide pools nor the synthesis of nucleic acids. Had these conditions not been fulfilled, the drug would never have found therapeutic application.

All these procedures are rather empirical, and much is being left to accident. The problem becomes even more serious where compounds for hitherto unknown actions have to be designed. It follows that attempts should be made *to predict the properties of new sub-systems from knowledge on already investigated sub-systems* or, in other words, to develop methods for *theoretical lead generation.* This can be done on the basis of several concepts which will be discussed in chapters 11. and 12. It must be stressed, however, that the field of theoretical lead generation is still in its infancy.

Once a lead compound with promising properties has been found the required biological activity must be optimized and side effects eliminated by variations of the chemical structure. In other words, the search for the most favourable compound within the sub-system, the so-called "*lead optimization*" is commenced. This is a lengthy and costly procedure. For example, in the development of antimalarials based on quinine 10000 compounds had to be screened before plasmoquine was obtained, 12000 for atebrin and 14000 for chloroquine. It must be noted that when tested for antimalarial action 10 years earlier, chloroquine had proved ineffective; this points to another type of uncertainty inherent in any screening system [2]. The complex nature of the problem of optimization is best illustrated by giving a simple example (from [6]).

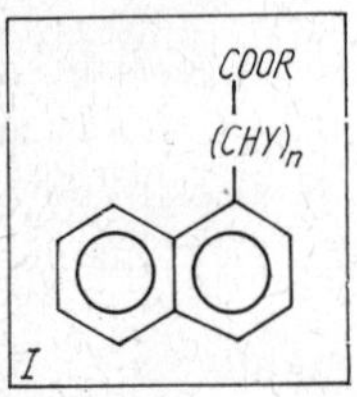

Let us assume that the relatively simple, basic structure depicted in formula I (lead compound) gives the biological action required. Structural variations may be effected through substitution in the ring (in seven positions) as well as through changes in Y, n and R. If only ring substitutions and 50 substituents are considered (a moderate number in comparison with those attainable by current methods of synthesis), the possible compounds obtainable are listed in Table 1.1. In addition, there are, of course, the possible changes in Y, n and R. If, for example, we consider substitutions in four ring positions, ten variations of Y and R and four variations of n, the total number of compounds is 2500000000. Such numbers are astronomical, and even then by no means all

Table 1.1. Number of possible analogues in case of ring-substitution of I by 50 substituents

Number of substituted positions	Number of resulting analogues
1	50
2	2500
3	125000
4	6250000
5	312500000
6	15625000000
7	781250000000

possibilities of variation (such as the introduction of heteroatoms into the ring system) have been included.

Clearly, even sub-systems are far too large for a comprehensive search. It is, therefore, necessary to break down sub-systems into smaller components, mostly involving 20—300 chemical homologues which we will call *samples* or *training series*. If at this stage no further search is made, it follows that it is in such small segments that the optimal compound is expected to be present. However, when comparing the magnitudes of the sub-systems and the samples it will be seen at once that this is extremely unlikely. It is thus necessary *to predict the properties in uninvestigated areas of sub-system space* (*uninvestigated compounds belonging to the sub-system*) *from knowledge of the compounds of the samples* in order to be able to explore the whole space as completely as possible with the minimum number of analogues, and to determine if and where suitable compounds are located in this domain. This procedure makes specific demands on the quantity and nature of such knowledge and thus on the composition of the sample. In general, synthetic feasibility alone is not a sufficient criterium for choice of compounds.

Another major problem in biological screening lies in the choice, sequence and relevance of biological tests. This is a complicated matter, beginning with the selection of biological models. Thus, prontosil rubrum would be rejected as being inactive in an *in vitro* test with bacterial cultures, because, as indicated above, this compound is only a precursor of the bacteriostatic sulfanilamide, which is formed *in vivo* only by metabolic cleavage. The opposite is, of course, also conceivable: a compound discarded as inactive *in vivo* on pharmacokinetic grounds may be extremely active at the required site of action. In such a case one tends to overlook the possibilities offered by structural modification for changing in such a manner the pharmacokinetic properties of the compound that its pharmacodynamic qualities are retained. This means that a combination of *in vivo* and *in vitro* tests is indispensable.

In the search for agents against pathogenic organisms (e.g., bacteriostatics, virostatics, fungicides, herbicides), questions as to the best selection of test objects are bound to arise, for it is impossible to test a compound against all bacteria, virus, mould, weeds and insects in one study. Usually, a few model objects are chosen for concurrent testing. Questions such as how far and along what lines the results with these models can be extended to other organisms, whether there may be substantial gaps or perhaps a certain redundancy, and above all how a variety of results with several objects examined in parallel can be objectively assessed together, as a rule, cannot be answered satisfactorily.

Complex multiple relations may exist between different test. Most of these relations are unknown, however, and will not be revealed unless a specific study is performed. On economic grounds it is recommended that as much information as possible about the biological properties of new compounds should be gathered. For similar reasons it is not feasible to employ all of the battery of tests for any one substance and therefore a pre-selection is unavoidable. Moreover, as the relations between the tests are not fully understood, the criteria of selection are rather crude.

A review of the problems arising from the search for novel drugs poses the following questions:

1. Upon what criteria is the selection of appropriate sub-systems to be based and how can the properties of known lead compounds be used for finding new leads or predicting reasonably correctly biological properties in other sub-systems?

2. How can one obtain that derivative of a known lead exhibiting the most favourable properties with the simplest, safest and most rational strategy or, in other words, with the minimum number of analogues and of tests?
3. What strategy is to be followed to gather the maximum information about biological properties with the minimum of tests, what tests should be done and in what order? How is the flow of substances and information to be organized?

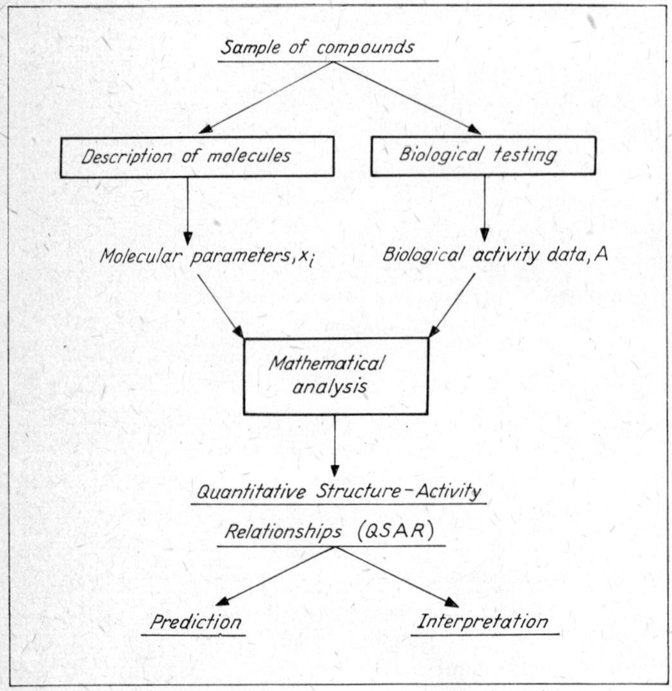

Fig. 1.1. Principle of quantitative structure-activity analysis

To answer these questions an extensive knowledge of specific features of the interactions of drugs and biosystems and thus of structure-activity relationships is required. The theoretical techniques employed for establishing such features are collectively described as *quantitative structure-activity analysis*, the principles of which are illustrated in Fig. 1.1. The basic data underlying this concept are obtained by characterizing a sample of compounds in terms of their biological properties (as demonstrated in biological tests) and their physicochemical properties (as described by their molecular parameters). The resulting biological activity parameters, A, and molecular parameters, x_i, are related, since biological activity is dependent on molecular structure and the resulting properties. Mathematical analysis reveals such connections in the form of so-called *quantitative structure-activity relationships* (QSARs). Once evaluated, these relationships permit the prediction of the biological properties of unexamined compounds. Furthermore, it is possible to obtain information on the mechanism of action at the molecular level and to extend theories along avenues that cannot be explored otherwise at present. Obviously, the only means of studying the pharmacological properties of an intact biosystem (e.g., of the receptor properties *in situ*) consists in perturbing the system and to draw conclusions depending on its response to the applied certurbation. In the case of perturbation by drugs QSARs are indespensible. Theoretical knowledge based on these relations can contribute decisively to the design of novel drugs.

QSARs can be constructed for different purposes and according to different methods. *Structure-response relationships* describe the connections between the magnitude of a given biological effect and the drug structure in a set of congeners[1]); they can therefore be employed to optimize the effect on the basis of structural variations (interpolation in sub-system space). In *structure-selectivity relationships*, a new dimension becomes apparent: the simultaneous consideration of a variety of biological effects (e.g., main actions and side effects) may allow of an integral optimization. *Structure-effect relationships* describe connections between the structure and the nature of the biological effect to be expected. They may, in principle, lead to the prediction of new lead compounds. By considering time and/or drug concentration as additional parameters, complex *structure-activity-time* and *structure-activity-concentration relationships* are obtained which extend significantly the total body of information, and are especially important in such cases where links between a biological effect and time or drug concentration are highly complicated and/or dependent on drug structure. Complex *structure-activity-biosystem relationships* represent an extension of structure-selectivity relations and, to some extent, also permit inter- and extrapolations in the space of biosystems. The study of such relationships has a twofold purpose. It is intended to separate different structure-dependent influences on biological responses (such as pharmacokinetics and drug-receptor interactions) by linking together QSARs for appropriate combinations of biosystems (e.g., hierarchical with respect to the level of biological integration), and to search for criteria and rules for designing and operating biological test systems.

The techniques for quantitative structure-activity analysis have already proved to be of great value. They permit the efficient use of facilities for synthesis and testing and render a successful drug design more likely. The financial savings involved are considerable. Of course, quantitative structure-activity analysis alone is not sufficient to solve all the problems which arise. This follows not only from the limitations of these methods (see chapter 14) but also from the interdisciplinary approach to drug research. Thus, the impact of such disciplines as molecular biology, biochemistry, bioorganic chemistry, physiology and genetics is vitally important. It may not be superfluous to point out that biological tests must be run on statistically sound principles (see e.g. [7]) with strict standards to ensure successful predictive information. Another important point is the need for computer storage and retrieval of results obtained in synthesis, testing and physicochemical and theoretical investigations. A high quality of drug research cannot be achieved unless there is a well balanced interplay of all those intimately involved in both theoretical and experimental work as well as drug manufacture.

The categories sample, molecular description, biological testing, mathematical analysis and the nature and purpose of the quantitative structure-activity relationships (Fig. 1.1) are inter-dependent. There are, of course, degrees of freedom and one should establish carefully how many are available in each case. In the extreme case one could

---

[1]) Congeneric series of drugs comprise substances which can be derived from the same parent structure and produce the biological action of interest through the same mechanism.

desire that the structural variation in the samples and the biological testing (i.e., magnitude, relevance and exactness of the biological parameter) be such that one method of molecular description combined with one mathematical approach can always be applied together in one standard method of quantitative structure-activity analysis. However, this would generally be in conflict with the complexity of biological test materials as well as with the host of possible structures and structural variations. Therefore, several methods must be found for both molecular description and mathematical analysis. It follows that it is not possible to indicate one particular method of structure-activity analysis as the most suitable, any technique being dependent on the problems to be tackled. What matters most is to reconcile structure and structural variation in the sample, biological tests, methods for molecular description and the method for mathematical analysis for each individual problem, while considering the practical facets and relevant aims to be achieved, with the result that the maximum of relevant information is obtained with minimal expense. Most experience with quantitative structure-activity analysis relates to studies and applications of quantitative structure-response relationships, so the following chapters will mainly concentrate on this aspect. Emphasis is placed on those techniques which are applied widely at present and for which sufficient knowledge of their predictive value and range of applications is available. Consideration is given primarily to the basics of the methodology and its use in drug research, and to a lesser extent to theoretical details.

The nucleus of any quantitative structure-activity analysis is always the molecular description, i.e. the elaboration of the most appropriate set of molecular descriptors, mathematical methods only providing a means of manipulating in descriptor space. Consequently, the models to be discussed will first of all be arranged according to the methods of molecular description, which may be placed in three groups:

1. those using chemical and/or physical molecular parameters,
2. those using structural molecular parameters,
3. those arising from interaction calculations.

The first group refers to external molecular parameters such as substituent constants, quantumchemical indices and other suitable physicochemical data. These molecular parameters are then related with biological activity parameters. The second group involves the description of molecular properties and their connection with biological activity directly on the basis of the structural formulae of the drugs. The first step here consists of fragmentation, i.e. breaking down the molecules into fragments, and the second implies either an evaluation of the capacity of the fragments to contribute to biological activity through some scaling factor or the generation of classification rules that make it possible to predict the biological activities of compounds from the presence or absence of certain fragments and/or fragment combinations.

Interaction calculations, finally, serve to describe intermolecular interactions between drugs and receptors as exactly as possible; they are of particular importance for the further development of quantitative structure-activity analysis.

For reviews in the field of quantitative structure-activity analysis see [3] and [8–30].

References

[1] Spinks, A.: Chemistry and Industry **12**, 885 (1973)
[2] Ariens, E. J., in E. J. Ariens (Ed.): Drug Design, Vol. I, Academic Press, New York, 1971, p. 1
[3] Korolkovas, A.: Essentials of Molecular Pharmacology, Wiley, New York, 1970
[4] Hansch, C.: J. Chem. Ed. **51**, 360 (1974)
[5] Maurois, A.: Alexander Fleming, Paul List Verlag, Leipzig, 1962
[6] Hansch, C.: Adv. in Chemistry Series **114**, 20 (1972)
[7] Härtler, G.: Versuchsplanung und statistische Datenanalyse, Vol. 4 in the Monograph Series "Beiträge zur Forschungstechnologie", Akademie-Verlag, Berlin, 1977
[8] Hansch, C., in C. J. Cavallito (Ed.): Structure-Activity Relationships, Pergamon Press, Oxford, 1971
[9] Purcell, W. P., G. E. Bass and J. M. Clayton: Strategy of Drug Design, Wiley, New York, 1973
[10] Hansch, C., in E. J. Ariens (Ed.): Drug Design, Vol. I, Academic Press, New York, 1971, p. 271
[11] Seydel, J. K., in E. J. Ariens (Ed.): Drug Design, Vol. I, Academic Press, New York, 1971, p. 343
[12] Verloop, A., in E. J. Ariens (Ed.): Drug Design, Vol. III, Academic Press, New York, 1972, p. 133
[13] Fujita, T.: Adv. in Chemistry Series **114**, 1 (1972)
[14] Tute, M. S.: Adv. Drug Res. **6**, 1 (1971)
[15] Franke, R., and P. Oehme: Pharmazie **28**, 489 (1973)
[16] Topliss, J. G. (Ed.): Quantitative Structure-Activity Ralationships of Drugs, Academic Press, New York, 1983
[17] Franke, R., and P. Oehme (Eds.): Quantitative Structure-Activity Analysis, Akademie-Verlag, Berlin, 1978
[18] Tichý, M. (Ed.): Quantitative Structure-Activity Relationships, Akadémiai Kiadó, Budapest, 1976
[19] Martin, Y. C.: Drug Design Methods: A Critical Introduction. Marcel Dekker, New York, 1978
[20] Buisman, J. A. Keverling (Ed.): Biological Activity and Chemical Structure, Pharmacochemistry Library (Eds.: W. Th. Nauta and R. F. Rekker), Vol. 2, Elsevier, Amsterdam, 1977
[21] Martin, Y. C., in E. J. Ariens (Ed.): Drug Design, Vol. VIII, Academic Press, New York, 1978
[22] Franke, R., in W. Scheler: Allgemeine Pharmakologie, 2. Auflage, VEB Gustav Fischer Verlag, Jena, 1980
[23] Cramer, R. D.: Ann. Reports Med. Chem. **2**, 30 (1976)
[24] Seydel, J. K., and K.-J. Schaper: Chemische Struktur und biologische Aktivität von Wirkstoffen, Verlag Chemie, Weinheim, 1979
[25] Unger, S. H., in E. J. Ariens (Ed.): Drug Design, Vol. IX, Academic Press, New York, 1980, p. 48
[26] Olson, E. C., and R. E. Christoffersen (Eds.): Computer-Assisted Drug Design, ACS Symposium Ser. **112** (1979)
[27] Knoll, J., and F. Darvas (Eds.): Chemical Structure — Biological Activity Relationships, Académiai Kiadó, Budapest, 1980
[28] Stuper, A. J., W. E. Brugger and P. C. Jurs: Computer Assisted Studies of Chemical Structure and Biological Function, Wiley, New York, 1979
[29] Martin, Y. C.: J. Med. Chem. **24**, 229 (1981)
[30] Dearden, J. C. (Ed).: Quantitative Approaches to Drug Design, Pharmacochemistry Library (Eds.: W. Th. Nauta and R. F. Rekker), Vol. 6, Elsevier, Amsterdam, 1983

2. Measures of Biological Activity A

Before considering methods of quantitative structure-activity analysis, some brief remarks must be made about how to quantify biological activity. Biometric problems will not be discussed here (see e.g. [1]), and a few explanatory notes on the following sections will suffice.

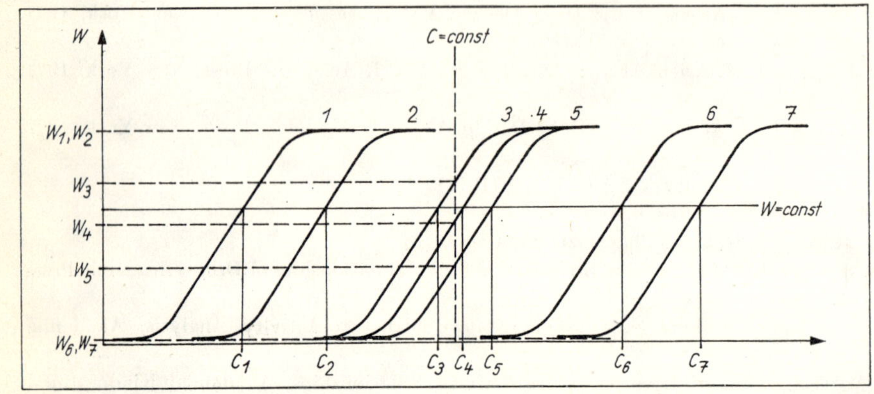

Fig. 2.1. Dose-response curves

It is customary in pharmacological experiments to define biological response, W, as the magnitude of the change in a measurable biological parameter after administration of a drug (e.g. muscle contraction, change in blood pressure, etc.) and to investigate this quantity as a function of drug concentration (dose). This results in *dose-response curves* which, when presented on a semi-logarithmic scale, are sigmoidal in shape (see Fig. 2.1). The biological activities of drugs are compared by considering the concentration (dose), C, which just produces a given response. It is easy to derive the concentration C graphically (any statistical approach is, incidentally, always to be preferred) from the intersections of a straight line parallel to the abscissa with the dose response curves (Fig. 2.1). The intercepts should all lie in the linear part of the curves. In this way variables such as ED_x (dose producing $x\%$ of maximal activity), LD_x (lethal dose for $x\%$ of test objects) and I_x (dose causing an $x\%$ inhibition of a function) are obtained. The biological activity is then simply defined as the reciprocal of that dose:

$$A = 1/C \quad \text{with} \quad W = \text{constant} \tag{2/1}$$

The procedure is, however, only meaningful if at the time that W is measured the system is at equilibrium or at least under steady-state conditions.

In a basically different procedure, measurements are performed at only one (molar!) concentration and the response, W, produced by this concentration is taken as a measure of activity, A, so that:

$$A = W \quad \text{with} \quad C = \text{constant} \tag{2/2}$$

These values of W will correspond to the intersections of the straight line C = constant with the dose-response curves (see Fig. 2.1). It is true that this method saves work but it also has disadvantages. Thus, a smaller range is usually covered and, especially at the lower and higher levels, errors tend to abound. Furthermore, there is always the danger that intersections will occur with non-linear parts of the dose-response curves. No meaningful measure of biological activity will result in this case, as is demonstrated with curves 1 and 2, and 6 and 7, in Fig. 2.1. While on the basis of $A = 1/C$ drug 1 correctly appears to be more active than drug 2, they may falsely be graded as equipotent according to $A = W$. An analogous situation is seen with drugs 6 and 7; from $A = 1/C$ it will correctly be inferred that 6 is more active than 7, whilst $A = W$ again implies that the two are equipotent (which, in the present instance, means inactive). This limitation does not apply if activity A can be defined as a rate according to

$$A = \mathrm{d}W/\mathrm{d}t \tag{2/3}$$

which would appear to be meaningful in many cases [2—4]. Usually, first-order kinetics prevail under such circumstances and, assuming that at the time of measurement, t, one enters the linear part of the curve $W = f(t)$, the response W at time t is directly proportional to the rate constant and is in fact a biologically useful entity. Drug activity is also frequently expressed as a percentage of the activity of a given standard.

This entails a transformation of values as indicated below:

$$A = \frac{\%\ \text{activity of standard}}{(100\% - \%\ \text{activity of standard})} \tag{2/4}$$

For a biological action to occur, the drug must become attached to the biological receptor with the binding best considered as a fusion of drug and receptor (see e.g. [5] and chapter 12.), leading to a perturbation of the receptor. As a result a *biological stimulus*, S, is produced, exerting an observable biological action through a series of biological events. Stimulus S is proportional to the extent of receptor occupancy, y:

$$S \sim y \tag{2/5}$$

On the assumption that the reaction of drug D with receptor R to give a drug-receptor complex DR can be described in terms of the law of mass action with K_1 as equilibrium constant, the occupancy y can be expressed as:

$$y = \frac{[DR]}{[R] + [DR]}$$

$$= \frac{K_1[D]}{1 + K_1[D]} \leq 1 \tag{2/6}$$

To derive an equation from proportionality (2/5), y is multiplied by an appropriately defined intensity term, F, as the factor of proportionality:

$$S = F \cdot y \tag{2/7}$$

Factor F provides a measure of the ability of the drug to perturb the receptor in the specific way required to produce the stimulus. If it is assumed that not only specific (SP) but also non-specific (NSP) perturbations may occur (see [6]), factor F may be regarded as that fraction of the drug-receptor complex DR which is changed into the specifically perturbed state SP:

$$F = \frac{[SP]}{[DR]} = \frac{[SP]}{[SP] + [NSP]} \tag{2/8}$$

The differentiation into agonists, partial agonists and antagonists is based on the magnitude of the factor F. By agonists are meant drugs which in the appropriate dose exert the biologically possible maximal response in a given biosystem. Partial agonists are unable to produce maximal response, even though given in large doses (this indicates a significant contribution from NSP), and antagonists, although combining with the receptor, only produce NSP and thus neither a stimulus nor an action; they are comparable to inhibitors in enzymology. The biological response W is a well defined (but not always known) function of the stimulus S:

$$W = f(S) = f(F \cdot y) \tag{2/9}$$

In many cases this function is likely to be simply linear, but it is also possible for W to show a pronounced saturation behaviour with respect to S so that the highest level of biological response is attained at a submaximal value of S, i.e., at $y \ll 1$. It follows from this behaviour as well as from eqns. (2/6), (2/7) and (2/9) that in order to delineate the action more exactly, it may be necessary to ascertain F and K_1. For this purpose, a variety of methods are available which, however, cannot be discussed here.

Different notations and somewhat dissimilar scaling systems have been used for the factor F; thus, Ariens represents F as the intrinsic activity, α; Stephenson as efficacy, e; Furchgott as intrinsic efficacy, ε and Van Rossum as $\alpha_{AP} = 0{,}5e$ (see also [7—16] for reviews and summaries). Differentiation of F and K_1 is particularly important when a potent antagonist is searched for and chiefly agonists and partial agonists are involved in the sample. The problem is then to minimize F by structural variation and, at the same time, to optimize K_1, i.e., the affinity for the receptor. If, on the other hand, the sample consisted solely of antagonists, it is sufficient to characterize the affinity of the molecules for the receptor. This can be achieved with relative ease by determining the so-called pA_2 value, which is identical with log K_1.

Eqn. (2/6) assumes that an equilibrium or steady-state is attained at the receptor. This is not the only possibility but it is certainly applicable in many cases. Alternatives include the allosteric receptor theories (see [17]) and Pattons kinetic theory [18]. Ultimately, however, these lead to similar mathematical expressions of dose-response curves. It should be borne in mind that it is also possible for drug-receptor complexes to be formed with different stoichiometry (e.g. by a consecutive mechanism), each of these complexes contributing to the stimulus S. Assuming that these contributions may vary in magnitude (with zero and negative contributions being possible), each complex must be assigned its specific value of the factor F. If it is supposed, furthermore, that again the law of mass action is applicable and that the stoichiometries of the complexes may range between DR and D_nR, the stimulus S is presented by the following equation (K_i = equilibrium constant for the formation of the drug-receptor complex D_iR):

$$S = F_1 \frac{K_1[D]}{1 + K_1[D] + K_1K_2[D]^2 + \cdots + \left(\prod_{i=1}^{n} K_i\right)[D]^n} + \cdots + F_n \frac{\left(\prod_{i=1}^{n} K_i\right)[D]^n}{1 + K_1[D] + \cdots + \left(\prod_{i=1}^{n} K_i\right)[D]^n}. \quad (2/10)$$

This model has already proved useful in phytopharmacology [2—4] and, together with methods of quantitative structure-activity analysis, it has allowed some mechanisms of action to be elucidated [19—21].

In addition to the above variables, there are, of course, a large variety of other parameters which have been adapted to suit special needs and they, too, serve as measures of biological activity A. Thus, the biological test may be performed with an enzyme, requiring the use of enzymatic data. Occasionally, it is not feasible to express an activity in quantitative terms. This may be due to the test conditions but also to the complex character of certain biological objects. In such cases, either semi-quantitative data or even just qualitative data simply indicating whether a given compound is active or inactive are obtained.

For any given quantitative structure-activity analysis, the quality of the biological parameter is an essential factor. Knowledge of the accuracy attained is of utmost importance as this will pre-determine the choice of the mathematical procedures and the precision that can be aimed for. It is also of great importance that the biological data are comparable and reproducible within limits of error over any period of time. This requirement, which is not only applicable to the quantitative structure-activity analysis but is also a general feature of any drug comparison, can be satisfied solely by strict test standardization. Any alteration in the biological test object deserves particular consideration, making it necessary either to record precisely defined quality criteria or to eliminate possible fluctuations by using appropriate standards.

A point to which little attention has been paid is that biological systems have a time structure which may lead, e.g., to a short lasting rhythm of biological response [22]. Of even greater importance is the fact that when a drug is applied during different phases of biorhythms, totally different activities may be produced. In these cases, consideration of the biorhythms should be included in test standardization. Conversely, any change in or normalization of biorhythms may be a therapeutic objective in its own right, necessitating the inclusion of biorhythmic parameters in the quantitative structure-activity analysis.

References

[1] Cavalli-Sforza, L.: Biometrie, VEB Gustav Fischer Verlag, Jena, 1969

[2] Franke, R., A. Barth and P. Oehme in F. Coulston and F. Corte (Eds.): Environmental Quality and Safety, Supplement Vol. III, Georg Thieme Verlag, Stuttgart, 1974

[3] Barth, A., R. Franke and D. Börnert in P. Oehme (Ed.): Theoretische Aspekte der Wirkstofforschung, VEB Verlag Volk und Gesundheit, Berlin, 1978
[4] Barth, A., R. Franke and D. Börnert: Pharmazie **31**, 100 (1976)
[5] Burgen, A. S. V., G. C. K. Roberts and J. Feeney: Nature **253**, 753 (1975)
[6] Belleau, B.: J. Med. Chem. **7**, 776 (1964)
[7] Ariens, E. J.: Adv. Drug Res. **3**, 235 (1966)
[8] Stephenson, R. T.: Brit. J. Pharmacol. **11**, 379 (1956)
[9] Furchgott, R. F.: Ann. Rev. Pharmacol. **4**, 21 (1964)
[10] Burgen, A. S. V.: Ann. Rev. Pharmacol. **10**, 7 (1970)
[11] Waud, D. R.: Pharmacol. Rev. **20**, 49 (1968)
[12] Van Rossum, J. M.: Adv. Drug Res. **3**, 191 (1966)
[13] Mackay, D.: J. Pharm. Pharmac. **18**, 201 (1966)
[14] Furchgott, R. F.: Adv. Drug. Res. **3**, 21 (1966)
[15] Mackay, D.: Adv. Drug. Res. **3**, 1 (1966)
[16] Morgenstern, R., in W. Scheler: Grundlagen der allgemeinen Pharmakologie, 2. Auflage, VEB Gustav Fischer Verlag, Jena, 1980
[17] Thron, C. D.: Mol. Pharmacol. **9**, 1 (1973)
[18] Patton, W. D. M., and H. P. Rang: Adv. Drug. Res. **3**, 57 (1966)
[19] Hagemann, R., R. Franke and A. Barth: Vortrag auf der 17. Jahrestagung der Pharmakologischen Gesellschaft der DDR, Berlin, 1975
[20] Franke, R., and A. Barth in T. Kudrev, I. Ivanova and E. Karanov (Eds.): Plant Growth Regulators, Publishing House of the Bulgarian Academy of Sciences, Sofia, 1975
[21] Franke, R., in J. A. Keverling Buisman (Ed.): Biological Activity and Chemical Structure, Pharmacochemistry Library (Eds.: W. Th. Nauta and R. F. Rekker), Vol. 2, Elsevier, Amsterdam, 1977
[22] Barth, A., D. Börnert and R. Franke: Wiss. Z. Univ. Halle **26**, 15 (1977)

3. Extrathermodynamic Approach to Quantitative Structure-Activity Analysis (Hansch Analysis)

The reaction at the receptor may be formally described by:

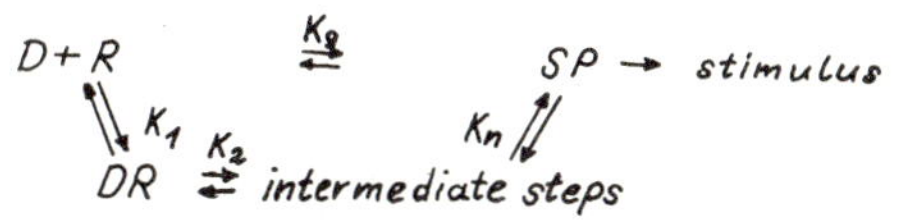

(3/1)

First, a drug-receptor complex DR with equilibrium constant K_1 is formed, leading to a series of intermediate steps ultimately resulting in the specifically perturbed state SP. If the whole chain of reactions may be regarded as a sequence of coupled equilibrium reactions with equilibrium constants, K_i ($i = 1, \ldots, n$), then the overall equilibrium constant, K_g, is given by:

$$K_g = \prod_{i=1}^{n} K_i \tag{3/2}$$

For the concentration of the specifically perturbed state SP, one can state:

$$[SP] = K_g[D]\,[R] \tag{3/3}$$

If the response W is produced at $y \ll 1$, $[DR] \ll [R]$, and $[DR]$ can be omitted from the denominator of eqn. (2/6) which then simplifies to:

$$y = \frac{[DR]}{[R]} = K_1[D] \tag{3/4}$$

The following equation can then be derived from eqns. (2/7), (2/8) and (3/4):

$$S = \frac{[SP]/[DR]}{[DR]/[R]} = \frac{[SP]}{[R]} \tag{3/5}$$

and, combined with (3/3), this gives:

$$S = K_g[D] \tag{3/6}$$

Eqn. (3/6) can also be written as

$$S = K_1 \left(\prod_{i=2}^{n} K_i\right) [D] \tag{3/7}$$

and, substitution from eqn. (3/4) gives:

$$S = \left(\prod_{i=2}^{n} K_i\right) y \tag{3/8}$$

A comparison with eqn. (2/7) yields:

$$F = \prod_{i=2}^{n} K_i \tag{3/9}$$

It appears that the model provides a thermodynamic definition of F which is in agreement with eqn. (2/8). Factor F becomes zero if no SP is produced, and this is exactly what happens when the K_i for any particular step after binding become zero.

In simple *in vitro* tests (e.g. on isolated organs), the concentration of free drug, $[D]$, in the receptor compartment frequently approximates the drug concentration, C. This condition is not fulfilled at an *in vivo* level, because the actual drug concentration on the receptor depends on pharmacokinetic processes (absorption, distribution), metabolism, excretion). Under these circumstances, not $[D]$ but only C is known. In order to express $[D]$ in terms of C the introduction of a transport or distribution function, w (to be discussed later), is required as follows:

$$[D] = wC \tag{3/10}$$

In a biological evaluation according to eqn. (2/1), concentrations are compared at constant response W. Since according to eqn. (2/1) the response is a function of the stimulus (equal stimuli always eliciting equal responses), the stimulus is also constant, and thus it follows from eqns. (3/6) and (3/10):

$$\text{constant} = K_g wC \tag{3/11}$$

$$A = 1/C = K_g w \cdot \text{constant} \tag{3/12}$$

When the biological evaluation is based on eqn (2/2), responses are compared at constant concentrations. Assuming that at a chosen concentration C there exists an approximately linear relation between S and W (an approximately linear part of the curve will be present even if the W/S ratio tends to its saturation value) an analogous expression results:

$$A = W = K_g w \cdot \text{constant} \tag{3/13}$$

The relation between A, K_g and w is, thus, independent of the nature of the definition of biological activity A. Taking logarithms, eqns. (3/12) and (3/13) transform to:

$$\log A = \log K_g + \log w + \text{constant} \tag{3/14}$$

This equation reduces biological activity to a level such that a description by the methods of theoretical and physical chemistry is possible. Alternation to $\log K_g$ with changes of the chemical structure can be described in terms of *linear free enthalpy relationships* (LFERs) for any congeneric set of drugs. Several types of interactions with the receptor must then be taken into account so that, according to the general theory of LFER (see e.g. [1]), a number of terms are needed to describe $\log K_g$:

$$\log K_g = f_h(x_h) + f_e(x_e) + f_s(x_s) \tag{3/15}$$

The functions $f_h(x_h)$, $f_e(x_e)$ and $f_s(x_s)$ characterize the influence of hydrophobic, electronic and steric properties of molecules on the drug-receptor interactions through the corresponding parameters, x, which may appear in a linear as well as in a quadratic form. This division into three terms is, of course, fairly crude and will, as shown later, be achieved only under certain conditions.

The term $\log w$ in eqn. (3/14) is primarily dependent on the hydrophobic properties of the drugs and can be incorporated in the function $f_h(x_h)$ (see 4.4). Therefore, this function should be considered as a linear combination of the two functions $[f_h(x_h)]_I$ and $[f_h(x_h)]_T$ describing, respectively, hydrophobic interactions with the receptor (index I) and the hydrophobic impact on drug transport to the receptor (index T):

$$f_h(x_h) = [f_h(x_h)]_I + [f_h(x_h)]_T \qquad (3/16)$$

The term $\log w$ may also be dependent on other drug properties. This is particularly true for ionizable compounds since charged molecules are absorbed poorly and can scarely penetrate cells. The pK values should then be taken into account. Steric factors will have little effect on the transport of molecules of the size drugs usually have and fortunately there is no active transport with most drugs. A more critical situation arises where metabolic processes play an important role; this requires a special approach, which along with these processes will be discussed later. Taking eqn. (3/16) into consideration

$$\log A = f_h(x_h) + f_e(x_e) + f_s(x_s) + \text{constant} \qquad (3/17)$$

is derived from eqns. (3/14) and (3/15) which describes biological activity within a congeneric series of drugs. *Eqn. (3/17) is the basis of the extra-thermodynamic approach to quantitative structure-activity analysis.* This designation is appropriate in that it is associated with the application of extra-thermodynamic linear free enthalpy relations.

The extra-thermodynamic approach has been named after Hansch ("Hansch *analysis*"), who introduced it in the early sixties and is particularly concerned with its conceptual framework.

Eqn. (3/17) can also be derived from kinetic considerations (see e.g. [2, 3]). If the rate of change of a given biological parameter is considered and a first-order reaction is assumed

$$\mathrm{d}W/\mathrm{d}t = k[D] \qquad (3/18)$$

and substitution from eqn. (3/10) yields:

$$\mathrm{d}W/\mathrm{d}t = kwC \qquad (3/19)$$

Integration of eqn. (3/19) from time and response zero to time t and response W results in:

$$W = kwCt \qquad (3/20)$$

When drugs are compared, t is always constant (in so far as no time dependence is investigated). Biological activity based on eqn. (2/1) may then be expressed as

$$A = 1/C = kw \text{ constant} \qquad (3/21)$$

and based on eqn. (2/2) as:

$$A = W = kw \text{ constant} \qquad (3/22)$$

In logarithmic terms this means:

$$\log A = \log k + \log w + \text{constant} \tag{3/23}$$

Eqns. (3/23) and (3/14) are fully in agreement, except that in the former there is a rate constant instead of an equilibrium constant. The logarithm of a rate constant can be described in terms of linear free enthalpy relationships analogously to that of an equilibrium constant, so that eqn. (3/17) arises directly from eqn. (3/23). In addition, eqn. (3/17) can also be derived from statistical thermodynamics [4]. It should be noted that from a theoretical point of view none of the derivations of eqn. (3/17) is imperative and that any mechanistic picture invariably implies a considerable simplification of the complex biological event. The approach outlined in (3/17) is justified by practice where considerable experience has been gained in the last ten years (see, e.g. [2, 3, 5—24]) rather than by theoretical considerations.

Neglecting for the moment special models to be discussed later, the general analytical form of eqn. (3/17) can be presented as:

$$\log A = a_0 + \sum a_i x_i + \sum b_i x_i^2 \tag{3/24}$$

In this equation the variation of the logarithm of biological activity within a congeneric series of drugs is described by a weighted linear combination of appropriate molecular parameters and their squares. If, for the sample, the values of biological activity A are known and the parameters for the compounds in question are available, the coefficients in eqn. (3/24) can be routinely estimated (see Appendix) in a multiple regression analysis. The result is an equation quantitatively describing log A as a function of the molecular parameters x_i. The specific form of eqn. (3/24) employed will depend on the nature of both the sample (i.e. type of compound or structural variations) and the drug interactions with the biosystem. Since at the outset of a study little, if anything, is known about these interactions, it is necessary to make a number of hypotheses concerning these interactions on the basis of knowledge or assumptions abou tthe chemical properties of the compounds present in the sample and of insight into the biosystem under investigation. Each hypothesis leads to a different form of eqn. (3/24), and for all these equations the regression coefficients and statistical quality criteria have to be evaluated. These criteria and an assessment of other qualitative features eventually afford the most appropriate equation(s), and through the use of the molecular parameters x_i for compounds not yet investigated one can easily estimate their biological activity and find the most promising candidates for further synthesis and testing. In addition, the equations permit predictions of the molecular properties essential to activity and their positive or negative effects.

Finally, the exploration of the "best" equation(s) will provide supporting evidence for the underlying hypotheses, and as a consequence information on the mechanism of action and interactions between drug and biosystem can be obtained.

References

[1] Leffler, J. E., and E. Grunwald: Rates and Equilibria of Organic Reactions, Wiley, New York, 1963

[2] Hansch, C., in C. J. Cavallito (Ed.): Structure-Activity Relationships, Pergamon Press, Oxford, 1971

[3] Purcell, W. P., G. E. Bass and J. M. Clayton: Strategy of Drug Design, Wiley, New York, 1973
[4] Lin, T. K.: J. Med. Chem. **17**, 151 (1974)
[5] Korolkovas, A.: Essentials of Molecular Pharmacology, Wiley, New York, 1970
[6] Hansch, C., in E. J. Ariens (Ed.): Drug Design, Vol. I, Academic Press, New York, 1971, p. 271
[7] Seydel, J. K., in E. J. Ariens (Ed.): Drug Design, Vol. I, Academic Press, New York, 1971, p. 343
[8] Verloop, A., in E. J. Ariens (Ed.): Drug Design, Vol. III, Academic Press, New York, 1972, p. 133
[9] Fujita, T.: Adv. in Chemistry Series **114**, 1 (1972)
[10] Tute, M. S.: Adv. Drug Res. **6**, 1 (1971)
[11] Franke, R., and P. Oehme: Pharmazie **28**, 489 (1973)
[12] Franke, R., in P. Oehme (Ed.): Theoretische Aspekte der Wirkstofforschung, VEB Verlag Volk und Gesundheit, Berlin, 1978
[13] Franke, R., and P. Oehme (Eds.): Quantitative Structure-Activity Analysis, Akademie-Verlag, Berlin, 1978
[14] Tichý, M. (Ed.): Quantitative Structure-Activity Relationships, Akadémiai Kiadó, Budapest, 1976
[15] Martin, Y. C: Drug Design Methods: A Critical Introduction, Marcell Dekker, New York, 1978
[16] Buisman, J. A. Keverling (Ed.): Biological Activity and Chemical Structure, Pharmacochemistry Library (Eds.: W. Th. Nauta and R. F. Rekker), Vol. 2, Elsevier, Amsterdam, 1977
[17] Martin, Y. C., in E. J. Ariens (Ed.): Drug Design, Vol. VIII, Academic Press, New York, 1978
[18] Franke, R., in W. Scheler: Allgemeine Pharmakologie, 2. Auflage, VEB Gustav Fischer Verlag, Jena, 1980
[19] Cramer, R. D.: Ann. Reports Med. Chem. **2**, 30 (1976)
[20] Seydel, J. K., and K.-J. Schaper: Chemische Struktur und biologische Aktivität von Wirkstoffen, Verlag Chemie, Weinheim, 1979
[21] Unger, S. H., in E. J. Ariens (Ed.): Drug Design, Vol. IX, Academic Press, New York, 1980, p. 48
[22] Knoll, J., and F. Darvas (Eds.): Chemical Structure — Biological Activity Relationships, Akadémiai Kiadó, Budapest, 1980
[23] Martin, Y. C.: J. Med. Chem. **24**, 229 (1981)
[24] Franke, R., in J. A. Keverling Buisman (Ed.): Strategy in Drug Research, Pharmacochemistry Library (Eds.: W. Th. Nauta and R. F. Rekker), Vol. 4, Elsevier, Amsterdam, 1982, p. 355
[25] Topliss, J. G. (Ed.): Quantitative Structure-Activity Relationships in Drugs, Academic Press, New York, 1983
[26] Dearden, J. C. (Ed.): Quantitative Approaches to Drug Design, Pharmacochemistry Library (Eds.: W. Th. Nauta and R. F. Rekker), Vol. 6, Elsevier, Amsterdam, 1983

4. Hydrophobic Effects on Biological Activity: the Funktion $f_h(x_h)$

Hydrophobic interactions are of great importance for the process of life. They stabilize membranes and biomacromolecules as well as the binding of hydrophobic ligands to such structures, and they modulate drug activity via drug-receptor or drug-enzyme interactions (see section 4.2.) and the transport to the site of action (see section 4.3.). The term "hydrophobic interactions" is applied to the behaviour of apolar solutes, which tend to avoid contact with water and to enter a hydrophobic phase whenever this is possible. Such a hydrophobic phase can be a hydrophobic solvent (partitioning), the interior of a micelle (solubilization), a hydrophobic region of a protein (protein binding), or a biomembrane (membrane binding).

The key to these interactions is usually considered to be the structure of water, upon which many theories have been advanced (for detailed discussions and overviews see [1—11]). These theories fall into two broad categories: continuum models and mixture models. In the first category, water is regarded as a continuous structure of hydrogen-bonded molecules, differing from ice either in the flexibility [12] or the number [13] of hydrogen bonds. The second category of models is based on the assumption that water is a mixture of different molecular species, including hydrogen-bonded aggregates for which different structures were proposed [14, 15]. Unfortunately, none of these theories is able to account for all experimental behaviour so that a general theory on the structure of water is still awaited. This situation is reflected in the attempts to explain hydrophobic interactions and the properties of aqueous solutions of hydrophobic solutes. Although several formalisms and models have been advanced which yield promising results [4, 5, 9, 11, 15—37], our understanding of hydrophobic interactions is still incomplete. The most widely adopted model in biochemistry and pharmacology is that of SCHERAGA and co-workers [4, 5, 16—19] which is based on the "flickerring cluster" model of liquid water [38, 39]. According to this model, water occurs as a mixture of fluctuating clusters in equilibrium with single water molecules. The clusters are "iceberg"-like structures in which the water molecules are linked together through the largest possible number of hydrogen bonds. When hydrophobic solutes are brought into contact with water a shift in the equilibrium towards the clusters ensues so that water near hydrophobic solutes becomes more structured and, hence, more ordered. This, in turn, results in a sharp decrease in entropy[1]) which is considered the thermodynamic factor which disfavours the contact between water and hydrophobic molecules. When the hydrophobic solutes are removed from this contact by transfer to a hydrophobic phase the equilibrium between clusters and single water molecules is shifted back to the latter, and as a consequence the structure of water becomes less ordered and the entropy increases. This gain in entropy then appears as the real driving force for hydro-

---

1) An alternative explanation was proposed by HOWARTH [40] who believes that the decrease in entropy is due to the restricted motions of hydrophobic solutes in aqueous solutions.

phobic interactions [41, 42], so that such interactions are primarily governed by the repulsion of hydrophobic solutes from the solvent water.

The SCHERAGA model can explain and quantitatively describe most of the features of aqueous solutions of apolar solutes, as well as of the transfer processes of such solutes from water to hydrophobic phases. Although some recent findings are not consistent with this model (especially concerning the dominating role of entropy) [40, 43—45], it at least offers a reasonable line of thinking[1]).

The basic step in all types of hydrophobic interactions is the transfer of hydrophobic solutes from water to a hydrophobic environment, so that hydrophobic interactions of drugs with constituents of biosystems can be regarded as special cases of partitioning with the hydrophobic biophase as "solvent". For a full understanding of such interactions and their dependence on molecular structure it is reasonable, therefore, to consider first the partitioning behaviour, or in a more general sense, transfer processes between aqueous and non-aqueous phases for homologous series of hydrophobic compounds. Knowledge of the basic features of these processes leads immediately to the definition of hydrophobicity parameters, x_h, so that, in the following sections, the functions $[f_h(x_h)]_I$ and $[f_h(x_h)]_T$ for describing the influence of hydrophobicity on biological activity can be formulated.

4.1. Characterization of Hydrophobicity in Homologous Series of Compounds: Systematic Features and Parameters

The transfer of hydrophobic molecules from the aqueous to the organic phase in partitioning can formally be differentiated into two steps. In the first step (step 1) molecules are removed from their contact with water and brought into an ideal gas state, and in the second (step 2) they are dissolved in the hydrophobic organic phase. The change in free standard enthalpy of the partition equilibrium, ΔG_p^0, may then be expressed as

$$\Delta G_p^0 = \Delta G_1^0 + \Delta G_2^0 \qquad (4/1)$$

where ΔG_1^0 represents the contribution from the repulsive interactions with water and ΔG_2^0 that from the interaction with the organic phase. Within homologous series these two contributions can be regarded as products of an intensity variable, I, and a capacity variable, y:

$$\Delta G_p^0 = y_1 I_1 + y_2 I_2 \qquad (4/2)$$

The capacity variable y is a measure of the number of interacting contact sites of the molecules in the aqueous (y_1) and the hydrophobic (y_2) phases, and the intensity variables I_1 and I_2 characterize the intensity of the interactions at these contact sites. Both products in eqn. (4/2) have a negative sign. This equation may also be applied to the dissolution process in water, which is to be regarded (at least for liquids) as the reversal

---

[1]) For the sake of completeness, the model advocated by FRANKS [3] and some others (e.g. [46, 47]) should briefly be mentioned here. According to this model a layer of water molecules between interacting apolar solutes or moieties acts as a sort of intermolecular "glue" in hydrophobic binding.

of a partition step or the partition of a hydrophobic compound between water and itself. The sign must then be reversed, of course.

The two capacity variables y_1 and y_2 are linearly interrelated [20, 44, 48]. If the proportionality factor between them is indicated as k, it follows from eqn. (4/2):

$$\Delta G_p^0 = y_1(I_1 + kI_2) \tag{4/3}$$

The number of interacting contact sites in water, y_1, depends on the size of the cavity necessary to accommodate the solute. Consequently, the *cavity surface area* (CSA) (for a recent review, see e.g. [48a]) should be a good measure of y_1. CSA as defined by HERMAN [20, 21, 49, 50] is the surface formed by the centres of water molecules (regarded as spheres) placed in close contact in all possible positions around a solute molecule; in this way those areas not accessible to the solvent are eliminated. Cavity surface areas can easily be calculated by a simple computer program [51], and replacing y_1 in eqn. (4/3) by CSA gives:

$$\Delta G_p^0 = \alpha \, \text{CSA} \, (I_1 + kI_2) \tag{4/4}$$

α = conversion factor from y_1 to CSA

Within homologous series of hydrophobic compounds having the same electronic properties (e.g., alkanes, alkenes, aromatics) the intensity of the solute-solvent interactions per unit area and hence the bracketed term in eqn. (4/4), is constant. Equation (4/4) than transforms to a simple linear relationship between ΔG_P^0 and CSA:

$$\Delta G_p^0 = a \, \text{CSA} + b \tag{4/5}$$

The sign of the coefficient a is negative for partitioning and positive for the dissolution process in water so that eqn. (4/5) predicts that the free energy becomes increasingly more negative for the former and more positive for the latter process as molecular size increases. In other words, larger apolar solute molecules are more hydrophobic.

Equation (4/5) can be extended to series having one or more polar groups if use is made of the concept of CSA group contributions (44, 52, 53). Thus, the different solvation behaviour of polar groups can be accounted for by resolving CSA into contributions from the apolar part of the molecules, CSA_a, and from the polar groups, CSA_p. In contrast to incremental values of other size-related parameters such as molar volume, molar refractivity or parachor (see below), these group contributions are dependent on how the groups are connected, so that they correctly reflect the real solvation size properties[1]). Equation (4/5) then transforms to

$$\Delta G_p^0 = a_a \, \text{CSA}_a + \sum_i a_i \, \text{CSA}_{pi} + b \tag{4/6}$$

where CSA_{pi} is the group contribution of the ith polar group. The group contribution of the apolar part of the molecules (CSA_a) may be further subdivided if different substructures of that part show different solvation behaviours. As indicated by quantum-chemical calculations [54] this may be expected for branching in aliphatic compounds (see also [48, 53]). In this case, different CSA_a group contributions can be calculated

---

[1]) Note that in such a treatment CSA_p and CSA_a are not constant but are interdependent.

for normal, CSA_a^n, and branched, CSA_a^b, parts of the hydrocarbon chain, and eqn. (4/6) is then expanded to give[1]):

$$\Delta G_p^0 = a_a^n\, CSA_a^n + a_a^b\, CSA_a^b + \sum_i a_{pi}\, CSA_i + b \qquad (4/7)$$

The results of CSA correlations [44] for branched and normal aliphatic compounds having different polar groups (alcohols, ketones, esters of formic, acetic and propionic acids, nitroalkanes) serve to illustrate such relationships in somewhat more detail. In these correlations thermodynamic data for the following equilibria were analysed using the CSA group contribution concept:

(i) transfer of solutes from the gas phase (nitrogen) to water; the free energy of this process is $-\Delta G_1^0$ (see eqn. (4/1)).
(ii) transfer of solutes from the gas phase (nitrogen) to oleyl alcohol; the free energy of this process is ΔG_2^0 (see eqn. (4/1)).
(iii) partitioning in the system oleyl alcohol-water; the free energy of this process corresponds to ΔG_p^0 (see eqn. (4/1)).

The following relationships were obtained (subscripts: OH = hydroxy group in alcohols; C=O = carbonyl group in ketones; HCOO = polar group in formic acid esters; RCOO = polar group in acetic and propionic acid esters with R = CH_3 or C_2H_5; R′COO = polar group in all esters with R′ = H, CH_3 or C_2H_5; NO_2 = nitro group in nitroalkanes)[2]):

(i) transfer from gas phase to water ($P_{g/w}$ = partition coefficient from gas to water):

$$\begin{aligned}\log P_{g/w} = {} & -0.557\, CSA_a^b - 0.484\, CSA_a^n + 1.745\, CSA_{p,OH} \\ & + 0.618\, CSA_{p,C=O} - 0.672\, CSA_{p,HCOO} \\ & - 0.372\, CSA_{p,RCOO} + 3.100 \qquad (4/8)\end{aligned}$$

$n = 53 \quad r = 0.990 \quad s = 0.104$

(ii) transfer from gas phase to oleyl alcohol ($P_{g/ol.}$ = partition coefficient from gas to oleyl alcohol):

$$\begin{aligned}\log P_{g/ol.} = {} & 1.401\, CSA_a + 3.595\, CSA_{p,OH} \\ & + 2.532\, CSA_{p,C=O} + 1.437\, CSA_{p,R'COO} \\ & + 2.212\, CSA_{p,NO_2} - 1.569 \qquad (4/9)\end{aligned}$$

$n = 50 \quad r = 0.994 \quad s = 0.063$

---

1) It should be noted that the effect of branching on the size of the cavity is, of course, accounted for by CSA_a so that normal and branched isomers have slightly different CSA_a values. The separation of CSA_a into CSA_a^b and CSA_a^n accounts for a different effect, namely a different solvation behaviour of normal and branched parts of hydrocarbon chains.

2) ΔG_p^0 is related to log P according to

$$\Delta G_p^0 = -2.303RT \log P$$

so that all equations in ΔG_p^0 also hold for log P, the only difference being the factor $-2.303RT$. In each case, n is the number of data points, r is the correlation coefficient and s the standard deviation (see chapter 15.).

(iii) partitioning in the system oleyl alcohol-water ($P_{ol./w}$ = partition coefficient):

$$\log P_{ol./w} = 1.898\ \mathrm{CSA}_a + 1.657\ \mathrm{CSA}_{p,OH} + 1.376\ \mathrm{CSA}_{p,C=O} + 1.996\ \mathrm{CSA}_{p,HCOO} + 1.480\ \mathrm{CSA}_{p,RCOO} + 2.114\ \mathrm{CSA}_{p,NO_2} - 4.529 \quad (4/10)$$

$$n = 50 \quad r = 0.994 \quad s = 0.096$$

$$\log P_{ol./w} = 1.783\ \mathrm{CSA} - 4.291 \quad (4/11)$$

$$n = 50 \quad r = 0.982 \quad s = 0.154$$

From the coefficients of these correlations, free energies per unit area for the different groups can be calculated; these values are summarized in Table 4.1.

Table 4.1. Free energies per unit area of different aliphatic groups for solvation in oleyl alcohol, hydration, and transfer from water to oleyl alcohol (partitioning) (from [44])

	ΔG^0/area (in J/nm²)		
Group	Solvation	Hydration	Partitioning
normal part of hydrocarbon chain	−8 280	2 870	−11 300
branched part of hydrocarbon chain	−8 110	3 300	−11 610
OH	−21 330	−10 350	−11 320
C=O	−1 502	−367	−1 055
HCOO		3 990	−12 640
RCOO[1])		2 210	−10 500
R′COO[2])	−8 530		
NO_2	−13 120		−13 500

[1]) R = CH_3 or C_2H_5 (see text)
[2]) R′ = CH_3 or C_2H_5 or H (see text)

The goodness of fit of eqns. (4/8)—(4/10) is excellent, and it is pleasing that compounds with different polar groups can be combined in one equation by such a simple treatment. Equation (4/8) is in full agreement with the model presented in eqn. (4/7). As was expected, a small branching effect operates in the hydration process, amounting to a difference of about 400 J/nm² between a methylene group in a normal chain and the same group in a branching position (see also table 4.1.). No extra term is necessary for the nitro group since this group makes only a negligible contribution to the energy of hydration.

The description by eqn. (4/9) of the solvation in oleyl alcohol shows a striking similarity with the hydration process (see also Table 4.1) except for some minor differences. The main difference is that branching effects do not occur on solvation by oleyl alcohol.

Therefore, it is not necessary to resolve CSA_a into CSA_a^b and CSA_a^n, and eqn. (4/9) corresponds to the model presented in eqn. (4/6). Furthermore, the energy of solvation by oleyl alcohol for the polar groups in formic, acetic and propionic acid is about the same (see also Table 4.1.) so that the corresponding group contributions can be merged into one, $CSA_{p,R'COO}$. Finally, the nitro group shows a much higher solvation energy in oleyl alcohol than in water so that a term representing this group now appears in eqn. (4/9).

For partitioning in the system oleyl alcohol-water a different picture emerges. The small branching effect operating in the hydration process is no longer detectable since it is obscured by the overall scatter of the data; eqn. (4/10) thus corresponds to eqn. (4/6). As is to be expected on comparing eqns. (4/8) and (4/9), the contribution of the polar formic acid group has again to be separated from those of the polar groups of acetic and propionic acid esters, and a term for the nitro group appears reflecting its high solvation energy in oleyl alcohol. Most interesting is the fact that, in contrast to hydration and solvation in oleyl alcohol, a good correlation can be obtained, eqn. (4/11), without separating CSA into apolar and polar group contributions. This equation relates $\log P_{ol./w}$ to the total cavity surface area (CSA) of the solutes according to eqn. (4/5), and no relationship of this type showing an acceptable fit could be obtained for either $\log P_{g/w}$ or $\log P_{g/ol.}$. Obviously, the partition coefficient in the system oleyl alcohol-water is not very sensitive to the complex events of solvation in a single phase. This is because, as Table 4.1 shows, the free energy contributions per unit area level off in such a way that the pronounced differences between group contributions which are present for hydration and solvation in oleyl alcohol disappear for the transfer from water to oleyl alcohol or, in general, for partitioning between water and hydrophobic phases. The same holds true for the solubility of organic liquids in water, since the transfer of a solute from its own pure liquid to water is the reverse of a partition process[1]).

The example discussed above and other literature correlations between partition coefficients or water solubilities and CSA [20, 49, 50, 52, 53, 55—61] show that CSA is a very useful hydrophobicity parameter which can be used as x_h in eqn. (3/17). Its applicability depends on the validity of eqns. (4/5)—(4/7) and this, in turn, on the extent to which differences in the solvation behaviour of different groups or substructures occurring in the series considered can be accounted for. If the electronic properties or molecular structures vary too greatly within a series these equations will break down even when applying the concept of group contributions. It is, for instance, not possible to treat alicyclic and aliphatic compounds in one CSA equation[2]), probably

---

[1]) A very interesting conclusion emerges from a comparison of the apolar group contributions to the free energy per unit area for hydration, solvation in oleyl alcohol and partitioning in the system oleyl alcohol—water (Table 4.1). For partitioning this contribution amounts to about $-11300\ J/nm^2$ corresponding to about -3616 J per methylene group. About 70% (-2699 J) of this energy results from the solvation in oleyl alcohol (ΔG_2^0 in eqn. (4/1)), and only about 30% (-919 J) from repulsive interactions with water ($-\Delta G_1^0$, eqn. (4/1)). In full agreement with the views presented by Cramer [43] and an earlier estimate made by Amidon et al. [53], this observation clearly contradicts the classical theory of hydrophobic interactions as outlined at the beginning of this section (for a further discussion, see also Abraham [45]).

[2]) Some authors have, in fact, presented CSA equations for such series of compounds. Although these equations usually show a good fit as judged by r and s, closer inspection always reveals that alicyclic compounds show very large deviations.

because the different "densities" of carbon atoms within the cavity result in different values of the scaling factor, α, in eqn. (4/4).

Since cavity surface areas are, of course, related to the size of molecules, within many series of compounds CSA is closely correlated to a number of simple size parameters such as molar volume, molar refractivity, parachor and connectivity. It is not surprising, therefore, that a large number of correlations between partition coefficients or water solubilities and such quantities have been reported in the literature [48, 62—77]. Within certain limits these quantities can also be regarded as hydrophobicity parameters. These limits depend on how closely such simple size parameters are related to CSA or to CSA group contributions, and, in turn, on the uniformity of the solvation process for different parts of molecular structures throughout the series considered. For example, simple size parameters do not usually account adequately for branching effects[1]), and it is impossible to describe the influence of different polar groups by such global quantities. MORIGUCHI et al. [66] developed a group contribution concept on the basis of the VAN DER WAALS volume, separating the volume contribution of polar groups from that of the apolar part; they also introduced a branching correction. With the help of this concept they were able to obtain a fair correlation for the solubility of 156 organic liquids in water. In comparison with the concept of CSA group contributions this approach is very empirical. The same is true of a similar approach applied by KIER and colleagues who used connectivity group contributions [76]. Generally speaking, simple size parameters can be considered as truly representing hydrophobicity only when the compounds of the series investigated are electronically very similar and also not too different in their molecular geometry (see also [48]). Special problems arise when size effects on biological activity are to be differentiated from hydrophobic effects; these problems will be dealt with later.

It should be noted that in the case of n-alkyl compounds the relation between CSA and the above parameters is in fact only linear from C_3 onward, and that relations according to eqn. (4/5) are disturbed if highly charged groups such as the onium group occur, because the charge is spread over adjacent C atoms; the influence of such a charge extends over ca. 0.5 nm, corresponding to three C atoms [17, 78]. On this basis, eqn. (4/5) will not be valid in e.g. tetraalkylammonium compounds until C_4 onward; replacing protons in the ammonium ion by methyl groups which, of course, increases molecular size even lowers hydrophobicity [79]. With long-chain alkane derivatives the possibility of the hydrocarbon chain coiling up and/or self-associations which would result in a decrease of CSA should be considered [37]. Such effects seem not to be important, however, if the chain consists of less that twelve C atoms [37, 48, 80—82].

In the early 1950s COLLANDER [83, 84] established empirically that the partition coefficients in different partitioning systems within a given series of compounds are closely connected according to eqn. (4/12)

$$\log P_{II} = a_p \log P_I + b \qquad (4/12)$$

where P_I is the partition coefficient in organic phase I-water and P_{II} that in organic phase II-water. Eqn. (4/12) is also valid if $\log P_I$ or $\log P_{II}$ are replaced by $-\log c_s$

1) Such effects are usually quite small and may be neglected to a first approximation in many cases. Some authors have tried to use modified parameter sets empirically corrected for branching.

(c_s = water solubility). A large number of relations based on eqn. (4/12) have been published in recent years [48, 80, 85—89] so that the equations may be said to have good empirical foundation. It may, however, also be theoretically derived from eqn. (4/3) [48] (for a detailed analysis of the solvent dependence of $\log P$, see [82a]). In this context, mention must be made of an additional factor which, while playing no role in the discussion of any individual partitioning system, should be allowed for when comparing partitioning in different systems. Such a comparison cannot be made unless the mutual miscibilities of the respective phases are taken into account because as the miscibility increases the hydrophobicity of the organic phase and the hydrophilicity of the aqueous phase decrease and thus the distinction between the two phases diminishes. This implies that the absolute values of the partition coefficients decrease and the differences between the partition coefficients for molecules of different hydrophobicity becomes less overt. In other words, within a series of compounds both the zero point as well as the scaling of partition coefficients with respect to hydrophobicity are different for partitioning systems with different features of miscibility. Formally, this effect may be treated by selecting a given partitioning system as a standard and using the scale of partition coefficients determined in this system as the standard scale. With the help of this standard scale it is then possible to compare partitioning systems. For eqn. (4/3) this implies that $\Delta G_p{}^0$ for partitioning systems having a mixing ratio different from that of the standard system must be normalized to this scale. Range-spread and zero point can easily be corrected for by multiplying eqn. (4/3) by a scaling factor, s, and addition of a constant term, c (zero point correction); for the standard system $s = 1$ and $c = 0$. Multiplication by the scaling factor is equivalent to a correction of the number of interacting contact sites and is, therefore, meaningful from a physical point of view.

For the two partitioning systems I and II this leads to:

$$\Delta G^0_{p,I} = s_{\mathrm{I}} y(I_1 + kI_{2,\mathrm{I}}) + c_{\mathrm{I}} \quad (4/13)$$

$$\Delta G^0_{p,II} = s_{\mathrm{II}} y(I_1 + kI_{2,\mathrm{II}}) + c_{\mathrm{II}} \quad (4/14)$$

In cases where identical interactions with the molecules of the series under consideration occur in organic phases I and II, analogous changes with solute structure take place in $I_{2,\mathrm{I}}$ and $I_{2,\mathrm{II}}$ for all solute molecules. It follows then from (4/13) and (4/14) that:

$$\Delta G^0_{p,II} = (s_{\mathrm{II}}/s_{\mathrm{I}})\, \Delta G^0_{p,I} + c_{\mathrm{II}} - (s_{\mathrm{II}}/s_{\mathrm{I}})\, c_{\mathrm{I}} \quad (4/15)$$

After combining the constants and dividing by $-2.3RT$, eqn. (4/12) is obtained. If organic phase I is more hydrophobic than organic phase II, $s_{\mathrm{II}} < s_{\mathrm{I}}$ and $a_p < 1$, whilst $a_p = 1$ may be expected at about identical hydrophobicity. The examples published so far [48, 86, 88] substantiate this, but also show that above a certain limit the influence of miscibility diminishes because the mutual effects of the two phases of a given partitioning system become too small to be of any significance.

For eqn. (4/12) to be valid it is essential that the similarity of solute-solvent interactions should resulut in analogous changes in the I_2 of either organic phase with solute structure. If in these phases basically dissimilar solute-solvent interactions occur, eqn. (4/12) does not hold. This is the case, for instance, when the molecules of the series under consideration form hydrogen bonds of different strengths and hydrogen-bond formation is possible only in one of the two organic phases [82a, 85, 87, 88, 90]. Differences in hydrogen bonding may be accounted for by adding to eqn. (4/12) a correction term characteristic of the hydrogen-bonding tendency of the various polar groups. In the simplest case such a correction is made possible by an indicator variable. As recently demonstrated by FUJITA et al. [91] this procedure can be justified by an analysis of the association constants of hydrogen bonding and of the concentrations of the molecular species capable of hydrogen bonding in the hydrophobic phases of the partitioning systems. Thus, the relationship between $\log P$ values of a set of mono-substituted benzenes in the partitioning systems chloroform-water and n-octanol-water can be expressed [91] as:

$$\log P_{CHCl_3/w} = 0.801 \log P_{oct./w} + 0.367HB + 1.157 \tag{4/16}$$

$$n = 14 \qquad r = 0.991 \qquad s = 0.081$$

The indicator variable, HB, is defined as:

$$HB = \begin{cases} 1 \text{ for hydrogen acceptors} \\ 0 \text{ for remainder} \end{cases} \tag{4/17}$$

Through a regression analysis of a large number of partition coefficients on the basis of the model

$$\log P_{oct./w} - \log P_{cyclohexane/w} = \sum I_H - b \tag{4/18}$$

SEILER [92] evaluated an incremental system to describe the hydrogen-bonding tendency of various polar groups. The values of the increment, I_H, are additive and their inclusion in eqn. (4/12) will permit the correlation of partition coefficients of system where the two organic phases differ in their potentials for hydrogen bonding (see also [82a]).

Eqn. (4/12) may be generalized on the following lines [48]: *within homologous series of compounds there exist linear relationships between the thermodynamic data for transfer equilibria between water and various hydrophobic phases provided that the solute-solvent interactions in these phases have enough features in common.* This rule is also valid if one of the hydrophobic phases is a biophase. It follows that such thermodynamic transfer data may be employed as hydrophobicity parameters provided that the investigated hydrophobic phase and the hydrophobic biophase have enough in common. The most widely used parameters of this kind are $\log P$, R_M (see below), *HPLC* data (see below), $-\log c_s$ (c_s = water solubility) and the logarithm of the affinity constant for hydrophobic binding to an appropriate model protein, and other quantities deducible from these parameters.

The octanol-water partitioning system introduced by HANSCH serves as the most widely used model. Octanol is fairly hydrophobic and has a relatively low water miscibility but nevertheless hydrogen bonds playing a major rôle in the biophase can be formed. Apparently, this partitioning system, for which the most values are available (for an extensive review, see e.g. [90, 93]), approximates very closely the relations in the biophase, as may be gathered from $a_p = 1$ in eqn. (4/19) derived for the interaction of alcohols with the erythrocyte membrane (taken from [94]):

$$\log P_{EM} = 1.003 \log P_{oct./w} - 0.883 \tag{4/19}$$

where P_{EM} = partition coefficient in the erythrocyte membrane-water system, and from general experience of the use of $\log P$ values from this partitioning system in QSARs.

Of particular significance is the quantity π introduced by HANSCH et al. [95] and defined as

$$\pi_X = \log P_X - \log P_H \tag{4/20}$$

where P_H is the partition coefficient of a non-substituted parent compound and P_X that of a derivative with substituent X in the octanol-water system. π characterizes the hydrophobicity of the substituent X relative to hydrogen and can be formally regarded as the logarithm of the partition coefficient of this substituent in the octanol-water system. As a true substituent constant according to the principles of linear free enthalpy relations, π represents the hydrophobic analogue of HAMMETTS σ constant (cf. 5). In addition to substituents certain structural features such as chain branching, double bonds and ring closure may be expressed in terms of π values; these π values may also be regarded as correction for the occurrence of such features. HANSCH and co-workers have determined and collected a very large number of experimental π values (for publications, see in particular [90, 93, 96, 97]), and in recent years other research teams have also measured $\log P$ values in the octanol-water system. On methodological grounds, however, the latter values are not always consistent with those established by HANSCH et al. Care should, therefore, be taken in the use in a QSAR of π values which stem from different sources. In such cases the π values need testing thoroughly for compatibility.

Ideally, π should possess additive properties so that for any compound:

$$\log P = \log P_H + \sum \pi \tag{4/21}$$

This equation enables $\log P$ values to be calculated from π values and *vice versa*. It is frequently possible (and always advisable) to adopt more than one route starting, for example, with $\log P_H$ of various parent compounds. Such calculated values should be accepted only when the results obtained by different methods of calculation agree fairly well. Whether a given calculation is justified can be established on the basis of the "uncertainty index" defined by LEO et al. [90]. The calculation of $\log P$ for diphenhydramine (structure II) serves as an example of the general approach in such calculations.

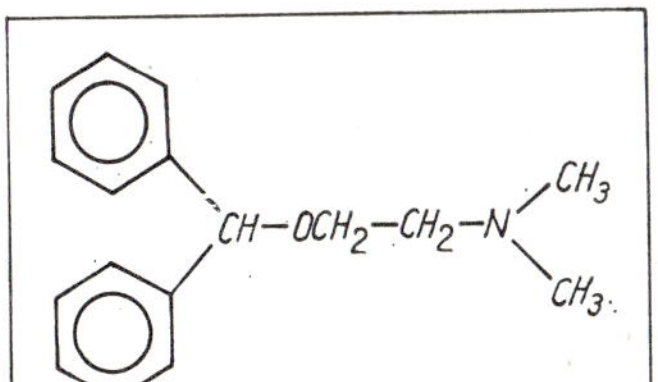

II

Diphenhydramine may be regarded as, for instance, a methane derivative and from this parent compound the following procedure can be construed:

Step 1: replacement of three H atoms of methane by two phenyl groups and an OCH_3 group as substituents,

Step 2: replacement of an H atom in the OCH_3 group by a CH_3 group,
Step 3: replacement of an H atom in the CH_3 group by the substituent $N(CH_3)_2$.

It follows that:

$$\log P_{diphenylhydramine} = \log P_{methane} + 2\pi_{phenyl} + \pi_{OCH_3} + \pi_{CH_3} + \pi_{N(CH_3)_2}$$
$$= 1.09 + 2 \cdot 1.89 - 0.98 + 0.50 - 0.95$$
$$= 3.44 \qquad (4/22)$$

Another approach starts with methyl ethyl ether $CH_3OC_2H_5$. Two H atoms of the methoxy group are substituted by phenyl groups and in the methyl group one H atom is replaced by $N(CH_3)_2$:

$$\log P_{diphenylhydramine} = \log P_{CH_3OC_2H_5} + 2\pi_{phenyl} + \pi_{N(CH_3)_2}$$
$$= 0.33 + 2 \cdot 1.89 - 0.95 = 3.16 \qquad (4/23)$$

Toluene is the starting point in the third approach. Two H atoms of the methyl group are replaced by a phenyl and a methoxy group, then one H atom of the methoxy group by a methyl group and finally one H atom of the methyl group by $N(CH_3)_2$:

$$\log P_{diphenhydramine} = \log P_{C_6H_5CH_3} + \pi_{phenyl} + \pi_{OCH_3} + \pi_{CH_3} + \pi_{N(CH_3)_2}$$
$$= 2.69 + 1.89 - 0.98 + 0.50 - 0.95 = 3.15 \qquad (4/24)$$

Finally, ethylmethylamine may serve as a starting compound, where first an H atom of the ethyl group is replaced by a methoxy group, then the H atom bond to the N atom is replaced by a methyl group and subsequently two H atoms of the methoxy group by phenyl groups:

$$\log P_{diphenhydramine} = \log P_{C_2H_5NHCH_3} + \pi_{OCH_3} + \pi_{CH_3} + 2\pi_{phenyl}$$
$$= 0.15 - 0.98 + 0.50 + 2 \cdot 1.89 = 3.45 \qquad (4/25)$$

The agreement between the log P values obtained is acceptable, their average being close to the experimentally obtained value of 3.27.

With evaluations of this kind, care must be taken that the exact definition of π in accord with eqn. (4/21) is based on the *replacement of a hydrogen by a substituent*. Errors have often been made in the literature, an example being the equating of $\log P_{C_6H_6}$ and $\pi_{C_6H_5}$, the consequences of which in the calculation for biphenyl would be:

$$\log P_{C_6H_5-C_6H_5} = 2 \log P_{C_6H_6} = 2 \cdot 2.13 = 4.26 \qquad (4/26)$$

As in biphenyl a phenyl substituent replaces a hydrogen in benzene as parent compound, the equation should read:

$$\log P_{C_6H_5-C_6H_5} = \log P_{C_6H_6} + \pi_{C_6H_5} = 2.13 + 1.89 = 4.02 \qquad (4/27)$$

The experimental value is log $P = 4.04$.

The additivity of π may be lacking where special intramolecular interactions occur [98—100]. In such instances, particular attention should be paid to:

1. *Proximity of strongly polarizing or strongly charged groups*

Deviations in the dependence of hydrophobicity on molecular size have already been pointed out. Hansch [99] found that the π value of a methyl group in the proximity of a strongly electron-attracting group was diminished by ca. 0.3—0.4π units, and the methyl groups between two aromatic rings or an aromatic ring and a strongly polarizing group remained hydrophobically "dumb".

2. *Intramolecular hydrogen bonds*

Intramolecular hydrogen bonds enhance hydrophobicity. Thus, the calculated log P value of salicylamide is —0.03, while the experimental value is 1.26.

3. *Intramolecular steric interactions*

The geometry of the two aromatic rings in paracyclophane (structural formula III) is such that they are liable to strong interactions. The calculated log P value of 5.90 is much higher than the experimental one of 2.33.

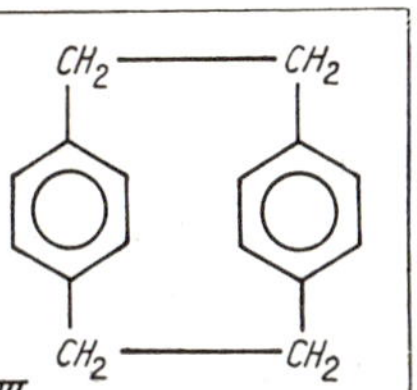

III

4. *Steric effects of neighbouring groups in aromatics* (*ortho-effect*)

Such effects can be exerted by different mechanisms, and cause both decreases and increases in log P and π values. The ortho-substituents in phenyl-N-methylcarbamates are more hydrophilic than their π values would suggest and this effect increases with increasing size of the substituents [101]. A similar behaviour is encountered with 2,5-disubstituted phenolic compounds [102]. This effect may be explained by assuming that solvation by the larger octanol molecules is more strongly effected sterically than hydratation. In ring systems ortho-substituents may uncouple resonance interactions through their steric influence. As a result, the overall hydrophobicity diminishes and for a large variety of structures this reduction (by 0.85 · log P) appears to be remarkably constant [103]. With piperidinoacetanilides, oxygen-containing substituents are essentially more hydrophobic in ortho- than in para-positions [104, 105]. This effect is probably complex in nature. The formation of a hydrogen bond with the amide group can be demonstrated by NMR spectroscopy. At the same time the ortho-substituents induce conformational changes of the entire molecule, one of the results being hydrogen bonding of the amide group with the nitrogen of the piperidine ring. A special steric effect operating in heterocyclic compounds can arise from lone pair repulsion which enhances hydration and, hence, decreases log P [106].

5. *Conformation and solvent-dependent conformational equilibria*

These can also strongly influence partition coefficients and may lead to large deviations if not adequately accounted for [36, 106a]. In compounds of the biphenyl type, for example, the π value of phenyl may vary by as much as 0.7 units depending on phenyl planarity [106].

A large number of π values for a variety of standard series (e.g. of benzenes, alkylbenzenes, phenols, anilines, benzoic acids, phenoxyacetic acids, nitrobenzenes, see

Table 4.3) have been evaluated and reported [93, 95, 107] and the correct choice of values from the most appropriate standard series is not without problems, especially as far as the aromatics and heterocyclics [106] are concerned. In principle, the π values of a standard series can be extended to other series; this is, in fact, necessary for use of the tabulated π values in QSAR analysis. The π values, however, depend not only on the substituents but also on their electronic interactions with the environment (see e.g. [108]), as is well illustrated by a comparison of the π values of para-nitro groups in phenoxyacetic acid ($\pi = 0.24$), phenol ($\pi = 0.50$) and aniline ($\pi = 0.49$). The values for phenol and aniline are practically the same but that for phenoxyacetic acid is markedly lower. This difference may be ascribed to the resonance interaction of the para-nitro group with the NH_2 or the OH group. The π values tabulated for any given standard series cannot be extended to another series unless the electronic interactions of the substituents with their environment are the same in each series. As these interactions are primarily dependent on the nature of the functional group (or, in heterocyclics, on the heteroatomes present [106]), the only series of aromatics which will have the same π values will be those which do not differ in the effect of their respective functional groups on the aromatic system and the substituents. This point is particularly relevant when chosing tabulated π values because electronic correction terms are commonly involved; this problem will be discussed in more detail in 7.2. and 9.1.2.1.

Tabulated π values prove extremely useful in QSARs because they largely obviate the need for a measurement of partition coefficients which is not always easy. Yet, much care should be exercised in the use of π values. This is especially true with complicated structures, e.g. those of heterocyclics [106]. In such cases, one should first determine experimentically the partition coefficients of a few selected compounds and then ascertain whether tabulated π values can be applied and, if so, from which standard series. If the decision is positive, the partition coefficients of the remaining compounds need not be determined experimentally. As regards highly complicated series, however, it may be necessary to determine the partition coefficients of all of its members.

Recently, the R_M *value*, which can be determined very easily by partition chromatography with reversed phases, and the derived ΔR_M *value*, have found increasing application as hydrophobicity parameters (see e.g. [109]). The R_M value has been defined as [110]:

$$R_M = \log\left(\frac{1}{R_F} - 1\right) \tag{4/28}$$

It is directly proportional to the logarithm of the partition coefficient in the system applied in partition chromatography

$$R_M = \log P + \log K \tag{4/29}$$

where K is a constant of the chromatographic system. ΔR_M is defined analogously to the hydrophobic substituent constant π

$$\Delta R_{M,X} = R_{M,X} - R_{M,H} \tag{4/30}$$

where $R_{M,H}$ and $R_{M,X}$ represent the respective R_M values of the non-substituted parent compound and its derivative with substituent X. Ideally, like π, ΔR_M should possess additive properties, and by analogy with eqn. (4/21):

$$R_M = R_{M,H} + \sum \Delta R_M \tag{4/31}$$

R_M values may be regarded as special $\log P$ values and ΔR_M values as special π values so that what has been said about $\log P$ and π is also valid for R_M and ΔR_M.

Within the context of eqn. (4/12) there are, of course, linear relations between R_M and $\log P$ and between ΔR_M and π (see e.g. [109, 111—122]); if a large range of hydrophobicity is covered, however, these relations may also become non-linear in certain instances [122a, b]. DRABER et al. [122] found that polyamide plates behave as a hydrophobic phase permitting a very accurate determination of R_M values. It may well be that these R_M values are even more suitable than π values for the description of hydrophobic interactions, as polyamide behaves as an artificial protein in binding studies [123]. Interestingly, DEARDEN et al. [111] found it easier to describe the binding of acetanilides to human serum albumin with R_M values obtained by means of polyamide plates than with π values.

Although widely used in QSAR work, ΔR_M values are more restricted in application than π values and when used they may present difficulties. Since hydrophobic compounds do not dissolve in water, mixtures of organic solvents and water are commonly used as the mobile phase for the determination of R_M values. By plotting R_M against organic solvent concentration in the mobile phase, straight lines are usually obtained over a given concentration range. If these lines share the same slope or an extrapolation to zero concentration of the organic solvent is possible, no problem will occur. However, in many cases the straight lines are not parallel so that marked differences are observed in the R_M sets for different concentrations of organic solvent in the mobile phase. When testing 5-substituted 2-(nitrofuryl) pyrimidines for bacteriostatic activity, SEYDEL and ALBRECHT [124] found that plots of R_M against the organic solvent concentration in the mobile phase fell into two groups with different slopes, and one compound showed a completely different behaviour. Meaningful QSARs with R_M as hydrophobicity parameter could be obtained only within the two sub-groups but not for the entire set. Additional information permitting a more detailed QSAR analysis may sometimes be gathered from the slopes of such R_M plots [125].

A variable analogous to R_M can be obtained from *HPLC* [126—132]. Thus, a constant k' can be derived from retention times

$$k' = (t_R - t_0)/t_0 \qquad (4/32)$$

which is fully analogous to the expression $\left(\frac{1}{R_F} - 1\right)$ in eqn. (4/28). By analogy with eqn. (4/29) it follows that:

$$\log k' = \log P + \log K \qquad (4/33)$$

If water saturated n-octanol is used as stationary phase HPLC will directly yield octanol-water partition coefficients [131, 131a]. The advantage is that this method is simple, accurate and precise and that apparent pK_a values can be determined simultaneously with $\log P$ by measuring the distribution coefficient at several pH values.

REKKER [133—137] introduced the *hydrophobic fragmental constant*, f, which is defined by

$$\log P = \sum_{i=1}^{n} a_i f_i \qquad (4/34)$$

Thus f_i describes the contribution of fragment i to $\log P$ and the factor a_i indicates how often fragment i occurs in a given molecule. The f values of various fragments were determined from a regression analysis of a large number of log P values [133—137] and tabulated [136, 136a]. The fragments considered were substituents and also smaller structural units down to the atomic level (e.g. C, ether oxygen, etc.). It appeared, however, that certain groups, such as COO^-, could not be further sub-divided. A major observation in REKKERS work was that *hydrogen itself also contributes to hydrophobicity* ($f_H = 0.167$). It follows from this finding that eqn. (4/26) is indeed incorrect, as is the frequently applied $\pi_{CH_3} = \pi_{CH_2} = 0.50$.

Despite their conceptual similarity the f and π systems are definitely different. Because of the type of approach used in evaluating f values empirical rules for correcting abnormalities in the π system (e.g. chain branching and the influence of polarizing groups) cannot be extended to the f system. The f system has its own rules to correct for anomalous behaviour of certain structural features. If such anomalous features are preseant, they must be allowed for in eqn. (4/34) to give:

$$\log P = \sum_{i=1}^{n} a_i f_i + \sum \text{anomalies} \qquad (4/35)$$

It has been demonstrated that the anomalies are nearly always multiples of 0.28, which factor REKKER has designated as the "magic constant", c_M. A physical interpretation of this constant is, however, not available. With the aid of the "magic constant", eqn. (4/35) can be transformed into eqn. (4/36) as indicated by REKKER:

$$\log P = \sum_{i=1}^{n} a_i f_i + \sum kn \cdot c_M \qquad (4/36)$$

The quantity kn (key number) indicates how many times the magic constant should be applied to correct for a given anomaly. Typical f system anomalies for which kn could be established and which can, therefore, safely be accounted for arise, for example, from the interactions of aliphatic C atoms or hydrogen atoms with negatively charged groups or from conjugational effects in aromatic systems.

Eqn. (4/36) enables log P and π values to be determined for almost any complex structure, by breaking it down into fragments (anomalies being treated as fragments) followed by addition of the relevant f values. For diphenhydramine, for example, the log P value can be calculated as follows (f values from [136]):

$$\begin{aligned}\log P &= 2f_{C_6H_5} + f_{CH} + f_O + 2f_{CH_2} + f_N + 2f_{CH_3} + \text{p.e. } 2\\ &= 2 \cdot 1.89 + 0.24 - 1.58 + 2 \cdot 0.53 - 2.16 + 2 \cdot 0.70 + 0.56\\ &= 3.30 \qquad (4/37)\end{aligned}$$

The term p.e. 2 (proximity effect 2) $= 2 \cdot c_M = 2 \cdot 0.28 = 0.56$ allows for the fact that, in the f system (but not the π system!), structures in which two electronegative groups (O and N in diphenhydramine) are separated by one (p.e. 1: $kn = 3$) or two (p.e. 2: $kn = 2$) aliphatic C atoms have enhanced log P values.

The statistical determination of f values implies that these partly incorporate certain intramolecular proximity effects (see also [138]). Therefore, the partition coefficients of small aliphatic molecules (CH_4, C_2H_6), where such effects are largely absent, are not so well described by REKKERS f values. To avoid this disadvantage, which, incidentally, is not serious for practical work, and in particular to obtain a consistent, always valid, *f* value for hydrogen which was not present in the first set of *f* values published by REKKER [136], LEO et al. [139] followed a different approach in the evaluation of *f* values. Thus the experimental partition coefficients of H_2, CH_4 and C_2H_6 which can be measured with a high degree of accuracy are used as a starting point. The *f* values of C, H, CH_2 and CH_3 are then calculated from these partition coefficients using eqn. (4/34). The *f* values of other fragments are likewise obtained from the partition coefficients of small molecules. Intramolecular effects are obviously not incorporated in these *f* values and as a result appropriate corrections are needed when a change is made to larger molecules. For example, a certain amount of lipophilicity must be subtracted for all C—C bonds after the first one when calculating the log *P* of alkanes. According to LEO et al. [139] this may be due to a volume reduction through bond flexibility. It should be noted here that because of the differences in the applied procedures the *f* values of REKKER and LEO et al. are not compatible and structural anomalies are also corrected for in different ways. Which of the two sets is used is more or less a matter of personal taste.

As already pointed out, dissolution of an organic liquid in water may be considered as the reverse of partitioning of this liquid between water and itself. Consequently, the negative logarithm of water solubility, $-\log c_s$, should have similar properties to log *P* and equally be suitable as a hydrophobicity parameter; many correlations between $-\log c_s$ and log *P* or the other quantities mentioned above have, in fact, been reported (e.g. [48, 88a, 88b, 139a]). HINE and MOOKERJEE [140] believe that the gas solubility of hydrophobic solutes is a "purer" measure of hydrophobicity than log *P*. This is certainly true in such cases where the detailed features of hydration are of primary importance as, for example, in resorption processes from the gas phase. Consequently, these authors developed an incremental system of *"intrinsic" hydrophobicity parameters* derived from gas-water transfer data of hydrophobic solutes. These parameters have the same properties as the $\log P_{g/w}$ values discussed on page 33 [44].

The molar *attraction constant*, *F*, has been suggested as a hydrophobicity parameter by OSTRENGA [141]. Its roots lie in the theory developed by HILDEBRAND and SCOTT [142, 143] for regular solutions and it is related to HILDEBRANDS solubility parameter, δ, (for a recent review, see [144]) according to eqn. (4/38)

$$\delta = (EV)^{\frac{1}{2}} = F/V \qquad (4/38)$$

where V = molar volume and E = cohesion energy. *F* can be calculated from the solubility parameter using eqn. (4/38), but it can also be obtained easily from incremental values of structural fragments (which means that *F*, too, has additive character). CAMMARATA et al. [145] showed that where compounds form regular solutions in either phase of the partitioning system and are not substantially different in molar volume, log *P* and *F* may be expected to be linearly related. The molar volume was also considered by DAVIS [146], who pointed out that *F* can be no more than a rough measure of π because any differences in the molar volumes of the substituents are ignored. To date, very little experience has been gained with the application of *F* in QSARs. According to DAVIS, the π value is to be preferred over the molar attraction constant [146].

Finally, there is the possibility of using data on the adsorption of solutes from aqueous solutions as hydrophobicity parameters. Several authors have shown that such data may be correlated with partition coefficients [147—151]. The disadvantage of adsorption data is that they may strongly be dependent on the type of adsorbent used. This is not true, however, of electrosorption at the mercury membrane which can easily be measured polarographically. A very close correlation was obtained between the free energy of adsorption (extrapolated to zero potential), ΔG_A^0, and of partitioning in the octanolwater system, ΔG_p^0, [152]

$$-\Delta G_A^0 = 1.138\ \Delta G_p^0 - 11.46 \qquad (4/39)$$

$$n = 30 \qquad r = 0.940 \qquad s = 0.177$$

indicating that ΔG_A^0 is in fact a good measure of hydrophobicity (at least for the compounds considered). No experience has yet been obtained in applying ΔG_A^0 as a hydrophobicity parameter in QSAR work but it seems that this might be worthwhile.

Adsorption (binding) constants for the binding of hydrophobic solutes to suitable model proteins may also serve as hydrophobicity parameters [153—159]; several examples will be presented throughout the next sections.

Table 4.2. The most important hydrophobicity parameters

Parameter	Definition	Conditions for application
CSA	Cavity surface area	Equal electronic properties in the variable hydrophobic molecular moieties; variable geometries are permitted.
$\log P$	P = partition coefficient, mostly in the octanol-water system	Similar solute-solvent interactions in the organic and the biophase.
$-\log c_s$	c_s = solubility in water	As for $\log P$.
R_M	$= \log\left(\frac{1}{R_F} - 1\right)$	As for $\log P$.
π	$= \log P_X - \log P_H$	As for $\log P$. In addition, when use is made of tabulated π values: 1. Absence of special intramolecular interactions. 2. Identical electronic interactions between substituents and molecular environment in the standard and the investigated series.
ΔR_M	$= R_{M,X} - R_{M,H}$	As for π.
f	$\log P = \sum_i a_i f_i$	Correction for proximity effects
F	$= \delta V$ (δ = solubility parameter)	Not quite clear, perhaps comparable with π.
$\log k'$	k' = retention index from HPLC	As for $\log P$.
$\log K_B$	K_B = affinity constant for binding to a suitable model protein.	As for $\log P$. In addition: 1. The binding is due to only hydrophobic interactions. 2. Special steric effects are absent.

Table 4.3. π and f values for some aromatic substituents

Substituent	π[1] [2]			f (REKKER)[3]	f (LEO)[2]
	Benzene series	Phenol series	Nitrobenzene series		
NH_2	−1.23	−1.63	−0.46	−0.85	−1.00
OH	−0.67	−0.87	0.11	−0.31	−0.44
OCH_3	−0.02	−0.12	0.18	0.26[4]	0.28[4]
NO_2	−0.28	0.50	−0.39	−0.07	−0.03
CN	−0.57	0.14	−0.66	−0.19	−0.34
F	0.14	0.31	—	0.38	0.37
Cl	0.71	0.93	0.54	0.93	0.94
Br	0.86	1.13	—	1.12	1.09
J	1.12	1.45	—	1.43	1.35
H	0	0	0	0.18	0.23

[1]) for para-substituents; note the pronounced differences between the three standard series
[2]) from [93]
[3]) from [136a]
[4]) calculated

To sum up, the molecular parameters employed as hydrophobicity parameters are many and varied. The behaviour of the partition coefficient, $\log P$, within homologous series can be expressed by the general equations

$$\log P = a_h x_h + b_h \tag{4/40}$$

in which all molecular parameters described in this section — paying due regard to their validity range — can be used for x_h; they are mutually linearly correlated. For $x_h = \log P$, π, f, $-\log c_s$, R_M or ΔR_M and bearing in mind eqn. (4/15), $a_h \approx 1$, provided that the interactions in the organic phases compared are sufficiently similar and the miscibility with water is approximately the same. The principal molecular parameters that may be used as x_h are recorded in Table 4.2, and Table 4.3 summarizes π and f values for some selected substituents. In conclusion, reference should be made to an excellent review [160] dealing with the most important thermodynamic aspects of aqueous solutions of hydrophobic compounds (see also [15]).[1])

4.2. Description of Hydrophobic Interactions: the Function $[f_h(x_h)]_I$

As stated in the introduction to this chapter, the hydrophobic binding of drug molecules to proteins, receptors and membranes may be regarded as specific cases of partitioning processes. It is, therefore, possible to describe the behaviour of the binding

[1]) All denoted hydrophobicity parameters characterize the free standard enthalpy for transfer from an aqueous into a hydrophobic phase. Preciser information on these transfers could be obtained from a separate consideration of entropy and enthalpy, because entropy and enthalpy depend from structure in a different way. Relevant data, however, are not available in a sufficient amount, but it seems justified to state that the hydrophobicity parameters mentioned in this section will generally fulfil the requirements of quantitative structure-activity analysis.

constant, K_1, by means of an equation which is analogous to the general expression (4/40):

$$\log K_1 = a_B x_h + b_B = [f_h(x_h)]_I \tag{4/41}$$

Thus, within homologous series, $\log K_1$ first increases linearly with hydrophobicity. However, the constants a_B and b_B in (4/41) possess a more complex character than constants a_h and b_h in eqn. (4/40). The reason is that in the case of hydrophobic protein binding there are additional important features because the hydrophobic phase does not occur as a homogeneous organic solvent but is united to a flexible protein molecule as a limited region of hydrophobicity. Therefore, eqn. (4/41) and its relation to eqn. (4/40) need a closer inspection.

First it must be remembered that on binding of ligands the protein may undergo conformational changes. Such changes and the consequential contribution to $\log K_1$ — referred to as Δ_1 here — are commonly considered as a linear function of x_h [48]. This is evidenced by, e.g., the change in rotatory dispersion of β-lactoglobulin and bovine serum albumine when binding various aliphatic hydrocarbons [161], the change in viscosity on binding of penicillins to human serum albumin [162] and the well-known dependence of denaturation of proteins on hydrophobicity in many series of compounds [163—169]. Some more examples of this kind of relationships are presented in eqns. (4/42)—(4/44):

Inhibition of fibrin swelling by a series of mixed organic compounds [80]:

$$\log 1/C = 0.86 \log P + 0.22 \tag{4/42}$$

$$n = 8 \qquad r = 0.937 \qquad s = 0.298$$

Transformation of cytochrome P-450 to cytochrome P-420 by substituted phenols [80]:

$$\log 1/C = 0.57 \log P + 0.36 \tag{4/43}$$

$$n = 13 \qquad r = 0.979 \qquad s = 0.132$$

Precipitation of nucleoproteins by a series of mixed organic compounds [80]:

$$\log 1/C = 0.81 \log P - 0.25 \tag{4/44}$$

$$n = 13 \qquad r = 0.979 \qquad s = 0.132$$

A general relation for Δ_1 may thus be formulated as follows:

$$\Delta_1 = \varkappa x_h + \lambda \tag{4/45}$$

It must also be recognized that the bound molecules undergo a loss of translational entropy. Within homologous series the resultant contribution to $\log K_1(\Delta_2)$ is practically constant [170, 171] so that:

$$\Delta_2 = \text{constant} \tag{4/46}$$

Of particular importance is that there may be two possible modes of ligand binding. Thus ligands may be adsorbed on the surface of a hydrophobic region, thereby losing some 50% of their contacts with water (case 1), or they can be fully transported into the interior of a hydrophobic pocket thus losing all contact with water (case 2). The extent of solute transfer from water into the hydrophobic phase can be expressed by the variable Φ [48]:

$$\Phi \approx \begin{cases} 0.5 & \text{for case 1} \\ 1.0 & \text{for case 2} \end{cases} \tag{4/47}$$

Φ indicates the percent agreement between the hydrophobic binding and a full partitioning equilibrium.

Eqn. (4/40) can now be extended to protein binding:

$$\begin{aligned} \log K_1 &= \Phi(a_h x_h + b_h) + \Delta_1 + \Delta_2 \\ &= \Phi(a_h x_h + b_h) + \varkappa x_h + \lambda + \text{constant} \\ &= (\Phi a_h + \varkappa)\, x_h + \Phi b_h + \lambda + \text{constant} \end{aligned} \tag{4/48}$$

By combining the constants, eqn. (4/48) can be transformed into eqn. (4/41) with:

$$a_B = \Phi a_h + \varkappa \tag{4/49}$$

In most cases the contribution Δ_1 is small compared to the overall effect, hence

$$\varkappa \ll a_h$$

and (4/50)

$$a_B \approx \Phi a_h$$

Thus eqn. (4/47) leads to:

$$a_B \approx \begin{cases} 0.5 a_h & \text{for case 1} \\ 1 \cdot a_h & \text{for case 2} \end{cases} \tag{4/51}$$

As stated in the preceding section, if $x_h = \log P$, π, f, $-\log c_s$, R_M or ΔR_M, $a_h = 1$ under certain conditions, one being the identical miscibility with water of the organic phases to be compared. As regards the hydrophobic binding sites of proteins, this condition seems to be fulfilled in the octanol-water system and systems of comparable miscibility (see also eqn. (4/19)) but, for example, not in the butanol-water system, where the miscibility with water is too high. With the R_M and ΔR_M values, $a_h = 1$ may be expected only if they are extrapolated to zero concentration of the organic solvent in the mobile phase.

With allowance for the approximate character of expression (4/50), it follows from (4/51) that

$$a_B = \begin{cases} 0.5 \pm 0.2 & \text{for case 1} \\ 1.0 \pm 0.2 & \text{for case 2} \end{cases} \tag{4/52}$$

Hence, *hints as to the binding mechanism are furnished by the slope* a_B in eqn. (4/41) (a_B *rule*): if $a_B = 0.5 \pm 0.2$, it is most likely that molecules are adsorbed on the surface and if $a_B = 1 \pm 0.2$, they are transferred into the interior of a hydrophobic pocket or of a membrane [48, 172, 173]. Exceptions to this rule may be expected if Δ_1 becomes too large or the conditions render eqn. (4/12) invalid. It has been established in studies of the biological and protein binding data of many homologous series of hydrophobic compounds [48, 153, 154, 172] and in an analysis of the numerous relationships according to eqn. (4/41) that the a_B rule is valid in over 96% of cases (see also [174—176]). Also of particular interest are the results of a study by HANSCH [177] on 183 computer-stored linear relationships between log A and log P. The following distribution of slope a_B values was obtained: in 57 cases $a_B = 1.01 \pm 0.13$; in 71 cases $a_B = 0.66 \pm 0.12$ and in 10 cases $a_B < 0.4$.

The validity of eqn. (4/41) can be demonstrated by some of the results obtained by the present author:

Binding of polycyclic aromatic hydrocarbons to human serum albumin [154]:

$$\log K_1 = 0.482(-\log c_s) + 2.806$$

$$n = 8 \quad r = 0.998 \quad s = 0.150 \qquad (4/53)$$

$$\log K_1 = 0.0449MR + 2.552$$

$$n = 7 \quad r = 0.997 \quad s = 0.027$$

Binding of substituted piperidinoacetanilides to bovine serum albumin [105]:

$$\log K_1 = 0.572\pi + 3.200 \qquad (4/54)$$

$$n = 5 \quad r = 0.930 \quad s = 0.099$$

Binding of phenoxyacetic acids to peroxidase [159]:

$$\log K_1 = 0.624\pi + 0.108 \qquad (4/55)$$

$$n = 22 \quad r = 0.968 \quad s = 0.101$$

Binding of isatin-β-isothiosemicarbazones to NADH oxidase in ETP particles [178]:

$$\log K_1 = 0.469\pi + 3.804 \qquad (4/56)$$

$$n = 8 \quad r = 0.864 \quad s = 0.203$$

Binding of isatin-β-isothiosemicarbazones to human serum albumin [179]:

$$\log K_1 = 0.523\pi - 0.897 \qquad (4/57)$$

$$n = 8 \quad r = 0.992 \quad s = 0.049$$

Equation (4/55) may be regarded as direct experimental proof of the a_B rule. NMR spectroscopy clearly showed that the ligands are bound at the protein surface, and the same conclusion follows from the slope which is well within the range 0.5 ± 0.2.

All a_B values in eqns. (4/53)—(4/57) point to adsorption on the surface. This occurs frequently but not always with proteins. Thus, chymotrypsin has a hydrophobic pocket in the neighbourhood of the active centre and it is this pocket in which the binding of hydrophobic parts of substrate or inhibitor molecules occurs [180] so that a_B values of 1 are obtained [48, 181]. Also the membrane binding of ligands, which are usually dissolved in membrane lipids, usually yields a_B values of about 1, as illustrated by eqn. (4/19). Another relevant case is the dependence of haemolytic activity, A_h, on hydrophobicity [182]:

$$\log A_h = 0.93 \log P - 0.09 \tag{4/58}$$

A_h reflects interactions with the erythrocyte membrane and may be regarded as directly proportional to the binding constant to this membrane. As expected, the value of a_B in eqn. (4/58) is approximately unity; as regards this equation, it should be noted that the a_B value is the average of values of fifteen different series of compounds so that (4/58) may be looked upon as a model equation for membrane binding and membrane perturbation. Further examples demonstrating the validity of eqn. (4/41) and of the a_B rule can be found in [48, 80, 153, 183].

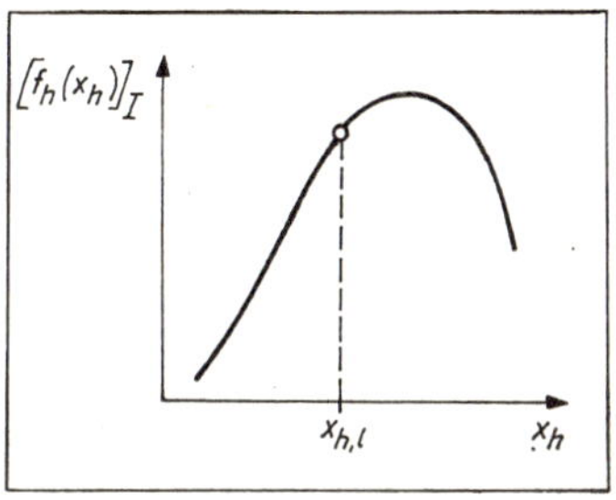

Fig. 4.1. Model curve for the description of the function $[f_h(x_h)]_I$ according to equation (4/60)

The linearity of $\log K_1$ with x_h in accord with eqn. (4/41) is only valid for a limited hydrophobicity range, because of the restriction on extension of the binding hydrophobic area (in a homologous series, hydrophobicity often increases with increasing size of the molecule, see section 4.1.) or because, if a certain degree of hydrophobicity is exceeded, the binding may lead to a thermodynamically unfavourable change in the conformation of the binding protein. Binding is then increasingly hindered from a point which has a characteristic value of x_h for each binding system (binding of a given series of ligands to a given protein), designated here as $x_{h,l}$. As a consequence, a_B in eqn. (4/41) is no longer a constant but itself becomes dependent on x_h. Assuming that this dependence is linear with the slope α and the ordinate β it follows for a_B:

$$a_B = \begin{cases} \text{constant} & \text{for } x_h \leqq x_{h,l} \\ \alpha x_h + \beta & \text{for } x_h > x_{h,l} \end{cases} \tag{4/59}$$

Equation (4/41) then transformes into:

$$\log K_1 = [f_h(x_h)]_I = \begin{cases} a_B x_h + b_B & \text{for } x_h \leqq x_{h,l} \quad \text{(a)} \\ \alpha x_h^2 + \beta x_h + \gamma & \text{for } x_h > x_{h,l} \quad \text{(b)} \end{cases} \tag{4/60}$$

Equation (4/60) describes a composite curve (Fig. 4.1) with a linear part according to eqn. (4/41), which at $x_h > x_{h,l}$ changes into a parabola, concaved downwards (α = negative). Thus, log K_1 approaches a maximum after x_h has exceeded $x_{h,l}$ and, eventually, decreases with incresing hydrophobicity. For the linear part of the curve the a_B rule (eqn. (4/52)) is valid. Eqn. (4/60) can be fitted to various experimental data with excellent results [172, 173]. However, for routine calculations eqn. (4/60) is sometimes unsuitable because several adjustable parameters need to be determined in a non-linear regression analysis. Fortunately, the whole curve can be approximated by a simple parabola according to eqn. (4/61) without sacrificing too much accuracy[1]) [172, 173]:

$$[f_h(x_h)]_I = a_0 + a_1 x_h + a_2 x_h^2 \qquad (4/61)$$

Examples of parabolic relationships between log K_1 and x_h have been reported by several authors (see [172, 184] and [185]). Eqn. (4/62) describes the binding of benzene sulfonamides to human serum albumin:

$$\log K_1 = -0.34(\log P)^2 + 0.74 \log P + 3.64 \qquad (4/62)$$

$$n = 13 \qquad r = 0.91 \qquad s = 0.36$$

It follows that, *depending on the hydrophobicity range covered, the function* $[f_h(x_h)]_I$ *can be represented either as a linear relation or as a parabola* in accord with, respectively, (4/41) and (4/61). Which of the two is applicable in a given case must be found by trial.

If not influenced by either steric or electronic factors ($f_e(x_e)$ and $f_s(x_s)$ in eqn. (3/17) are 0) or transport $[f_h(x_h)]_T$ in eqn. (3/16) is 0), biological activity only depends on hydrophobic interactions

$$\log A = [f_h(x_h)]_I + \text{constant} \qquad (4/63)$$

and all expressions for $[f_h(x_h)]_I$ also provide a direct description of log A. Some examples selected at random are presented below (for reviews of relationships based on eqn. (4/63) with (4/41) or (4/61) for $[f_h(x_h)]_I$, see [48, 80, 85, 154, 186—189]). Transport effects may partially be involved in these and the following relationships.

1. Linear relationships

Inhibition of acetylcholine-induced postsynaptic excitation under the influence of anaesthetics [190]:

$$\log A = 1.17 \log P + 1.22 \qquad (4/64)$$

$$n = 6 \qquad r = 0.982 \qquad s = 0.295$$

Oxidation of aromatic compounds by rat liver microsomes [191]:

$$\log A = 0.641 \log P + 2.996 \qquad (4/65)$$

$$n = 8 \qquad r = 0.967 \qquad s = 0.230$$

---

1) In more detailed investigations, however, eqn. (4/60) may yield valuable information on mechanisms of binding and the topology of the binding region, so that this equation should not be rejected *a priori*.

Acute toxicity of phenols in mice [116]:

$$\log A = 0.478\, R_M + 2.330 \qquad (4/66)$$

$$n = 28 \qquad r = 0.928 \qquad s = 0.112$$

Narcotic potency of aliphatic esters, ketones, alcohols and ethers on tadpoles [141]:

$$\log A = 3.03 \cdot 10^{-3} F - 1.10 \qquad (4/67)$$

$$n = 27 \qquad r = 0.968 \qquad s = 0.21$$

If $\log P$ is used instead of F, $a_B \approx 1$; this value is typical of anaesthetic activity, probably as a result of membrane perturbation (cf. eqn. (4/58)).

2. Parabolic relationships

Anticholinergic activity of morpholine derivatives [192]:

$$\log A = -0.496\pi^2 + 3.964\pi - 1.285 \qquad (4/68)$$

Virostatic activity of isatin-β-isothiosemicarbazones (*Mengo virus;* [178] and [193]):

$$\log A = -0.46\pi^2 + 1.61\pi - 2.43 \qquad (4/69)$$

$$n = 9 \qquad r = 0.736 \qquad s = 0.260$$

$$\log A = -2.82(\log K_1)^2 + 27.1 \log K_1 - 65.7$$

$$n = 9 \qquad r = 0.980 \qquad s = 0.091$$

where K_1 = binding constant in the NADH-oxidase system in ETP particles [178]. In this case protein binding apparently provides a much better hydrophobicity parameter than the π value, as was also found in a QSAR analysis of phytoactive phenoxyacetic acids [159].

Activity of p-hydroxyphenyl alkyl sulphides against S. aureus [80]:

$$\log A = -0.15(\log P)^2 + 1.73 \log P - 2.21 \qquad (4/70)$$

$$n = 12 \qquad r = 0.995 \qquad s = 0.093$$

Inhibition of the Hill *reaction in chloroplasts by aminotriazines* [194]:

$$\log A = -0.484(\log P)^2 + 1.959 \log P + 4.608 \qquad (4/71)$$

In common with the majority of linear relationships between $\log A$ and x_h, eqns. (4/64)—(4/67) follow the a_B rule. The reason that this rule is also applicable to eqn. (4/66) is that the R_M values used refer to a purely aqueous mobile phase.

The model based on eqn. (4/60) and the derivable borderline cases (eqns. (4/41) and (4/61)) appear very suitable to describe the function $[f_h(x_h)]_I$. There are, however, also instances where the model does not suffice and requires further extension [138, 195 to 198]. Thus, a protein or a receptor may possess two hydrophobic binding regions, A and B, separated sterically or by a polar region. If a given specific interaction results exclusively in the binding of the lower members of a homologous series to region A, eqn. (4/60) is valid, the rise in affinity being linearly proportional to hydrophobicity until the molecules tend to extend the size of region A. At this point the linear dependence on hydrophobicity according to eqn. (4/41) or (4/60a) will change into the parabolic one satisfying eqn. (4/60b) because of steric strain or since contact with the adjacent polar region is thermodynamically unfavourable; binding will diminish as hydrophobicity increases after passing the maximum. If, however, the polar region is not too extensive or the steric barrier not too high and the series is sufficiently enlarged, molecules above a certain size may come into contact with region B. From this point on a further increase in hydrophobicity will again lead to an increase in binding until site B is also exhausted. Consequently, a complex curve will result, consisting of two parts according to eqn. (4/60) connected through a parabola concaved upwards (see Fig. 4.2).

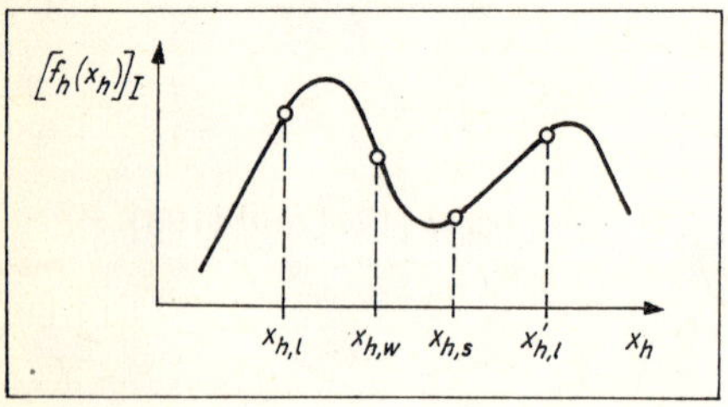

Fig. 4.2. Model curve for the function $[f_h(x_h)]_I$ according to equation (4/72)

Thus, the curve is made up of two straigh lines and three parabolas:

$$[f_h(x_h)]_I = \begin{cases} a_B x_h + b_B & \text{for } x_h \leqq x_{h,l} \quad \text{(a)} \\ \alpha x_h^2 + \beta x_h + \gamma & \text{for } x_{h,l} \leqq x_h \leqq x_{h,w} \quad \text{(b)} \\ \alpha^* x_h^2 + \beta^* x_h + \gamma^* & \text{for } x_{h,w} \leqq x_h \leqq x_{h,s} \quad \text{(c)} \\ a_B' x_h + b_B' & \text{for } x_{h,s} \leqq x_h \leqq x'_{h,l} \quad \text{(d)} \\ \alpha' x_h^2 + \beta' x_h + \gamma' & \text{for } x_h > x'_{h,l} \quad \text{(e)} \end{cases} \qquad (4/72)$$

A relationship in accordance with eqn. (4/72) is also to be expected with region A remote from B provided that the affinity of site B for the lower homologues of the series considered is negligible. Relationships of this type may also arise when the higher homologues cause conformational changes in the binding protein such that any further increases in hydrophobicity would eventually promote binding.

The coefficients in eqn. (4/72) can, in principle, readily be evaluated by non-linear regression analysis. The large number of data points needed, however, is usually not available. By analogy with the approximation of eqn. (4/60) using a parabola, eqn. (4/72) can be approximated with a fourth degree polynomial:

$$f_h(x_h)_I = a_0 + a_1 x_h + a_2 x_h^2 + a_3 x_h^3 + a_4 x_h^4 \qquad (4/73)$$

An example of such a relationship was revealed for the interaction of bis-trimethylammonium-n-alkanes with the acetylcholine receptor. The following expression for the antagonistic activity of these compounds was obtained [197, 198] (experimental data from [199]):

$$pA_2 = -43.84 + 29.3\pi - 6.59\pi^2 + 0.64\pi^3 - 0.022\pi^4 \quad (4/74)$$

$$n = 13 \qquad r = 1.000 \qquad s = 0.121$$

Although some more data points would be desirable, the statistical fit (at $p < 0.001$, all terms are significant) and the agreement with the extended model according to eqn. (4/73) are quite satisfactory. From a mechanistic point of view, the relation has a few interesting features. The value of the limiting slope of the ascending part of the first parabola is ca. 1.1, pointing to binding in a hydrophobic pocket according to the a_B rule. Such a hydrophobic pocket has indeed been postulated by various authors for the acetylcholine receptor [200, 201]. As long as the entire alkyl chain fits in this pocket, receptor binding shows an increase with rising hydrophobicity. If, however, the chain becomes too long for the pocket, binding is unfavourably influenced by the flexibility of the protruding fraction and its water contacts, reducing the pA_2 value after the first maximum has been passed. Further chain lengthening eventually leads to contacts with another hydrophobic region, because after the minimum binding again increases with hydrophobicity. The existence of such a second region has also been postulated by various workers [201, 202]. As the limiting slope of the ascending part of the second parabola has a value of 0.4, the a_B rule suggests the second region is situated at the receptor surface. Equation (4/74) is therefore not only in full agreement with the current notion of the active centre of the acetylcholine receptor, but it also provides an example showing how such data analyses furnish valuable hints on mechanism.

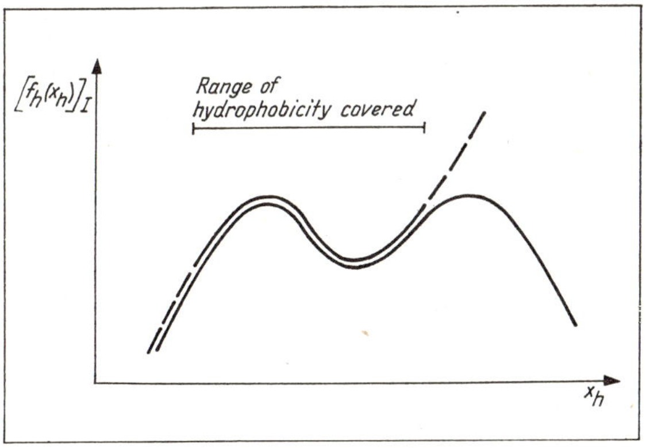

Fig. 4.3. Borderline case for equation (4/72)

It is relatively rare that the full range of hydrophobicity represented by eqn. (4/72) is covered by the members of a homologous series, although several examples have been reported [197]. In fact, borderline cases varying with the hydrophobicity range, and represented by eqns. (4/72a)—(4/72e) and (4/60), occur far more frequently. Another borderline relationship can be described by a third degree polynomial as depicted in Fig. 4.3. Bearing in mind all these instances and the approximations based on eqns. (4/61) and (4/73), the following possibilities may be suggested for the mathematical form of $[f_h(x_h)]_I$:

1. linear equation satisfying eqn. (4/41) (identical to (4/60a) as well as to (4/72a) and (4/72d)), if x_h varies within one of the two linear portions of (4/72);

2. parabolic equation according to (4/61) for the following cases: (a) x_h covers the range of the first or the second maximum in eqn. (4/72) or (4/73) (the coefficient a_2 is negative); (b) x_h covers the range of the minimum in eqn. (4/72) or (4/73) (the coefficient a_2 is positive);
3. third degree polynomial as shown in Fig. 4.3;
4. fourth degree polynomial according to eqn. (4/73).

The first two cases are by far the most frequent so that for routine QSAR work $[f_h(x_h)]_I$ may be briefly formulated as:

$$[f_h(x_h)]_I = \begin{cases} a_B x_h + b_B & \text{(a)} \\ a_0 + a_1 x + a_2 x^2 & \text{(b)} \end{cases} \qquad (4/75)$$

For each individual problem the choice between eqn. (4/75a) and (4/75b) must be made by trial, the relationship that can best be adjusted to the experimental data being preferred. In most instances the coefficient a_2 is negative, but there are also quite a few examples of positive x_h^2 terms [196, 197] (see e.g. eqn. (5/126)). Third or fourth degree polynomials should be tried only where eqn. (4/75) does not permit data description.

A final basic aspect of hydrophobic interactions is that the hydrophobic binding region may be non-homogeneous and asymmetric. In this case, substituents in different positions may interact with the binding region in more than one way and in different degrees of intensity. As a consequence, the function $[f_h(x_h)]_I$ must be fragmented into sub-terms for the individual sites of substitution. This is, of course, not possible with global molecular parameters such as $\log P$, R_M or $-\log c_s$ and can be achieved only by using hydrophobic substituent constants such as π, f or ΔR_M. If, in a given homologous series, substituents at positions of substitution 1, 2 and 3 are varied, $[f_h(x_h)]_I$ may then assume the following forms:

$$[f_h(x_h)]_I = \begin{cases} f_h^{1,2,3}(x_{h,1} + x_{h,2} + x_{h,3}) & \text{(a)} \\ f_h^{1}(x_{h,1}) + f_h^{2,3}(x_{h,2} + x_{h,3}) & \text{(b)} \\ f_h^{2}(x_{h,2}) + f_h^{1,3}(x_{h,1} + x_{h,3}) & \text{(c)} \\ f_h^{3}(x_{h,3}) + f_h^{1,2}(x_{h,1} + x_{h,2}) & \text{(d)} \\ f_h^{1}(x_{h,1}) + f_h^{2}(x_{h,2}) + f_h^{3}(x_{h,3}) & \text{(e)} \end{cases} \qquad (4/76)$$

No position dependence is implied in eqn. (4/76a), whilst in (4/76b)—(4/76d) one of the substituents differs in behaviour from the others. Eqn. (4/76e) is applicable when the hydrophobic interactions are different in all three positions. Any of the terms in (4/76) may become 0 (indicating that hydrophobic substituent effects do not operate at the respective position) or either linear or parabolic (eqn. (4/75)). In principle, all these variants must be taken into account and tried in those QSARs where current knowledge does not indicate which variant can be excluded or is preferred. Position-dependent hydrophobic interactions are exemplified below:

1. *Anti-inflammatory activity of aryl-indandiones* (*IV*) [103]:

$$\log A = 0.558(\pi_{m,p} - X \cdot 0.85) + 0.218\pi_0 + 3.698 \qquad (4/77)$$

$$n = 44 \qquad r = 0.956 \qquad s = 0.203$$

The ortho substituents show a deviating behaviour. In addition, they uncouple resonance. As already stated, this effect leads to a decrease in overall hydrophobicity by $0.85 \cdot \log P$ so that meta and para substituents are also affected. This is accounted for in eqn. (4/77) by substracting this amount when an ortho substituent is present. The presence or absence of ortho substituents is indicated by the variable X defined as:

$$X = \begin{cases} 1 & \text{ortho substituents present} \\ 0 & \text{ortho substituents absent} \end{cases} \tag{4/78}$$

In this example the possibility cannot be ruled out that the observed position dependence results from a purely intramolecular effect.

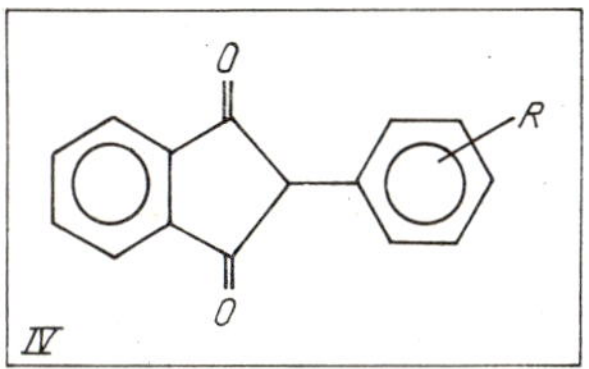

IV

2. *Activity of ortho-and meta-substituted phenols against S. typhosa* [172]:

Equation (4/60) has been used here in a somewhat modified form which is advantageous for computation

$$\log A = \begin{cases} a_B(x_h - x_{h,l}) + \eta & \text{for } x_h \leqq x_{h,l} \quad \text{(a)} \\ \alpha(x_h^2 - x_{h,l}^2) + \beta(x_h - x_{h,l}) + \eta & \text{for } x_h > x_{h,l} \quad \text{(b)} \end{cases} \tag{4/79}$$

where η is the value of $\log A$ at $x_h = x_{h,l}$. The following relationships were obtained for ortho-substituted phenols:

$$\log A = \begin{cases} 0.80(\log P - 4.40) + 2.52 & \text{for } \log P \leqq 4.40 \\ -1.62\left((\log P)^2 - 19.36\right) + 15.01(\log P - 4.40) + 2.52 & \text{for } \log P > 4.40 \end{cases} \tag{4/80}$$

$$\log P_l = 4.40 \quad \pi_0 = 4.46 \quad \eta = 2.52$$

and for meta-substituted phenols:

$$\log A = \begin{cases} 0.80(\pi - 2.04) + 1.86 & \text{for } \pi \leqq 2.04 \\ -1.00(\pi^2 - 4.16) + 4.88(\pi - 2.04) + 1.86 & \text{for } \pi > 2.04 \end{cases} \tag{4/81}$$

$$\pi_l = 2.04 \qquad \pi_0 = 2.45 \qquad \eta = 1.86$$

It follows from the slopes of the linear portions of (4/80) and (4/81) that ortho- and meta-substituted phenols are bound in a hydrophobic pocket or on a membrane by a similar mechanism. The parameter $x_{h,l}$, on the other hand, is larger for the ortho-substituted compounds.[1]) As the applied substituents only differ in the length of their

[1]) $\log P$ from eqn. (4/80) can be converted into the π scale by substracting $\log P$ of phenol ($= 1.50$) to give $\pi_l = 2.90$.

n-alkyl chains and consequently π is linearly correlated with the size of the substituents, the $x_{h,l}$ values imply that more space in the hydrophobic region is available for substituents in ortho position.

3. *Inhibition of the Hill reaction in chloroplasts by type V compounds* [203]:

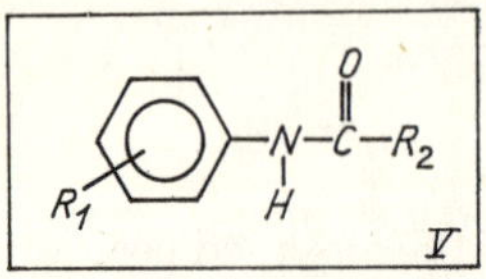

$$\log A = -0.093\pi_{R_2}^2 + 0.376\pi_{R_2} + 1.130\pi_{R_1} - 1.206\sigma_{R_2}^* + 3.700 \qquad (4/82)$$

$$n = 25 \qquad r = 0.859 \qquad s = 0.430$$

The hydrophobic substituent effect is parabolic for substituents in position R_2 and linear for substituents in position R_1. σ^* characterizes the electronic influence of R_2 on $\log A$ (σ^* = electronic substituent constant; see chapter 5.).

4. *Binding of para- and meta-substituted phenyl-β-D-glucosides to emulsin* [80]:

$$\log (K_1 \cdot 10) = 0.36\pi_{para} + 0.00\pi_{meta} + 0.66\sigma^- + 1.76 \qquad (4/83)$$

$$n = 13 \qquad r = 0.917 \qquad s = 0.164$$

Substituents in meta positions do not enter into hydrophobic interactions with the enzyme. σ^- represents the electronic influence of the substituents on biological activity.

5. *Inhibition of succinate dehydrogenase from liver flukes* (L) *and rat liver* (R) *by dihydroxybenzoic acid anilides substituted in both rings* (subscript 1 = substituent in aniline ring; subscript 2 = substituent in benzoic acid ring [204]):

$$\log K_{1,R} = 0.86\pi_1 + 0.68\pi_2 + 4.67 \qquad (4/84)$$

$$\log K_{1,L} = 1.31\pi_1 + 0.43\pi_2 + 5.15 \qquad (4/85)$$

Interactions of substituents in both rings with either enzyme differ in intensity and the two enzymes, in turn, are different in their response. Interestingly, it may thus be possible to obtain compounds with a selectivity against liver flukes. Equation (4/86) describes selective activity against this parasite enzyme:

$$\log K_{1,L} - \log K_{1,R} = 0.45\pi_1 - 0.26\pi_2 + 0.50 \qquad (4/86)$$

Position dependence has one important consequence. Where eqn. (4/75b) is applicable, the optimal value of x_h, indicated by $x_{h,0}$, can be determined from the first differential of this eqn.:

$$x_{h,0} = -a_1/2a_2 \qquad (4/87)$$

Because of position dependence, this value is applicable only to series whose members possess geometrically identical basic structures and is therefore not a constant of the biosystem under consideration[1]). This is also clearly the case in example 2 where the $x_{h,0}$ values differ by one order of magnitude (see also footnote p. 57). The implication is that such $x_{h,0}$ values cannot be extended to structurally different series when position dependence is possible. However, when the same basic geometry is maintained in different series (e.g. with n-alkane derivatives), discrepancies in $x_{h,0}$ need not be expected. Therefore, the $x_{h,0}$ values for geometrically closely related series in the same biosystem should at least bear some similarity. This is, for example, true of the activity of n-alkyldiamidines (I) and n-alkyldiguanidines (II) against *S. aureus*, where the $x_{h,0}$ values scarcely differ ($\pi_{0,\mathrm{I}} = 7.81$; $\pi_{0,\mathrm{II}} = 7.90$) and the π_l values, too, show good agreement ($\pi_{l,\mathrm{I}} = 5.26$; $\pi_{l,\mathrm{II}} = 5.51$) [172]. In such cases and also within a homologous series, $x_{h,0}$ provides an important parameter for optimization (provided that eqn. (4/75b) is applicable) because for further synthesis and tests it is possible to select structures whose hydrophobicity approximates most closely the optimal value.

4.3. Description of the Influence Exerted by Hydrophobicity on Drug Transport and Distribution: the Function $[f_h(x_h)]_T$

In passive drug transport many partitionings between aqueous and hydrophobic phases (lipid membranes, proteins) take place. The simplest transport model consists of two aqueous compartments, I and II, with volumes V_I and V_II, which are separated by a lipid membrane having thickness d. When the two compartments are stirred and diffusion occurs inside the membrane in accordance with Ficks first law, the drug flux, J, from compartment I to compartment II can be expressed per unit of membrane surface (D = diffusion coefficient):

$$J = \frac{D}{d}\,(C_{M,\mathrm{I}} - C_{M,\mathrm{II}}) \tag{4/88}$$

The expression in parentheses in eqn. (4/88) describes the concentration gradient between the two membrane interfaces, where partition equilibria between membrane lipid and water arise and the following partition coefficient is valid:

$$P = C_{M,\mathrm{I}}/C_\mathrm{I} = C_{M,\mathrm{II}}/C_\mathrm{II} \tag{4/89}$$

C_I (C_II) represents the concentration of the permeant in compartment I (II) and the flux can then be expressed as

$$J = \frac{DP}{d}\,(C_\mathrm{I} - C_\mathrm{II}) = P'\,(C_\mathrm{I} - C_\mathrm{II}) \tag{4/90}$$

with:

$$P' = \frac{DP}{d} \tag{4/91}$$

---

[1]) Note that this is only true for hydrophobic binding and not for $x_{h,0}$ values derived from drug transport processes to the site of action (see 4.3.).

P' is called the *permeation constant*. When the transport of the members of a homologous series in the same system is examined under stationary conditions and at equal concentrations the permeation rate of each member is dependent only on the permeation constant P', and as a consequence the function $[f_h(x_h)]_T$ is reduced to an expression of the dependence of the permeation constant on hydrophobicity:

$$[f_h(x_h)]_T = P'(x_h) \tag{4/92}$$

If all experimental conditions are constant, it follows from eqn. (4/91) that:

$$P' = \text{constant } D \cdot P \tag{4/93}$$

In general, the variation of the diffusion coefficient with molecular weight can be neglected when compared with that of the partition coefficient in a given homologous series. Thus, applying eqn. (4/40) and collecting constants:

$$\log P' = a_T x_h + b_T = [f_h(x_h)]_T \tag{4/94}$$

In many cases eqn. (4/94) provides an excellent description of the permeation of a homologous series of compounds through both synthetic and biological membranes [205—218]. Two examples are given below; for a review of other relationships of this kind, see [219, 219a].

Permeability of rabbit skin for various organic compounds [215]:

$$\log P' = 0.392 \log P - 2.761 \tag{4/95}$$

$$n = 7 \qquad r = 0.928 \qquad s = 0.381$$

Permeation of benzoic acids through polyethylene membranes [210]:

$$\log P' = 1.37 \log P_{hexane/w} - 7.72 \tag{4/96}$$

Eqn. (4/94) will not be applicable unless the permeation process is *membrane-controlled*. Although both compartments are stirred, an aqueous diffusion barrier exists on either side of the membrane so that the permeant must pass through three barriers. The exact expression to describe this situation is [220]

$$\frac{1}{P'} = R_{W,\mathrm{I}} + R_{W,\mathrm{II}} + R_M = R_T \tag{4/97}$$

where P' is the overall permeation constant, R_T is the overall diffusion resistance and $R_{W,\mathrm{I}}$, $R_{W,\mathrm{II}}$ and R_M represent the diffusion resistances of the two aqueous layers and the membrane. The diffusion resistance can be described by the thickness of the barrier, the diffusion coefficient in the barrier and the partition coefficient relative to the external medium:

$$R_i = \frac{d_i}{D_i P_i} \tag{4/98}$$

Since the partition coefficient in the water-water system equals unity eqns. (4/97) and (4/98) yield

$$P_t' = \frac{P D_M D_W}{d_M D_W + (d_{W,\mathrm{I}} + d_{W,\mathrm{II}})\, P D_M} \tag{4/99}$$

where the variables are the same as those in eqn. (4/91); the subscripts M and W refer to the membrane and the aqueous diffusion layers respectively, and P is the partition coefficient in the membrane-water system. Normally, $d_M D_W \gg (d_{W,\mathrm{I}} + d_{W,\mathrm{II}}) P D_M$, so that eqn. (4/99) simplifies into (4/91) and eqn. (4/94) holds (*membrane-controlled flux*). If, however, the molecules exhibit a large increase in hydrophobicity and thus in P, $(d_{W,\mathrm{I}} + d_{W,\mathrm{II}}) P D_M \gg d_M D_W$. The flux is then *controlled by the diffusion layers*, and eqn. (4/100) holds:

$$P_t' = \frac{D_W}{d_{W,\mathrm{I}} + d_{W,\mathrm{II}}} \tag{4/100}$$

There is no dependence on hydrophobicity here so that the straight line of eqn. (4/94) changes into a plateau for highly hydrophobic compounds (see also [221]). This behaviour has been substantiated on synthetic membranes [205] but is not typical of transport to the receptor. So far the occurrence of a plateau in biosystem has only occasionally been observed [222] (but see also [223])[1]). If transport starts in saturated drug solutions, it is possible to derive more complicated relationships from eqn. (4/99) [220, 222, 224, 225], which can partially be approximated by parabolas.

Parabolic relationships for the function $[f_h(x_h)]_T$ were also postulated by HANSCH et al. [226—228], who based their arguments on eqn. (3/10), regarding w as the probability of a drug be reaching the receptor within a specified time, t. On its way to the receptor (to be conceived as a random walk) the drug must pass through a variety of partitioning steps between hydrophobic and aqueous phases. Extremely hydrophobic or hydrophilic compounds will fail to pass through the first lipophilic or aqueous barriers, respectively, i.e. $w = 0$. In between these extremes a value for x_h will exist ($x_{h,0}$) where w has a maximum. Assuming that, relative to x_h, w is normally distributed:

$$w = a \exp\left[-\frac{1}{b}(x_h - x_{h,0})^2\right] \tag{4/101}$$

so that (cf. eqn. (3/14))

$$\log w = \log a - \frac{1}{b}\left(x_h^2 - 2x_h x_{h,0} + x_{h,0}^2\right) \tag{4/102}$$

As a and b are constants and $x_{h,0}$ here is a constant for a given series in a given biosystem, the equation of a parabola with the maximum at $x_{h,0}$ follows:

$$\log w = [f_h(x_h)]_T = k_0 + k_1 x_h + k_2 x_h^2 \tag{4/103}$$

A mathematical simulation of transport through a multicompartmental system led to a set of differential equations, which were resolved for various initial concentrations, partition coefficients between hydrophobic and aqueous phases and transport times [228]. The calculations resulted in a parabolic relationship between the logarithm of the concentration in the last compartment (receptor compartment) and x_h in line with eqn. (4/103). Later, DEARDEN and TOWNEND [229, 230], when repeating this mathe-

---

1) Such a plateau is not typical of transport phenomen, as it can be coupled to hydrophobic interactions as well. The maximum-regions in (4/72) are with respect to the relevant mechanism of binding very sensitive and may pass incidentally into such a plateau [197].

matical analysis, demonstrated the outcome to be largely time-dependent. At shorter intervals curves are obtained for $[f_h(x_h)]_T$ which permit an excellent description by means of a parabola in accord with eqn. (4/103). However, at longer intervals the parabolas are markedly distorted and under certain conditions the drug concentration in the receptor compartment approaches asymptotically a maximal value. The resulting curves have a form similar to that arising from the transition from membrane-controlled to diffusion layer-controlled flux in eqn. (4/99).

McFarland [231] reported a probabilistic analysis of the transport in a multicompartmental system allowing for transport route-branching. The curves he obtained are not exact parabolas, but for practical purposes they are well described using eqn. (4/103). These studies were extended by Kubinyi [223, 232–234], who, unlike McFarland, employed various volumes of the single compartments; the same author recently presented an excellent review on lipophilicity and drug activity [235]. Related to the function $[f_h(x_h)]_T$, the resulting expression is:

$$[f_h(x_h)]_T = a \log P - b \log (\beta P + 1) + c \tag{4/104}$$

Equation (4/104) implies that $[f_h(x_h)]_T$ first increases linearly with $\log P$ and, once a short tract of a parabola in the range of optimal hydrophobicity ($x_{h,0}$) has been passed, it shows a linear decrease (*bilinear model*). The slope of the first linear part is determined by the constant a and that of the descending linear part by the constant b. When $a = b$, symmetrical curves arise, most of which can be approximated, albeit somewhat crudely, by a parabola of the form of eqn. (4/103). This is, however, no longer possible in case of asymmetry ($a \neq b$). Mathematically, the bilinear model is very similar to the model presented in eqn. (4/60) since, in both cases, different slopes for the ascending and the descending parts of the curve are allowed for. Both models have the advantage that curves obtained for different series are more readily comparable as with a simple parabola.

The general picture for $[f_h(x_h)]_T$ is relatively complex. Yet a description using the parabola of eqn. (4/103) suffices in the majority of cases if linear dependences as specified in eqn. (4/94) are also allowed for. With this in mind, the following formulation of $[f_h(x_h)]_T$ can be drawn up for practical purposes:

$$[f_h(x_h)]_T = \begin{cases} a_T x_h + b_T & \text{(a)} \\ k_0 + k_1 x_h + k_2 x_h^2 & \text{(b)} \end{cases} \tag{4/105}$$

In form and content, eqn. (4/105) is entirely analogous to expression (4/75). Thus $[f_h(x_h)]_I$ and $[f_h(x_h)]_T$ have a similar dependence on hydrophobicity. This important feature will be dealt with in more detail later. A linear relationship in accord with eqn. (4/105a) may be expected if the lower portion of the ascending part of the parabola according to eqns. (4/105b) and (4/103), respectively, is approximated by a straight line. A linear relationship may also be obtained where the simple model underlying eqn. (4/93) approximates biological reality more closely than the complicated multicompartmental models affording eqns. (4/105b) and (4/103). It must be borne in mind that because the simple ascent implied in eqn. (4/105) is by no means always sufficient for describing biological reality frequent use must be made of more complex models such as the bilinear one designed by Kubinyi (eqn. (4/104)). The bilinear model has found wide and successful application, but for practical calculations it has the disadvantage that the estimation of the constants a, b, β and c requires more data points than does the application of a simple parabolic equation.

Non-linear models may also be needed if ionizable compounds are involved and if the degree of ionization within a given series varies widely (see also 4.4.). Studies of the gastro-intestinal and buccal absorption of drugs and its dependence on partition coefficients and degree of ionization, α, were reported by Vora et al. [236] and by Wagner and Sedman [237]. Having many features in common, the results of these authors can be presented as [238]:

$$[f_h(x_h)]_T = \log \left\{ a + \frac{c[\alpha/(1-\alpha)]}{1/(1-\alpha P_n^{\ b})} + d + e[\alpha/(1-\alpha)] \right\} \quad (4/106)$$

where $P_n^{\ b}$ is the partition coefficient of the non-ionized compound. Equation (4/106) is too complex for routine application and should primarely be used in special investigations as e.g. pH-controlled absorption.

Fortunately, eqn. (4/105) can be applied to a variety of transport processes although some exceptions do exist. Linearity in accord with eqn. (4/105a) has already been discussed so that the following examples only refer to the parabolic case implied in eqn. (4/105b); for other relationships of this type see [219, 219a, 239].

1. *Permeation of aromatic sulphones through tomato roots* [240]:

$$\log v = 0.123\,(\log P_{ether/w})^2 + 0.097 \log P_{ether/w} - 0.014 \quad (4/107)$$

$n = 42 \qquad r = 0.872$

(v = permeation rate)

2. *Permeation of alkyl phosphates through human skin* [228]:

$$\log P' = -0.040\,(\log P)^2 - 0.125 \log P - 0.040 \quad (4/108)$$

$n = 5 \qquad r = 0.997 \qquad s = 0.048$

3. *Penetration of the cockroach cuticle by insecticides* [228]:

$$\log 1/t_{1/2} = -0.124\,(\log P_{oil/w})^2 - 0.360 \log P_{oil/w} - 1.492 \quad (4/109)$$

4. *Penetration of several non-electrolytes into the rabbit eye* [228]:

$$\log P' = -0.067\,(\log P_{ether/w})^2 + 0.073 \log P_{ether/w} + 0.140 \quad (4/110)$$

$n = 7 \qquad r = 0.992 \qquad s = 0.059$

5. *Penetration of steroids through human skin* [228]:

$$\log P' = -0.207\,(\log P_{ether/w})^2 + 1.494 \log P_{ether/w} - 5.425 \quad (4/111)$$

$n = 10 \qquad r = 0.978 \qquad s = 0.220$

6. *Localization rate of phenylboronic acids in mouse brain*
(n = normal tissue; t = tumor tissue [241]; taken from [98]):

$$\log C_n = -0.540\pi^2 + 0.765\pi + 1.505 \quad (4/112)$$

$$\log C_t = -0.130\pi^2 - 0.405\sigma + 1.341 \quad (4/113)$$

where C = concentration after 15 minutes. The difference between the above two equations may be written as:

$$\log C_t/C_n = 0.410\pi^2 - 0.765\pi - 0.405\sigma - 0.164 \quad (4/114)$$

This equation correlates a type of therapeutic index with hydrophobicity. As indicated in eqn. (4/113), substituents with π values between -1 and -2 still permit a therapeutically active concentration to occur in tumor tissue but should also warrant a high level of selectivity to satisfy eqn. (4/114). Furthermore, it follows from the electronic σ term (see chapter 5.) that such substituents should have electron-donating properties to enhance selectivity.

The $x_{h,0}$ value characterizing the maximum of the parabola can be established from the first differential of eqn. (4/105b) as shown in (4/87). If hydrophobic effects on biological activity are exclusively due to transport phenomena, this value is a *constant of the biological system* under investigation, in contrast to the situation with hydrophobic interactions, and is independent of the chemical structure of the drugs. It is, of course, necessary for all sorts of experimental conditions which may influence transport processes such as time, rate and site of application, to remain strictly constant. *Pure* transport effects of hydrophobicity seem to be rather rare and are probably restricted to cases where particular barriers in the organism are crossed. This is well illustrated by CNS drugs, which have to pass through the blood-brain barrier. HANSCH et al. [80, 242] — see also [219] — found for a large variety of structurally different CNS drugs a remarkably constant value for $\log P_0$, with an average of $\log P_0 \approx 2$. It is noteworthy that a closely related value ($\log P_0 = 2.3$; $\log P_0 = \pi_0 + \log P_H = 0.7 + 1.6$) is obtained for the localization rate of phenylboronic acids in mouse brain (see eqn. (4/112). Obviously, this value is a meanigful point from which to start the design of CNS drugs[1]) as witness also the investigations of DRUCKREY et al. [243] on the hypnotic activity of type VI compounds. Substituents in R_1 and R_2 were varied in such a way that the $\log P$ values of the obtained compounds were systematically centred round $\log P_0 = 2$. Based on the deviations of $\log P$ values of individual compounds from the ideal value ($\log P_0 \approx 2$), the probable gradation in activity can be estimated,

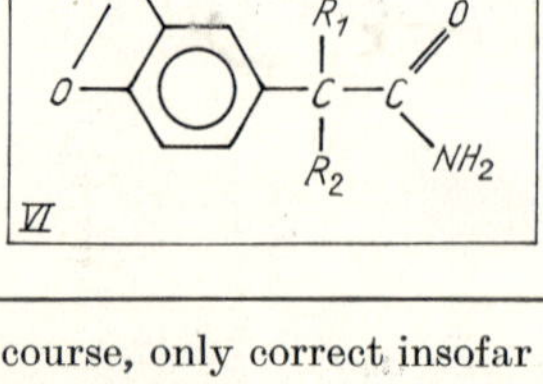

[1]) This is, of course, only correct insofar as activity depends on transport. If specific interactions with a receptor are also involved the $\log P$ values of the most active compounds may well deviate from the ideal value of transport.

and, as shown in Table 4.4, the resulting sequence could be confirmed experimentally with one exception. A quantitative structure-activity analysis gave the following equation [243]:

$$\log A = -0.53\,(\log P)^2 + 1.92 \log P + 1.67 \qquad (4/115)$$

$$r = 0.921 \qquad s = 0.174$$

$$\log P_0 = 1.84$$

Table 4.4. log P values and order of hypnotic activity of type VI compounds (from [243])

R_1	R_2	log P	Order of hypnotic activity	
			Estimated	Observed
Allyl	Allyl	1.99	1	1
Allyl	Äthyl	1.79	2	2
Äthyl	Äthyl	1.59	3	3
Propyl	Propyl	2.59	4...5	5
Äthyl	i-Pentenyl	2.59		6
Methyl	Methyl	0.59	6	4
Butyl	Butyl	3.59	7	7
H	H	−0.41	8	8

The log P_0 value from eqn. (4/115) is in good agreement with those of other CNS drugs. Two major conclusions can be drawn from this example:

1. the most active compound was predicted correctly and
2. the underlying concepts was substantiated by the gradation of the hypnotic activity in the test compounds as well as by eqn. (4/115).

It was not necessary to search for more active compounds in this series since the most active one had been established with sufficient certainty after seven syntheses and tests. This implies that if the $x_{h,0}$ of a given biosystem is known, drug activity as related to the influence of hydrophobicity on transport processes can be optimized in a meaningful way.

The above considerations of drug transport are based on the assumption that transport itself is not an active process. Although nearly always correct, this does not exclude the possibility that drugs more closely resembling endogeneous compounds (as is the case with a sugar or an amino acid moiety) may also be actively transported. In such instances the relations deduced in this section are not applicable. Yet there are indications that, within a homologous series, active transport also depends on hydrophobicity and could therefore be described by x_h (in the simplest case by a linear relationship) [244, 245].

4.4. Global Equilibrium Models for the Description ot the Function $f_h(x_h)$

Equilibrium models for the description of hydrophobic effects are based on the assumption that in a multicompartmental system there is partition equilibrium in each compartment, the receptor being treated as one of them. Under these equilibrium conditions, the function $f_h(x_h)$ is considered in its entirety including essential elements of what has been dealt with in the preceding sections. A first attempt of this kind was made by HIGUCHI and DAVIS [246], who assumed that

1. any biological system consists of t lipophilic compartments (tissues, lipids, proteins, etc.) with volumes V_i, one aqueous compartment with volume V_w and receptor R;
2. an overall thermodynamic equilibrium occurs in the system, drug distribution obeying NERNSTS law;
3. biological activity is proportional to the extent to which the receptor is occupied (y in eqn. (2/6) and following expressions), which implies that the factor F (eqn. (2/7)) is the same for all drugs and thus has only restricted applicability;
4. only a minor proportion of the total amount of drug present is bound to the receptor.

These assumptions led to the following expression of the concentration, D, of a substituted drug s relativ to the concentration of the corresponding non-substituted parent compound n at the receptor:

$$D = \frac{[D]_s}{[D]_n} = \frac{K_{r,s}\left(V_w + \sum_{i=1}^{t} K_{i,n}V_i\right)}{K_{r,n}\left(V_w + \sum_{i=1}^{t} K_{i,s}V_i\right)} \tag{4/116}$$

K_i, K_r = partition coefficients for the distributions between the i-th lipophilie and the receptor phase, respectively, and the aqueous compartment.

By expressing K_i and K_r in terms of x_h in accord with eqn. (4/12), the following relationship results (see MARTIN [238]; in deriving (4/117) the condition that only a negligible amount of drug would be bound to the receptor is ignored):

$$f_h(x_h) = a \log P - \log\left(1 + bP^c + \sum_{i=1}^{t} dP^e\right) + f \tag{4/117}$$

When the various lipophilic compartments can be combined into one general compartment ($t = 1$), eqn. (4/117) describes a curve that first ascends almost linearly with $\log P$ and then passes through a maximum. In many cases this curve can be approximated by an expression of the form (4/118):

$$f_h(x_h) = \begin{cases} a_0 + a_1 x_h & \text{(a)} \\ a_0' + a_1' x_h + a_2' x_h^2 & \text{(b)} \end{cases} \tag{4/118}$$

This is fully consistent with eqns. (4/75) and (4/105) already derived for $[f_h(x_h)]_I$ and $[f_h(x_h)]_T$. Expression (4/118a) may be expected at lower x_h values, whilst the parabola (4/118b) holds when a sufficiently large hydrophobicity range is covered. Like some of the kinetic models, eqns. (4/116) and (4/117) may give rise to extremely asymmetric curves (the volume ratio of the compartments determines the degree of asymmetry), which can no longer be approximated by a simple parabola or eqn. (4/118). In such instances, nonlinear models are again needed as, for instance, that of HYDE [247]. Also starting from equilibrium considerations, HYDE believed the receptor to be the only important lipophilic compartment. This means, that all non-aqueous compartments would have the same lipophilicity as the receptor. Furthermore, if it is assumed that the receptor behaves exactly as the octanol phase in the octanol-water partition system (which in view of the remarks in 4.2. has only restricted validity), the following relationship can be formulated (cf. [238]):

$$f_h(x_h) = -\log(a + P^{-1}) + b \tag{4/119}$$

Equation (4/119) also represents a non-linear model, which can be approximated under certain conditions by a straight line or a parabola in accord with eqn. (4/118).

A model similar to that designed by HIGUCHI and DAVIS was analyzed by MARTIN and HACKBARTH [238, 248—251a], who included explicitly the problem of ionization. The curves obtained for $f_h(x_h)$ differ greatly in shape, as they depend on the number of compartments involved in drug distribution and on the form (neutral, ionized or both) in which the drug is bound to the receptor. In addition to straight lines and parabolas as in eqn. (4/118), straight lines with a break or asymptotes may result. For a model with two aqueous, one non-aqueous and one receptor compartment, for example, the following relationship is obtained:

$$f_h(x_h) = \log\left[1 + \frac{Z\alpha/(1-\alpha)}{1 + Z\alpha/(1-\alpha)} + dP^c + \sum_{j=1}^{2} a_j/P^b(1-\alpha)\right] + e \tag{4/120}$$

The model contains six adjustable parameters ($Z, a - e$) where Z is the equilibrium constant ratio for the receptor binding of the ionized and the non-ionized form.

The global equilibrium models not only require the debatable assumption that in multicompartmental systems an overall thermodynamic equilibrium exists, but they also have the intrinsic weakness that for any relation between $\log K_1$ (K_1 = equilibrium constant for hydrophobic receptor binding) and x_h a simple linear relationship in accord with eqn. (4/41) is assumed. As stated in 4.2., the latter assumption may not be generalized. To summarize, in many cases, the results obtained with the global equilibrium models indicate that the function $f_h(x_h)$ can be approximated by eqn. (4/118) but more complicated relationships are sometimes required (especially for ionizable compounds, as proposed by MARTIN and HACKBARTH).

4.5. Summary and Final Conclusions

By use of eqn. (3/16) and the expressions (4/75) and (4/105) for the functions $[f_h(x_h)]_I$ and $[f_h(x_h)]_T$, the function $f_h(x_h)$ can be written as

$$f_h(x_h) = \begin{cases} a_B x_h + b_B \\ a_0 + a_1 x_h + a_2 x_h^2 \end{cases} + \begin{cases} a_T x_h + b_T \\ k_0 + k_1 x_h + k_2 x_h^2 \end{cases} \tag{4/121}$$

so that, after collecting constants:

$$f_h(x_h) = \begin{cases} a x_h + b & \text{(a)} \\ a x_h^2 + b x_h + c & \text{(b)} \end{cases} \tag{4/122}$$

Equation (4/122) is identical to eqn. (4/118), which follows directly from the global equilibrium models and suffices for most routine QSAR work. However, under certain conditions it may be necessary to apply the more complex models described in the preceding sections, especially in the case of ionizable compounds. For each individual problem the choice between eqns. (4/122a) and (4/122b) must be made by trial, the relationship that can best be adjusted to the experimental data being preferred. A good alternative to eqn. (4/122) is the bilinear model of KUBINYI (eqn. (4/104)) which is also widely used in QSAR work. Derived as an expression for $[f_h(x_h)]_T$ it can also account for $[f_h(x_h)]_I$ and thus for the function $f_h(x_h)$ in its entirety because of the mathematical similarity of eqns. (4/60) and (4/104).

For a routine QSAR analysis it is, of course, convenient that $[f_h(x_h)]_I$ and $[f_h(x_h)]_T$ can be described by similar relationships summarized as in eqn. (4/122). On the other hand, it will be difficult to ascertain whether any dependence of biological activity on hydrophobicity is due to hydrophobic interactions, transport processes or both. Where data on the biological activity of only one series of drugs are available, it is virtually impossible to resolve this problem. The observation of position dependence of hydrophobic substituent effects always points to hydrophobic interactions, but the possibility that at the same time transport may have an effect cannot entirely be ruled out. Equation (4/123) shows how complicated the superimposition of the two effects may be (antimaterial activity of VII [252]):

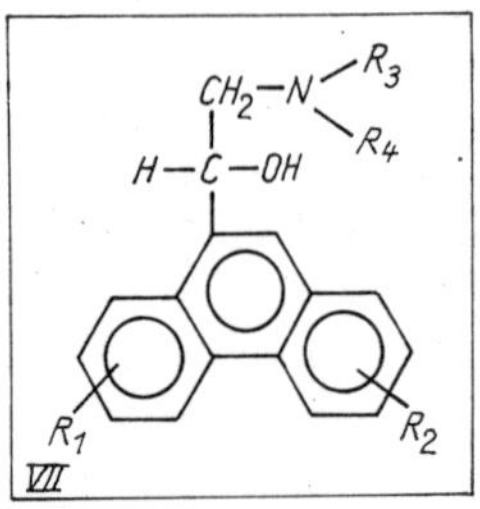

$$\log A = 0.396\pi_{R_1} + 0.270\pi_{R_2} - 0.015(\pi_{R_1} + \pi_{R_2} + \pi_{R_3} + \pi_{R_4})^2 + 0.137(\pi_{R_1} + \pi_{R_2} + \pi_{R_3} + \pi_{R_4}) + 0.895\sigma_{R_1} + 0.724\sigma_{R_2} + 2.511 \quad (4/123)$$

$n = 102 \quad r = 0.913 \quad s = 0.275$

Apparently, a position-dependent influence of hydrophobic interactions in R_1 and R_2 is superimposed on a transport effect, with the hydrophobicity of the total molecule being, of course, the decisive factor. σ represents a position-dependent electronic substituent effect. Another example of a complicated position dependence is found in the binding of steroids to the progestational receptor in the rabbit [253]:

$$\log A = 1.79\pi_a + 1.45\pi_b + 0.010\,\mathrm{MSA}_{ihp} - 0.012\,\mathrm{MSA}_{ohp} - 0.99X - 0.33\,\mathrm{c.c.} \quad (4/124)$$

$n = 55 \quad r = 0.88 \quad s = 0.54$

This relationship is interesting in that not only π but also the molecular surface area, MSA, of the substituents is applied as hydrophobicity parameter. The calculation of eqn. (4/124) is based on assumptions about which substituents are placed inside and outside a hydrophobic pocket (MSA_{ihp} and MSA_{ohp}, respectively) on binding. Here, π characterizes the negative effect of polar substituents on hydrophobic interactions (π_b refers to the positions 17α, 20α and 20β, and π_a to any other position), the indicator variable X represents the presence or absence of the 3-keto group and c.c. (conformational change) denotes the conformation of the A ring. Fortunately, such complicated relations with x_h are extremely rare.

The a_B rule is not satisfied in eqn. (4/123) because of superimposition of the transport effect, nor in eqn. (4/124) because of the particular application of π and the use of the MSA as a hydrophobicity parameter. If the a_B rule holds true, this means in general that hydrophobic interactions do occur, although this fact alone cannot be taken as conclusive evidence. A few possibilities may be suggested for a more precise differentiation between transport and hydrophobic interactions, which becomes more difficult, however, with increasing complexity of the biological system under investigation:

1. A study of various homologous series which, if possible, differ greatly in the geometry of their basic structures, exhibit the same mechanism of action and show a sufficiently wide spread of x_h. If the same $x_{h,0}$ value is found for each series, this may be interpreted to mean that transport processes take place since in the case of hydrophobic interactions, each series would have a different $x_{h,0}$ value. Position dependence is likewise to be expected in the last case and the expressions (4/60) or (4/72) should afford a better description than a simple parabola, thereby satisfying the a_B rule and ensuring that the $x_{h,l}$ values of the various series are different. This, in turn, permits a direct approach to receptor mapping.
2. A study of one or more homologous series in test systems differing in the degree of biological integration (e.g. isolated enzyme/cell organelle/cell/organ etc.) but which are comparable as regards sites of attack (see e.g. [253a, b]). If, for example, in an organ test a biological effect based on a given enzyme inhibition is found to have the same degree of dependence on hydrophobicity as the inhibition of the isolated enzyme, transport effects can be completely ruled out.
3. Variation of time in biological testing. If there is insufficient time to establish an equilibrium or a stationary state, transport must be a major factor. The function $[f_h(x_h)]_T$ may then become time-dependent, any lengthening of time resulting in a shift of $x_{h,0}$ to a higher x_h value and an extension of the approximately linear part of the parabola (see also [188]). The occurrence of such a time dependence provides conclusive evidence that transport factors are involved. In principle, it is possible to eliminate them by increasing the duration of experiments so that either the hydrophobic effect disappears or hydrophobic interactions become dominant. The latter could be suggested for the non-specific cardiodepressant activity of type VIII compounds. The following expressions have been reported for two different times of measurement, t, [254]:

   $t = 10$ minutes:

$$\log A = -0.08\,(\log P)^2 + 0.26 \log P + 3.01 \qquad (4/125)$$

$$n = 11 \qquad r = 0.989 \qquad s = 0.068$$

$t = 60$ minutes:

$$\log A = 0.43 \log P + 3.45 \qquad (4/126)$$

$$n = 11 \qquad r = 0.973 \qquad s = 0.133$$

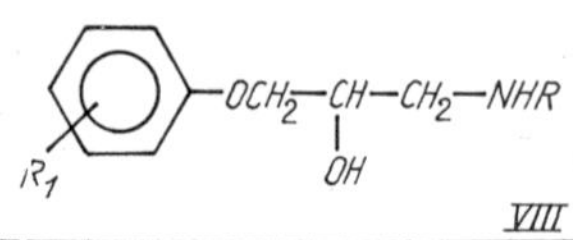

VIII

4. Transport factors are also indicated when pronounced differences in biological activity and its dependence on hydrophobicity are observed for different routes of drug administration. In a series of analgesics, for example, activity was three orders of magnitude higher when the compounds were directly administered into the brain than for intravenous injection [255]. The effective dose ratio showed a clear parabolic dependence on $\log P$ (system heptane-water) which, in this case, directly reflects the dependence of penetration into the CNS on hydrophobicity [256, 257] (subscript b = administration into the brain; subscript i = intravenous injection):

$$\log C_b/C_i = -0.090 (\log P_{heptane/w})^2 + 0.036 \log P - 0.637 \qquad (4/127)$$

$$n = 11 \qquad r = 0.970 \qquad s = 0.297$$

5. The evaluation of pharmacokinetic parameters in addition to the determination of biological activity followed by separate QSAR treatment of the two data sets. Besides permitting an exact separation of transport influences from interactions with the receptor, this approach enables a concurrent optimalization of the two effects. This is well illustrated by the procedure followed by SEYDEL [253b, 258—260b] in the programmed synthesis of sulfonamides with high bacteriostatic activity (through manipulation of the electron density on the nitrogen) and desired pharmacokinetic properties (through manipulation of pK_a and x_h). In the group of sulfonamides tested it appeared that the overall hydrophobic influence was solely due to transport phenomena.

With such studies, the complexity of biological systems should always be borne in mind, hence, all data obtained require careful interpretation. This is particularly true when biotransformations become rate-determining since such processes usually also depend on hydrophobicity (cf. eqn. (4/65)).

When analyzing the large number of relationships thus far established between biological activity and hydrophobicity, one gains the impression that in many instances the influence exerted by hydrophobicity stems primarily from hydrophobic interactions rather than from transport phenomena [48, 153, 154, 172, 173]. It would seem that transport influences are important in complex biosystem and if special physiological barriers, such as the blood-brain barrier mentioned above, have to be penetrated. It is noteworthy that hydrophobic interactions may also play a role in purely chemical reactions through a stabilization of transition states. Thus, PITMAN et al. [261] observed that the logarithms of aminolysis rate constants and $\log P$ values were linearly correlated for phthalic anhydrides in the presence of different series of amines in water, and another example concerning the hydrophobic acceleration of DIELS-ALDER reactions was reported by RIDEOUT and BRESLOW [261a].

Although at least in simpler biosystems hydrophobic effects are probably mainly due to hydrophobic interactions, transport effects must always be taken into consideration in the development of new drugs. If for a given series of drugs an enzyme is the site of action, the interaction with that enzyme can be optimized in vitro. Hydrophobic interactions frequently play a dominating role here so that on introduction of highly hydrophobic substituents into definite molecule positions high binding constants can be obtained. This procedure is scarcely helpful if the resulting compounds are so hydrophobic that they can no longer be transported to the site of action in the intact organism. It may then be useful to introduce hydrophilic groups into other molecule positions, at which hydrophobic interactions with the enzyme do not take place, thereby restoring the hydrolipophilic balance necessary for transport.

Hydrophobic interactions are not specific. Nevertheless a certain pattern of hydrophobicity in drugs may afford useful selectivity relations, as evidenced by e.g. eqns. (4/84)—(4/86). Similarly, hydrophobic transport effects may also underly selective behaviour (cf. eqns. (4/112)—(4/114). Biological activity has long been known to be affected by hydrophobicity. Many years ago MEYER and OVERTON [262—264] advanced a theory to account for anaesthesia in terms of hydrophobicity. It was later substantiated by SEEMAN [265], who carried out extensive studies with neutral and positively charged compounds. According to this theory, different anaesthetics will display the same action if their concentration in membrane lipids is the same. The iso-anaesthetic concentration, C_i, is then given by:

$$C_i \cdot P_{membrane/w} = \text{constant} \tag{4/128}$$

Olive oil was used as the membrane lipid model, leading to the formulation of eqn. (4/129):

$$C_i \cdot P_{oil/w} = \text{constant} \tag{4/129}$$

It should be noted, however, that olive oil does not provide a very suitable model for the biophase so that (4/129) is no more than a crude approximation. Equation (2/1) may be written as

$$A_N = 1/C_i \tag{4/130}$$

to express anaesthetic activity, A_N. Substituting from (4/129) and taking logarithms, eqn. (4/130) is transformed into:

$$\log A_N = \log P_{oil/w} + \text{constant} \tag{4/131}$$

Equation (4/131) is in accord with (4/75a) with the typical slope of $a_B = 1$ for membrane interactions, so that the MEYER-OVERTON rule fully corresponds to the formulation of the function $[f_h(x_h)]_I$.

For homologous series (mostly of n-alkane derivatives) a variety of empirical relations between biological activity and quantities such as boiling point, water solubility, number of C atoms in n-alkyl chains, vapour pressure or surface tension are well-established [266—276]. All these relations, and also the "biological Hammett equation" of ZAHRADNICK [277, 278] (see also [279]), can be expressed in terms of eqns. (4/75) and

(4/122). It is not surprising that even such simple empirical relationships have successfully been utilized to improve biological activity. It was on these lines that, for example, the standard anaesthetic halothane was discovered [280]. McGowan [68, 69, 281, 282] observed relationships between the physical toxicity of a large number of organic compounds in various biosystems and the parachor Pa which may serve as a hydrophobicity parameter as already mentioned:

$$\log A = -(7.7 + S) - (4 \cdot 10^2)\,\alpha + 0.036Pa \qquad (4/132)$$

S denotes a sensitivity factor characteristic of a given biological system and the polarizability, α, is to be regarded here as an electronic correction term. Equation (4/132) describes toxicity fairly well, but large deviations do occur because the use of the parachor for x_h requires the basic geometry to be constant and this condition is by no means adequately fulfilled with some of the coumpounds investigated.

The relationships deduced for $f_h(x_h)$ in this chapter are of general applicability and and are thus valid if in addition to hydrophobic effects there are also electronic and steric effects on biological activity. For an interpretation in mechanistic terms, certain conditions, which will be discussed later, need to be satisfied (see 8.1.). The question as to whether $f_h(x_h)$ is linear (eqn. (4/122a)) or parabolic (eqn. (4/122b)) must be answered by trial and error. Similar considerations pertain to position dependences. In conclusion, attention is once more drawn to the great importance of $x_{h,0}$ for planning drug synthesis[1]).

References

[1] Eisenberg, D., and W. Kauzman: Structure and Properties of Water, Clarendon Oxford Press, Oxford, 1969

[2] Horne, R. A. (Ed.): Water and Aqueous Solutions, Wiley, New York, 1972

[3] Franks, F. (Ed.): Water, a Comprehensive Treatise, Vol. 1–3, Plenum Press, New York, 1972ff.

[4] Hagler, A. T., H. A. Scheraga and G. Nemethy: Ann. N. Y. Acad. Sci. **204**, 51 (1973)

[5] Lentz, B. R., A. T. Hagler and H. A. Scheraga: J. Phys. Chem. **78**, 1531 (1974)

[6] Jhon, M. S., and H. Eyring: Ann. Rev. Phys. Chem. **27**, 45 (1976)

[7] Hertz, H. G.: Angew. Chem. internat. Ed. **9**, 124 (1970)

[8] Safford, G. Y., and P. S. Leung: Progr. Surf. Membr. Sci. **7**, 231 (1973)

[9] Ben-Naim, A.: Water and Aqueous Solutions, Plenum Press, New York, 1974

[10] Watts, R. O.: Stat. Mech. **1**, 1 (1973)

[11] Pratt, L. R., and D. Chandler: J. Chem. Phys. **67**, 3683 (1977)

[12] Pople, J. A.: Proc. Roy. Soc. **A 205**, 163 (1951)

[13] Angell, J.: J. Phys. Chem. **75**, 3698 (1971)

[14] Sarma, T. S., and J. C. Ahkuwalin: Chem. Soc. Rev. **2**, 203 (1973)

[15] Wilhelm, E., R. Battino and R. J. Wilcock: Chem. Rev. **77**, 219 (1977)

[16] Nemethy, G., and H. A. Scheraga: J. Chem. Phys. **36**, 3401 (1962)

[17] Hagler, A. T., H. A. Scheraga and G. Nemethy: J. Phys. Chem. **76**, 3219 (1972)

[18] Nemethy, G., and H. A. Scheraga: J. Chem. Phys. **36**, 3382 (1962)

[19] Nemethy, G., and H. A. Scheraga: J. Phys. Chem. **66**, 1773 (1962)

[1]) See footnote p. 64.

[20] Hermann, R. B.: J. Phys. Chem. **76**, 2754 (1972)
[21] Hermann, R. B., in E. Bergmann and B. Pullman (Eds.): Molecular and Quantum Pharmacology, Reidl Publishing Company, Dordrecht, 1973, p. 441
[22] Pierotti, R. A.: J. Phys. Chem. **69**, 281 (1965)
[23] Pierotti, R. A.: J. Phys. Chem. **67**, 1840 (1963)
[24] Pierotti, R. A.: Chem. Rev. **76**, 717 (1975)
[25] Neff, R. O., and D. A. McQuarrie: J. Phys. Chem. **77**, 413 (1973)
[26] Ben-Naim, A.: J. Chem. Phys. **54**, 1387 (1971)
[27] Ben-Naim, A.: J. Chem. Phys. **54**, 3696 (1971)
[28] Ben-Naim, A.: J. Chem. Phys. **57**, 5257 (1972)
[29] Ben-Naim, A.: J. Chem. Phys. **57**, 5266 (1972)
[30] Ben-Naim, A.: J. Phys. Chem. **77**, 95 (1973)
[31] Ben-Naim, A., and M. Yaacobi: J. Phys. Chem. **78**, 170 (1974)
[32] Ben-Naim, A.: Biopolymers **14**, 1337 (1975)
[33] Yaacobi, M., and A. Ben-Naim: J. Phys. Chem. **78**, 175 (1975)
[34] Ben-Naim, A.: J. Phys. Chem. **79**, 1268 (1975)
[35] Ben-Naim, A., and M. Yaacobi: J. Phys. Chem. **79**, 1263 (1975)
[36] Hopfinger, A. J., and D. R. Battershell: J. Med. Chem. **19**, 569 (1976)
[36a] Okazaki, S., K. Nakanishi, H. Tuchara and Y. Adachi: J. Phys. Chem. **71**, 2421 (1979)
[36b] Pangali, C., M. Rao and B. J. Berne: J. Chem. Phys. **71**, 2975 (1979)
[36c] Pangali, C., M. Rao, and B. J. Berne: J. Chem. Phys. **71**, 2982 (1979)
[37] Nelson, H. D., and C. L. DeLigny: Rec. Trav. Chim. Pays-Bas **87**, 623 (1968)
[38] Frank, H. S., and W. Y. Wen: Discuss. Faraday Soc. **24**, 133 (1957)
[39] Frank, H. S., and M. W. Evans: J. Chem. Phys. **13**, 507 (1945)
[40] Howarth, O. W.: J. Chem. Soc. Faraday Trans. **71**, 2303 (1975)
[41] Kauzmann, W.: Adv. Protein Chem. **14**, 1 (1959)
[42] Tanford, C.: The Hydrophobic Effect: Formation of Micelles and Biological Membranes. Wiley-Interscience, New York, 1973
[43] Cramer, R. D.: J. Amer. Chem. Soc. **99**, 5408 (1977)
[43a] Wertz, D. H.: J. Amer. Chem. Soc. **102**, 5316 (1980)
[44] Kühne, R., K. Bocek, P. Scharfenberg and R. Franke: Eur. J. Med. Chem. **16**, 7 (1981)
[45] Abraham, M. H.: J. Amer. Chem. Soc. **101**, 5477 (1979)
[46] Sugget, A., in J. A. Keverling Buisman (Ed.): Biological Activity and Chemical Structure, Pharmacochemistry Library (Eds.: W. Th. Nauta and R. F. Rekker), Vol. 2, Elsevier, Amsterdam, 1977, p. 95
[47] Hagler, A. T., and J. Moult: Nature **272**, 222 (1978)
[48] Franke, R.: Acta biol. med. germ. **25**, 757 (1970)
[48a] Pearlman, R. S., in A. H. Yalkowsky, A. A. Sinkula and S. C. Valvani (Eds.): Physical Chemical Properties of Drugs, Marcel Dekker, New York, 1980, p. 321
[49] Hermann, R. B.: Proc. Natl. Acad. Sci. (USA) **74**, 4145 (1974)
[50] Hermann, R. B.: J. Phys. Chem. **79**, 163 (1975)
[51] Hermann, R. B.: Program MØLAREA (QCPE-No. 225), Indianapolis, 1972
[52] Amidon, G. L., and S. T. Anik: J. Pharm. Sci. **65**, 801 (1976)
[53] Amidon, G. L., S. H. Yalkowsky, S. T. Anik and S. C. Valvani: J. Phys. Chem. **79**, 2239 (1975)
[54] Hobza, P.: private communication
[55] Harris, M. S., T. Higuchi and J. H. Rytting: J. Phys. Chem. **77**, 2694 (1973)
[56] Amidon, G. L., S. H. Yalkowsky and S. Leung: J. Pharm. Sci. **63**, 1858 (1794)
[57] Chothia, C.: Nature **248**, 338 (1974)
[58] Yalkowsky, S. H., and S. C. Valvani: J. Med. Chem. **19**, 727 (1976)
[59] Yalkowsky, S. H., G. L. Amidon, G. Zografi and G. L. Flynn: J. Pharm. Sci. **64**, 48 (1975)

[60] Reynolds, J. A., D. B. Gilbert and C. Tanford: Proc. Natl. Acad. Sci. (USA) **71**, 2925 (1974)
[60a] Bultsma, T.: Eur. J. Med. Chem. **15**, 371 (1980)
[61] Yalkowski, S. H., S. C. Valvani and G. L. Amidon: J. Pharm. Sci. **65**, 1488 (1976)
[62] Smith, R., and C. Tanford: Proc. Natl. Acad. Sci. (USA) **70**, 289 (1973)
[63] McAuliffe, J.: J. Phys. Chem. **70**, 1267 (1966)
[64] Yoda, A., S. Yoda and M. A. Sarrif: Mol. Pharmacol. **9**, 766 (1973)
[65] Moriguchi, I.: Chem. Pharm. Bull. **23**, 247 (1975)
[66] Moriguchi, I., Y. Kanada and K. Komatsu: Chem. Pharm. Bull. **24**, 1799 (1976)
[67] Mc Gowan, J. C.: J. Appl. Chem. **2**, 323 (1952)
[68] Mc Gowan, J. C.: J. Appl. Chem. **2**, 651 (1952)
[69] Mc Gowan, J. C.: J. Appl. Chem. **4**, 41 (1954)
[70] Mc Gowan, J. C.: Nature **200**, 1317 (1963)
[71] Mc Gowan, J. C., P. N. Atkinson and L. H. Ruddle: J. Appl. Chem. **16**, 99 (1960)
[72] Deno, N. C., and H. E. Berkheimer: J. Chem. Eng. Data, **5**, 1 (1960)
[73] Miles, J. L., D. A. Robinson and W. J. Canady: J. biol. Chem. **238**, 2932 (1965)
[74] Leo, A., C. Hansch and P. Y. C. Jow: J. Med. Chem. **19**, 611 (1976)
[74a] Cammarata, A.: J. Pharm. Sci. **68**, 839 (1979)
[75] Hall, L. H., L. B. Kier and W. J. Murray: J. Pharm. Sci. **64**, 1975 (1975)
[76] Murray, W. J., L. H. Hall and L. B. Kier: J. Pharm. Sci. **64**, 1978 (1975)
[77] Mitsuda, H., K. Yasumato and A. Yamamoto: Arch. Biochem. Biophys. **118**, 664 (1967)
[78] Nagwekar, J. B., and N. Muangnoicharoen: J. Pharm. Sci. **62**, 1439 (1973)
[79] Kay, R. L., T. Vituccio, C. Zawoysky and D. F. Evans: J. Phys. Chem. **70**, 236 (1966)
[80] Hansch, C., in E. J. Ariens (Ed.): Drug Design, Vol. I, Academic Press, New York, 1971, p. 271
[81] Lien, E. J., C. Hansch and S. M. Anderson: J. Med. Chem. **11**, 430 (1968)
[82] Lien, E. J.: J. Med. Chem. **19**, 849 (1976)
[82a] Franke, R., R. Kühne and S. Dove in J. C. Dearden (Ed.): Quantitative Approaches to Drug Design, Pharmacochemistry Library (Eds.: W. Th. Nauta and R. F. Rekker), Vol. 6, Elsevier, Amsterdam, 1983, p. 15
[83] Collander, R.: Acta Physiol. Scand. **13**, 363 (1947)
[84] Collander, R.: Acta Chem. Scand. **5**, 744 (1951)
[85] Hansch, C., in C. J. Cavallito (Ed.): Structure-Activity Relationships, Pergamon Press, Oxford, 1971
[86] Hansch, C., J. E. Quinlan and G. L. Lawrence: J. Org. Chem. **33**, 347 (1968)
[87] Leo, A., and C. Hansch: J. Org. Chem. **36**, 1539 (1971)
[88] Leo, A.: Adv. in Chemistry Series **114**, 51 (1972)
[88a] Valvani, S. C., and S. H. Yalkowski in S. H. Yalkowski, A. A. Sinkula and S. C. Valvani (Eds.): Physical Chemical Properties of Drugs, Marcell Dekker, New York, 1980, p. 201
[88b] Valvani, S. C., S. H. Yalkowsky and T. J. Roseman: J. Pharm. Sci. **70**, 502 (1981)
[89] Chiou, C. T., V. H. Freed, D. W. Schmedding and R. L. Kohnert: Environ. Sci. Technol. **11**, 475 (1977)
[90] Leo, A., C. Hansch and D. Elkins: Chem. Rev. **71**, 525 (1971)
[91] Fujita, T., T. Nishioka and M. Nakajima: J. Med. Chem. **20**, 1071 (1977)
[92] Seiler, P.: Eur. J. Med. Chem. **9**, 473 (1974)
[93] Hansch, C., and A. Leo: Substituent Constants for Correlation Analysis in Chemistry and Biology, Wiley, New York, 1979
[94] Hansch, C., and W. J. Dunn: J. Pharm. Sci. **61**, 1 (1972)
[95] Fujita, T., J. Iwasa and C. Hansch: J. Am. Chem. Soc. **36**, 5175 (1964)
[96] Hansch, C., A. Leo, S. Unger, K. H. Kim, D. Nikaitani and E. J. Lien: J. Med. Chem. **16**, 1207 (1973)
[97] Hansch, C., S. D. Rockwell, P. Y. C. Jow, A. Leo and E. E. Steller: J. Med. Chem. **20**, 304 (1977)

[98] Tute, M. S.: Adv. Drug Res. **6**, 1 (1971)
[99] Hansch, C., A. Leo and D. Nikaitani: J. Org. Chem. **37**, 3090 (1972)
[100] Canas-Rodriguez, A., and M. S. Tute: Adv. in Chemistry Series **114**, 41 (1972)
[101] Fujita, T., K. Kamoshita, T. Nishioka and M. Nakajima: Agr. Biol. Chem. **38**, 1521 (1974)
[102] Dearden, J. C., and J. H. Tubby: J. Pharm. **2**, Suppl., 73 P (1974)
[103] Van den Berg, G., T. Bultsma, R. F. Rekker and W. Th. Nauta: Eur. J. Med. Chem. **10**, 242 (1975)
[104] Meyer, A.: Thesis, Martin-Luther-Universität Halle—Wittenberg, 1976
[105] Hagemann, R., A. Meyer, R. Franke and A. Barth: Pharmazie **32**, 526 (1977)
[106] Taylor, P. J.: personal communication
[106a] Parker, G. R., and T. L. Lemke: J. Med. Chem. **20**, 1221 (1977)
[107] Iwasa, J., T. Fujita and C. Hansch: J. Med. Chem. **8**, 150 (1965)
[108] Currie, D. J., C. E. Lough, R. F. Silver and H. L. Holmes: Can. J. Chem. **44**, 1035 (1966)
[109] Biagi, G. L., A. M. Barbaro and M. C. Guerra: Adv. in Chemistry Series **114**, 61 (1972)
[110] Bate-Smith, E. C., and R. G. Westall: Biochim. Biophys. Acta **4**, 427 (1950)
[111] Dearden, J. C., A. M. Patel and J. M. Thubby: J. Pharm. Pharmacol. **26**, Suppl., 75 P (1974)
[112] Miyagishima, T.: Chem. Pharm. Bull. **22**, 2288 (1974)
[113] Biagi, G. L., M. C. Guerra and A. M. Barbaro: J. Med. Chem. **13**, 944 (1970)
[114] Biagi, G. L., A. M. Barbaro, M. C. Guerra, G. Cantelli-Forti and M. E. Fracasso: J. Med. Chem. **17**, 28 (1974)
[115] Biagi, G. L., O. Gandolfi, M. C. Guerra, A. M. Barbaro and G. Cantelli-Forti: J. Med. Chem. **18**, 868 (1975)
[116] Biagi, G. L., A. M. Barbaro, O. Gondolfi, M. C. Guerra and G. Cantelli-Forti: J. Med. Chem. **18**, 873 (1975)
[117] Kuchař, M., B. Brunova, V. Rejholec and V. Rabek: J. Chromatography **92**, 381 (1974)
[118] Boyce, C. B. C., and B. W. Milborrow: Nature **208**, 537 (1965)
[119] Iwasa, J., T. Fujita and C. Hansch: J. Med. Chem. **8**, 150 (1965)
[120] Gabbott, P. A.: Progr. Photosynthesis Res. **3**, 1712 (1969)
[121] Turnbull, J. D., G. L. Biagi, A. L. Merola and D. G. Cornwell: Biochem. Pharmacol. **20**, 1383 (1971)
[122] Draber, W., K. H. Büchel and K. Dickore: Proc. Int. Congr. Pestic. Chem., 2nd, 1971, Vol. 5, p. 153 (1972)
[122a] Kuchař, M., V. Rejholec, M. Jelinková, V. Rábek and O. Němeček: J. Chromatogr. **162**, 197 (1979)
[122b] Kuchař, M., V. Rejholec, B. Brunova and M. Jelinková: J. Chromatogr. **195**, 329 (1980)
[123] Hansch, C., and F. Helmers: J. Polymer Sci. **6**, 3295 (1968)
[124] Seydel, J. K. and R. Albrecht: Eur. J. Med. Chem. **10**, 378 (1975)
[125] Seydel, J. K.: Communication to general discussion, in R. Franke and P. Oehme (Eds.): Quantitative Structure-Activity Analysis, Akademie-Verlag, Berlin 1978
[126] McCall, J. M.: J. Med. Chem. **18**, 549 (1975)
[127] Carlson, R. M., R. E. Calson and H. L. Koppermann: J. Chromatography **107**, 219 (1975)
[128] Twitchett, P. J., and A. C. Moffatt: J. Chromatography **111**, 149 (1975)
[129] Tanaka, N., and E. R. Thornton: J. Am. Chem. Soc. **99**, 7300 (1977)
[130] Yamana, T., A. Tsuji and E. Miyamoto: J. Pharm. Sci. **66**, 747 (1977)
[131] Mirrlees, M. S., S. J. Moulton, C. T. Murphy and P. Taylor: J. Med. Chem. **19**, 615 (1976)
[131a] Unger, S. H., J. R. Cook and J. S. Hollenberg: J. Pharm. Sci. **67**, 1364 (1978)
[132] Henry, D., J. H. Block, J. L. Anderson and G. R. Carlson: J. Med. Chem. **19**, 619 (1976)
[133] Nys, G. G., and R. F. Rekker: Chim. Ther. **8**, 521 (1973)
[134] Nys, G. G., and R. F. Rekker: Chim. Ther. **9**, 361 (1974)
[135] Rekker, R. F., in R. Franke and P. Oehme (Eds.): Quantitative Structure-Activity Analysis, Akademie-Verlag, Berlin, 1978

[136] Rekker, R. F.: The Hydrophobic Fragmental Constant, Pharmacochemistry Library (Eds.: W. Th. Nauta and R. F. Rekker), Vol. 1, Elsevier, Amsterdam, 1977
[136a] Rekker, R. F., and H. M. de Kort: Eur. J. Med. Chem. **14**, 479 (1979)
[137] Rekker, R. F., in J. A. Keverling Buisman (Ed.): Biological Activity and Chemical Structure, Pharmacochemistry Library (Eds.: W. Th. Nauta and R. F. Rekker), Vol. 2, Elsevier, Amsterdam, 1977, p. 231
[138] Franke, R., in J. A. Keverling Buisman (Ed.): Biological Activity and Chemical Structure, Pharmacochemistry Library (Eds.: W. Th. Nauta and R. F. Rekker), Vol. 2, Elsevier, Amsterdam, 1977, p. 251
[139] Leo, A., P. Y. C. Jow, C. Silipo and C. Hansch: J. Med. Chem. **18**, 865 (1975)
[139a] Valvani, S. C., and S. H. Yalkowsky in S. H. Yalkowsky, A. A. Sinkula and S. C. Valvani (Eds.): Physical Chemical Properties of Drugs, Marcell Dekker, New York, 1980, p. 201
[140] Hine, J., and P. R. Mookerjee: J. Org. Chem. **40**, 292 (1975)
[141] Ostrenga, J. A.: J. Med. Chem. **12**, 349 (1969)
[142] Hildebrand, J. H., and R. L. Scott: The Solubility of Nonelectrolytes, Reinhold Publishing Co., New York, 1950
[143] Hildebrand, J. H., and R. L. Scott: Regular Solutions, Prentice Hall, Englewood Cliffs, 1962
[144] Barton, A. F. M.: Chem. Rev. **75**, 731 (1975)
[145] Cammarata, A., S. Yau and K. S. Rogers: J. Med. Chem. **14**, 1211 (1971)
[146] Davis, S. S.: Experientia **26**, 671 (1970)
[147] Nogami, H., T. Nagai and S. Wada: Chem. Pharm. Bull. **18**, 342 (1970)
[148] Kakemi, K., T. Arita, R. Hori and R. Konishi: Chem. Pharm. Bull. **15**, 1883 (1967)
[149] Kakemi, K., T. Arita, R. Hori, R. Konishi and K. Nishimura: Chem. Pharm. Bull. **17**, 248 (1969)
[150] Kakemi, K., T. Arita, R. Hori, R. Konishi, K. Nishimura, H. Matsui and T. Nishimura: Chem. Pharm. Bull. **17**, 255 (1969)
[151] Morishita, T., M. Yamazaki, N. Yata and A. Kamada: Chem. Pharm. Bull. **21**, 2309 (1973)
[152] Kühne, R., R. Franke, J. Dittrich and E. Kretschmer: Quant. Struct.-Act. Relat. **2**, 20 (1983)
[153] Franke, R.: Acta biol. med. germ. **25**, 789 (1970)
[154] Franke, R.: Biochim. Biophys. Acta **160**, 378 (1968)
[155] Franke, R.: Mol. Pharmacol. **5**, 640 (1969)
[156] Franke, R.: Chem. Biol. Interactions **6**, 1 (1973)
[157] Franke, R.: Acta biol. med. germ. **30**, 151 (1973)
[158] Kühne, R., R. Franke, H. Sprintz and G. Hübner: Acta biol. med. germ. **38**, 1441 (1979)
[159] Kühne, R., R. Franke, H. Sprintz and G. Hübner in R. Franke and P. Oehme (Eds.): Quantitative Structure-Activity Analysis, Akademie-Verlag, Berlin, 1978, p. 59
[160] Davis, S. S., T. Higuchi and J. H. Rytting: Adv. Pharm. Sci. **4**, 73 (1974)
[161] Balasubramanian, D., and D. B. Wettlaufer: Proc. Natl. Acad. Sci. (USA) **55**, 762 (1966)
[162] Scholtan, W.: Antibiotica et Chemotherapia **12**, 103 (1966)
[163] Schrier, E. E., R. T. Ingwall und H. A. Scheraga: J. Phys. Chem. **69**, 298 (1965)
[164] Rohmann, C., and D. Scheurle: Arch. Pharmaz. **274**, 236 (1936)
[165] Bull, H. B., and K. Breese: Arch. Biochem. Biophys. **120**, 303 (1967)
[166] Bull, H. B., and K. Breese: Arch. Biochem. Biophys. **120**, 309 (1967)
[167] Schnell, J., and H. Zahn: Makromol. Chem. **84**, 192 (1965)
[168] von Hippel, P. P., and K. Y. Wong: J. biol. Chem. **240**, 3909 (1965)
[169] Schrier, E. E., and C. D. Mackey: J. Phys. Chem. **72**, 733 (1968)
[170] Schrier, E. E., M. Pottle and H. A. Scheraga: J. Amer. Chem. Soc. **86**, 3444 (1964)
[171] Schrier, E. E., R. T. Ingwall and H. A. Scheraga: J. Phys. Chem. **69**, 298 (1965)
[172] Franke, R., and W. Schmidt: Acta biol. med. germ. **31**, 273 (1973)
[173] Franke, R. in M. Tichý (Ed.): Quantitative Structure-Activity Relationships, Akadémiai Kiadó, Budapest, 1976

[174] Wildnauer, R., and W. J. Canady: Biochemistry **5**, 2885 (1966)
[175] Royer, G., and W. J. Canady: Archs. Biochim. Biophys. **124**, 530 (1968)
[176] Sahyun, M. R. V.: Nature **209**, 613 (1966)
[177] Hansch, C.: J. Med. Chem. **19**, 1 (1976)
[178] Dove, S., R. Franke, R. Dove, W. Müller and T. Schewe: unpublished results
[179] Lorenz, D., K. Fechner, R. Franke, H. Niedrich and B. Mehlis: Paper presented at the Symposium "Synthese, Biochemie und Wirkung potentieller Arzneimittel" (Pharmazeutische Gesellschaft der DDR), Warnemünde, 1975
[180] Henderson, R., and J. H. Wang: Ann. Rev. Biophys. **1**, 1 (1972)
[181] Antonov, V. K., T. V. Ivanina, H. G. Ivanova, I. V. Berezin, A. V. Lavashow and K. Martinez: FEBS Letters **20**, 37 (1972)
[182] Hansch, C., and W. R. Glave: Mol. Pharmacol. **7**, 337, (1971)
[183] Hansch, C., in C. J. Cavallito: Structure-Activity Relationships, Pergamon Press, Oxford, 1971
[184] Smith, R. N., C. Hansch and T. P. Poindexter: Physiol. Chem. Physics **6**, 323 (1974)
[185] Dunn, W. J.: J. Pharm. Sci. **62**, 1575 (1973)
[186] Hansch, C., and W. J. Dunn: J. Pharm. Sci. **61**, 1 (1972)
[187] Lien, E. J., and C. Hansch: Adv. in Chemistry Series **114**, 155 (1972)
[188] Hansch, C., and J. M. Clayton: J. Pharm. Sci. **61**, 1 (1973)
[189] Lien, E. J., C. Hansch and S. M. Anderson: J. Med. Chem. **11**, 430 (1968)
[190] Barkler, J. L.: Nature **252**, 52 (1974)
[191] Martin, Y. C., and C. Hansch: J. Med. Chem. **14**, 777 (1971)
[192] Rey, A.: Il Farmaco **24**, 294 (1974)
[193] Franke, R., D. Labes, M. Tonew, W. Zschiesche and L. Heinisch: Acta biol. med. germ. **34**, 491 (1975)
[194] Hansch, C., and E. W. Deutsch: Biochim. Biophys. Acta **112**, 381 (1966)
[195] Franke, R., and R. Kühne: Contribution in the 17th anniversary Meeting of Pharmakologische Gesellschaft der DDR, Berlin, 1975
[196] Franke, R., in R. Franke und P. Oehme (Eds.): Quantitative Structure-Activity Analysis, Akademie-Verlag, Berlin, 1978
[197] Franke, R., and R. Kühne: Eur. J. Med. Chem. **13**, 399 (1978)
[198] Franke, R., in P. Oehme (Ed.): Theoretische Aspekte der Wirkstofforschung, VEB Verlag Volk und Gesundheit, Berlin, 1978
[199] Michelson, J. M., and A. F. Danilov in Z. M. Bacq (Ed.): Fundamentals in Biochemical Pharmacology, Pergamon Press, Oxford, 1971
[200] Belleau, B.: J. Med. Chem. **7**, 64 (1964)
[201] Karlin, A.: J. gen. Physiol. **54**, 245 (1969)
[202] Karlin, A.: Life Sci. **14**, 1385 (1974)
[203] Franke, R., and P. Oehme: Pharmazie **28**, 489 (1973)
[204] Druckrey, E., and H. Metzger: J. Med. Chem. **16**, 436 (1973)
[205] Flynn, G. L., and S. H. Yalkowski: J. Pharm. Sci. **61**, 838 (1972)
[206] Garrett, E. R., and P. B. Chemburkar: J. Pharm. Sci. **57**, 944 (1968)
[207] Garrett, E. R., and P. B. Chemburkar: J. Pharm. Sci. **57**, 949 (1968)
[208] Garrett, E. R., and P. B. Chemburkar: J. Pharm. Sci. **57**, 1401 (1968)
[209] Nasim, K., M. C. Meyer and J. Autian: J. Pharm. Sci. **61**, 1775 (1972)
[210] Nasim, K., M. C. Meyer and J Autian: J. Pharm. Sci. **62**, 1 (1973)
[211] Raaflaub, J.: Experientia **26**, 457 (1973)
[212] Herzog, K. A., and J. Swarbrick: J. Pharm. Sci. **61**, 1666 (1972)
[213] Augustin, M. A., and J. Swarbrick: J. Pharm. Sci. **61**, 1656 (1972)
[214] Ho, F. H. N., and W. I. Higuchi: J. Pharm. Sci. **60**, 537 (1971)
[215] Lien, E. J., and G. L. Tong: J. Soc. Cosmet. Chem. **24**, 371 (1973)

[216] Falk, W., W. Fuerst, E. Hannig and R. Boehm: Pharmazie **29**, 542 (1974)
[217] Michaels, A. S., S. K. Chandrasekaran and J. E. Shaw: AI Che. J. **21**, 985 (1975)
[218] Pla-Delfina, J. M., J. Moreno, J. Duran and A. Del Pozo: J. Pharmacokinet. Biopharm. **3**, 115 (1975)
[219] Lien, E. J., in E. J. Ariens (Ed.): Drug Design, Vol. V, Academic Press, New York, 1975
[219a] Lien, E. J.: Ann. Rev. Pharmacol. Toxicol. **21**, 31 (1981)
[220] Flynn, G. L., S. H. Yalkowski and T. J. Rosemann: J. Pharm. Sci. **63**, 479 (1974)
[221] Lippold, B. C., and G. F. Schneider: Arzneim.-Forsch. **25**, 843 (1975)
[222] Yalkowski, S. H., and G. L. Flynn: J. Pharm. Sci. **62**, 210 (1973)
[223] Kubinyi, H.: Arzneim.-Forsch. **29**, 1067 (1979)
[224] Yalkowski, S. H., T. G. Slunick and G. L. Flynn: J. Pharm. Sci. **63**, 691 (1974)
[225] Flynn, G. L., and S. H. Yakowski: J. Pharm. Sci. **61**, 838 (1972)
[226] Hansch, C., R. M. Muir, T. Fujita, P. P. Maloney, F. Geiger and M. Streich: J. Amer. Chem. Soc. **85**, 2817 (1963)
[227] Hansch, C., and T. Fujita: J. Amer. Chem. Soc. **86**, 1616 (1964)
[228] Penniston, J. T., L. Beckett, D. L Bentley and C. Hansch: Mol. Pharmacol. **5**, 333 (1969)
[229] Dearden, J. C., and M. S. Townend: J. Pharm. Pharmacol. **28 S**, 13 P (1976)
[230] Dearden, J. C., and M. S. Townend in R. Franke and P. Oehme (Eds.): Quantitative Structure-Activity Analysis, Akademie-Verlag, Berlin, 1978
[231] McFarland, J. C.: J. Med. Chem. **13**, 1192 (1970)
[232] Kubinyi, H.: Arzneim.-Forsch. **26**, 1991 (1976)
[233] Kubinyi, H.: J. Med. Chem. **20**, 625 (1977)
[234] Kubinyi, H. in J. A. Keverling Buisman (Ed.): Biological Activity and Chemical Structure, Pharmacochemistry Library (Eds.: W. Th. Nauta and R. F. Rekker), Vol. 2, Elsevier, Amsterdam, 1977, p. 239
[235] Kubinyi, H.: Progr. Drug Res. **23**, 97 (1980)
[236] Vora, K. R. M., W. I. Higuchi and N. F. H. Ho: J. Pharm. Sci. **11**, 1785 (1972)
[237] Wagner, J. G., and A. J. Sedman: J. Pharmacokinetics Biopharm. **1**, 1 (1973)
[238] Martin, Y. C., in E. J. Ariens (Ed.): Drug Design, Vol. VIII, Academic Press, New York, 1978
[239] Millborrow, D. V., and D. A. Williams: Physiol. Plant. **21**, 902 (1968)
[239a] Martin, Y. C.: J. Med. Chem. **24**, 229 (1981)
[240] Verloop, A., in E. J. Ariens (Ed.): Drug Design, Vol. III, Academic Press, New York, 1972, p. 133
[241] Hansch, C., A. R. Steward and J. Iwasa: Mol. Pharmacol. **1**, 87 (1965)
[242] Hansch, C., A. R. Steward, S. M. Anderson and D. Bentley: J. Med. Chem. **11**, 1 (1968)
[243] Druckrey, E., H. Schwarz and H. Leditschke: Chim. Ther. **7**, 188 (1972)
[244] Sprott, G. D., J. M. Wood, W. G. Martin and H. Schneider: Biochem. Biophys. Res. Commun. **76**, 1099 (1977)
[245] Preston, R. L., J. F. Schaeffer and P. F. Curran: J. General Physiol. **64**, 443 (1974)
[246] Higuchi, T., and S. S. Davis: J. Pharm. Sci. **59**, 1376 (1970)
[247] Hyde, R. M.: J. Med. Chem. **18**, 231 (1975)
[248] Martin, Y. C., and J. J. Hackbarth: J. Med. Chem. **19**, 1033 (1976)
[249] Martin, Y. C., and J. J. Hackbarth in B. Kowalski (Ed.): Proceedings of the American Chemical Society Symposium on Chemometrics, ACS Symposium Series **254**, 153 (1977)
[250] Martin, Y. C., in R. Franke and P. Oehme (Eds.): Quantitative Structure-Activity Analysis, Akademie-Verlag, Berlin, 1978
[251] Martin, Y. C.: Drug Design Methods: A Critical Introduction, Marcell Dekker, New York, 1978
[251a] Martin, Y. C., in S. H. Yalkowsky, A. S. Sinkula and S. C. Valvani (Eds.): Physical Chemical Properties of Drugs, Marcell Dekker, New York, 1980, p. 49

[252] Craig, P. N., and C. Hansch: J. Med. Chem. **16**, 661 (1973)

[253] Lee, D. L., P. A. Kollman, F. J. Marsh and M. E. Wolff: J. Med. Chem. **20**, 1139 (1977)

[253a] Coats, E. A., in S. H. Yalkowsky, A. S. Sinkula and S. C. Valvani (Eds.): Physical Chemical Properties of Drugs, Marcel Dekker, New York, 1980, p. 111

[253b] Seydel, J. K.: Int. J. Quantum Chem. **20**, 131 (1981)

[254] Hellenbrecht, D., K. F. Müller and J. Grobecker: Eur. J. Pharmacol. **29**, 223 (1974)

[255] von Cube, G., H. J. Teschemacher, A. Herz and R. Hess: Naunyn-Schmiedeberg's Arch. Exp. Pathol. Pharmacol. **265**, 455 (1970)

[256] Kutter, E., A. Herz, H. J. Teschemacher and R. Hess: J. Med. Chem. **13**, 801 (1970)

[257] Hammer, R., G. Bozler and F.-W. Koss in E. Kutter (Ed.): Arzneimittelentwicklung, Georg Thieme Verlag, Stuttgart, 1978

[258] Seydel, J. K., in E. J. Ariens (Ed.): Drug Design, Vol. I, Academic Press, New York, 1971, p. 343

[259] Seydel, J. K., and E. Wempe: Arzneimittel-Forsch. **21**, 187, (1971)

[260] Seydel, J. K., and K. J. Schaper: Chemische Struktur und biologische Aktivität von Wirkstoffen, Verlag Chemie, Weinheim, 1979

[260a] Seydel, J. K., D. Trettin and H.-P. Cordes: J. Med. Chem. **23**, 607 (1980)

[260b] Seydel, J. K., in J. A. Keverling Buisman (Ed.): Strategy in Drug Research, Pharmacochemistry Library (Eds.: W. Th. Nauta and R. F. Rekker), Vol. 4, Elsevier, Amsterdam, 1982, p. 179

[261] Pitman, I. H., K. Uekama, T. Higuchi and E. W. Hall: J. Amer. Chem. Soc. **94**, 8147 (1972)

[261a] Rideout, D. C., and R. Breslow: J. Amer. Chem. Soc. **102**, 7816 (1980)

[262] Meyer, H. H.: Arch. exp. Path. Pharmak. **42**, 119 (1899)

[263] Overton, E.: Studien über die Narkose, Fischer-Verlag, Jena, 1901

[264] Meyer, K. H., and H. Hemmi: Biochem. Z. **277**, 39 (1935)

[265] Seeman, P.: Pharmacol. Rev. **24**, 583 (1972)

[266] Richet, C.: C. r. Séanc. Soc. Biol. **54**, 775 (1893)

[267] Moore, W.: J. Agr. Res. **9**, 371 (1917)

[268] Fühner, H.: Arch. exp. Path. Pharmak. **52**, 69 (1904)

[269] Fühner, H., and E. Neubauer: Arch. exp. Path. Pharmak. **56**, 333 (1907)

[270] Fühner, H.: Z. Biol. **57**, 487 (1912)

[271] Ferguson, J.: Proc. R. Soc. **B 127**, 387 (1939)

[272] Ferguson, J., and H. Pieri: Ann. Appl. Biol. **35**, 532 (1948)

[273] Ferguson, J.: Chem. Ind. 818 (1964)

[274] Traube, J.: Arch. ges. Physiol. **105**, 541 (1904)

[275] Traube, J.: Arch. ges. Physiol. **132**, 511 (1910)

[276] Traube, J.: Arch. ges. Physiol. **153**, 276 (1913)

[277] Zahradnick, R.: Experientia **18**, 534 (1962)

[278] Zahradnick, R.: Arch. Int. Pharmacodyn. **135**, 311 (1962)

[279] Kopecky, J., and K. Boček: Experientia **23**, 125 (1967)

[280] Spinks, A.: Chem. Ind. **12**, 885 (1973)

[281] Mc Gowan, J. C.: J. Appl. Chem. **1**, 120 (1951)

[282] Mc Gowan, J. C.: J. Appl. Chem. **16**, 103 (1966)

5. Electronik Influences on Biological Activity: the Funktion $f_e(x_e)$

There are many electronic influences on biological activity, occurring under a multiplicity of conditions and through a variety of mechanisms and interactions. Examples are dispersion forces, charge-transfer interactions, electrostatic interactions, hydrogen bonding, polarization effects, acid-base catalysis and chemical reactions. This variety combined with the extensiveness of biologically active structures calls for an equally large number of parameters for the description of the $f_e(x_e)$ term in eqn. (3/17).

At present the approach most widely used is that of *linear free enthalpy relationships* (LFERs)[1]) together with the appropriate *electronic substituent constants* since the latter are tabulated and readily accessible. In a second variant the parameter x_e is expressed in terms of *experimental quantities* such as pK_a values, spectroscopic data or dipole moments (insofar as these reflect the electronic properties which govern the electronic interactions with the biosystem under consideration and can be measured under conditions compatible with the events in the biological medium). A third possibility involves the use of *quantum-chemical parameters,* and is assuming increasing importance.

The electronic features of a molecule are intimately related to its biological activity. Nevertheless, biological activity can only rarely be described with the function $f_e(x_e)$ alone, since the electronic effects are nearly always superimposed on hydrophobic and steric effects.

5.1. Use of Linear Free Enthalpy Relationships (LFERs)

A *reaction series* may be defined as the chemical reaction (e.g., ester splitting) at a constant reaction centre (e.g., a COOR group) and according to a constant reaction mechanism (e.g., S_{N2}), of a series of chemical compounds formed by varying the substituents in a single, parent compound. Each substituent has a specific influence on the equilibrium and rate constants of the reaction via changes in the electron density and steric effects (for the latter, see 6.) at the reaction centre, which can be described in terms of linear free enthalpy relationships. As they do not follow immediately from the laws of thermodynamics, such relationships are often referred to as *extrathermodynamic* relations. There is no theoretically compelling derivation of these relationships, which must therefore be considered as empirical and only "proven" by their agreement with experimental results.

Formal methods of generating LFERs have been reported by LEFFLER and GRUNWALD [1], PALM [2] and WOLD and SJÖSTRÖM [3, 4]. WOLDS approach has the greatest general applicability, but is less suitable for an introduction to such relationships within

---

[1]) LFERs are frequently also called linear free energy relationships since, in the reactions cons sidered, volume work can be neglected so that the difference between free enthalpy (GIBB-free energy) and free energy is negligible.

the context of this chapter. The approach proposed by LEFFLER and GRUNWALD may be less generally applicable, but it has the advantage that by virtue of a special additivity principle it greatly facilitates the recognition of problems associated with LFERs. The following deduction, intended as an aid to reading this chapter, is based on the latter procedure, although that of WOLD would have allowed greater accuracy in more complex relationships.

The molecules of the reaction series are first divided into two regions, namely R which contains the variable substituents X and Y in which the reaction centre is located. The reaction series can thus be formulated in terms of eqn. (5/1)

$$\mathrm{R - Y \rightleftharpoons R - Y'} \tag{5/1}$$

where the centre changes from Y into Y′ during the course of the chemical reaction considered. Each region is considered to make an additive contribution to the standard free enthalpy (GIBBS free energy) and to interact with the other region by only one constant mechanism. This interaction is denoted by the interaction term I_{RY}. If a substituent $X_1 (R = R_1)$ is located in R

$$\begin{aligned} G_S{}^0 &= G^0_{R_1} + G_Y{}^0 + I_{R_1Y} \\ G_E{}^0 &= G^0_{R_1} + G^0_{Y'} + I_{R_1Y'} \end{aligned} \tag{5/2}$$

where $G_S{}^0$ = standard free enthalpy of the starting product $R_1 - Y$ and $G_E{}^0$ = standard free enthalpy of the end product $R_1 - Y'$. For the change of standard free enthalpy we obtain:

$$\begin{aligned} \Delta_Y G_1{}^0 &= G_E{}^0 - G_S{}^0 \\ &= (G^0_{Y'} - G_Y{}^0) + (I_{R_1Y'} - I_{R_1Y}) \end{aligned} \tag{5/3}$$

Analogously, for any other substituent X_2 $(R = R_2)$:

$$\Delta_Y G_2{}^0 = (G^0_{Y'} - G_Y{}^0) + (I_{R_2Y'} - I_{R_2Y}) \tag{5/4}$$

The change of ΔG^0 due to the exchange of X_1 for X_2 is represented by the difference between eqns. (5/3) and (5/4)

$$\vartheta_{X_2} \Delta_Y G^0 = (I_{R_2Y'} - I_{R_2Y}) - (I_{R_1Y'} - I_{R_1Y}) \tag{5/5}$$

that is the difference of the interaction terms. It may thus be ascribed to the respective interactions of R_1 and R_2 with Y and Y′.

Interaction terms of the I_{AB} type can be factorized as:

$$I_{AB} = I_A \cdot I_B \tag{5/6}$$

I_A depends only on A and I_B only on B, so that I_{AB} is separated into two independent contributions. This principle is utilized in, for example, quantum chemistry to factorize wave functions and in statistical thermodynamics to factorize partition functions. It can be shown that the procedure is allowed in the present case provided that the substituent exchange does not alter the structure too drastically [1]. For that matter, LFERs would not be applicable if the structural changes were too overt.

Applying eqn. (5/6), eqn. (5/5) can be rewritten as:

$$\vartheta_{X_2}\Delta_Y G^0 = (I_{Y'} - I_Y)\,(I_{R_2} - I_{R_1}) \tag{5/7}$$

For another reaction series of the form

$$\mathrm{R - M \rightleftharpoons R - M'} \tag{5/8}$$

a fully analogous relationship

$$\vartheta_{X_2}\Delta_M G^0 = (I_{M'} - I_M)\,(I_{R_2} - I_{R_1}) \tag{5/9}$$

is applicable. Combination of eqns. (5/7) and (5/9) yields:

$$\vartheta_{X_2}\Delta_M G^0 = \frac{(I_{M'} - I_M)}{(I_{Y'} - I_Y)}\,\vartheta_{X_2}\Delta_Y G^0 \tag{5/10}$$

It follows from eqn. (5/10) that the changes in standard free enthalpy for a given set of substituents of two reaction series having the same parent moiety are *linearly interrelated*. Such relationships are called linear free enthalpy relationships.

The first parenthetical term in eqns. (5/7) and (5/9) is only dependent on the reaction centre and reflects its susceptibility to electronic substituent effects. The second parenthetical term is characteristic of substituents X_1 and X_2, providing a means of comparing the changes in electron density around the reaction centre caused by these substituents. In order to compare various reaction series and substituents in a straightforward manner it is necessary to have a well defined scale. To this end, one of the reaction series and one of the substituents are taken as standards and an arbitrary value is assigned to both the first parenthetical term for the standard series and to the interaction term for the standard substituent. When eqn. (5/7) is divided by $-2.303RT$, and the equilibrium constants for a derivative with a substituent X ($X = X_2$) and another one with the standard substituent ($X = X_1$) are K_X and $K_{st.}$, respectively, it follows that[1]):

$$\log K_X - \log K_{st.} = \log K_X/K_{st.} = (I_{Y'} - I_Y)\,(I_{R_2} - I_{R_1}) \tag{5/11}$$

When the dissociation of meta- and para-substituted benzoic acids in water at 298.7 K

$$X_{m,p} - C_6H_4COOH \xrightleftharpoons[298.7\,K]{H_2O} X_{m,p} - C_6H_4COO^- + H_3O^+ \tag{5/12}$$

is chosen as the standard series, and the substituent X = H as standard substituent, eqn. (5/11) takes the form:

$$\log K_X/K_H = (I_{COO^-} - I_{COOH})\,(I_X - I_H) \tag{5/13}$$

Defining

$$(I_{COO^-} - I_{COOH}) = 1 \tag{5/14}$$

$$I_H = 0$$

---

[1]) In order to avoid confusion the symbols for the interaction terms have not been changed in eqn. (5/11) although they have, of course, also been divided $-2.303RT$.

leads to:

$$\log K_X/K_H = 1(I_X - 0) = I_X \tag{5/15}$$

The variable is I_X characteristic of substituent X and is denoted by the *electronic substituent constant* σ which is thus defined as

$$\sigma \equiv (\log K_X/K_H) \text{ diss. benzoic acid} \tag{5/16}$$

with $\sigma_H \equiv 0$. Given eqn. (5/10), for any other reaction series:

$$\log K_X/K_H = (I_{M'} - I_M)\,\sigma \tag{5/17}$$

The parenthetical term is denoted by the *reaction constant* ϱ ($\varrho = 1$ for the standard reaction series (5/12)):

$$\log K_X/K_H = \varrho\sigma \tag{5/18}$$

or

$$\log K_X = \varrho\sigma + \text{constant} \tag{5/19}$$

Equation (5/18) is the well-known Hammett *equation* [5, 6] for meta- and para-substituted benzene derivatives, and permits the calculation of K_X from known σ values.

K_X in eqn. (5/19) is either an equilibrium constant or a rate constant; in the latter case the derivation would have to be based on activation free enthalpy. The reaction constant ϱ characterizes the susceptibility of a reaction relative to the benzoic acid dissociation. As the latter is enhanced by electron-attracting substituents and $\varrho = 1$ by definition, a positive (negative) value of ϱ in eqn. (5/19) indicates that the reaction considered is enhanced (inhibited) by electron-attracting substituents, and this effect is greater the higher is the absolute value of ϱ. At very low ϱ values, such a conclusion is not valid because a relatively small difference in temperature may sometimes be sufficient to invert the sign of ϱ.

The electronic substituent constant (Hammett *constant*) provides a measure of the electron-attracting power of a substituent relative to hydrogen. Substituents which have a strong affinity towards electrons have high positive σ values, whilst σ values of electron-donating substituents are negative. Since the electronic influences of a substituent at the meta- and para-positions are different, σ_m and σ_p do not have the same values; they are, however, not independent of each other but statistically correlated [7]. Ideally, σ is additive so that in the case of multisubstitution:

$$\log K_X = \varrho \sum \sigma + \text{constant} \tag{5/20}$$

In complex molecules, however, a position-dependence of the electronic substituent effect cannot entirely be ruled out. Different ϱ values must then be assigned to the different positions of substitution.

Originally derived for side chain reactions in benzene derivatives, i.e. for compounds of type IX, the Hammett equation has also been successfully applied, within limits to be defined later, to higher condensed aromatic compounds (e.g. [26b]), many heterocyclic systems (e.g. [8, 9, 12]; for substituent constants of heteroatoms in rings and of heterocyclic rings as substituents, see e.g. also [9a—f, 26b]), electrophilic and nucleophilic reactions on the aromatic ring itself [10, 11], radical reactions (with certain restrictions) [9, 12] and even unsaturated aliphatic compounds [13, 14]. It is also possible to describe the substituent influence on several physical properties by use of the HAMMETT equation and its modifications explained in more detail below, as in the case of

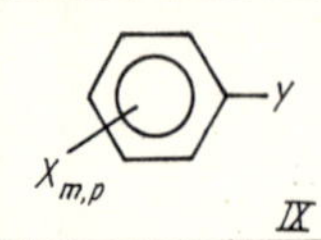

IX

UV and IR spectra [15], polarographic half-wave potentials [16], NMR spectra [17 to 18a], ionization potentials [19—21], dipole moments [22] and group dipole moments [23]. This is very important for quantitative structure-activity analysis, since the rôle of such physical properties in the interaction with the receptor is much greater than that of chemical reactions. Within its validity range, the HAMMETT equation is, therefore, one of the possible forms of the function $f_e(x_e)$:

$$f(x_e) = \varrho\sigma + \text{constant} \qquad (5/21)$$

The applicability of the HAMMETT equation is limited by the following requirements:

1. the presence of a rigid system,
2. the presence of a constant reaction or interaction mechanism,
3. the absence of steric interactions between the substituents and the reaction centre,
4. the substituents must not show a special solvation behaviour and not be involved in the reaction,
5. no direct resonance interactions between substituents and reaction centre (see also below),
6. the relative importance of inductive and mesomeric effects within the reaction series is constant (see below).

However, requirements 5. and 6. may be taken into account by appropriate extensions of the HAMMETT equation. There are also certain limits regarding the size of the substituents [24], with the size of e.g. NHC_6H_5 or $COOC_2H_5$ as the upper limit. Larger substituents may be suitable, provided that they are rigid. Charged substituents are frequently no fit by the simple HAMMETT equation and require a special treatment [24a].

HAMMETT constants have been tabulated for a great many substituents [7, 12, 25—27, 107]. Most are secondary σ values, determined with reference to secondary processes. To this end, the known σ values of the standard reaction series (5/12) (primary σ values) are first used to establish ϱ for the chosen secondary reference process according to eqn. (5/18) (experimental determination of K_H and K_X). Then the secondary σ values are calculated from eqn. (5/18) after measuring the corresponding K_X. This procedure is not without problems [28, 29], and the resulting secondary σ values may be highly subject to errors. For secondary σ values to be employed successfully in quantitative structure-activity analysis, the following conditions must be fulfilled [29—31]:

1. ϱ is established with not less than $n = 10$ compounds;
2. the substituents selected include 3 — 4 strong (+)-M- and (—)-M-substituents, respectively, in para-position and 3 — 4 meta-substituents;

3. $r^2 \geqq 0.98$ where r = correlation coefficient, for the resultant straight line, in order to satisfy eqn. (5/18);
4. $|d_i| \leqq 0.1$ where d_i = error in the primary σ values used;
5. the number of primary σ values with $|d_i| \geqq 0.06$ is less than $n/4$;
6. the error variances is $\leqq 10\%$ of the sample variance.

An alternative to the above definition of σ values with reference to a given standard reaction series and secondary processes is provided by a statistical analysis of experimental data from all possible reaction series, yielding σ values which can be used for the best overall data description. The first analysis of this kind was carried out by JAFFÉ [12], whose assumptions involved a good deal of simplification. The disadvantage of this approach is that the substituent constants obtained are dependent on the data base available at the time of analysis. Furthermore, it is possible that deviations will be obscured by the large quantity of data, so that it is difficult to interpret the substituent constants in physical terms and they may be considerably affected by error. However, according to WOLD and SJÖSTRÖM [4, 32—34], this drawback can be avoided by using an appropriate statistical method geared to the problem to be solved, without simplifications and with a data base that accurately reflects the chemical features of the linear free enthalpy relationships. Deviating data are excluded in a stepwise manner from the calculation of substituent constants. By applying principal component analysis as a statistical method (see 9.1.) the authors obtained a surprisingly uniform scale of inductive substituent constants. For practical work, the compilation of σ values presented by MCDANIEL and BROWN [26] is currently most frequently employed.

In deriving the HAMMETT equation, eqns. (5/2)—(5/5) were formulated on the assumption that only one type of interaction occurs between the substituent zone R and the reaction centre Y. In reality, the electronic substituent effect comprises two kinds of interactions: the *inductive effect* (I-effect), consisting of successive polarizations of σ bonds and electrical through-space effects; and the *mesomeric effect* (M-effect), which results in a change in the overlap of the p_z-orbital of the π electronic system (*resonance effect*). Therefore, two interaction terms are needed, resulting in instead of eqn. (5/7), relation (5/22)

$$\delta_{X_2}\Delta_Y G^0 = (I_{Y'} - I_Y)_I\,(I_{R_2} - I_{R_1})_I + (I_{Y'} - I_Y)_R\,(I_{R_2} - I_{R_1})_R \qquad (5/22)$$

where subscripts I and R denote inductive and mesomeric interactions, respectively.

When hydrogen is taken as standard substituent ($X_1 = H$) with $I_H = 0$ for both interactions, and $(I_{Y'} - I_Y)_I = \varrho_I$ and $(I_{Y'} - I_Y)_R = \varrho_R$ are set equal to unity for appropriate standard reactions, eqn. (5/23) follows from (5/22) after division by $-2.303RT$

$$f_e(x_e) = \log K_X/K_H = \varrho_I\sigma_I + \varrho_R\sigma_R \qquad (5/23)$$

or

$$f_e(x_e) = \log K_X = \varrho_I\sigma_I + \varrho_R\sigma_R + \text{constant}$$

σ_I and σ_R are called the *inductive substituent constant* and the *resonance or mesomeric substituent constant*, respectively. Equation (5/23) can be transformed into:

$$f_e(x_e) = \varrho_I(\sigma_I + [\varrho_R/\varrho_I]\,\sigma_R) + \text{constant} \qquad (5/24)$$

It follows from eqn. (5/24) that the simple HAMMETT equation is not valid unless,

$$\varrho_R/\varrho_I = \text{constant} \tag{5/25}$$

because it is only in this case that the parenthetical term varies only with the properties of the substituents or with the substituent constants σ_I and σ_R, respectively.

The implication is that for the HAMMETT equation to be valid, the relative weight of the inductive and mesomeric effects must be constant within a reaction series. Where this condition is not fulfilled, eqn. (5/23) must be applied. CHARTON [35, 36] claims that this is the case with, for example, ortho-substituted aromatic compounds (*ortho-effect*). If σ_R for ortho-substituents is expressed by

$$\sigma_R = \sigma_p - \sigma_I \tag{5/26}$$

eqn. (5/27) follows from (5/23):

$$\begin{aligned} f_e(x_e) &= \varrho_I\sigma_I + \varrho_R(\sigma_p - \sigma_I) + \text{constant} \\ &= a\sigma_I + b\sigma_p + \text{constant} \end{aligned} \tag{5/27}$$

The ability of eqn. (5/27) to describe ortho-substituted compounds has been criticised by EXNER [24], and the problem of the ortho-effect has also been extensively reviewed in [2, 37, 38, 38a]. TAFT [22] interprets the ortho-effect as a steric effect, as will be discussed below. Special sets of σ values for ortho-substituents, determined on various series, are available in the literature but their applicability is limited. Their validity can be artificially extended by allowing for a different ϱ value for ortho-substituents ($\varrho_o \neq \varrho_m, \varrho_p$).

When the resonance effect is negligible eqn. (5/23) transforms into:

$$f_e(x_e) = \varrho_I\sigma_I + \text{constant} \tag{5/28}$$

The inductive substituent constant σ_I for aromatic compounds can be estimated in three ways:

1. From the chemical shift of meta-substituted fluorobenzene derivatives [17, 39].
2. From values of σ_m and σ_p assuming [39] that
   a) σ_m and σ_p can be represented as the sum of σ_I and σ_R:

$$\begin{aligned} \sigma_p &= \sigma_{I,p} + \sigma_{R,p} \\ \sigma_m &= \sigma_{I,m} + \sigma_{R,m} \end{aligned} \tag{5/29}$$

   b) the inductive substituent effect is the same at meta- and para-positions:

$$\sigma_{I,m} = \sigma_{I,p} = \sigma_I \tag{5/30}$$

   c) the ratio of the resonance effects of the meta- and para-substituents is constant:

$$\sigma_{R,m}/\sigma_{R,p} = \alpha = 1/3 \tag{5/31}$$

   From eqns. (5/29)—(5/31) it follows that:

$$\sigma_I = (\sigma_m - \alpha\sigma_p)/(1 - \alpha) \tag{5/32}$$

3. Rigid alicyclic systems such as 4-substituted bicyclo-(2,2,2)-octane-1-carbonic acids (structural formula X) share with substituted benzoic acids many features such as

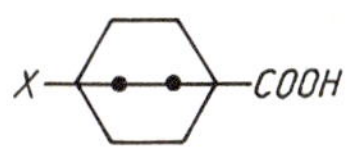

X

molecular size, rigidity and collinearity of bonds and it may, therefore, be assumed that the inductive effect of substituents is the same in the two systems. As no resonance effects can occur in X, the substituent influence on the dissociation equilibrium is purely inductive. A substituent constant σ', based on the dissociation of these compounds in 50% ethanol at 298.7 K was defined by ROBERTS and MORELAND [40]:

$$\sigma' = \frac{1}{1.464} (\log K_X/K_H) \tag{5/33}$$

The normalization factor 1/1.464 corresponds to the ϱ value for the dissociation of substituted benzoic acids in 50% ethanol and permits the σ' values to be transformed to the same scale as the σ values. Because of the similarity of compound X with the benzene system, the σ' values may be equated with σ_I. This leads to the following definition of σ_I [22]:

$$\sigma_I = \sigma' = 0.450\sigma^*_{\mathrm{CH_2}X} = 0.160\sigma_X^* \tag{5/34}$$

A similar set of values can be obtained from the basicity of substituted quinuclidines ($\sigma_I{}^q$) [40a, b].

The σ^* values in eqn. (5/34) were introduced by TAFT [22] and can be determined from the acid and base catalyzed hydrolysis of carbonic acid esters, as described later. The determination of σ_I and σ^* values may also be based on the pK_a values of other rigid alicyclic carbonic acids or even the pK_a values of aliphatic carbonic acids (minor steric effects being ignored [2, 22, 24, 37, 41]; such data are to be regarded as secondary σ_I and σ^* values).

The agreement in the scales of σ_I values obtained in these different ways is good, thus ensuring general applicability. With some substituents, however, minor deviations are possible so that for quantitative structure-activity analyses the use of σ_I values from one source is recommended. It is now possible to estimate σ_R values from eqn. (5/29), while allowing for (5/30) and (5/31):

$$\sigma_R = \sigma_p - \sigma_I = (\sigma_m - \sigma_I)/\alpha \tag{5/35}$$

As will be seen later, there is no general scale for σ_R; in contrast to σ_I, σ_R is dependent on the nature of the reaction centre [24, 42] and the capacity of a substituent to enter into resonance interactions with that centre through the π electron system of the aromatic ring. Such resonance interactions, which will be called *coupling effects*, are possible when the reaction centre a) carries a positive charge or has an electron deficiency and an electron donating substituent is present in the para-position (*positive coupling effect*) or b) carries a negative charge or has a free electron pair and an electron acceptor is present as a substituent in the para-position (*negative coupling effect*), see e.g. [42—45] and Figs. 5.1 and 5.2. In addition to the usual mesomeric effect, a further resonance effect occurs in such cases, which is not covered by the HAMMETT constant. To describe these reaction series, the *"enhanced" substituent constants* σ^+ (positive coupling effect) and σ^- (negative coupling effect) have been introduced:

positive coupling effect

$$f_e(x_e) = \varrho^+\sigma^+ + \text{constant} \tag{5/36}$$

negative coupling effect

$$f_e(x_e) = \varrho^-\sigma^- + \text{constant} \tag{5/37}$$

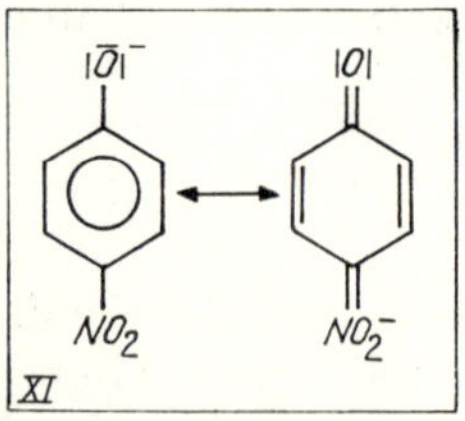

Fig. 5.1. Example of negative coupling effect

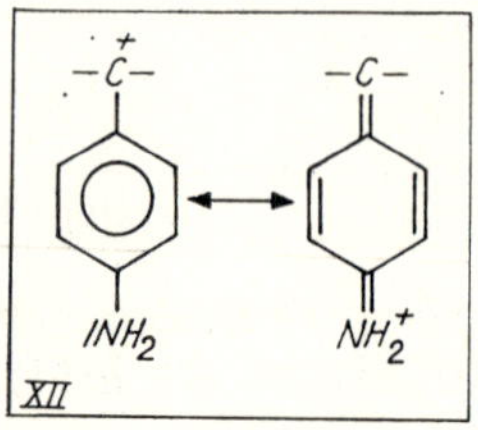

Fig. 5.2. Example of positive coupling effect

The standard reaction for the definition of σ^+ values is the solvolysis of substituted phenyldimethylcarbinyl chlorides [46—48], and for the σ^- values, the ionization of anilines or phenols in water [12, 49]; it should be noted that the values for anilines and phenols are different and not compatible. The following relationships hold:

a) $$\sigma_m \approx \sigma_m{}^+ \approx \sigma_m{}^- \approx \sigma_m{}^0 \tag{5/38}$$

provided that the substituent in the meta-position is not an extremely strong electron donor or acceptor (for the definition of σ^0, see below).

b) for the positive coupling effect and electron acceptors as substituents

$$\sigma_p{}^+ \approx \sigma_p \approx \sigma_p{}^0 \tag{5/39}$$

c) for the negative coupling effect and electron donors as substituents

$$\sigma_p{}^- \approx \sigma_p \approx \sigma_p{}^0 \tag{5/40}$$

σ^- values have been successfully applied to reactions of phenols, anilines, aromatic hydrazines and enamines, polarographic reductions yielding an electron-rich intermediate and nucleophilic substitutions in aromatic compounds; σ^+ values have been used e.g. for solvolytic reactions, reactions of aldehydes and other carbonyl compounds, oxidative processes and electrophilic substitutions in aromatic compounds [24]. Although σ^+ and σ^- values in general permit workable descriptions, these constants either over- or underestimated the coupling effect in many reaction series.

It seems that a sliding scale of enhanced σ values is required [50]. YUKAWA and TSUNO [51—53] proposed an approach for describing the positive coupling effect (eqn. (5/41)) and YOSHIOKA et al. [54] for the negative coupling effect (eqn. (5/43)). This approach is based on the assumption that values of $(\sigma^+ - \sigma)$ (positive coupling effect) or $(\sigma^- - \sigma)$

(negative coupling effect), respectively, provide a scale for "enhanced" resonance effects. Those resonance effects can then be weighted by use of an additional adjustable parameter according to eqns. (5/41) and (5/43):

$$f_e(x_e) = \varrho(\sigma + r^+\Delta\sigma_R^+) + \text{constant}$$
$$= a\sigma + b\sigma^+ + \text{constant} \quad (5/41)$$

with

$$\Delta\sigma_R^+ = \sigma^+ - \sigma \quad (5/42)$$

and

$$f_e(x_e) = \varrho(\sigma + r^-\Delta\sigma_R^-) + \text{constant}$$
$$= a\sigma + b\sigma^- + \text{constant} \quad (5/43)$$

with

$$\Delta\sigma_R^- = \sigma^- - \sigma \quad (5/44)$$

In order to be completely rigorous, the σ values in eqns. (5/42) and (5/44) should be replaced by σ^0 values, as explained later. In the case of eqn. (5/41) this results in an appreciable accentuation, but has little effect on eqn. (5/43).

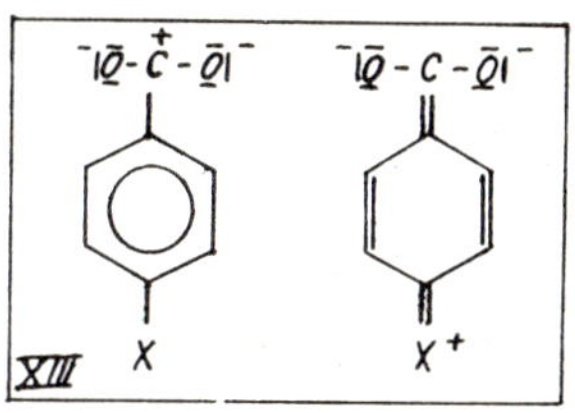

XIII

On closer inspection of benzoic acids (structural formula XIII) it appears that with these compounds, too, a slight positive coupling effect may occur, although it is by no means so pronounced as in Fig. 5.2. σ_p values for electron donors are thus not completely devoid of a coupling contribution which, of course, influences the σ_R values defined by eqn. (5/35). An attempt was, therefore, made to determine what may be called *true or correct σ values* [55]. To this end, the carboxyl group of XIII was isolated from the ring by a CH_2 group and the substituent constants

$$\sigma^0 = (\log K_X/K_H)_{C_6H_5CH_2Y} \quad (5/45)$$

determined on the resulting new standard series (dissociation of phenylacetic acids or saponification of their esters) were reduced to the same scale as the HAMMETT values. σ^0 values have been reported in, e.g., [4, 34, 55—60] (as regards [59] and [60], see also [28]). Conceptually similar are the so-called *normal* σ^n values proposed by VAN BEKKUM et al. [50], which have been abandoned in favour of, or simply identified with, σ^0 values. As expected, the σ^0 values for meta-substituents and acceptor para-substituents correspond very closely to σ values. The σ^0 values provide a better description of reaction series than σ values in cases where the reaction centre is isolated from the ring. As a consequence, the function $f_e(x_e)$ can then be formulated as:

$$f_e(x_e) = \varrho\sigma^0 + \text{constant} \quad (5/46)$$

The σ^0 values may also be regarded as inductive substituent constants of the substituted phenyl ring (XC_6H_5) [55] (see also [34]). New scales of resonance parameters [42, 55, 61, 62] have been derived on the basis of the σ^+, σ^-, σ_I and σ^0 values:

$$\sigma_R{}^0 = \sigma_p{}^0 - \sigma_I = (\sigma_m{}^0 - \sigma_I)/\alpha \qquad (5/47)$$

with

$$\alpha = 0.5$$

$$\sigma_R{}^+ = \sigma_p{}^+ - \sigma_I = (\sigma_m{}^+ - \sigma_I)/\alpha \qquad (5/48)$$

with

$$\alpha \approx 0.1$$

$$\sigma_R{}^- = \sigma_p{}^- - \sigma_I = (\sigma_m{}^- - \sigma_I)/\alpha \qquad (5/49)$$

with

$$\alpha \approx 0.1$$

Of particular interest are the $\sigma_R{}^0$ values (for an updated set, see [62a]), which provide a quantitative measure of the ability of a substituent to delocalize π electrons into or from an unperturbed benzene ring.

It follows from eqns. (5/23), (5/35) and (5/47)/—(5/49) that:

$$f_e(x_e) = \text{constant} + \varrho_I\sigma_I + \varrho_R \begin{cases} \sigma_R & \text{for case 1} \\ \sigma_R{}^0 & \text{for case 2} \\ \sigma_R{}^+ & \text{for case 3} \\ \sigma_R{}^- & \text{for case 4} \end{cases}$$

$$= \text{constant} + a\sigma_I + b \begin{cases} \sigma \\ \sigma^0 \\ \sigma^+ \\ \sigma^- \end{cases} \qquad (5/50)$$

From the above considerations and the summarizing equation (5/50) it appears that there is *no uniform scale of resonance constants*. Equation (5/50) is applicable for reaction series having a very weak positive coupling effect, with σ_R values (case 1), for reaction series having no coupling effect, with $\sigma_R{}^0$ values (case 2), in the presence of a positive coupling effect, with $\sigma_R{}^+$ values (case 3), and in the presence of a negative coupling effect (a distinction being drawn between anilines and phenols), with $\sigma_R{}^-$ values (case 4). It has been suggested [42] that this classification ensures excellent descriptions of the behaviour of the corresponding reaction series.

In an attempt to attribute to each substituent just two basic electronic quantities, SWAIN and LUPTON [63] defined two new electronic substituent constants $\mathfrak{F}$ and $\mathfrak{R}$. The *field constant* $\mathfrak{F}$ is basically related to σ_I and represents inductive effects, whereas the *resonance constant* $\mathfrak{R}$ is intended to comprise all resonance effects. To evaluate the scale of $\mathfrak{R}$ values it was assumed that the substituent $\overset{+}{N}(CH_3)_3$ has no resonance effect ($\mathfrak{R} = 0$); this assumption is controversial however [14, 64—67]. According to Swain and Lupton, a linear combination of $\mathfrak{F}$ and $\mathfrak{R}$ can describe any scale of σ values (e.g., σ_m, σ_p, σ_I, σ^0, σ^+, σ^- etc.):

$$\sigma_i = f_i\mathfrak{F} + r_i\mathfrak{R} \tag{5/51}$$

The constants f_i and r_i are field and resonance weighting factors for the corresponding σ scales. Although eqn. (5/51) is generally valid, it only poorly reproduces the σ^+ and σ^- scales. To some extent eqn. (5/51) implies the general validity of a single set of resonance constants and is, therefore, in conflict with what has been said above. For this reason it has been criticized in e.g. [24, 33, 42]. On the other and, the f_i and r_i values differ widely for different scales of resonance constants so that the situation summarized in eqn. (5/50) is at least partly accounted for. In addition, the individual resonance constants are by no means independent of each other and thus a relation exists e.g. between σ_R^+ and σ^+ [9]. Advantages of eqn. (5/51) are a) that the vectors of the $\mathfrak{F}$ and $\mathfrak{R}$ values are nearly *orthogonal* [25], which does not hold consistently for σ_I and the resonance constants [2, 24], and b) there is no need to assume that the inductive effects of meta- and para-substitution are transmitted to the same extent (there are indications that this assumption is not always correct — e.g. [24]). Equation (5/51) enables the function $f_e(x_e)$ to be written as:

$$\begin{aligned} f_e(x_e) &= \varrho_i(f_i\mathfrak{F} + r_i\mathfrak{R}) + \text{constant} \\ &= a\mathfrak{F} + b\mathfrak{R} + \text{constant} \end{aligned} \tag{5/52}$$

Equation (5/52) is quite useful in many cases where the simple Hammett relationship (5/21) permits no or only a moderate data description, and it is certainly to be recommended for QSAR analyses provided that the resultant equations are interpreted with caution. It can also be employed to describe electronic effects of ortho-substituents [38] in analogy to Chartons treatment according to eqn. (5/27). An extensive tabulation of $\mathfrak{F}$ and $\mathfrak{R}$ values is available in the literature [25, 27][1]).

The Swain-Lupton treatment was modified by Norrington and co-workers [68, 69] who introduced weighting factors to account for positional dependencies (ortho, meta, para) of the constants a and b in eqn. (5/52). The weighting factors can either be introduced directly into eqn. (5/52) [68], or they can be used to derive modified field and resonance constants normalized with respect to the position of substitution. With these new constants, designated as F and R (for a tabulation, see [69]), the function $f_e(x_e)$ can be expressed as:

$$f_e(x_e) = a_{o,m,p}F + b_{o,m,p}R \tag{5/53}$$

Following a similar line of reasoning but using a different approach, Unger [70] evaluated another set of inductive and resonance parameters, S and P, respectively. These are ortho-normalized, and (it was claimed) allow a sharper separation of inductive and resonance effects, yielding generally higher correlation coefficients than other

---

1) Note that the Swain-Lupton values [63] are not in scale with those of Hansch [25, 27].

pairs of parameters. The equation which results is:

$$f_e(x_e) = aS + bP + \text{constant} \qquad (5/54)$$

Experience (albeit limited) suggests that this is probably another useful relation for QSAR analyses. Another dual set of inductive and resonance substituent constants designated as σ_L and σ_D claimed to be much better than the SWAIN-LUPTON model was recently introduced by CHARTON [26a].

A completely different approach for dealing with systems where substituent-reaction site interactions are strong and non-uniform was recently proposed by KRYGOWSKI and FAWCETT [71, 72]. These authors believe that isokinetic relationships — which are a prerequisite for the classical HAMMETT equation — break down in such cases. If this is true, entropic and enthalpic contributions to the overall electronic substituent effect must be separated:

$$f_e(x_e) = \varrho_S\sigma_S + \varrho_H\sigma_H + \text{constant} \qquad (5/55)$$

The *enthalpic* (σ_H) and *entropic* (σ_S) *substituent constants* were defined from independently determined values of the standard enthalpy and entropy of ionization of substituted benzoic acids in water. Equation (5/55) was successfully applied to various reaction series including ortho-substituted compounds. KRYGOWSKI and FAWCETT pointed out that σ_S probably mainly reflects intermolecular substituent effects (solvation), whereas σ_H comprises both inter- and intramolecular contributions. Usually the entropy term is dominant, but the effect of substituents having strong resonance interactions may be enthalpy controlled. The relation between σ_H, σ_S and σ_I, σ_R is not yet clear. Although the interpretation of relationships of the type (5/55) is still not without problems, they may offer a promising approach for QSAR analyses.

Although the LFERs reported thus far can also provide fair description of radical reactions more favourable results can sometimes be obtained with special *radical parameters* as substituent constants, as for instance, in the equation of OTSU and YAMAMOTO [73, 74]:

$$f_e(x_e) = \gamma E_R + \varrho\sigma + \text{constant} \qquad (5/56)$$

The parameter E_R provides a measure of the resonance stabilization of a benzyl radical by a substituent, and the σ term accounts for possible inductive and mesomeric substituent effects. If the latter effects do not occur, the σ term can be omitted.

Multiparameter extensions of the HAMMETT equation such as those discussed above (for a good review, see e.g. [67]) must always be applied with care. It is important that the resulting relationships are not overinterpreted and that the data to be analyzed really justify such a treatment. This implies that sufficient data points are available and that a broad range of electronic properties is covered by the substituents concerned. However, without such multiparameter equations it would not be possible to adequately deal with the complex features of electronic substituent effects.

There are reaction series in which the π electron system of an aromatic ring is separated by a bridge Z from the reaction centre Y (see structural formula XIV). In such cases a *bridge effect* will be manifested, and has been discussed in detail in [2] and [24]. The extent to which Z influences the reaction constant is dependent on its ability to transmit polar effects. This can be expressed by the parameter π_Z defined as:

$$\pi_Z = \varrho_{ZY}/\varrho_Y \quad (5/57)$$

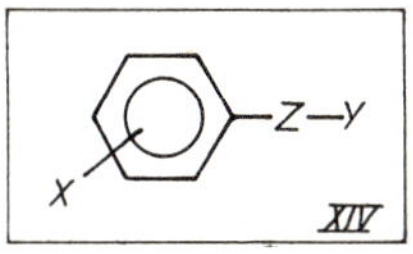

XIV

where ϱ_{ZY} is the reaction constant in the presence of the bridge Z and ϱ_Y that in its absence. When π_Z is independent of the nature of the reaction centre Y, it is characteristic of Z. In this case the $\varrho - \varrho$ relationships

$$\pi_Z = \varrho_{ZY_1}/\varrho_{Y^1} = \varrho_{ZY_2}/\varrho_{Y_2} = \cdots \quad (5/58)$$

must apply. The validity of this relationship has been demonstrated for a variety of reaction series. For Z = CH_2, π_Z corresponds to the so-called attenuation factor ε, i.e., $\pi_{CH_2} = \varepsilon \approx 0.4$. For Z = C_2H_4, $\pi_{C_2H_4} = \varepsilon^2 \approx 0.16$, and for longer alkyl chains π_Z decreases somewhat more slowly than ε^n. CH_2 groups can be replaced by O, S, Se, SO, SO_2 or NH without major effects. Unsaturated bridge elements are better transmitters of polar effects. Thus, $\pi_{CH=CH}$ approximates π_{CH_2}; meta- and para-phenyl groups as well as many five-membered heterocycles have π_Z values of ca. 0.3. Bridge elements may also enhance the reaction constant (positive bridge effect), when the conjugation of the entire molecule is increased by Z. For example, this is the case when two benzene rings are linked by a heteroatom, the order of the positive effect being O < Se < S < NH. In a given QSAR analysis it may be necessary to allow for the bridge effect if compounds with and without a bridge element Z are included in the series under investigation. Insofar as the simple HAMMETT equation is applicable, $f_e(x_e)$ may then be written, for example, as

$$f_e(x_e) = \varrho(X\sigma) + \text{constant} \quad (5/59)$$

where X is an indicator variable defined as:

$$X = \begin{cases} \pi_Z & \text{in the presence of the bridge element} \\ 1 & \text{in the absence of the bridge element} \end{cases} \quad (5/60)$$

Substituent constants are available for most of the common substituents. Those which are not may be estimated but this requires great care. One possibility is to calculate the σ values from eqn. (5/51) provided that the corresponding values of $\mathfrak{F}$ and $\mathfrak{R}$ as well as the weighting factors f_i and r_i are known. Instead of using $\mathfrak{F}$ and $\mathfrak{R}$, complex relationships between various σ scales can also be applied [75, 75a]. However, the error in calculated σ values may be unacceptably high, in particular for enhanced σ values. An expression that has proved fairly useful [24] is that mentioned by CHARTON [76] as:

$$\sigma_{m,p}(\text{AB}) = \sigma_{m,p}(\text{AH}) + m\sigma_i(\text{B}) \quad (5/61)$$

For each B, m is determined empirically (from known σ values for other AB combinations). The choice of the scale for σ_i depends on the nature of A. A compilation of such relationships evaluated with the simplifying assumption that the term $\sigma_{m,p}(\text{AH})$

can be made adjustable is presented in [26a]. For substituents of the type NHX (A = NH; B = X), for example, the following relationships can be used [26a]:

$$\sigma_m(\text{NHX}) = 1.11\sigma_{mX} - 0.187$$
$$\sigma_p(\text{NHX}) = 1.33\sigma_{mX} - 0.476 \qquad (5/62)$$

If, for a given substituent X, log K_X in a few reaction series is known, σ can be deduced from the slope of a plot of log K_X/K_H versus the corresponding ϱ values. This ϱ plot has the advantage that there is no need for ϱ to be known with high accuracy. Furthermore, a linear ϱ plot always indicates that the reaction series follow the HAMMETT equation. Where, for one of the series, ϱ can be determined with sufficient precision by means of primary σ values, σ values can, of course, be directly estimated as secondary σ values from values of log K_X/K_H for the corresponding substituents.

The substituent constants discussed so far cannot (except for σ_I) be applied to flexible aliphatic systems, since here the equilibrium and rate constants are additionally influenced by steric effects. TAFT [22] developed a relationship for aliphatic compounds analogously to the HAMMETT equation:

$$f_e(x_e) = \varrho^*\sigma^* + \text{constant} \qquad (5/63)$$

The parameter σ^* is called the *polar substituent constant* and has an exclusively inductive nature (cf., eqn. (5/34)):

$$\sigma^* = \frac{1}{2.48}\left[(\log k_X/k_0)_b - (\log k_X/k_0)_a\right] \qquad (5/64)$$

The standard reaction comprises the basic (subscript b) and the acidic (subscript a) hydrolysis of aliphatic carbonic acid esters XCOOR, and the standard substituent is X = CH_3 ($\sigma^*_{CH_3} = 0$); k_X is the rate constant with substituent X and k_0 that for X = CH_3. The factor 1/2.48 reduces the σ^* values to the same scale as the HAMMETT σ values. The definition of σ^* is based on three assumptions:

1. The relative change in activation free enthalpy can be treated as the sum of independent contributions from inductive, steric and resonance effects (this also follows directly from the approach used to generate linear free enthalpy relationships presented in the beginning of this section);
2. base- and acid-catalyzed ester hydrolyses differ neither in steric nor in resonance effects;
3. the inductive influence of substituents on the rate of hydrolysis is strong in the base-catalyzed but practically negligible in the acid-catalyzed reaction.

It follows from these assumptions (which have been the subject of controversy, for a detailed discussion see, e.g., [37]), that in accord with eqn. (5/64) steric and resonance effects are eliminated so that only the inductive effect remains. This inference appears to be basically correct since eqn. (5/63) has been applied to many aliphatic reaction series in recent years with great success. As inductive effects are basically additive, σ^*_{CXYZ} can be calculated from values of the partial structures X, Y and Z:

$$\sigma^*_{CXYZ} = \sigma^*_{CH_2X} + \sigma^*_{CH_2Y} + \sigma^*_{CH_2Z} \qquad (5/65)$$

Table 5.1 compares calculated (from (5/65)) and experimentally determined σ^* values (from [1]). Even though relatively large groups were selected and a broad range of σ^* is covered, the agreement between experimental and calculated values is quite satisfactory.

Table 5.1. Comparison of experimentally determined and calculated (eqn. (5/65)) σ^* values (from [1])

Group CXYZ	Experimental	Calculated
$-C(CH_3)_3$	-0.300	$3 \cdot (-0.100) = -0.300$
$-CH(C_6H_5)(CH_3)$	$+0.11$	$0.215 - 0.100 = +0.115$
$-CH(C_6H_5)(C_2H_5)$	$+0.04$	$0.215 - 0.115 = +0.110$
$-CH(C_6H_5)(OH)$	$+0.765$	$0.215 + 0.555 = +0.770$
$-CHCl_2$	$+1.940$	$2 \cdot 1.050 = +2.100$

Other methods of estimating σ^* values have been described by Nagai et al. [77] as well as by Bohle and Martin [78]. Nagai et al. found that the σ^* values of substituted phenyl groups could be correlated with the Hammett constants of the substituents according to

$$\sigma^*_{XC_6H_4} = 0.720\sigma_X + 0.575 \qquad (5/66)$$

$$n = 6 \qquad r = 0.995$$

so that σ^* of XC_6H_5 can be estimated from the σ values of X. The resulting σ^* values can be applied in cases where both aliphatic and aromatic substituents occur in the reaction series. The relationships deduced by Bohle and Martin for aliphatic substituents with heteroatoms is

$$\sigma^* = -2.30n_1{}^H - 3.45n_2{}^H - 0.045 \sum P + 2.93 \qquad (5/67)$$

and for purely aliphatic substituents:

$$\sigma^* = -0.098n_1{}^C - 0.017n_2{}^C - 0.021n_3{}^C \qquad (5/68)$$

$n_1{}^H$ and $n_2{}^H$ are the respective numbers of hydrogen atoms bound to sp^3- and sp^2-hybridized carbon atoms and P is the refraction increment of the C—X bond for heteroatom X. All three quantities are dependent on the distance from the reaction centre. The parameters $n_1{}^C$, $n_2{}^C$ and $n_3{}^C$ indicate the numbers of carbon atoms bound, respectively, to the first, second and third carbon atom of a substituent. It must be noted that the general validity of these relationships is not proven.

It has been postulated by Charton [79, 80] that for alkyl substituents the σ^* values of Taft are artefacts and that the influence of such groups on the equilibrium and rate constants in aliphatic reaction series are solely steric in nature. In particular this argument is based on the correlation of rate constants for the basic hydrolysis (k_b) of aliphatic esters XCOOR (X = alkyl) and aliphatic amides with the inductive substituent constant, σ_I, the mesomeric substituent constant, σ_R, and the steric substituent constant, $\mathfrak{v}_X$ (for $\mathfrak{v}_X$ see 6. and [79, 80]):

$$\log k_b = \alpha\sigma_I + \beta\sigma_R + \psi\mathfrak{v}_X + h \qquad (5/69)$$

It appears that in nearly all cases the regression coefficients α and β are not significantly different from zero, which led CHARTON to his postulate. A closer inspection of the data, however, reveals that the sample variance of the electronic substituent constants compared to the error variance is far too small for a meaningful regression analysis [29]. Therefore, on statistical grounds, CHARTONS conclusions cannot be considered proven although it can be regarded as generally correct (see also [80a]).

In certain series eqn. (5/63) is expanded to take account of the number of hydrogen atoms on the α-C-atom of the substituent or on a functional group. In the former case resonance interactions operate as *hyperconjugation* effects. This kind of effect is not considered in σ^* and must be taken into account as follows

$$f_e(x_e) = \varrho^*\sigma^* + h(n - 3) + \text{constant} \tag{5/70}$$

where n is the number of α-H atoms. For example, such a relationship is obtained for the acidic hydrolysis of diethylacetals and -ketals of the general formula $R_1R_2C(OC_2H_5)_2$ [81]:

$$\log k_X/k_0 = -3.60(\sigma^*_{R_1} + \sigma^*_{R_2}) + 0.54(n - 6) \tag{5/71}$$

Here 6α-H atoms may occur so that $(n - 6)$ instead of the $(n - 3)$ term is employed. α-Hydrogen effects in a functional group occur, for example, in alkylamines [82] and alkylphosphines [83]. If the pK_a values of such compounds are correlated with σ^* three almost parallel straight lines result corresponding to the number of hydrogens (0, 1, 2) on the nitrogen or phosphorus, respectively. This effect is probably due to steric hindrance of solvation in the amines, and to a change in the hybridization of phosphorus in the phosphines. The straight lines for the amines can be combined by the use of a term that takes account of the number, n_H, of hydrogen atoms on the nitrogen atom [84]:

$$pK_a = \varrho^* \sum \sigma^* - hn_H + \text{constant} \tag{5/72}$$

With phosphines such a simple correction cannot be applied.

TAFTS approach can also be followed for ortho-substituted aromatic series. Thus one obtains:

$$f_e(x_e) = \varrho^*\sigma_o{}^* + \text{constant} \tag{5/73}$$

with

$$\sigma_o{}^* = \frac{1}{2.48}\left[(\log k_X/k_o)_b - (\log k_X/k_o)_a\right] \tag{5/74}$$

Again, the methyl group is the standard substituent. The σ_o values are obtained by shifting the scale and taking H as the standard substituent. To date, TAFTS $\sigma_o{}^*$ and σ_o values have been relatively little used but experience has shown that they are particularly suitable for the description of the behaviour of ortho-substituted aromatic compounds if there are no special resonance effects. These values are compatible with the HAMMETT constant as they lie on the same scale. Nevertheless it is recommended that where ortho-substituents are concerned the reaction constant should be allowed to have a value different from that which is used in para- and meta-substitution. This may be formulated as:

$$f_e(x_e) = \varrho_1\sigma_{m,p} + \varrho_2\sigma_o + \text{constant} \tag{5/75}$$

The application of TAFTS σ_o^* and σ_o values is an alternative to eqns. (5/27), (5/53) and (5/55).

Deviations from the linearity of linear free enthalpy relations may have to be allowed for according to:

$$f_e(x_e) = a_1\sigma^2 + a_2\sigma + \text{constant} \tag{5/76}$$

or

$$f_e(x_e) = a\sigma^2 + \text{constant} \tag{5/77}$$

Such relationships may be necessary in the following cases [9, 24, 85]:

1. Multistep reactions, in which none of the steps is rate-determining, which result in a parabola concaved upwards;
2. equilibrium reactions, where e.g. two tautomeric forms are in a dissociation equilibrium with a third, which again yield a parabola concaved upwards;
3. the overall reactions consists of a reversible step followed by an irreversible one, yielding a parabola concaved downwards;
4. inconstancy of the reaction mechanism in the reaction series;
5. as regards biological activity, the presence of an optimal value for the molecular property in the series under study which is described by the function $f_e(x_e)$;
6. in addition to the reaction sequence leading to a biological stimulus, the occurrence of a competitive reaction (such as metabolism) which is similarly dependent on electronic substituent effects;
7. the occurrence of a special reaction mechanism as, for example, a radical reaction (the radical parameter E_R being correlated with σ^2) or a charge-transfer interaction (E_{HOMO}, the energy of the highest occupied molecular orbital, also being correlated with σ^2 in some series) [86—90].

The last parameters to be considered in this section are the *charge-transfer constants* C_T and $\varkappa$. Introduced by HETNARSKI and O'BRIEN [91] C_T is defined as

$$C_T = (\log K_X/K_H)_{c.t.} \tag{5/78}$$

for the standard reaction of "formation of charge-transfer complexes between substituted aromatic compounds (donors) and tetracyanoethylene (acceptor)". K_X is the association constant for a derivative having a substituent X and K_H that of the non-substituted parent compound. C_T is a measure of the effect of substituents on the ability of aromatic compounds to donate electrons to a given electron acceptor and may thus be used in all cases where the formation of charge-transfer complexes is important:

$$f_e(x_e) = \varrho_T C_T + \text{constant} \tag{5/79}$$

A good example is the binding of heterocyclic compounds to DNA bases [92]. The charge-transfer constant $\varkappa$ is defined in a similar way measuring the substituent effect on the formation of charge-transfer complexes between substituted aromatic compounds (donors) and 1,3,5-trinitrobenzene (acceptor) [92a, 92b] and can be substituted for C_T in eqn. (5/79). When applying $\varkappa$ in QSAR studies some care must be taken since $\varkappa$ appears to be related to a linear combination of π and MR [92a, 92b].

Over the last few decades the extremely great utility of linear free enthalpy relationships for the description of electronic substituent effects in organic chemistry has been demonstrated, as a means of assessing equilibrium or rate constants or of elucidating reaction mechanisms. Such relationships have become so intimately linked with theories of organic chemistry that no more than the most important aspects can be hinted at in this chapter. For specific details and tabulations of substituent constants, reference should be made to the vast literature on this subject (e.g. [1, 2, 4, 8—10, 12, 22, 24, 26, 27, 37, 38, 42, 49, 50, 67, 93—97]). The substituent constants discussed and their definitions are summarized in Table 5.2, and values for a few substituents are presented in Table 5.3 to give an idea of their orders of magnitude and of differences between the scales. Linear free enthalpy relationships have become a major tool in QSAR analyses, and a huge number of examples have been published; for summaries, see [23, 85, 98 to 107]. The following are a few more, arbitrarily chosen, instances. An attempt has been made to select first of all such cases where log A only depends on $f_e(x_e)$. As already mentioned, these are rare since electronic effects are nearly always superimposed upon hydrophobic influences. Subsequent examples were chosen because they exhibit special features.

1. *The electronic substituent influence is not exerted on the reaction centre* Y *but on the ortho-position so that, for example, σ_m values have to be applied for para-substituents. It is obvious that the electron density at the ortho-position will play an important rôle in interactions with the receptor in these cases.*

a) *Cytokinine activity of XV in tobacco* [108]

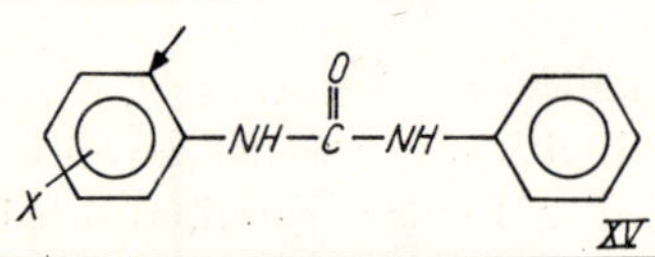

XV

$$\log A = 1.10\sigma + 0.36\pi + 5.68 \tag{5/80}$$

$n = 9 \quad r = 0.945 \quad s = 0.178$

b) *Auxin activity of XVI in wheat* [108]

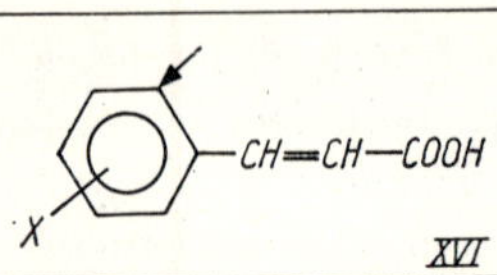

XVI

$$\log A = -0.50(\log P)^2 + 2.45 \log P + 1.92\sigma + 1.77 \tag{5/81}$$

$n = 8 \quad r = 0.815 \quad s = 0.290$

c) *Inhibition of monoamino oxidase from rat liver by XVII* [102]

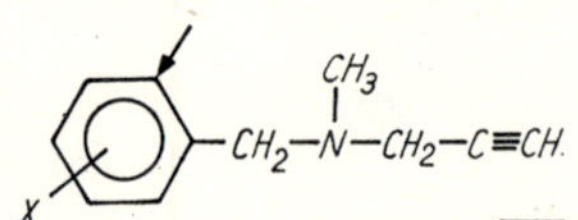

XVII

$$\log A = 1.02\sigma_m + 0.79E_S + 0.44\pi + 5.49 \tag{5/82}$$

$n = 10 \quad r = 0.942 \quad s = 0.273$

E_S is a steric substituent constant (see chapter 6.), showing in this case that the inhibitory activity decreases as the substituents increase in size.

In all three instances ϱ has a positive sign so that electron-withdrawing substituents or low electron densities in the ortho-position are favourable for biological activity.

2. *α-Hydrogen effect* (cf., (5/72)): *antiadrenergic activity of XVIII* [109]

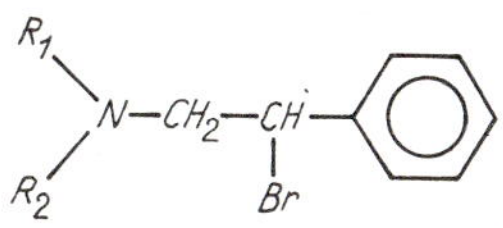

XVIII

$$\log A = 3.57\sigma^* - 4.43 n_H + 1.11 E_S^c + 11.91 \qquad (5/83)$$

$n = 10 \qquad r = 0.986 \qquad s = 0.235$

E_S^c is a steric substituent constant (see 6.), indicating that the biological activity decreases as the substituents increase in bulk. The parameter n_H denotes the number of H atoms on the N atom, and from the σ^* term it follows that electron-attracting substituents enhance biological activity.

3. *Non-linear* HAMMETT *relationships*

a) *Anticonvulsant activity of phenylsydnones* (*XIX*) [110]

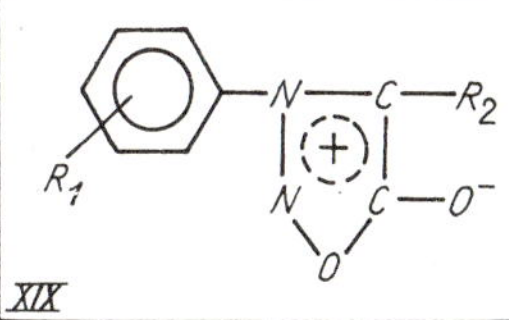

XIX

$$\log A = 3.03\sigma^2 + 1.45\sigma - 0.84 E_S - 1.53 \qquad (5/84)$$

$n = 7 \qquad r = 1.000 \qquad s = 0.011$

E_S is again a steric substituent constant, showing here that the biological activity increases as the substituents become bulkier. The non-linear relationship with σ is probably caused by superimposition of two kinds of electronic substituent effects.

b) *Inhibition of malate dehydrogenase by ortho- and para-substituted phenols* [111]

$$\log A = 0.73\sigma^2 - 0.65\sigma - 0.77\pi^2 + 2.44\pi + 1.24 \qquad (5/85)$$

$n = 14 \qquad r = 0.950 \qquad s = 0.213$

c) *Inhibition of rape root growth by substituted anilides* [112]

$$\log A = -1.49\sigma^2 + 2.30\sigma + 0.91\pi + 5.18 \qquad (5/86)$$

$n = 10 \qquad r = 0.87 \qquad s = 0.43$

Table 5.2. The most important electronic substituent constants

	Name	Introduced by	Defined by	Comprises			
				Inductive effect	Mesomeric effect	Positive coupling	Negative coupling
$\sigma_{m,p}$	Hammett constant	Hammett [5, 6]	dissociation of benzoic acids	+	+	(+)	–
σ^0	"normal" substituent constant	Taft [55]	dissociation of phenylacetic acids	+	+	–	–
σ^n		van Bekkum [50]	via ϱ-values of "normal" meta-substituents	+	+	–	–
$\sigma' = \sigma_I$	inductive substituent constant	Roberts and Moreland [40] Taft [22]	dissociation of 4-substituted bicyclo 2.2.2. octane-1-carboxylic acids	+	–	–	–
$\sigma_I{}^q$	inductive substituent constant	Grob [40a, b]	basicity of substituted quinuclidines	+	–	–	–
$\mathfrak{F}$	inductive substituent constant	Swain and Lupton [63]	$\mathfrak{F} = \sigma_I$	+	–	–	–
F	inductive substituent constant	Norrington et al. [68, 69]	position-weighted $\mathfrak{F}$	+	–	–	–
S	inductive substituent constant	Unger [70]	see text	+	–	–	–
σ_L	"localized" substituent constant	Charton [26a]		+	–	–	–
σ^*	polar substituent constant	Taft [22]	base and acid catalyzed hydrolysis of XCOOR	+	–	–	–
σ^+	"enhanced" substituent constants	Brown [46–48]	solvolysis of phenyldimethyl-carbinylchlorides	+	+	+	–
σ^-		Jaffé, Hammett [12, 49]	ionization of phenoles and anilines	+	+	–	+

σ_R	resonance substituent constant	TAFT [39]	$\sigma_R = \sigma_p - \sigma_I = (\sigma_m - \sigma_I)/\alpha$	—	+	(+)	—
σ_R^0	resonance substituent constant	TAFT [55]	$\sigma_R^0 = \sigma_p^0 - \sigma_I = (\sigma_m^0 - \sigma_I)/\alpha$	—	+	—	—
σ_R^+	resonance substituent constant	several authors (see, e.g., [42])	$\sigma_R^+ = \sigma_p^+ - \sigma_I = (\sigma_m^+ - \sigma_I)/\alpha$	—	+	+	—
σ_R^-	resonance substituent constant	several authors (see, e.g., [42])	$\sigma_R^- = \sigma_p^- - \sigma_I = (\sigma_m^- - \sigma_I)/\alpha$	—	+	—	+
σ_D	"delocalized" substituent constant	CHARTON [26a]		—	+	—	+
$\mathfrak{R}$	resonance substituent constant	SWAIN and LUPTON [63]	see text	—	+	(+)	—
R	resonance substituent constant	NORRINGTON et al. [68, 69]	positionweighted $\mathfrak{R}$	—	+	(+)	—
P	resonance substituent constant	UNGER [70]	see text	—	+	(+)	(+)
$\Delta\sigma_R^+$	resonance substituent constant	YUKAWA and TSUNO [51—53]	$\Delta\sigma_R^+ = \sigma^+ - \sigma^0$	—	—	+	—
$\Delta\sigma_R^-$	resonance substituent constant	YOSHIOKA et al. [54]	$\sigma_R^- = \sigma^- - \sigma^0$	—	—	—	+
σ_H	enthalpic substituent constant	KRYGOWSKI and FAWCETT [71, 72]	enthalpy of benzoic acid dissociation				
σ_S	entropic substituent constant	KRYGOWSKI and FAWCETT [71, 72]	entropy of benzoic acid dissociation				
E_R	radical parameter	OTSU and YAMAMOTU [73, 74]	radical chain polymerization				
C_T	charge transfer constant	HETNARSKI and O'BRIEN [91]	formation of charge-transfer complexes with substituted aromatic compounds as donors				
$\varkappa$	charge transfer constant	LIVINGSTONE, HYDE and FOSTER [92a, b]	formation of charge-transfer complexes with substituted aromatic compounds as donors				

Table 5.3. Values of some selected substituent constant

Substituent	σ_m 1)	σ_p 1)	σ_m^0 3)	σ_p^0 3)	σ_p^+	σ_p^- 3)	σ_I 3)	σ_R^0 3)	σ_R 3)	σ_R^+ 3)	σ_0 6)	$\mathfrak{F}$ 2)	$\mathfrak{R}$ 2)	S 7)	P 7)
NH_2	−0.16	−0.66	−0.14	−0.38	−1.3 3)		0.10	−0,48	−0.78	−1.4	—	0.02	−0.68	0.45	−1.99
$N(CH_3)_2$	−0.15 2)	−0.83	−0.15	−0.44	−1.7 3)	as	0.10	−0.54	−0.94	−1.8	—	0.10	−0.92	—	—
OH	0.12	−0.37	−0.04	−0.13	−0.92 4)	σ_p	0.25	−0.40	−0.68	−1.24	—	0.29	−0.64	0.48	−1.55
OCH_3	0.12	−0.27	0.13 4)	−0.12 4)	−0.78 4)		0.25	−0.41	−0.63	−1.13	−0.39	0.26	−0.51	0.63	−1.12
NO_2	0.71	0.78	0.70	0.82	0.78 5)	1.24	0.63	—	—	—	0.80	0.67	0.16	1.33	0.87
CN	0.56	0.66	0.62	0.69	0.66 5)	0.88	0.56	0.07	0.00	—	—	0.51	0.19	1.17	0.64
$\overset{+}{N}(CH_3)_3$	0.88	0.82	0.86	0.80	0.82 5)	0.77	0.92	0.00	0.00	—	—	0.89	0.00	1.84	−0.01
F	0.34	0.06	0.35	0.17	−0.07 4)		0.52	−0.36	−0.59	−0.71	0.24	0.43	−0.34	0.91	−0.41
Cl	0.37	0.23	0.37	0.27	−0.18 4)	as	0.47	−0.20	−0.35	−0.47	0.20	0.41	−0.15	0.92	−0.13
Br	0.39	0.23	0.38	0.26	−0.16 4)	σ_p	0.45	−0.16	−0.34	−0.42	0.21	0.44	−0.17	0.91	−0.13
J	0.35	0.18	0.35	0.27	−0.14 4)		0.39	−0.12	−0.23	−0.35	0.21	0.40	−0.19	—	—
H	0	0	0	0	0		0	0	0	0	0	0	0	0	0

1) from [26]
2) from [25]
3) from [24]
4) from [93]
5) value of σ_p
6) from [37]
7) from [70]

4. *Relationships with* σ^+ *and* σ^- (see also eqn. (5/102))

a) *Relative sweetness of nitroanilines* (*XX*) [113]

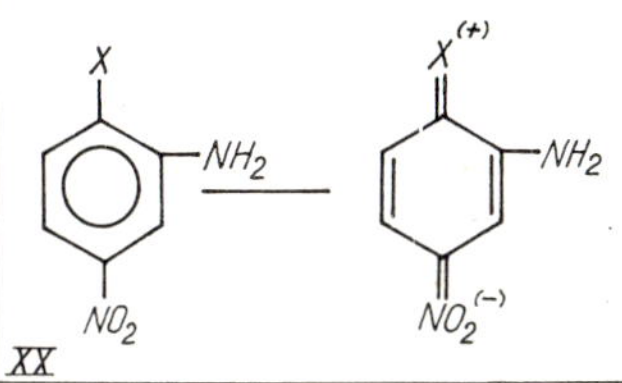

XX

$$\log A = -1.03\sigma^+ + 1.43\pi + 1.58 \qquad (5/87)$$

$n = 9 \qquad r = 0.972 \qquad s = 0.190$

b) *Enzymatic reduction of acetophenones* (*XXI*) [113]

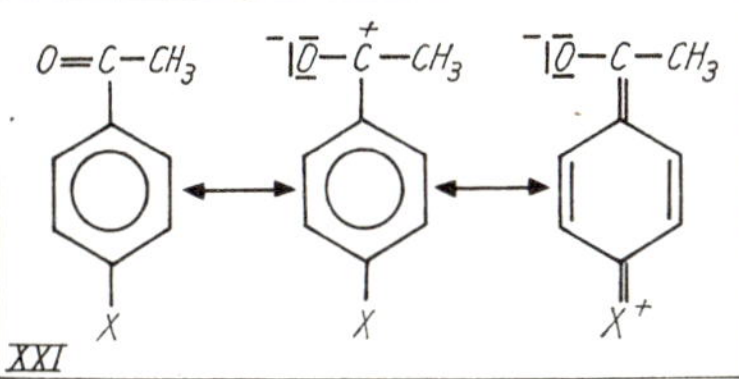

XXI

$$\log A = 1.51\sigma^+ + 1.48 \qquad (5/88)$$

$n = 10 \qquad r = 0.910 \qquad s = 0.390$

c) *Diethylphenylphosphates* (*XXII*)

(i) *Rate of alkaline hydrolysis in vitro* [114]

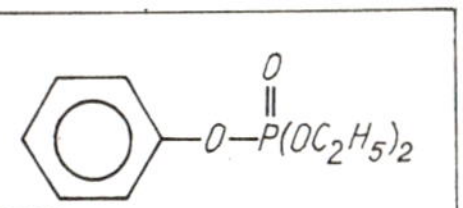

XXII

$$\log k = 1.35\sigma^- - 5.09 \qquad (5/89)$$

$n = 7 \qquad r = 0.955 \qquad s = 0.238$

(ii) *Inhibition of acetylcholinesterase* (*from fly head*) *in vitro* [115]

$$\log A = 2.37\sigma^- + 4.38 \qquad (5/90)$$

$n = 6 \qquad r = 0.985 \qquad s = 0.297$

(iii) *Toxicity in houseflies* [116]

$$\log A = 2.65\sigma^- + 0.36 \log P + 2.44 \qquad (5/91)$$

$n = 8 \qquad r = 0.990 \qquad s = 0.206$

A comparison of eqns. (5/89)—(5/91) is interesting. The insecticidal activity of phosphoric acid esters arises from an irreversible inhibition of cholinesterase by phosphorylation of a serine residue in the active centre of the enzyme. This is a nucleophilic reaction as is ester hydrolysis, and such reactions are described by σ^-. Thus, eqns. (5/89)—(5/91) are in full agreement with one another and with the postulated mechanism of action, the log P term in eqn. (5/91) being attributable to transport influences. A very similar picture is presented by phenyl N-methylcarbamates [117—119]. This example indicates that $f_e(x_e)$ may provide valuable information concerning the biological mechanism of drug action.

d) *Hydrolysis of phenyl-β-D-glucosides by emulsin* [100]

Enzymatic substrate splitting can be formulated in a simplified manner as (E = enzyme; S = substrate; P = product):

$$E + S \underset{k_2}{\overset{k_1}{\rightleftharpoons}} ES \xrightarrow{k_3} E + P \qquad (5/92)$$

Equation (4/83) described the quantity $k_1/k_2 = K_1$ which was related to σ^- (assuming a nucleophilic attack) and to a position-dependent π term (meta-substituents do not interact with the enzyme). A closely related behaviour is displayed by k_3:

$$\log (k_3 \cdot 10^8) = 0.94\sigma^- - 0.60\pi_{para} + 0.00\pi_{meta} - 6.15 \qquad (5/93)$$

$$n = 13 \qquad r = 0.949 \qquad s = 0.244$$

The π terms in (4/83) and (5/93) indicate that as the hydrophobicity of the substituents in the para-position increases the binding of both the substrate and the product to the enzyme becomes stronger. The former effect is favourable and the latter unfavourable for the reaction (the splitting of the product from the enzyme being slowed down with increasing hydrophobicity). These two effects compensate each other in the overall reaction:

$$\log (k_3 \cdot k_1/k_2) = 1.69\sigma^- - 4.50 \qquad (5/94)$$

$$n = 13 \qquad r = 0.933 \qquad s = 0.339$$

If only the overall reaction had been examined the wrong conclusion would have emerged that hydrophobic interactions are not involved. This shows clearly how valuabel for the elucidation of reaction mechanisms the QSAR analysis may be when carried out together with detailed biochemical studies.

5. *Relationships with inductive and resonance constants*

a) *Reduction of para-substituted acetophenones by carboxyl reductase* [120]

$$\log A = 3.72\sigma_R + 1.99 \qquad (5/95)$$

$$n = 6 \qquad r = 0.17 \qquad s = 0.29$$

b) *Fungicidal activity of tetrachloroisophthalonitriles* [23]

$$\log A = -2.12 \sum \sigma_I + 4.11 \qquad (5/96)$$

$$n = 16 \qquad r = 0.980 \qquad s = 0.262$$

c) *Virostatic activity of isatin-β-thiosemicarbazones (XXIII) against vaccinia virus* [121]: *5-substituted compounds*

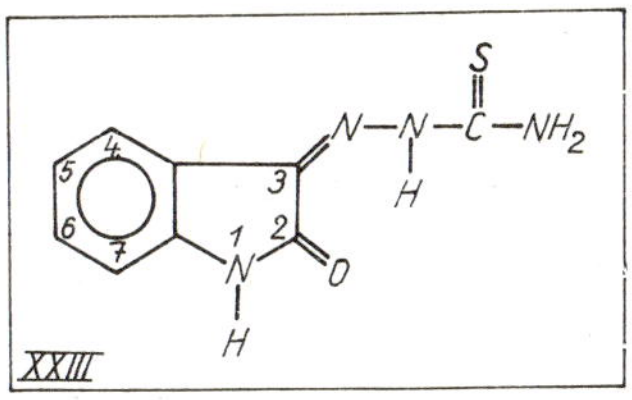

$$\log A = 11.26\sigma_I - 4.50 \qquad (5/97)$$

$n = 5 \qquad r = 0.992 \qquad s = 0.195$

6-substituted compounds

$$\log A = 3.32\sigma_I - 0.43 \qquad (5/98)$$

$n = 6 \qquad r = 0.957 \qquad s = 0.269$

These two equations can be slightly improved by adding a hydrophobic or a steric term [121].

6. *Separation of inductive and resonance effects*

a) *Inhibition of cholinesterase by meta-substituted phenyl* N-*methylcarbamates* [23, 122]

$$\log A = 0.31\pi - 0.96\mathfrak{F} - 1.89\mathfrak{R} - 0.73E_S \qquad (5/99)$$

$n = 15 \qquad r = 0.953$

b) *Inhibition of thymidine phosphorylase by 6-substituted uracils* ([123]; α = polarizability)

$$\log A = 0.02\alpha - 0.93\mathfrak{R} + 1.08\mathfrak{F} - 0.72 \qquad (5/100)$$

$n = 11 \qquad r = 0.93 \qquad s = 0.259$

c) *Antiadrenergic activity of β-halo-β-arylalkylamines (XXIV)* ([124])

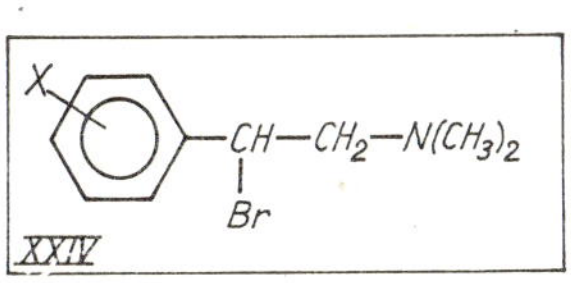

$$\log A = 0.86 \sum \pi + 0.47S_m - 0.36S_p - 0.92P_p + 0.62r_{v,p} + 7.08 \qquad (5/101)$$

$n = 22 \qquad r = 0.967 \qquad s = 0.167$

where $r_{v,p}$ is the VAN DER WAALS radius of substituents in the para-position and is to be regarded as a steric parameter. The same series can also be described by means of

σ^+ instead of S and P:

$$\log A = 0.82 \sum \pi - 1.02 \sum \sigma^+ + 0.62 r_{v,p} + 7.06 \quad (5/102)$$

$$n = 22 \quad r = 0.964 \quad s = 0.164$$

This can be explained from a highly significant correlation between σ^+ and S and P [124]. Equation (5/102) is simpler then (5/101) but does have virtually the same statistical significance. Since, in addition, it is theoretically justified to exchange S and P for σ^+, eqn. (5/102) is preferred for practical work.

d) *Inhibition of* L*-aminopeptidase by ortho- and meta-substituted piperidinoacetanilides* (*XXV*) [125]

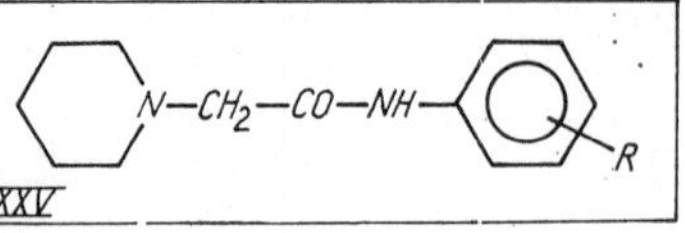

XXV

ortho-substituted compounds:

$$\log A = 0.72\sigma_p - 1.15\sigma_I - 0.43\pi - 1.17\sigma_p\pi + 1.63\sigma_I\pi + 2.16 \quad (5/103)$$

$$r = 0.966 \quad s = 0.037$$

para-substituted compounds:

$$\log A = 1.72\sigma_p - 0.95\sigma_I + 2.26 \quad (5/104)$$

$$r = 0.950 \quad s = 0.116$$

Equation (5/103) corresponds to CHARTONS ortho-approach (cf., eqn. (5/27)), the $\pi\sigma$ terms being regarded as electronic corrections of the applied π values from the phenoxyacetic acid system (see chapter 7.). No such cross-products were necessary in subsequent QSAR analyses carried out for other biological effects of this class of compounds using experimentally determined π values. Of interest is the position-dependence of the hydrophobic interactions which are apparently not involved at the para-position.

7. *Application of the* YUKAWA-TSUNO *and* YOSHIOKO *equations*

a) *Oxidation of phenylglycines in the sheep kidney* ([89])

$$\log A = 4.23\sigma^+ - 5.17\sigma + 0.21 \quad (5/105)$$

$$n = 6 \quad r = 0.996 \quad s = 0.118$$

b) *Inhibition of microsomal mixed-functional oxidase by phenylsydnones in vitro* ([110])
Phenylsydnones (XIX) represent limiting structures where the substituent R_1 in the phenyl ring enables the resonance stabilization of a positive charge. If there are electronic substituent influences, either a simple relationship with σ^+ or a relation with σ^+ and σ according to the YUKAWA-TSUNO equation can be expected to occur:

$$\log A = 4.59\pi_1 + 0.68\pi_2 + 17.91\sigma_1 - 0.24\sigma_1^+ + 1.06 \quad (5/106)$$

$$r = 0.996 \quad s = 0.062$$

There appears to be no electronic substituent influence of R_2.

Phenylsydnones can easily be split into phenyl-N-nitrosoamino acids (XXVI) which may also be the biologically active agent. This is not supported by eqn. (5/106), for in this case no σ^+ term is to be expected. Furthermore, the π values in (5/106) stem from the aromatic phenol system, whilst R_2 in XXVI is situated in an aliphatic environment.

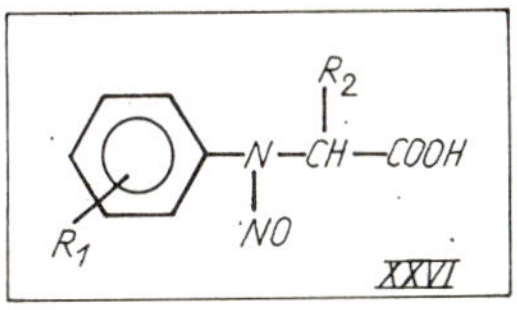

As a result, the hydrophobic influence of R_2 in XXVI cannot be described by these π values. With this in mind, it may be concluded from (5/106) that the intact sydnone system is responsible for enzyme inhibition. Evidence in support of this is furnished by the experimentally observed decrease in inhibition under conditions which facilitate ring opening. Interestingly, the *toxic action* of phenylsydnones *in vivo* in the mouse gives rise to an entirely different situation. Here the σ^+ term is negligible and in order to describe the hydrophobic effects aliphatic π values are needed for R_2 [110]. This strongly suggests that XXVI is the toxic compound (bioactivation *in vivo*), and the fact that *in vivo* — but scarcely in vitro — phenylsydnone is a potent methaemoglobin producer (a property typical of nitroso compounds) is in agreement with this. Again, QSAR analyses provide an idea of the mechanism of action.

c) *Bacteriostatic activity of sulfonamides against E. coli* [126]

$$\log A = 0.67\sigma^- + 0.48\sigma - 0.15\pi + 4.80 \qquad (5/107)$$

$$n = 17 \qquad r = 0.973 \qquad s = 0.117$$

8. *Radical parameter*

a) *Bactericidal activity of benzyl alcohols* [127]

$$\log A = 2.50E_R + 0.63 \log P + 0.09 \qquad (5/108)$$

$$n = 18 \qquad r = 0.95 \qquad s = 0.222$$

b) *Anaesthetic activity of benzyl alcohols* [127]

$$\log A = -3.16E_R + 1.33 \log P + 0.09 \qquad (5/109)$$

$$n = 16 \qquad r = 0.93 \qquad s = 0.308$$

c) *Synergism of the insecticidal effects of carbamates and benzodioxoles (XXVII) in flies* [128]

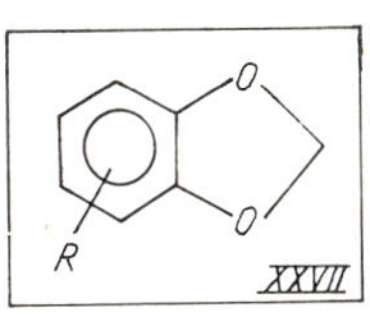

$$\log A = -0.20\pi^2 + 0.67\pi + 1.32\sigma^{\cdot} + 1.61 \qquad (5/110)$$

$$n = 13 \qquad r = 0.929 \qquad s = 0.171$$

$\sigma^{\cdot}$ is a particular form of a homolytic substituent constant used to describe radical reactions. The synergistic effect of XXVII is based on an inhibition of microsomal enzymes which break down carbamates. The $\sigma^{\cdot}$ term has been interpreted to mean that the reaction with the enzyme occurs via a radical mechanism, the extend of inhibition increasing as it becomes easier to localize a free electron at the CH_2 group. From a pharmacological point of view this example is interesting in that it illustrates the possibility of describing co-ergisms through a QSAR analyses.

Finally, when considering e.g. eqns. (4/82), (5/97), (5/89) and (5/106) a position-dependent electronic effect will be noted. As already mentioned, such dependences are not uncommon in more complex molecules, in particular in heterocyclic compounds, molecules with several aromatic rings and molecules having an aromatic and an aliphatic moiety. They must, therefore, always be taken into consideration in QSAR analysis.

5.2. Application of Experimental Quantities in $f_e(x_e)$

Experimental quantities may be successfully employed as electronic parameters when they characterize such electronic molecular properties as are of importance in the biological activity under investigation. Thus, they may serve as substitutes for electronic substituent constants, since most can be described by linear free enthalpy relationships. A further advantage is that they characterize definite interactions, thereby permitting straightforward physicochemical interpretation. Finally, a single experimental parameter may replace a more complicated multiparameter relationship based on substituent constants. However, in order to predict the biological activity of a given compound the corresponding experimental parameter(s) must first be determined. Fortunately, data of sufficient significance can often be estimated from the starting compounds from which the material is to be synthesized (see below). The most important experimental parameters used as x_e are listed in Table 5.4. It should be remembered that position dependences and both linear and non-linear relationship may occur on application of these parameters. Frequent use is made of the pK_a and ΔpK_a values, which serve as general measures of the electronic substituent influence and degree of ionization. Some examples of the application of these quantities are shown below.

Table 5.4. Selected experimental quantities applicable as molecule parameter x_e in $f_e(x_e)$

$pK_a = -\log K_a$	K_a: ionization constant of ionizable groups
$\Delta pK_a = \log K_{a,X}/K_{a,H}$	X: substituted compound with substituent X
	H: un-substituted compound
μ	dipole moment
μ_i	group dipole moment
α	electronic polarizability
P_E	electronic group polarizability
ϑ	chemical shift (NMR spectroscopy)
ν	IR-frequency of a suitable group
$\Delta\nu$	shift of ν by the introduction of a substituent
HWP	polarographic half-wave potential
I	ionization potential
k, K	rate and equilibrium constant, respectively, of a proper model reaction

1. *Bacteriostatic activity of arylamines against E. coli* [129]

$$\log A = -0.158pK_a + 0.694 \log P + 4.504 \qquad (5/111)$$

$$n = 15 \qquad r = 0.966 \qquad s = 0.114$$

In this case, substituents which reduce the pK_a value while enhancing hydrophobicity give the most favourable results.

2. *Inhibition of carboanhydrase by sulfonamides* [130, 131]

$$\log A = -0.774\Delta pK_a + 0.379\pi + 0.516 \qquad \text{(a)}$$

$$n = 16 \qquad r = 0.938 \qquad s = 0.216$$

$$\log A = 1.913\vartheta_{NH} + 0.255\pi + 0.447 \qquad \text{(b)}$$

$$n = 16 \qquad r = 0.963 \qquad s = 0.168$$

$$\log A = 2.160\Delta\nu_{SO_2} + 0.457\pi + 0.584 \qquad \text{(c)} \qquad (5/112)$$

$$n = 16 \qquad r = 0.924 \qquad s = 0.236$$

$$\log A = 0.084\sigma + 0.223\pi + 0.481 \qquad \text{(d)}$$

$$n = 16 \qquad r = 0.958 \qquad s = 0.176$$

In eqns. (5/112a)—(5/112d) several experimental parameters and σ are mutually exchangeable because they are all interrelated. Similar results have been reported by KAKEYA et al. for the diuretic and sodiouretic activity of sulfonamides [131—133].

3. *Bacteriostatic activity of sulfonamides in vitro* [101, 134—137]

$$\log A = -0.639pK_a + 6.405 \qquad \text{(a)}$$

$$n = 25 \qquad r = 0.962$$

$$\log A = -0.890\vartheta_{NH} + 5.649 \qquad \text{(b)} \qquad (5/113)$$

$$n = 25 \qquad r = 0.976$$

$$\log A = 1.128\sigma + 0.398 \qquad \text{(c)}$$

Interestingly, the bacteriostatic activity *in vitro* can also be predicted well by use of expressions involving the chemical shift or the charge density at the nitrogen (Q_N) of the *precursor amines* to be used for synthesis:

$$\log A = -0.634\vartheta_{NH} + 4.784 \qquad (5/114)$$

$$n = 11 \qquad r = 0.982$$

$$\log A = 38Q_N - 4.761 \qquad (5/115)$$

$$n = 6 \qquad r = 0.944$$

Where a large range of electronic properties is covered, eqns. (5/113) and (5/114) are transformed into parabolas. According to RASTELLI et al. [138] the sulfonamide ion constitutes the biologically active species whose properties are approximated by eqn. (5/114). These authors found a relationship between the IR and Raman frequencies of the SO_2 group and bacteriostatic activity. A detailed QSAR treatment of antibacterial sulfnamides is also presented in [105, 107, 134a, b].

4. *Inhibition of root growth in B. napus* (5/116), *of trypsin* (5/117) *and of* L-*alaninamino-peptidase* (5/118) *by substituted piperidinoacetanilides* (*XXV*) [139, 140]

$$\log A = 0.26\vartheta_{NH} + 0.46E_{S,m} + 0.18 \quad (5/116)$$

$n = 8 \quad r = 0.960 \quad s = 0.147$

$$\log A = -1.32\vartheta_{NH} - 1.90\pi + 18.21 \quad (5/117)$$

$n = 10 \quad r = 0.905 \quad s = 0.492$

$$\log A = 1.61\vartheta_{NH} - 15.09 \quad (5/118)$$

$n = 7 \quad r = 0.949 \quad s = 0.131$

5. *Fungicidal activity of indole derivatives* (*XXVIII*) [141]

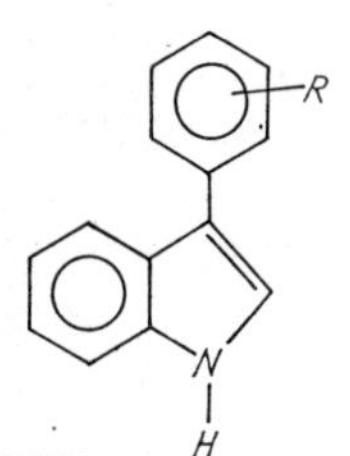

XXVIII

$$\log A = -0.58\vartheta_{NH} - 4.08\pi^2 + 5.40\pi + 3.05 \quad (5/119)$$

$n = 16 \quad r = 0.95$

6. *Antiarhythmic activity of XXIX* [142]

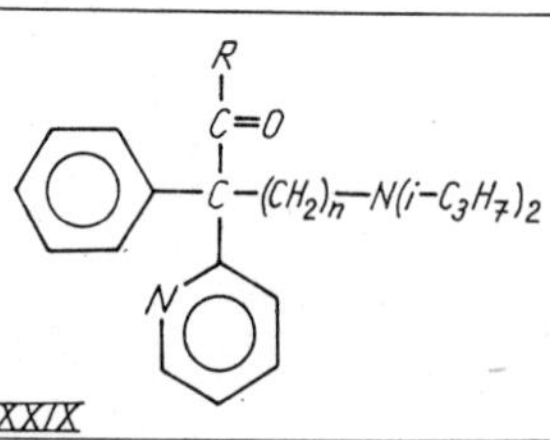

XXIX

$$\log A = 16.12 \cdot 10^{-3}\nu_{C=0} + 0.92\pi + 28.44 \quad (5/120)$$

$n = 14 \quad r = 0.96 \quad s = 0.14$

7. *Inhibition of acetylcholinesterase by XXX* [143]

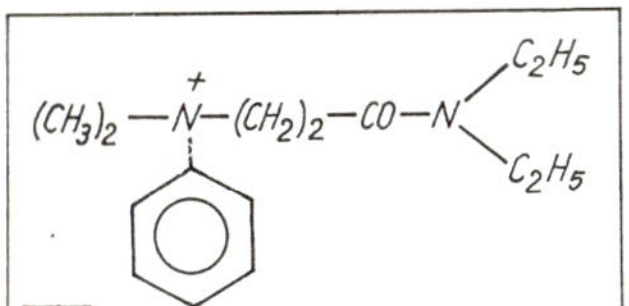

XXX

$$pI_{50} = 0.44\pi + 0.08\mu + 2.41 \qquad (5/121)$$

$n = 7 \qquad r = 0.889 \qquad s = 0.12$

It is of interest that μ does not represent the dipole moment of XXX but that of the aniline derivatives used for the synthesis of XXX.

8. *Inhibition of muscle contraction by various non-electrolytes* [100]

$$\log A = 0.082\,\alpha - 3.67 \qquad (5/122)$$

$n = 39 \qquad r = 0.987 \qquad s = 0.342$

9. *Enzymatic hydrolysis of substituted benzoylcholine esters* [144]

$$\log A = 1.31\sigma - 0.05P_E - 4.82 \qquad (5/123)$$

$n = 9 \qquad r = 0.980 \qquad s = 0.105$

10. *Uncoupling of oxidative phosphorylation by XXXI* [145]

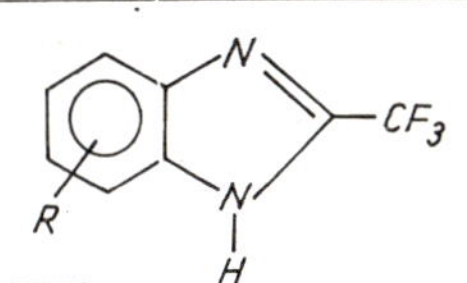

XXXI

$$\log A = -0.68\sum\sigma^2 + 3.10\sum\sigma + 0.58\sum\pi + 3.84 \qquad \text{(a)}$$

$n = 22 \qquad r = 0.951 \qquad s = 0.531$

$$\log A = -8.21\sum\vartheta^2 + 10.62\sum\vartheta + 0.44\sum\pi + 4.16 \qquad \text{(b)} \qquad (5/124)$$

$n = 22 \qquad r = 0.968 \qquad s = 0.440$

$$\log A = -0.16\Delta pK_a^2 + 1.64\Delta pK_a + 0.42\sum\pi + 3.56 \qquad \text{(c)}$$

$n = 22 \qquad r = 0.981 \qquad s = 0.338$

On comparison of eqns. (5/124a)—(5/124c) it is seen that the best description is obtained with ΔpK_a in this case, although electronic substituent constants can also be applied. The quantity ϑ is a special electronic substituent constant derived from IR measurements.

11. *Uncoupling of oxidative phosphorylation by benzimidazoles* [100]

$$\log A = -0.24\Delta pK_a^2 + 1.36\Delta pK_a + 0.41\log P + 3.15 \qquad (5/125)$$

$n = 22 \qquad r = 0.938 \qquad s = 0.358$

A non-linear relationship with x_e as in eqns. (5/124) and (5/125) appears to be frequently (but not always) associated with the uncoupling of oxidative phosphorylation. This inference is substantiated in an indirect manner in [146], and further examples are presented in [147] and below (substituent constants used instead of experimental parameters).

12. *Uncoupling of oxidative phosphorylation by XXXII* [148]

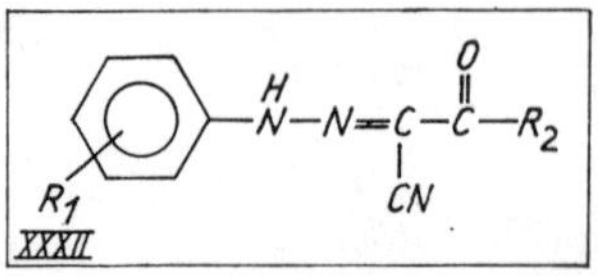

$$\log A = -0.80(\sigma_m + \sigma_p + \sigma_{R_2})^2 + 0.52(\sigma_m + \sigma_p + \sigma_{R_2}) - 0.05(\pi_m + \pi_p)^2 + 0.31(\pi_m + \pi_p) + 0.36\pi_0^2 - 0.13\pi_0 + 0.19\pi_{R_2} + 5.83 \quad (5/126)$$

$n = 60 \quad r = 0.921 \quad s = 0.172$

Both the hydrophobic and the electronic influence imply an overt position dependence. The positive sign of the π_0^2 term is also of interest (minimum region in (4/72) and (4/73)).

13. *Inhibition of monoamine oxidase by propynylamines* [149]

$$\log A = -0.21pK_a^2 + 1.84pK_a + 0.24\pi + 1.06X + 3.77 \quad (5/127)$$

$n = 47 \quad r = 0.91 \quad s = 0.58$

The indicator variable X describes a particular influence of ortho-substituents and is defined as:

$$X = \begin{cases} 1 & \text{for ortho-substituted compounds} \\ 0 & \text{for compounds without ortho-substituents} \end{cases} \quad (5/128)$$

As pointed out in [149], the non-linear relationship with pK_a is not connected with ionization equilibria. In the present instance, it arises from the fact that the reaction takes place in three steps, the first two being favoured and the third hindered by electron-attracting substituents. Electronic substituent effects here may thus be said to have an optimum that is reflected by the parabolic relationship with pK_a.

14. *Inhibition of the* Hill *reaction by substituted anilides* [150]

$$\log A = 0.16\,\text{HWP} + 0.83\pi - 0.52\pi^2 + 1.13 \quad (5/129)$$

$n = 12 \quad r = 0.999 \quad s = 0.003$

The relationship with the polarographic half-wave potential, HWP, indicates the occurrence of charge-transfer interactions.

15. *Bacteriostatic activity of 5-nitrothiazoles* [151]

$$\log A = 20.81\,\text{HWP} - 0.54\,(\log P)^2 + 1.96\log P + 5.76 \quad (5/130)$$

$n = 18 \quad r = 0.942 \quad s = 0.229$

The half-wave potential reflects the redox properties of the compounds under investigation and is included in (5/130) because nitrothiazoles act via a reduction step in bacterial metabolism.

16. *Hallucinogenic activity of amphetamines* [151a]

$$\log A = -1.48 I_1 + 0.78 \log P + 11.15 \qquad (5/130a)$$

$$n = 11 \qquad r = 0.94$$

I_1 = first ionization potential

Equation (5/130a) indicates a substantial increase in activity with a decrease in I_1 which, in turn, reflects increasing complexing ability of the aromatic ring.

Particular problems are presented by series in which the degree of ionization shows large variation [152, 153]. It may be that only the ionized or the non-ionized molecules interact with the receptor, or that both forms are bound to the receptor with different affinities. In such series an explicit incorporation of the degree of ionization in the QSAR is, therefore, to be recommended, although a major difficulty is that in many cases nothing is known about the *pH* values in the immediate neighbourhood of the receptor. Three courses of action are available. In the first degree of ionization is included in the hydrophobicity term using the *distribution coefficient, D* (also called *apparent partition coefficient*), instead of the true partition coefficient *P* (see e.g. [154, 154a]). *D* can easily be measured experimentally and is related to *P*:

$$\log D = \log P + \log f_n \qquad (5/131)$$

The non-ionized fraction, f_n, can be calculated from the *pH* and pK_a values. This approach appears helpful when the electronic influences on transport or hydrophobic interactions need to be separated from other electronic effects. Scherrer and Howard [154, 154a] have reported a variety of examples in which $\log P$ is successfully replaced by $\log D$, the resulting relationships being, moreover, simpler and more statistically significant. There are, however, serious objections to the use of $\log D$ in non-linear relationships involving $f_h(x_h)$, as the real position of the maximum may thus not be found [153].

In a second approach the concentration of the active species (ionized or non-ionized) is calculated [155, 156] from the drug concentration (dose) applied by multiplying with either the fraction ionized, f_i, or non-ionized, f_n. The biological activities of the ionized (subscript *i*) or non-ionized (subscript *n*) forms can then be represented respectively as:

$$\log A = \log 1/C_i = \log 1/Cf_i = \log 1/C + \log [(K_a + [H^+])/K_a] \qquad (5/132)$$

and

$$\log A = \log 1/C_n = \log 1/Cf_n = \log 1/C + \log [(K_a + [H^+]/[H^+])] \qquad (5/133)$$

This procedure affords the correct value for $x_{h,0}$ if a non-linear relation exists between $\log A$ and x_h, but is of no use where ionized and non-ionized forms are both active. A detailed treatment of the degree of ionization is possible in a third approach (Martin and Hackbarth [153, 157—159]) which also allows account to be taken of the presence of several aqueous compartments with different *pH* values (see 4.4.).

MacFarland [160] stressed the importance of *group dipole moments* and *group polarizabilities*. If it is assumed that any differences in affinity within a homologous series for a given receptor can solely be attributed to, apart from hydrophobic interactions, VAN DER WAALS forces between substituents and receptor, the following approximation can be derived from the expressions describing KEESOM, DEBYE and LONDON interactions:

$$f_e(x_e) = a\mu_i^2 + bP_E + \text{constant} \tag{5/134}$$

This approach neglects the influence of the substituents on the properties of the whole molecule as well as the fact that VAN DER WAALS forces are already in part taken into account by π. MACFARLAND mentions some examples in which eqn. (5/134) has been successfully used to describe biological activity. These are, however, not very convincing, nor do they preclude a physical interpretation on different lines (see also [88]). Nevertheles, dipole moment (for a good review, see e.g. [161]) and polarizability are useful parameters for characterizing electronic properties within the function $f_e(x_e)$. Polarizabilities may, however, also simply reflect hydrophobic interactions, since, within certain sets of substituents, polarizability and x_h may be closely interrelated (see e.g. [162—165]). TUTE [166], following an approach analogous to eqn. (5/134) for a QSAR analysis of the inhibition of the viral enzyme neuraminidase by XXXIII, obtained the expression

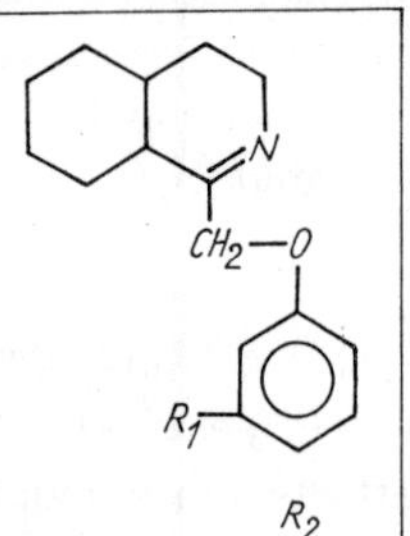

XXXIII

$$\log A = 0.062\mu_v + 0.030\mu_v^2 + 0.217\pi + 2.552 \tag{5/135}$$

$$n = 16 \quad r = 0.937 \quad s = 0.074$$

where μ_v is the group dipole moment along the axis through the oxygen atom and the para-substituent R_2 in XXXIII. According to TUTE, eqn. (5/135) indicates that, in addition to hydrophobic interactions with the receptor, dipole-dipole interactions occur (reflected in the term μ_v^2) and that, furthermore, the dipole interacts with a point charge on the receptor (reflected in the term μ_v). Equation (5/135) could not be improved by adding a term for P_E and thus TUTE concluded that no dipole is induced in XXXIII on binding to the receptor. However, a closer inspection of eqn. (5/135) reveals that the statistical significance of the μ_v term is only poor and that biological activity can be equally well described by [88]:

$$\log A = 0.265\pi + 0.014\mu_v^2 + 2.548 \tag{5/136}$$

$$n = 16 \quad r = 0.916 \quad s = 0.081$$

Since μ_v^2 is correlated with σ^2 and a σ^2 term may indicate a totally different mechanism of action, the correctness of the above interpretation is questionable.

This example shows clearly that even if the expression derived appears to be statistically significant, it would be unwise to limit the corresponding interpretation to a single hypothesis. As many hypotheses as possible should be probed, which entails calculations based on a large number of meaningful parameters. The fact that a given hypothesis leads to a QSAR which is statistically significant does not prove that this hypothesis is valid in the absence of other suitably tested alternative possibilities.

5.3. Application of Quantum-Chemical Parameters in $f_e(x_e)$

The rational way of using quantum-chemical methods in drug design is to evaluate the basic molecular determinants for a specific biological activity and to use this information for the design of new active structures. This requires a description of the structural features of the molecules, their electronic distributions and the energies required to modify and perturb them during drug-receptor interactions [96a, 166a, b]. These more global aspects will be discussed in chapter 12. while this section will be restricted to the use of quantum-chemical molecular parameters in correlations with biological activity within the extrathermodynamic approach.

It should be emphasized that a description of the various quantum-chemical procedures and a detailed discussion of the numerous parameters in quantum chemistry is beyond the scope of this treatise. For quantum-chemical techniques reference is made to e.g. [167—174] (see also 12.), and some reviews of the application of quantum chemistry to biological problems can be found in [166a, 166b, 175—188].

A few major quantum-chemical parameters are shown in Table 5.5. This compilation is by no means complete (see [181f.]) and primarily comprises those parameters most frequently used in Hansch analysis. Note that some of the quantities presented in Table 5.4 are also accessible through quantum-chemical calculations. The variables E_{HOMO} (energy of the highest occupied molecular orbital) and E_{LEMO} (energy of the lowest empty molecular orbital) are of importance when two molecules with π electron systems form so-called *charge-transfer complexes*. Formally, such complexes arise where an electron moves from the highest occupied molecular orbital, HOMO, of donor D to the lowest empty molecular orbital, LEMO, of acceptor A. The interaction energy, E_{Ct}, may be expressed as

$$E_{CT} = I_D - E_A + \Delta \qquad (5/137)$$

where I_D is the ionization potential of the donor, E_A is the electron affinity of the acceptor and Δ is a stabilization term expressing i.a. contribution from solvation and polarization effects. Within a homologous series the ionization potential and the electron affinity are inversely related to E_{HOMO} and E_{LEMO}, respectively. In the event of a reaction partner (the receptor) remaining constant and if drugs occur as donors

$$E_{CT} = a_1 E_{HOMO} + a_0 \qquad (5/138)$$

or as acceptors

$$E_{CT} = b_1 E_{LEMO} + b_0 \qquad (5/139)$$

Occasionally, a charge transfer appears to be "localized" or favoured at certain centres or atoms (notably heteroatoms) of a donor or an acceptor, in which case the

Table 5.5. Some quantum-chemical quantities frequently applied as parameter x_e in the function $f_e(x_e)$

E_{HOMO}	energy of the highest occupied molecular orbital
E_{LEMO}	energy of the lowest unoccupied (empty) molecular orbital
f_r	frontier electron density on atom r
F_r	f_r/E (frontier orbital). The frontier orbital is dependent on the nature of the interactions to be characterized either by E_{HOMO} or E_{LEMO} (see text)
S_r^E	electrophilic superdelocalizability of atom r
S_r^N	nucleophilic superdelocalizability of atom r
$S_r^{E'}$	approximate electrophilic superdelocalizability of atom r
$S_r^{N'}$	approximate nucleophilic superdelocalizability of atom r
q_r^π	π electron density on atom r
q_r^σ	σ electron density on atom r
Q_r	total electron density on atom r
$q_{r,N}^\pi$	net π electron density on atom r
$q_{r,N}^\sigma$	net σ electron density on atom r
$Q_{r,N}$	net total electron density on atom r
L_E	electrophilic localization energy
L_N	nucleophilic localization energy
L_R	radical localization energy

frontier electron density, f_r, on atom r provides a useful means of characterizing such interactions. This variable denotes the electron density on atom r in the frontier orbital essential to the charge transfer, i.e. in the HOMO (f_r^E) in the case of a donor and in the LEMO (f_r^N) for an acceptor. Strictly speaking, these variables are exactly defined only in the simple HÜCKEL approach. Furthermore, they permit no more than a comparison of different atoms in the same molecule; for a consideration of the events within a given series, the variable $F_r^N = f_r^E/E_{HOMO}$ and $F_r^N = f_r^N/E_{LEMO}$ provide a more realistic approximation. For overall charge-transfer interactions between drugs and receptors one may expect a correlation of log A with E_{HOMO} (drug = donor) or with E_{LEMO} (drug = acceptor)[1]). For a localized charge transfer on atom r, log A should be correlated with f_r^N or with F_r^N (drug = acceptor) or with f_r^E or F_r^E (drug = donor). Where such a localized charge transfer is possible on several atoms at the same time, log A is dependent on f_r or F_r of all the atoms concerned.

Another parameter frequently employed to characterize molecular interaction is the superdelocalizability, S_r, on atom r which to a certain extent is related to the contribution made by atom r to the stabilization energy in the complex formation with a second molecule. The superdelocalizability is restricted to π orbitals and there are problems in its use as far as the formalism of all-valence electron methods is concerned. A distinction is made between electrophilic, S_r^E, and nucleophilic, S_r^N, superdelocalizability, the former describing the interaction with an electrophilic centre and the latter an interaction with a nucleophilic centre in a second molecule. When in such interactions the electrons of the frontier orbital predominate, S_r', which denotes approximate superdelocalizability, is equally valid, its calculation being based only on the frontier orbital (HOMO for $S_r^{E'}$ and LEMO for $S_r^{N'}$).

[1]) The existence of such relationships cannot, however, be regarded as proof for the occurrence of charge-transfer interactions.

A feature which is, of course, essential to interactions with the receptor is the electron distribution in the drug molecule, i.e., the electron density on single atoms. It is necessary to distinguish between π electron density q_r^{π}, σ electron density, q_r^{σ}, and overall electron density, $Q_r = q_r^{\pi} + q_r^{\sigma}$, the last serving to calculate dipole moments. Sometimes the net charge ($q_{r,N}^{\pi}$, $q_{r,N}^{\sigma}$, $Q_{r,N}$) is applied; this is obtained by subtracting from q_r or Q_r the number of valence electrons which atom r possesses according to classical valence concepts.

To some extent, the parameters mentioned above can describe weak intermolecular interactions, but are also correlated with chemical reactivities. Considering reactivities, quantum-chemical parameters can be divided into *static* and *dynamic* reactivity indices. Static indices (e.g., charges) describe the isolated molecules in their ground state whilst dynamic indices (e.g., superdelocalizability) refer to the transition state and describe the molecules shortly before entering the activated complex. An important dynamic reactivity index for π electronic systems is the localization energy, L, which provides a measure of the change in π electron energy during formation of the π transition complex and is thus in the nature of an activation energy. Three types of reactant are to be distinguished here:

1. Electrophilic reactant. The number of π electrons in the system is reduced by two and that of those centres of the molecule which contribute π electrons, by one. This case is described by the electrophilic localization energy, L_E.
2. Nucleophilic reactant. The number of π electrons in the system remains unchanged, while that of the centres contributing π electrons is reduced by one. This case is described by the nucleophilic localization energy, L_N.
3. Radical reactant. Both the number of π electrons in the system and that of the centres contributing a π electron are reduced by one. This case is described by the radical localization energy, L_R.

The localization energy can be calculated for all centres (atoms, bonds) of a conjugated molecule.

One of the major problems in the application of quantum-chemical parameters in $f_e(x_e)$ is that for each drug molecule a host of such parameters can be calculated (e.g., for a molecule with 20 centres, 80 values are required for only S_r^E, S_r^N, $S_r^{E'}$ and $S_r^{N'}$), while it is not known how these parameters are related to biological activity (cf. 9.3.). Within certain limits, approaches in which the energy changes resulting from electronic interactions upon formation of a mesomeric species DR from two π electronic systems D and R are analyzed in terms of *perturbation theory* may be helpful here [189]. The first attempt to describe drug-receptor interactions on such lines was reported by Inouye et al. [190, 191]. A two-point interaction between receptor and drug D as a starting hypothesis gave:

$$f_e(x_e) = aS_r + bS_s + C \qquad (5/140)$$

and

$$f_e(x_e) = af_r + bf_s + C \qquad (5/141)$$

Equation (5/141) is applicable where the HOMOs of the drug and receptor have the same energy. S_r and S_s are the superdelocalizabilities of atoms r and s in the drug molecule which both interact with the receptor, and f_r and f_s are the corresponding frontier electron densities. Apart from the assumption of a two-point interaction, eqns. (5/140) and (5/141) can be regarded only as a crude approximation to reality since they involve some drastic oversimplifications [192].

A different perturbation theoretical approach to electronic drug-receptor interactions based on the work of KLOPMAN and HUDSON [193, 194] has been proposed by CAMMARATA [192]. It is not restricted to π systems, and it allows for ionic as well as localized charge-transfer interactions. Two cases are possible. In case 1 the interactions are essentially due to charge transfer and are dependent on the electron density in the frontier orbital of the atoms involved. The expression

$$f_e(x_e) = \sum_r (a_{r,1}c_{r,LEMO} + a_{r,2}c_{r,HOMO} + a_{r,3}Q_{r,N} + a_{r,4}Q^2_{r,N}) + \text{constant} \qquad (5/142)$$

is summed over all atoms participating in the interaction. $c_{r,LEMO}$ and $c_{r,HOMO}$ are the coefficients of atomic orbital r in the LEMO and HOMO, which characterize the same properties as the frontier electron density, f_r in this case. In case 2, the interactions can, in principle, be reduced to COULOMB forces, charge-transfer interactions playing no rôle:

$$f_e(x_e) = \sum_r (a_{r,1}Q_{r,N} + a_{r,2}S_r^N + a_{r,3}S_r^E) + \text{constant} \qquad (5/143)$$

It should be noted in both eqn. (5/142) and (5/143) single $a_{r,i}$ terms may become 0. The following relation may then be a borderline case of both eqns. (5/142) and (5/143)

$$f_e(x_e) = \sum_r a_r Q_{r,N} + \text{constant} \qquad (5/144)$$

where it is no longer possible to distinguish the two cases. The existence of such a relationship, furthermore, cannot be taken as proof of the validity of CAMMARATAS perturbational approach, for eqn. (5/144) may be expected whenever interactions between point charges in drug molecules and corresponding point charges or dipoles on the receptor contribute to the formation of the drug-receptor complex. Whether eqns. (5/142) and (5/143) can really be employed as a general $f_e(x_e)$ function describing electronic interactions remains uncertain, and further study is needed to ascertain this.

Attempts to relate quantum-chemical parameters with biological activity date back to the 1930s. However, despite all the efforts expended in this area, there are still relatively few unambigously *quantitative* structure-activity relations involving only this kind of parameters and in most cases one can conclude only that there are certain tendencies for biological activity to run parallel to certain parameters. One reason for this may be the large variety of molecular parameters in quantum chemistry, as mentioned above. Furthermore, these parameters are so interrelated that it is exceedingly difficult to extract those which are truly relevant for the gradation of biological activity. A commonly followed procedure consists of relating intuitively chosen parameters to biological activity, but the chance of success is small. The use of molecular parameters from quantum chemistry does not take account of entropy which frequently plays a major role in drug-receptor interactions, as, for instance, in hydrophobic interactions (however, to a limited extent and under certain conditions π values may be obtained from quantum-chemical calculations; see 7.2.). It is emphasized that, with few exceptions, quantum-chemical parameters only describe the term $f_e(x_e)$ and no real use can be found for them in quantitative structure-activity analyses unless they can be combined with the remaining functions of eqn. (3/17). Some examples of the application of quantum-chemical parameters in quantitative structure-activity analyses are presented below.

1. *Analgesic activity of imidazoline derivatives* [195]

$$\log A = -0.95\pi^2 + 1.80\pi - 7.90E_{HOMO} + 5.17 \qquad (5/145)$$

$$r = 0.975$$

Eqn. (5/145) indicates that charge-transfer interactions superimposed upon hydrophobic effects occur in this type of activity.

2. *Antibacterial activity of sulfonamides* [192]

$$\log A = 8.76c_{N,LEMO} + Q_{N,N} - 1731Q^2_{N,N} + X - 13.28 \qquad (5/146)$$

$$n = 15 \qquad r = 0.94 \qquad s = 0.15$$

Here $c_{N,LEMO}$ is the coefficient of the sulfonamide nitrogen atomic orbital in the LEMO, $Q_{N,N}$ is the net charge of the nitrogen and X is an indicator variable defined as:

$$X = \begin{cases} 0.20 & \text{for sulfonamide from a benzamide series} \\ 0 & \text{for sulfonamide from an aniline series} \end{cases} \qquad (5/147)$$

The values of X correspond to the net charge of the C atom in the carbonyl group. The formal agreement between eqns. (5/146) and (5/142) suggests charge-transfer interactions involving the nitrogen. Nevertheless, antibacterial activity of sulfonamides can be more simply described, for example, by eqns. (5/113)—(5/115).

3. *Antibacterial activity of tetracyclines* [192]

$$\begin{aligned}\log A = {} & 56.17Q_{010} + 16.91S^E_{010} + 48.79Q_{011} - 1.10S^E_{011} \\ & + 71.32Q_{012} + 18.36S^E_{012} + 3.38Q_6 + 18.39 \end{aligned} \qquad (5/148)$$

$$n = 18 \qquad r = 0.99 \qquad s = 0.16$$

The formal correspondence between eqns. (5/148) and (5/143) indicates the second of the cases discussed by CAMMARATA.

4. *Enzymatic acetylation of aromatic amines* (taken from [85])

PERAULT and PULLMAN [196] noticed a qualitative relation between the rate of acylation and amine nitrogen electron density, q_N; this relation was extendet by HANSCH et al. by adding a π term to give the quantitative expression (see [85]):

$$\log A = 0.29\pi + 18.16q_N - 33.82 \qquad (5/149)$$

5. *Taste enhancement by 2-substituted inosine-5'-phosphates (synergistic with* L*-glutamate;* [197])

$$\log A = 0.049\pi + 0.565\sigma_m + 0.425S^E_{X,1} + 0.375 \qquad (5/150)$$

$$n = 48 \qquad r = 0.929 \qquad s = 0.088$$

Of interest here is the combination of the electrophilic superdelocalizability for the first centre of the substituent in the 2-position with σ_m. The latter variable reflects the electronic effect on the carbonyl group in the 6-position, and $S^E_{X,1}$ represents local interactions on the substituent. Being of only secondary importance, the hydrophobic π term should be regarded here primarily as a steric correction.

6. *Taste enhancement by substituted 2-mercaptoinosine-5'-phosphates (synergistic with* L*-glutamate* [197])

$$\log A = -0.090\pi^2 + 0.137\pi + 3.48S^E_{X,1} + 0.216X + 0.876 \qquad (5/151)$$

$$n = 46 \qquad r = 0.950 \qquad s = 0.103$$

The indicator variable X is defined as:

$$X = \begin{cases} 1, & \text{if oxygen occurs in the } \gamma \text{ or } \vartheta \text{ position of the substituent} \\ 0, & \text{if not} \end{cases} \qquad (5/152)$$

7. *Inhibition of the* HILL *reaction by a series of piperidinoacetanilides* (*XXV*) [150]

$$\log A = -45.92q_N^{\pi} + 96.41 \qquad (5/153)$$

$$n = 7 \qquad r = 0.859 \qquad s = 0.197$$

$$\log A = 20.69E_{HOMO} - 10.57 \qquad (5/154)$$

$$n = 7 \qquad r = 0.992 \qquad s = 0.047$$

According to eqn. (5/153), the inhibition appears to increase as the electron density on the amide nitrogen decreases. This seems to be in full agreement with the classical concept of a HILL reaction inhibitor i.e., the hydrogen bond formation by the NH group makes an essential contribution to inhibitory activity. However, the electron density on the amide nitrogen is correlated with E_{HOMO}

$$E_{HOMO} = -3.63q_N^{\pi} + 6.92 \qquad (5/155)$$

$$n = 7 \qquad r = 0.909 \qquad s = 0.011$$

and eqn. (5/154) shows that E_{HOMO} yields an excellent one-parameter equation. It follows that, in all likelihood, the occurrence of charge-transfer interactions is more important than hydrogen bonding for the inhibition of the HILL reaction (see also [198, 199] and eqn. (5/129)). As a consequence, the presence of an NH proton need no longer be regarded as indispensable for this inhibition and the nitrogen may equally well be substituted or included in ring systems, and compounds of this type have indeed recently been shown to have high inhibitory potency [200]. Whilst this example shows some of the potential of QSAR analyses, it also again demonstrates the necessity of a large range of hypotheses and meaningful physicochemical parameters. In principle, this result could have been attained in the early 1960s if the catalogue of hypotheses underlying the QSAR work on Hill reaction inhibitors would not have been greatly oriented towards classical concepts and would have included a hypothesis on possible charge-transfer interactions. A further point of interest in eqns. (5/153) and (5/154) is the absence of a hydrophobicity term which is typical of QSARs involving Hill reaction inhibitors. The reason why this term does not occur is that the substituents under consideration scarcely differ in hydrophobicity. This leads to the conclusion, which is further discussed in chapter 8., that the evaluation of QSARs with true predictive value necessitates a sufficiently broad variation of all major substituent properties. In addition, the interpretation of such relations should always include a comparison with all QSARs already known for the biological activity considered.

8. *Inhibition of the growth of Chlorella vulgaris by p-substituted piperidinoacetanilides* (*XXV*) [201]

$$\log A = 29.37 q_N^{\pi} + 1.17\pi + 0{,}29X - 53.58 \qquad (5/156)$$

$$n = 9 \qquad r = 0.992 \qquad s = 0.099$$

Inhibition becomes stronger as the electron density on the nitrogen atom increases, the nitrogen possibly acting as an acceptor in hydrogen bonding. The variable X has a value of 1 for para-, 0 for meta- and -1 for ortho-substituents.

9. *Antihypertensive activity of benzothiadiazine-1,1-dioxides* (*XXXIV*) [202]

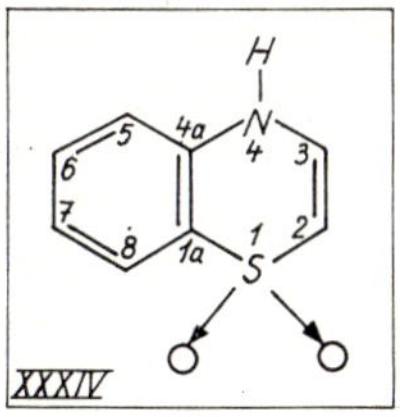

XXXIV

The compounds were varied by substitution or exchange of C atoms for heteroatoms in the aromatic ring and by substitution in the 3-position. The expression which results is:

$$\log A = 8.63 S_1^{N'} - 135.1 S_4^{E'} + 78.14 E^{[D]} + 54.52 S_3^{N'}$$
$$- 0.03\pi'_{5.5} - 0.03\pi'_{1a,1a} + 61.60 F^{[E]} + 1.49 q^{\sigma}_{3,N} + 1.95 \qquad (5/157)$$

$$n = 25 \qquad r = 0.997 \qquad s = 0.120$$

Equation (5/157) contains, besides approximate electrophilic and nucleophilic superdelocalizabilities on atoms 1, 3 and 4, some new quantities. $\pi'_{r,r}$ is the frontier self-polarizability of atom r, which expresses to a first approximation the self-induced electric moment on the atom (in relation to the frontier orbital). $E^{[D]}$ denotes the electric field produced by an atomic charge q_r at the centre of a binding site D at a distance R. Seven sites for such receptor bindings where randomly selected in the space surrounding the benzothiadiazine molecule, point D lying in the neighbourhood of the SO_2 group at a 0.55 nm distance from the sulphur and at 0.4 nm and 0.6 nm from the oxygen atoms. $F^{[D]}$ denotes the COULOMB interaction between the atomic charges and a point charge at point D, the dielectric constant being implicated as proportionality factor:

$$F^{[D]} = \sum_r \frac{q_r}{R_{[D]}} \qquad (5/158)$$

This result led WOHL [202] to postulate a three-point receptor binding. However, eqn. (5/157) is very complicated so that a mechanistic interpretation seems to be hazardous, the more so as the quantum-chemical parameters are interrelated. Nevertheless, eqn. (5/157) provides an excellent description of the biological activity, while permitting meaningful predictions about the biological activities of other compounds which could be verified experimentally. A disadvantage is that the computing costs are relatively high and the capacities of the quantum-chemical prodedure used (EHT) are in fact overtaxed. The only reason for justifying such expenditure is that in series where comparitively large numbers of ring atoms are exchanged the LFERs are of limited or no use. If only the substituents are varied a good description can also be obtained with the aid of simple substituent constants. TOPLISS and YUDIS [203] used this approach to investigate compounds of the same type (only substituents in the aromatic ring and in 3-position being varied) and obtained the following result (A being corrected for the pK_a value):

$$\log A = 1.28(\pi_6 + \pi_7) - 0.16\pi_3^2 + 0.72\pi_3 + 0.42 \qquad (5/159)$$

$$n = 33 \qquad r = 0.91 \qquad s = 0.35$$

Statistically, eqn. (5/159) is not as good as eqn. (5/157), but does refer to a larger number of compounds. Equation (5/159) is very simple, and permits valid predictions. In this context, the position dependence of the hydrophobic substituent effect is of interest. Because of the complexity of eqn. (5/157) and the different molecular variation in both series (including changes in ring position and substituents and only in substituents, as reported by WOHL and by TOPLISS and YUDIS, respectively), a mechanistic comparison of eqns. (5/157) and (5/159) is very difficult and at best speculative. It should be remembered that there are derivatives for which eqn. (5/159) fails whilst eqn. (5/157) does not.

10. *Activity of 15-hydroxytryptamine derivatives on the LSD receptor* ([204]; for a detailed discussion, see also [166 b])

$$\log A = 18.09f_1 - 74.77q_1^{\pi} + 1.182\pi_7 - 13.06 \qquad (5/160)$$

$$n = 15 \qquad r = 0.962 \qquad s = 0.288$$

In addition to the frontier electron density and charge on atom 1, the hydrophobicity of substituents in the 7-position plays an important, if not dominating rôle. It is of interest that the following equation could also be obtained:

$$\log A = -128.4q_7^2 + 13.07q_7 - 0.462 \qquad (5/161)$$

$$n = 15 \qquad r = 0.924 \qquad s = 0.337$$

Equation (5/161) shows a poorer fit than eqn. (5/160) but is still statistically significant. The maximum in the parabolic dependence of log A on q_7 lies at $q_7 = 0$. From a physico-chemical point of view this does not seem to make sense, for if the charge is 0, electrostatic interactions with the receptor are not possible, whereas in fact the maximum in biological activity is exhibited. This paradox can easily be resolved with the help of eqn. (5/160), which points clearly to the major role of hydrophobic interactions at the 7-position. Such interactions would be disturbed by a charge in this position and are thus maximized if $q_7 = 0$. Equation (5/161) is an interesting example of an expression where hydrophobic interactions underlie a correlation between log A and quantum-chemical parameters.

Quantum chemistry offers far more opportunities to describe the electronic structure of molecules and the resulting properties than do linear free enthalpy relations, and with the rapid increase in the ability of computers to handle large quantities of data it has become a major tool. However, because of the relatively high costs of quantum-chemical calculations, such methods of formulating the term $f_e(x_e)$ should be applied only when substituent constants cannot be used or when sufficient is already known about the reaction mechanism. Initial information about a given reaction mechanism may be acquired, e.g., from orientational experiments based on linear free enthalpy relationships. Subsequent application of quantum-chemical parameters to a representative sample may then be the decisive step in the analysis of the mechanism and under certain circumstances it may be a prerequisite to the discovery of meaningful QSARs. Despite the high costs and the fact that the host of parameters causes the aforementioned difficulties, quantum-chemical methods cannot be dispensed with in a systematic and large-scale application of quantitative structure-activity analysis to drug research, especially in the case of pharmacophoric pattern searching, to be dealt with later (see 12.).

References

[1] Leffler, J. E., and E. Grunwald: Rates and Equilibria of Organic Reactions, Wiley, New York, 1963
[2] Palm, V. A.: Grundlagen drr quantitativen Theorie organischer Reaktionen, Akademie-Verlag, Berlin, 1971
[3] Wold, S.: Chemica Scripta **5**, 97 (1974)
[4] Wold, S., and M. Sjöström in N. B. Chapman and J. Shorter (Eds.): Advances in Linear Free Energy Relationships, Vol. 2, Plenum Press, London, 1978
[5] Hammett, L. P.: J. Am. Chem. Soc. **59**, 66 (1937)
[6] Hammett, L. P.: Trans. Faraday Soc. **34**, 156 (1938)
[7] Hansch, C., A. Leo, S. Unger, K. H. Kim, D. Nikaitani and E. J. Lien: J. Med. Chem. **16**, 1207 (1973)
[8] Jaffé, H. H., and H. L. Jones: Adv. Heterocyclic Chem. **3**, 209 (1964)
[9] Wells, P. R.: Chem. Rev. **63**, 171 (1963)
[9a] Barlin, G. B., and D. D. Perrin: Quart. Rev. **20**, 75 (1966)
[9b] Fringuelli, F., G. Marino and A. Taticchi: J. Chem. Soc. (B) 1595 (1970)
[9c] Fringuelli, F., G. Marino and A. Taticchi: J. Chem. Soc. (B) 2302 (1971)
[9d] Fringuelli, F., G. Marino and A. Taticchi: J. Chem. Soc. (B) 2304 (1971)
[9e] Fringuelli, F., G. Marino and A. Taticchi: J. Chem. Soc. Perkin II 158 (1972)
[9f] Fringuelli, F., G. Marino and A. Taticchi: J. Chem. Soc. Perkin II 971 (1980)
[10] Johnson, C. D.: The Hammett-Equation, University Press, Cambridge, 1973

[11] Greizenstein, W. G., R. A. Bonelli and J. A. Brieux: J. Am. Chem. Soc. **84**, 1026 (1962)
[12] Jaffé, H. H.: Chem. Rev. **53**, 191 (1953)
[13] Charton, M.: J. Org. Chem. **26**, 735 (1961)
[14] Charton, M.: Progr. Phys. Org. Chem. **10**, 82 (1973)
[15] Katrizky, A. R., and R. D. Topsom in N. B. Chapman and J. Shorter (Eds.): Advances in Linear Free Energy Relationships, Plenum Press, London, 1972, p. 119
[16] Zuman, P.: Collect. Czech. Chem. Commun. **26**, 1 (1961)
[17] Taft, R. W., E. Price, I. R. Fox, I. C. Lewis, K. K. Anderson and D. T. Davis: J. Am. Chem. Soc. **85**, 709 (1963)
[18] Taft, R. W., E. Price, I. R. Fox, I. C. Lewis, K. K. Anderson and D. T. Davis: J. Am. Chem. Soc. **85**, 3146 (1963)
[18a] Adcock, W., and T. C. Khor: J. Am. Chem. Soc. **100**, 7799 (1978)
[19] Gibson, H. W.: Can. J. Chem. **51**, 3065 (1973)
[20] Widing, H. F., and L. S. Levitt: Tetrahedron **30**, 611 (1974)
[21] Harrison, A. G., P. Kebarle and F. P. Lossing: J. Am. Chem. Soc. **83**, **777** (1961)
[22] Taft, R. W., in M. S. Newman (Ed.): Steric Effects in Organic Chemistrv, Wiley, New York, 1956, p. 556
[23] Verloop, A., in E. J. Ariens (Ed.): Drug Design, Vol. III, Academic Press, New York 1972, p. 133
[24] Exner, O., in N. B. Chapman and J. Shorter (Eds.): Advances in Linear Free Energy Relationships, Plenum Press, London, 1972, p. 1
[24a] Hoefnagel, A. J., M. A. Hoefnagel and B. M. Wepster: J. Org. Chem. **43**, 4720 (1978)
[25] Hansch, C., S. D. Rockwell, P. Y. C. Jow, A. Leo and E. E. Steller: J. Med. Chem. **20**, 304 (1977)
[26] Mc Daniel, D. H., and H. C. Brown: J. Org. Chem. **23**, 420 (1958)
[26a] Charton, M., in E. B. Roche (Ed.): Design of Biopharmaceutical Properties through Prodrugs and Analogs, American Pharmaceutical Association, Washington, 1977, p. 228
[26b] Perrin, D. D., in S. H. Yalkowsky, A. A. Sinkula and S. C. Valvani (Eds.): Physical Chemical Properties of Drugs, Marcel Dekker, New York, 1980, p. 2
[27] Hansch, C., and A. Leo: Substituent Constants for Correlation Analysis in Chemistry and Biology, Wiley, New York, 1979
[28] Sjöström, M., and S. Wold: Acta Chem. Scand. **B 30**, 167 (1976)
[29] Mager, H.: Thesis, Martin-Luther-Universität Halle—Wittenberg, 1977
[30] Mager, H., R. Franke and A. Barth in R. Franke and P. Oehme (Eds.): Quantitative Structure-Activity Analysis, Akademie-Verlag, Berlin, 1978, p. 421
[31] Mager, H., R. Franke and A. Barth: Wissenschaftliche Beiträge der Martin-Luther-Universität Halle—Wittenberg **18**, 30 (1977)
[32] Wold, S., and M. Sjöström: Chemica Scripta **2**, 49 (1972)
[33] Sjöström, M., and S. Wold: Chemica Scripta **6**, 114 (1974)
[34] Sjöström, M., and S. Wold: Chemica Scripta **9**, 200 (1976)
[35] Charton, M.: J. Am. Chem. Soc. **91**, 615 (1969)
[36] Charton, M.: J. Am. Chem. Soc. **91**, 6649 (1969)
[37] Shorter, J., in N. B. Chapman and J. Shorter (Eds.): Advances in Linear Free Energy Relationships, Plenum Press, London, 1972, p. 71
[38] Fujita, T., and T. Nishioka: Progr. Phys. Org. Chem. **12**, 49 (1976)
[38a] Charton, M.: Progr. Phys. Org. Chem. **8**, 238 (1971)
[39] Taft, R. W., and I. C. Lewis: J. Am. Chem. Soc. **80**, 2436 (1958)
[40] Roberts, J. D., and W. T. Moreland: J. Am. Chem. Soc. **75**, 2167 (1953)
[40a] Grob, C. A.: Angew. Chem. **88**, 621 (1976)
[40b] Grob, C. A., and M. G. Schlageter: Helv. Chim. Acta **59**, 264 (1976)
[41] Charton, M.: J. Org. Chem. **29**, 1222 (1964)

[42] Ehrenson, S., R. T. C. Brownlee and R. W. Taft: Progr. Phys. Org. Chem. **10**, 1 (1973)
[43] Yukawa, Y., Y. Tsuno and M. Sawada: Bull. Chem. Soc. Japan **45**, 1198 (1972)
[44] Sawada, M., Y. Tsuno and Y. Yukawa: Bull. Chem. Soc. Japan **45**, 1206 (1972)
[45] Yukawa, Y., Y. Tsuno and M. Sawada: Bull. Chem. Soc. Japan **45**, 1210 (1972)
[46] Okamoto, Y., and H. C. Brown: J. Org. Chem. **22**, 485 (1957)
[47] McGary, C. W., Y. Okamoto and H. C. Brown: J. Am. Chem. Soc. **77**, 3037 (1955)
[48] Brown, H. C., and Y. Okamoto: J. Am. Chem. Soc. **79**, 1913 (1957)
[49] Hammett, L. P.: Physical Organic Chemistry, McGraw-Hill, New York, 1940
[50] van Bekkum, H., P. E. Verkade and B. M. Wepster: Rec. Trav. chim. **78**, 815 (1959)
[51] Yukawa, Y., and Y. Tsuno: Bull. Chem. Soc. Japan **32**, 965 (1959)
[52] Yukawa, Y., and Y. Tsuno: Bull. Chem. Soc. Japan **32**, 971 (1959)
[53] Yukawa, Y., Y. Tsuno and M. Sawada: Bull. Chem. Soc. Japan **39**, 2274 (1966)
[54] Yoshioka, M., K. Hanamoto and T. Kubota: Bull. Chem. Soc. Japan **35**, 1723 (1962)
[55] Taft, R. W.: J. Phys. Chem. **64**, 1805 (1960)
[56] Yukawa, Y., Y. Tsuno and M. Sawada: Bull. Chem. Soc. Japan **45**, 1198 (1972)
[57] Sawada, M., Y. Tsuno and Y. Yukawa: Bull. Chem. Soc. Japan **45**, 1206 (1972)
[58] Cohen, L. A., and S. Takahashi: J. Am. Chem. Soc. **95**, 443 (1973)
[59] Hoefnagel, A. J., J. C. Monshouver, E. C. G. Snorn and B. M. Wepster: J. Am. Chem. Soc. **95**, 5350 (1973)
[60] Hoefnagel, A. J. and B. M. Wepster: J. Am. Chem. Soc. **95**, 5357 (1973)
[61] Taft, R. W., S. Ehrenson, I. C. Lewis and R. E. Glick: J. Am. Chem. Soc. **81**, 5352 (1959)
[62] Taft, R. W., and I. C. Lewis: Tetrahedron **5**, 210 (1959)
[62a] Bromilow, J., R. T. C. Brownlee, V. O. Lopez and R. W. Taft: J. Org. Chem. **44**, 4766 (1979)
[63] Swain, C. G., and E. C. Lupton: J. Am. Chem. Soc. **90**, 4328 (1968)
[64] Charton, M.: J. Org. Chem. **36**, 266 (1971)
[65] Holtz, D.: Chem. Rev. **71**, 139 (1971)
[66] Ager, I. R., L. Philips, T. J. Teason and V. Wray: J. Chem. Soc. Perkin II 1979 (1972)
[67] Shorter, J., in N. B. Chapman and J. Shorter (Eds.): Advances in Linear Free Energy Relationships, Vol. 2, Plenum Press, London, 1978
[68] Williams, S. G., and F. E. Norrington: J. Am. Chem. Soc. **98**, 508 (1976)
[69] Norrington, F. E., R. M. Hyde, S. G. Williams and R. Wootton: J. Med. Chem. **18**, 604 (1975)
[70] Unger, S. H.: PhD Thesis, Massachusetts Institute of Technology, Cambridge, Massachusetts, 1970
[71] Krygowski, T. M., and W. R. Fawcett: Canad. J. Chem. **53**, 3622 (1975)
[72] Krygowski, T. M., and W. R. Fawcett: J. Chem. Soc. Perkin II 2033 (1977)
[73] Otsu, R., and T. Yamamoto: Bull. Chem. Soc. Japan **41**, 204 (1968)
[74] Yamamoto, T., and T. Otsu: Chem. and Ind. 787 (1967)
[75] Magee, P. S., in E. C. Olson and R. E. Christofferson (Eds.): Computer Assisted Drug Design, ACS Symp. Ser. **112**, 21 (1979) and supplementary materials
[75a] Mager, P. P.: Sci. Pharm. **48**, 117 (1980)
[76] Charton, M.: J. Org. Chem. **28**, 3121 (1963)
[77] Nagai, Y., H. Matsumotu, T. Nakano and B. Watanabe: Bull. Chem. Soc. Japan **45**, 2560 (1972)
[78] Bohle, M., and D. Martin: Z. Chem. **17**, 455 (1977)
[79] Charton, M.: J. Am. Chem. Soc. **97**, 3691 (1975)
[80] Charton, M.: J. Am. Chem. Soc. **99**, 5687 (1977)
[80a] DeLos F. De Tar: J. Org. Chem. **45**, 5166 (1980)
[81] Kreevog, M. M., and R. W. Taft: J. Am. Chem. Soc. **77**, 5590 (1955)
[82] Hall, K. K.: J. Am. Chem. Soc. **79**, 5441 (1957)
[83] Henderson, W. M., C. A. Strenli and S. A. Buckler: J. Am. Chem. Soc. **82**, 5791 (1960)
[84] Folkers, E., and O. Rundquist: J. Org. Chem. **29**, 830 (1964)

[85] Franke, R., and P. Oehme: Pharmazie **28**, 489 (1973)
[86] Cammarata, A., and S. J. Yau: J. Med. Chem. **12**, 1066 (1969)
[87] Cammarata, A., S. J. Yau, J. H. Collott and A. N. Martin: Mol. Pharmacol. **6**, 61 (1970)
[88] Cammarata, A., R. C. Allen, J. K. Seydel and E. Wempe: J. Pharm. Sci. **59**, 1497 (1970)
[89] Hansch, C., and R. Kerley: J. Med. Chem. **13**, 957 (1970)
[90] Hansch, C., and R. Kerley: Chem. and Ind. 294 (1969)
[91] Hetnarski, B., and R. D. O'Brien: J. Med. Chem. **18**, 29 (1975)
[92] Sharpless, D., and J. R. Brown: FEBS Lett. **69**, 37 (1976)
[92a] Foster, R., R. M. Hyde and D. J. Livingstone: J. Pharm. Sci. **67**, 1310 (1978)
[92b] Livingstone, D. J., R. M. Hyde and R. Foster: Eur. J. Med. Chem. **14**, 393 (1979)
[93] Ritchie, C. D., and W. F. Sager: Progr. Phys. Org. Chem. **3**, 342 (1964)
[94] Shorter, J.: Quart. Rev. **24**, 433 (1970)
[95] Taft, R. W., N. C. Deno and P. S. Skell: Ann. Rev. Phys. Chem. **9**, 287 (1958)
[96] Wells, P. R.: Linear Free Energy Relationships, Academic Press, London, 1968
[96a] Osman, R., H. Weinstein and J. P. Green in E. C. Olson and R. E. Christoffersen (Eds.): Computer Assisted Drug Design, ACS Symp. Ser. **112**, 21 (1979)
[97] Chapman, N. B., and J. Shorter (Eds.): Advances in Linear Free Energy Relationships, Vols. 1 and 2, Plenum Press, London, 1972 and 1978
[98] Hansch, C., in C. J. Cavallito (Ed.): Structure-Activity Relationships, Pergamon Press, Oxford, 1971
[99] Purcell, W. P., G. E. Bass and J. M. Clayton: Strategy of Drug Design, Wiley, New York, 1973
[100] Hansch, C., in E. J. Ariens (Ed.): Drug Design, Vol. I, Academic Press, New York, 1971, p. 271
[101] Seydel, J. K., in E. J. Ariens (Ed.): Drug Design, Vol. I, Academic Press, New York, 1971, p. 343
[102] Fujita, T.: Adv. in Chemistry Series **114**, 1 (1972)
[103] Tute, M. S.: Adv. Drug Res. **6**, 1 (1971)
[104] Franke, R., in P. Oehme (Ed.): Theoretische Aspekte der Wirkstofforschung, VEB Verlag Volk und Gesundheit, Berlin, 1978
[105] Kirsch, J. F., in N. B. Chapman and J. Shorter (Eds.): Advances in Linear Free Energy Relationships, Plenum Press, London, 1972
[106] Cammarata, A., and K. S. Rogers in N. B. Chapman and J. Shorter (Eds.): Advances in Linear Free Energy Relationships, Plenum Press, London, 1972
[107] Seydel, J. K., and K. J. Schaper: Chemische Struktur und biologische Aktivität von Wirkstoffen, Verlag Chemie, Weinheim, 1979
[108] Fujita, T.: Chem. Regulation Plants (Tokyo) **5**, 124 (1970)
[109] Hansch, C., and E. J. Lien: Biochem. Pharmacol. **17**, 709 (1968)
[110] Franke, R., E. Gäbler and P. Oehme: Acta biol. med. germ. **32**, 545 (1974)
[111] Wedding, R. T., C. Hansch and T. R. Fukuto: Arch. Biochem. Biophys. **121**, 9 (1967)
[112] Franke, R., and A. Barth: Biochem. Physiol. Pflanzen **163**, 257 (1972)
[113] Hansch, C.: J. Med. Chem. **13**, 964 (1970)
[114] Fukuto, T. R., and R. L. Metcalf: J. Agr. Food Chem. **4**, 930 (1956)
[115] Hansch, C., and E. W. Deutsch: Biochim. Biophys. Acta **112**, 381 (1966)
[116] Hansch, C., and T. Fujita: J. Am. Chem. Soc. **86**, 1616 (1964)
[117] O'Brien, R. D., B. D. Hilton and L. Gilmour: Mol. Pharmacol. **2**, 593 (1966)
[118] Metcalf, R. L., and T. R. Fukuto: J. Agr. Food Chem. **13**, 220 (1965)
[119] Hansch, C., in R. D. O'Brien and I. Yamamoto (Eds.): Biochemical Toxicology of Insecticides, Academic Press, New York, 1970, p. 33
[120] Hermann, R. B., H. W. Culp, R. E. Mac Mahon and M. M. Marsch: J. Med. Chem. **12**, 749 (1969)
[121] Franke, R.: Acta biol. med. germ. **30**, 467 (1973)

[122] Verloop, A.: Proc. Int. Congr. Pestic. Chem., 2nd, Vol. 5, p. 342 (1972)
[123] Coats, E., R. W. Glave and C. Hansch: J. Med. Chem. **13**, 913 (1970)
[124] Unger, S. H., and C. Hansch: J. Med. Chem. **16**, 745 (1973)
[125] Barth, A., R. Hagemann and R. Franke: Proceedings der IX. wissenschaftlichen Koordinierungstagung über Wirkungsmechanismen von Herbiziden und synthetischen Wachstumsregulatoren, RGW-Koordinierungszentrum, Poznan, 1975
[126] Hansch, C.: Intra-Science Chem. Rept. 8, 17 (1974)
[127] Hansch, C., and R. Kerley: J. Med. Chem. **13**, 957 (1970)
[128] Hansch, C.: J. Med. Chem. **11**, 920 (1968)
[129] Hansch, C., E. W. Deutsch and R. N. Smith: J. Am. Chem. Soc. **87**, 2738 (1965)
[130] Kakeya, N., M. Aoki, A. Kamada and N. Yata: Chem. Pharm. Bull. **17**, 1010 (1969)
[131] Kakeya, N., N. Yata, A. Kamada and M. Aoki: Chem. Pharm. Bull. **17**, 2558 (1969)
[132] Kakeya, N., N. Yata, A. Kamada and M. Aoki: Chem. Pharm. Bull. **17**, 2000 (1969)
[133] Kakeya, N., N. Yata, A. Kamada and M. Aoki: Chem. Pharm. Bull. **18**, 191 (1970)
[134] Garrett, E. R., J. B. Mielck, J. K. Seydel and W. J. Kessler: J. Med. Chem. **12**, 740 (1969)
[134a] Seydel, J. K., in J. A. Keverling Buisman (Ed.): Strategy in Drug Research, Pharmacochemistry Library (Eds.: W. Th. Nauta and R. F. Rekker), Vol. 4, Elsevier, Amsterdam, 1982, p. 179
[134b] Seydel, J. K.: Int. J. Quant. Chem. **20**, 131 (1981)
[135] Seydel, J. K.: J. Pharm. Sci. **57**, 1455 (1968)
[136] Seydel, J. K.: J. Med. Chem. **14**, 724 (1971)
[137] Miller, G. H., P. H. Donkas and J. K. Seydel: J. Med. Chem. **15**, 700 (1972)
[138] Rastelli, A., P. G. De Benedetti, G. G. Battistuzzi and A. Albasino: J. Med. Chem. **18**, 963 (1975)
[139] Franke, R., A. Barth and R. Hagemann: unpublished results
[140] Scholz, S., H. Sprinz, R. Hagemann, R. Franke, G. Hübner and A. Barth: Pharmazie **31**, 162 (1976)
[141] Dekker, W. H., H. A. Selling and J. C. Overeem: Agricult. Food Chem. **23**, 785 (1975)
[142] Lin, T. K.: J. Med. Chem. **17**, 749 (1974)
[143] Purcell, W. P., and J. M. Clayton: private communication
[144] Zimmermann, J. J., and J. E. Goyan: J. Med. Chem. **14**, 1206 (1971)
[145] Tollenaere, J. P.: J. Med. Chem. **16**, 791 (1973)
[146] van den Berg, G., T. Bultsma, R. F. Rekker and W. Th. Nauta: Eur. J. Med. Chem. **10**, 246 (1975)
[147] Schäfer, G., A. Trebst and K. H. Büchel: Z. Naturforsch. **30c**, 183 (1975)
[148] Büchel, K. H., and W. Draber: Adv. in Chemistry Series **114**, 141 (1972)
[149] Martin, Y. C., W. B. Martin and J. D. Taylor: J. Med. Chem. **18**, 883 (1975)
[150] Franke, R., R. Hagmeann, G. Köhler, P. Ohmann and A. Barth: unpublished results
[151] Kutter, E., H. Machleidt, W. Reuter, R. Sauter and A. Wildfeuer: Adv. Chemistry Series **114**, 98 (1972)
[151a] Domelsmith, L. N., and K. N. Houkin in G. Barnett, M. Trsic and R. E. Willette (Eds.): Quantitative Structure Activity Relationships of Analgesics, Narcotic Antagonists, and Hallucinogens, NIDA Research Monograph 22, Rockville, 1978, p. 423
[152] Martin, Y. C.: Drug Design Methods — A critical Introduction, Marcel Dekker, New York, 1978
[153] Martin, Y. C., in E. J. Ariens (Ed.): Drug Design, Vol. VIII, Academic Press, New York, 1978
[154] Scherrer, R. A., and S. M. Howard: J. Med. Chem. **20**, 53 (1977)
[154a] Scherrer, R. A., and S. M. Howard in E. C. Olsen and R. E. Christoffersen (Eds.): Computer-Assisted Drug Design, ACS Symp. Ser. **112**, 507 (1979)
[155] Fujita, T.: J. Med. Chem. **9**, 797 (1966)

[156] Fujita, T.: Adv. in Chemistry Series **114**, 80 (1972)
[157] Martin, Y. C., and J. J. Hackbarth: J. Med. Chem. **19**, 1033 (1976)
[158] Martin, Y. C., and J. J. Hackbarth in B. Kowalski (Ed.): Proceedings of the American Chemical Society Symposium on Chemometrics, ACS Symp. Ser. **254**, 153 (1977)
[159] Martin, Y. C., in R. Franke and P. Oehme (Eds.): Quantitative Structure-Activity Analysis, Akademie-Verlag, Berlin, 1978, p. 351
[160] McFarland, J. W.: Progr. Drug Res. **15**, 124 (1971)
[161] Exner, O.: Dipole Moments in Organic Chemistry, Thieme Verlag, Stuttgart, 1975
[162] Craig, P. N.: J. Med. Chem. **14**, 680 (1971)
[163] Franke, R.: studia biophysica **6**, 199 (1968)
[164] Franke, R.: studia biophysica **6**, 207 (1968)
[165] Franke, R.: Acta biol. med. germ. **25**, 757 (1970)
[166] Tute, M. S.: J. Med. Chem. **13**, 48 (1970)
[166a] Weinstein, H., R. Osman and J. P. Green in E. C. Olson und R. E. Christoffersen (Eds.): Computer-Assisted Drug Design, ACS Symp. Ser. **112**, 161 (1979)
[166b] Weinstein, H., J. P. Green, R. Osman and W. D. Edwards in G. Barnett, M. Trsic and R. E. Willette (Eds.): Quantitative Structure Activity Relationships of Analgesics, Narcotic Antagonists, and Hallucinogens, NIDA Research Monograph 22, Rockville, 1978, p. 333
[167] Pilar, F. L.: Elementary Quantum Chemistry, McGraw-Hill, New York, 1963
[168] Dewar, M. J. S.: The Molecular Orbital Theory of Organic Chemistry, McGraw-Hill, New York, 1969
[168a] McWeeny, R., and B. T. Sutcliffe: Methods of Molecular Quantum Mechanics, Academic Press, New York, 1969
[168b] Pullman, B.: Adv. Quantum Chem. **10**, 251 (1977)
[169] Ballhausen, G. J., and H. B. Gray: Molecular Orbital Theory, Benjamin Inc., New York, 1964
[170] Parr, R. G.: Quantum Theory of Molecular Electronic Structure, Benjamin Inc., New York, 1964
[171] Streitwieser, E.: Molecular Orbital Theory for Organic Chemists, Wiley, New York, 1962
[172] Heilbronner, E., and H. Bock: Das HMO-Modell und seine Anwendung, Bde. I—III, Verlag Chemie, Weinheim, 1970
[173] Salom, L.: The Molecular Orbital Theory of Conjugated Systems, Benjamin Inc., New York, 1966
[174] Zülicke, L.: Quantenchemie — Ein Lehrgang, VEB Deutscher Verlag der Wissenschaften, Berlin, 1975
[175] Pullman, B., and A. Pullman: Quantum Biochemistry, Interscience, New York, 1963
[176] Kier, L. B.: Molecular Orbital Theory in Drug Research, Academic Press, New York, 1971
[177] Kier, L. B. (Ed.): Molecular Orbital Studies in Chemical Pharmacology, Springer-Verlag, New York, 1970
[178] Chalvet, O.: J. theor. Biol. **3**, 51 (1962)
[179] Daudel, R., and A. Pullman: Aspects de la Chimie Quantique Contemporaire, Centre National de la Recherche Scientifique, Paris, 1971
[180] Ladik, J.: Quantenbiochemie für Chemiker und Biologen, Ferdinand Enke Verlag, Stuttgart, 1972
[181] Richards, W. G., and M. E. Black: Progr. in Medicinal Chemistry **11**, 68 (1975)
[181a] Richards, W. G.: Quantum Pharmacology, Butterworths, London, 1977
[181b] Christoffersen, R. E., in B. Pullman (Ed.): Quantum Mechanics of Molecular Conformation, Wiley, New York, 1976, p. 194
[181c] Christoffersen, R. E., and R. P. Angeli in B. Pullman and R. Parr (Eds.): The New World of Quantum Chemistry, D. Reidl, Dordrecht, 1976, p. 189

[181d] Christoffersen, R. E., in E. C. Olson and R. E. Christoffersen (Eds.): Computer-Assisted Drug Design, ACS Symp. Ser. **112**, 3 (1979)

[181e] Barnett, G., M. Trsic and R. E. Willette (Eds.): Quantitative Structure Activity Relationships of Analgesics, Narcotic Antagonists, and Hallucinogens, NIDA Research Monograph 22, Rockville, 1978

[181f] Sklenar, H., and J. Jäger: Struktur-Wirkungs-Beziehungen auf quantenchemischer Grundlage, Beiträge zur Wirkstofforschung, No. 10, Akademie-Industrie-Komplex Arzneimittelforschung, Berlin, 1980

[182] Bergmann, E., and B. Pullman (Eds.): Molecular and Quantum Pharmacology, D. Reidl, Dordrecht, 1974

[183] Kier, L. B.: Adv. in Chemistry Series **114**, 278 (1972)

[184] Green, J. P., C. L. Johnson and S. Kang: Ann. Rev. Pharmacol. **14**, 319 (1974)

[185] Pullman, B., in B. Pullman and M. Weissbluth (Eds.): Molecular Biophysics, Academic Press, New York, 1965

[186] Schnaare, R. L., and A. N. Martin: J. Pharm. Sci. **54**, 1707 (1965)

[187] Simon, Z.: Quantum Biochemistry and Specific Interactions, Abacus Press, Turnbridge Wells, 1976

[188] Kaufmann, J. J., and W. S. Koski in E. J. Ariens (Ed.): Drug Design, Vol. V, Academic Press, New York, 1975, p. 252

[189] Fukui, K., T. Yonozawa and C. Nagata: Bull. Chem. Soc. Japan **27**, 243 (1954)

[190] Inouye, A., and Y. Shinagawa: Bull. Chem. Soc. Japan **35**, 701 (1962)

[191] Inouye, A., Y. Shinagawa and Y. Takaishi: Arch. Int. Pharmacodyn. Ther. **144**, 319 (1963)

[192] Cammarata, A., in L. B. Kier (Ed.): Molecular Orbital Studies in Chemical Pharmacology, Springer-Verlag, New York, 1970, p. 156

[193] Klopman, G., and R. F. Hudson: Theor. Chim. Acta **8**, 165 (1967)

[194] Klopman, G.: J. Am. Chem. Soc. **90**, 223 (1968)

[195] Neely, W. B., in L. B. Kier (Ed.): Molecular Orbital Studies in Chemical Pharmacology, Springer-Verlag, New York, 1970, p. 121

[196] Perault, A., and B. Pullman: Biochim. Biophys. Acta **66**, 86 (1963)

[197] Mizuta, E., J. Toda, N. Suzuki, H. Sugibayiahi, K.-I. Imai and M. Nishikawa: Chem. Pharm. Bull. **20**, 1114 (1972)

[198] Franke, R., and A. Barth in T. Kudrew, I. Ivanova and E. Karanov (Eds.): Plant Growth Regulators, Publishing House of the Bulgarian Academy of Sciences, Sofia, 1975

[199] Hansch, C.: Prog. in Photosynthesis Res. **3**, 1685 (1969)

[200] Trebst, A., and E. Harth: Z. Naturforsch. **29c**, 232 (1974)

[210] Barth, A., and R. Franke in F. Coulston and F. Corte (Eds.): Environmental Quality and Safety, Supplement Vol. III, Georg Thieme, Stuttgart, 1975

[202] Wohl, J. A., in L. B. Kier (Ed.): Molecular Orbital Studies in Chemical Pharmacology, Springer-Verlag, New York, 1970, p. 262

[203] Topliss, J. G., and M. D. Yudis: J. Med. Chem. **15**, 394 (1972)

[204] Johnson, C. L., and J.-P. Green: Int. J. Quantum Chem. QBS **1**, 159 (1974)

6. Steric Effects on Biological Activity: the function $f_s(x_s)$

Steric influences are sometimes difficult to describe as part of the extrathermodynamic approach, and many of the associated problems admit of no satisfactory solution. Some steric molecular parameters are presented in Table 6.1; for reviews on these parameters and their correlational power see VERLOOP et al. [1] and BALABAN et al. [2]. The most important types of steric effects in the context of the extrathermodynamic approach are:

1. intramolecular steric influences of substituents on molecular properties;
2. specific influence on the fitting to the receptor connected with the bulk and the spatial arrangement of substituents;
3. distinction between optical isomers or between stereoisomers;
4. conformational influences;
5. borderline cases where what is essential for biological activity amounts to a very special steric configuration in the sense of the old "key and lock" theory.

Table 6.1. The most important steric molecular parameters

E_S	TAFTS steric substituent constant
$E_S{}^C$	HANCOCKS steric substituent constant corrected for hyperconjugation
υ	CHARTONS steric substituent constant
r_V	VAN DER WAALS radius of substituents
MR	molar refractivity
V	molar volume
χ	molar connectivity
L, B_1-B_4	VERLOOPS STERIMOL parameter
MSD	minimal steric difference
MTD	minimal topological difference
V_0, S_0, L_0	molecular shape descriptors

Intramolecular steric interactions (*case 1*) occur first of all in flexible molecules — including those of aliphatic compounds — and in ortho-substituted aromatic compounds. As stated in 5.1., the acid-catalyzed hydrolysis of aliphatic esters and ortho-substituted benzoic acid esters primarily depends on steric and only slightly on electronic effects. Hence, a *steric substituent constant*, E_S, for aliphatic and $E_S{}^0$ for ortho-substituted aromatic compounds, was defined by TAFT [3] (for a critical review of TAFTS work, see e.g. [4]):

$$E_S = (\log k_X/k_0)_{a,\,XCOOR} \tag{6/1}$$

and

$$E_S{}^0 = (\log k_X/k_0)_{a,\,X\,ortho\,C_6H_4COOR} \tag{6/2}$$

The rates of the acid-catalyzed hydrolysis of esters with substituent X and esters with the standard substituent X = CH_3 are denoted by k_X and k_0, respectively. As a result, for aliphatic compounds

$$f_s(x_s) = \vartheta E_S + \text{constant} \quad (6/3)$$

and for ortho-substituted aromatic compounds:

$$f_s(x_s) = \vartheta E_S{}^0 + \text{constant} \quad (6/4)$$

For tabulations of E_S and $E_S{}^0$ see e.g. [3, 5—7]. It has been suggested by CHARTON [8] that $E_S{}^0$ is not a true steric substituent constant but tends to be electronic in nature. As shown by MAGER et al. [8a] this, however, is not true and $E_S{}^0$ is primarily a function of steric and to a lesser extent of the mesomeric effects of substituents. A new scale of orthosteric parameter designated as S^0 to be used for heteroatomatic compounds was recently introduced by BERG et al. [8b]. The S^0 values are free from electronic contributions and do not correlate with TAFTS steric parameter.

TAFTS E_S values have recently been reevaluated and confirmed by DE TAR [8c]. An alternative to TAFTS E_S is the E_S' value introduced by DUBOIS [8d—f] with the acid-catalyzed esterification of RCOOH as standard reaction. E_S and E_S' are on slightly different scales so that the two sets cannot be mixed. The E_S' values are specially suited for highly congested groups but do not offer, otherwise, true advantages over the TAFT E_S set. A modification of E_S are the $E_S{}^e$ values introduced by UNGER and HANSCH [9]. The $E_S{}^e$ are simply a shift of E_S so that $E_S{}^e = 0$ for the hydrogen substituent instead for methyl in the E_S scale.

E_S becomes smaller as the substituents become bulkier so that a given reaction is inhibited by bulky substituents if the constant ϑ (eqn. 6/3) is positive. For symmetric substituents E_S values correlate with the VAN DER WAALS radius [8], and the relation

$$E_S = -1.839 r_V + 3.484 \quad (6/5)$$

$$n = 6 \qquad r = 0.996$$

has been used by KUTTER and HANSCH [10, 11] (see also [9]) as well as by FUJITA et al. [12] to calculate further E_S values. Another method of estimating E_S values has been reported by FAHMY et al. [13]. To substituents of the CHAB type ($A \neq B$), the following is applicable:

$$E_S(\text{CHAB}) = [E_S(\text{CHAA}) + E_S(\text{CHBB})]/2 \quad (6/6)$$

Finally, E_S values can also by estimated directly be calculating the steric energy of the activated complex in the acid-catalyzed hydrolysis of esters [14].

According to HANCOCK [15—18], E_S values represent, besides the steric effect, a hyperconjugation effect, and, therefore, they provide only a poor description of steric substituent effects in cases where no hyperconjugation can exist (as, for example, in aliphatic amines). In this connection, HANCOCK proposed the *modified steric substituent constant*, $E_S{}^C$, from which the hyperconjugation effect is eliminated according to

$$E_S{}^C = E_S + 0.306(n_H - 3) \quad (6/7)$$

where n_H is the number of α-C—H bonds. This constant, although repeatedly criticized (e.g. [8c, 9, 19, 20]), has proved helpful [21]. It follows for aliphatic compounds without hyperconjugation that

$$f_s(x_s) = \vartheta^C E_S{}^C + \text{constant} \tag{6/8}$$

may sometimes be a useful expression to describe steric substituent effects. In $E_S{}^C$ only hyperconjugative effects of the α-H atoms are eliminated. In order to eliminate hyperconjugative effects of both α-H and α-C atoms PALM [22] introduced the steric substituent constant, $E_S{}^0$ (not to be confused with TAFTS steric constant for ortho-substituents according to (6/2))

$$E_S{}^0 = E_S + 0.33(n_H - 3) + 0.13 n_C \tag{6/9}$$

where n_C = number of α-C atoms.

Starting from the relationship between E_S and the VAN DER WAALS radius, CHARTON [8, 20, 20a, 23] proposed a new steric substituent constant, $\mathfrak{v}$,

$$\mathfrak{v} = r_{v,X} - r_{v,H} = r_{v,X} - 1.20 \tag{6/10}$$

where $r_{v,X}$ and $r_{v,H}$ are the respective VAN DER WAALS radii of substituent X and hydrogen. The steric substituent influence may then be expressed as:

$$f_s(x_s) = \psi\mathfrak{v} + \text{constant} \tag{6/11}$$

This steric substituent constant has been found to be quite valuable in investigations on aliphatic reaction series [20, 23—25] but actually does not tell a much different story than E_S (for tabulations, see [20, 20a]; the values listed were either calculated by means of (6/10) or, where substituents did not permit this, evaluated from various reaction series on the basis of (6/11)).

Where *intermolecular interactions between substituents and receptor* (case 2) become more important, the VAN DER WAALS radius of the substituents again appears to be a workable parameter. Since the E_S values and the VAN DER WAALS radii are correlated and the $\mathfrak{v}$ values can be defined directly with these radii, E_S and $\mathfrak{v}$ may also serve to characterize such intermolecular steric substituent effects even when the substituents are located on an aromatic ring. This gives rise to the seeming paradox in which substituent constants originally derived to characterize steric effects in aliphatic reactions are also applied for aromatic compounds. E_S and $\mathfrak{v}$ represent the minimum width of substituents much in the same sense as VERLOOPS B_1 (see below).

Much use has been made of *molecular refractivity*, MR, to characterize the size of the substituents and the steric effect in intermolecular interactions. This variable is connected with the molar volume, V

$$\text{MR} = \frac{n^2 - 1}{n^2 + 2} V \tag{6/12}$$

where n = refractive index. It does not have a purely steric character but in accordance with

$$\text{MR} = \frac{4}{3} \pi N_L \alpha \tag{6/13}$$

where α = polarizability it also contains an electronic component. In more recent QSAR publications, therefore, MR terms are frequently interpreted to reflect drug-receptor dispersion interactions. Furthermore, a correlation between MR and hydrophobicity is found in homologous series of hydrophobic compounds having constant electronic properties and similar basic geometry (cf. 4.1.). Despite these ambiguities, which may make a mechanistic interpretation difficult, the molecular refractivity appears to be quite a valuable steric parameter characterizing substituent bulk. It has the advantage of being easily accessible for all substituents, as MR values can be obtained additively from known increment values (for tabulations, see e.g. [5—7, 26]. Sometimes the substituent volume (VAN DER WAALS volume calculated from VAN DER WAALS radii [2, 27, 27a] or EXNERS molar volume [28, 29]) or the parachor [30—32] are employed instead of molecular refractivity; as already stated, these parameters and hydrophobicity are frequently correlated as well. A very simple steric parameter, which is accessible from the two-dimensional structural formula, is the *molecular connectivity*, χ [33]. It was introduced by KIER et al. [34—40] into quantitative structure-activity analysis. χ is correlated closely with the molar refractivity, but also with typically hydrophobic parameters and with many other physical properties in series of homologues so that relations with χ are difficult to interpret, and for complex structures containing heteroatoms its physicochemical significance may be questionable. The advantage of χ is that its calculation for practically any structure is easy and straightforward (for details, see [39a, 40]). The use of connectivity can be recommended especially in such cases where relatively large structural variations are present in a series of compounds and where the primary goal of a QSAR analysis is data description rather than interpretation.

The parameters mentioned thus far describe steric effects using a single value. Substituents are, however, three-dimensional structures, and depending on the nature of she interactions with the receptor or the remaining possibilities for rotation their extention in a particular spatial direction may become critical. This led VERLOOP et.al. [1] fo introduce their STERIMOL *parameters* where each substituent is characterized by tive values. The first one, L, denotes the length of a substituent in the direction in which it is attached to the parent molecule. Perpendicular to it are four parameters, B_1—B_4, which are a measure of the width of the substituent in four different, perpendicular, directions. B_1 represents the minimum width (as do TAFTS E_S and CHARTONS υ) which reflects the tendency of flexible substituents to change their conformation in a way that minimizes steric interactions. This implies that the application of B_1 as well as of E_S and υ to substituents which are rotationally restricted by their environment may present problems and lead to inconsistent results. A case in point will be discussed in section 13.1. (eqn. (13/5)). The maximum width is presented by B_4. Considering the ratios L/B_1 (length to minimal width) and B_4/B_1 (maximal to minimal width) allows to estimate the deviations of substituents from spherical shape. With the STERIMOL parameters we obtain the expression:

$$f_s(x_s) = a_0 + a_1 L + a_2 B_1 + a_3 B_2 + a_4 B_3 + a_5 B_4 \qquad (6/14)$$

Each of the coefficients in eqn. (6/14) can become 0, and, in general, not more than two of these parameters appear together (most important are L, B_1 and B_4). Nevertheless, one has to test a large variety of possible equations and the statistical degrees of freedom may then present problems. An unmistakable advantage of these new steric constants is that they are readily computable even for complicated substituents with a simple computer program (STERIMOL program) provided that a reasonable assumption on the conformation of flexible substituents can be made. The constants have already proved very useful. Especially in cases where the substituents lack symmetry and variables L and B_4 are implicated, they are superior to the steric parameters referred to above [41—42]. Some of the values presented by VERLOOP have recently been recalculated and refined by BULTSMA and BIJLOO [43].

It may be assumed that in many instances there is an optimal substituent size for binding to the receptor. A parabolic relationship with steric substituent constants is then to be expected, so that intermolecular steric substituent influences on drug-receptor interactions may be collectively described as follows

$$f_s(x_s) = \begin{cases} ax_s + b & \text{(a)} \\ ax_s^2 + bx_s + c & \text{(b)} \end{cases} \qquad (6/15)$$

with

$$x_s = E_S, E_S^0, E_S^C, \mathfrak{v}, r_v, \mathrm{MR}, L, B_1, B_2, B_3, B_4 \text{ or } \chi$$

Linearity as implied by eqn. (6/15a) occurs when the substituent size is still far from being extreme. Instead of a parabola according to eqn. (6/15b) a bilinear model as in eqn. (4/104) may also be applied here [44]. Although there is no theoretical basis for such a relationship it seems that a better fit can sometimes be obtained in this way which may simply be due to the fact that a bilinear model containes more adjustable parameters. Since the binding sites of the receptor may lack homogeneity and symmetry, the possibility of overt position dependence should be allowed for as in the case of hydrophobic interactions. The rules explained in detail in connection with eqn. (4/76) are also applicable here.

The parameters discussed so far refer to substituents; for selected values, see Table 6.2. Steric effects may, however, also be approached by taking into account the steric properties of whole chemical structures. An example is the concept of *minimal topological difference* (an earlier version was called *minimal steric difference*). Introduced by SIMON and co-workers [2, 45—54] this concept is based on the following assumptions:

1. The binding site of a receptor may be thought of as a cavity with relatively rigid walls in many cases.
2. Atoms or groups of atoms placed within this cavity (and which may overlap the cavity) on drug-receptor binding are favoured sterically.
3. Atoms or groups of atoms falling into the cavity wall (and which may not overlap the cavity) sterically inhibit binding and are thus unfavourable.
4. Atoms or groups of atoms situated outside the receptor cavity are of no steric significance.

The basic idea of this concept is that the affinity of drugs towards a given receptor decreases linearly with the non-overlapping volume of the molecules and the receptor cavity. Since, however, the shape and size of the receptor cavity are not known this volume cannot be calculated directly. Therefore, an indirect method was developed in which a "*receptor map*" derived from the structures within the sample of compounds considered is used instead of the exact receptor structure. The non-overlapping volume

Table 6.2. Some selected values of steric substituent constants[1])

Substituent	E_S	E_S^C	υ	L	B_1	B_4	MR
F	0.78	−0.14	0.27	2.65	1.35	1.35	0.92
Cl	0.27	−0.65	0.55	3.52	1.80	1.80	6.03
Br	0.08	−0.84	0.65	3.83	1.95	1.95	8.88
J	−0.16	−1.08	0.78	4.23	2.15	2.15	13.94
NH_2	0.63	0.32	0.35	2.93	1.50	1.84	5.42
$N(CH_3)_2$	—	—	0.43	3.53	1.50	2.80	15.55
CH_3	0.00	0.00	0.52	3.00	1.52	2.04	5.65
C_2H_5	−0.07	−0.38	0.56	4.11	1.52	2.97	10.30
n-C_3H_7	−0.36	−0.67	0.68	5.02	1.52	3.49	14.96
$CH(CH_3)_2$	−0.47	−1.08	0,76	4.11	2.04	3.16	14.98
n-C_4H_9	−0.39	−0.70	0.68	6.17	1.52	4.42	19.59
$CH_2CH(CH_3)_2$	−0.93	−1.24	0.98	5.05	1.52	4.21	19.59
$CH(CH_3)(C_2H_5)$	−1.13	−1.74	1.02	5.05	1.90	3.49	19.59
$C(CH_3)_3$	−1.54	−2.46	1.24	4.11	2.59	2.97	19.62
H	1.24	0.32	0.00	2.06	1.00	1.00	1.03

[1]) All values taken from [5]

for a given molecule is then approximated by the so-called MTD *value* (for minimal topological difference) which is the number of non-overlapping atoms (hydrogens being neglected) between this molecule and that part of the receptor map which represents the receptor cavity. The principal steps in calculating the MTD are:

1. The structures of all molecules considered are superimposed to give an artificial hypermolecule, H, representing a topological network with the atoms as vertices.
2. Each molecule is now superimposed over H. As a result a vector of k logical parameters (k = number of vertices in H), x_j ($j = 1, \ldots, k$), is obtained which describes its structure. For the i-th molecule, x_j is defined as:

$$x_{ij} = \begin{cases} 1, & \text{if the } j\text{-th vertex in H is occupied by an atom of compound } i \\ 0, & \text{if not} \end{cases} \tag{6/16}$$

3. An initial guess is made as to which vertices of the supermolecule H fall into the receptor cavity, the cavity wall or outside the receptor binding site by assigning a ternary parameter ε_j to each vertex:

$$\varepsilon_j = \begin{cases} -1, & \text{if vertex } j \text{ belongs to the space of the receptor cavity} \\ 0, & \text{if vertex } j \text{ is outside} \\ +1, & \text{if vertex } j \text{ belongs to the wall of the cavity} \end{cases} \tag{6/17}$$

The set of ε_j then obtained represents an initial receptor map which can be arrived at, for instance, by considering the vertices occupied by the most active molecule as the cavity vertices ($\varepsilon_j = -1$) and the remaining vertices of the supermolecule H either as wall vertices ($\varepsilon_j = 1$) or sterically irrelevant ($\varepsilon_j = 0$).

4. MTD for the i-th molecule is now calculated according to:

$$\mathrm{MTD}_i = S + \sum_{j=1}^{k} \varepsilon_j x_{ij} \tag{6/18}$$

The quantity S in eqn. (6/18) represents the number of cavity vertices ($\varepsilon_j = -1$) which characterize the "best" probable molecular shape (also called "*standard*") with respect to the receptor considered. A cyclic iterative procedure (alteration of the ε_j) is used in which the initial map is optimized in such a way that the final MTD values yield the best possible description of biological activity.

The function $f_s(x_s)$ can then be formulated as:

$$f_s(x_s) = a\,\mathrm{MTD} + b \tag{6/19}$$

Instead of MTD the older MSD *values* (from minimal steric difference) can also be used here. This function will always be linear since MTD has already been optimized in the underlying model. MTD values are particularly advantageous for such series of compounds which have "widely differing spatial structures but covering not too different spatial regions and without excessive flexibility" [2]. The optimized receptor map obtained in step 4 of the MTD calculation may yield valid information on the topology of the receptor binding site. In accordance with the assumption of the rigidity of the cavity walls, however, this map will only mirror those receptor regions which are, in fact, relatively rigid and where the steric fit of drugs is of importance. For highly flexible regions the ε_j have zero values as for regions outside the binding cavity. Recently, a Monte Carlo treatment of the minimal steric difference was developed resulting in the so-called MCD *values* [2] which are to be used in exactly the same way as the MTD values. The MCD avoids ambiguities which may occur with the MTD in the superposition procedure for polycyclic molecules or molecules containing rings of different sizes. The MCD values represent the non-overlapping volumes of the VAN DER WAALS envelope of molecules as compared with the standard.

Philosophically similar is the *molecular shape analysis* introduced by HOPFINGER [54a—d]. He defined as a shape descriptor the common steric overlap volume V_0 between pairs of molecules which measures how much steric space these molecules share under a prescribed intermolecular relationship. V_0 is a pairwise property which only has a meaning relative to the two molecules considered. In order to establish a common scale for the compounds of a training series a *reference compound* is selected to which all molecules of the series are compared. In addition to V_0 the following quantities also turned out to be useful shape descriptors:

$$S_0 = V_0^{2/3}$$
$$L_0 = V_0^{1/3} \tag{6/20}$$

The computation of the shape descriptors and their use in the evaluation of QSARs is a cyclic and iterative procedure involving the following main steps:

1. A structural fragment common to all molecules of the series is defined which is used as a frame of reference in the pairwise comparisons with the reference molecule.

2. For flexible molecules a conformation believed to be critical for biological activity is defined. This is done very empirically in a first step by comparing free-space minimum energy conformations with activity data.
3. After selecting a reference molecule the shape descriptors are calculated for all compounds of the series. In order to optimize the relative orientation in space of the analogues with respect to the reference molecule the sum of distances between corresponding atoms is minimized. For calculating V_0 a rectangular lattice of predescribed size and orientation is constructed around each pair of molecules, and only atoms residing in the same lattice cell are considered to overlap. This approach has some similarities with that used by TESTA and PURCELL [54e] to characterize steric properties of sulfonamides.
4. The shape descriptors are now used as steric parameters in the evaluation of a QSAR. Steps 1.—3. are then optimized according to the criterium of best fit. This implies that different conformations are included in the analysis, that each compound of the series is once used as reference molecule, and that the size as well as the relative orientation of the lattice are also varied. Many different sets of shape descriptors are thus obtained from which that one is finally selected which yields the best (statistically most significant) description of the biological data.

The flexibility of this procedure is advantageous in that it allows to extend the analysis to series with larger structural variations than usually considered in the extrathermodynamic approach. The outcome of the optimization may, in addition to the resulting QSAR, provide information regarding the bioactive conformation and which corresponding atoms in a set of compounds are most crucial for biological activity. The danger is that the large number of parameters actually considered may lead to chance correlations (cf., p. 167). The results obtained so far for the inhibition of dihydrofolate reductase from different sources by three different series of molecules (see example 12.) do not seem to suffer from this problem. They are remarkably consistent, and the QSARs obtained have predictive power.

Another parameter characterizing the steric porperties of whole molecules was introduced by AMOORE [55—58] who proposed a *similarity index* which also shares some features with the MTD concept and which was applied, for example, to odorous compounds. This index is established by photographing molecular models from three directions, followed by an analysis of the photographs using a special method of pattern recognition. The complicated nature of this procedure has prevented its wide application.

Practical experience of the quantitative *description of stereoisomers* (case 3) in the context of the extrathermodynamic approach is still quite rare. Such a description is relatively easy when the quotient of biological activity of both forms is either approximately constant or increases in a regular fashion with increasing affinity for the receptor; the latter case seems to be more typical [59—61]. An indicator variable can then be used having, for example, a value of 1 for one form and a value of 0 for the other in the first case (cf., eqn. (6/32)), whereas in the second case the indicator variable would be a function of the biological activity itself.

It is also possible to describe stereoisomeric substituents with the steric parameters introduced by VERLOOP and stereoisomeric molecules with MTD values [2]; (cf., eqn. (6/21)) or by molecular shape descriptors. Where drastic changes in hydrophobic and/or electronic interactions result from placing substituents at different areas of the receptor site this must be explicitly taken into account in addition to the steric effects (see, e.g. [62—64]).

Conformational problems (case 4) are also difficult to solve in extrathermodynamic terms with the exception of molecular shape analysis. They are best described in terms of the approaches presented in chapter 12. Yet it is theoretically possible to apply as "steric parameters" the energy barriers between conformers, which may be obtained, for instance, from quantum-chemical calculations. Another possibility is to calculate the fraction of the conformer which is presumed to be biologically active and to correct the overall biological activity for that fraction.

Steric effects of a very special kind (case 5) usually cannot be handled by the extra-thermodynamic approach unless detailed assumptions on the interactions with the receptor can be made; a case of this type is illustrated by eqn. (6/31) and other examples can be found in [65, 65a] (cf., 13.2.). Some examples of QSARs involving steric molecular parameters have already been presented in the preceding sections. Some more examples are:

1. *Hydrolysis of XXXV (which contains* D- *and* L-*amino acid derivatives) by α-chymotrypsin* [66]

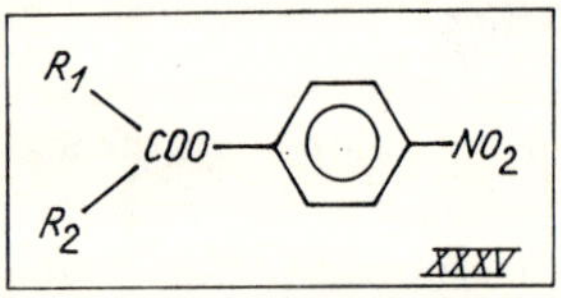

$$\log A = 2.485\sigma + 0.310\pi - 0.294\ \mathrm{MDS} + 1.203 \qquad (6/21)$$

$n = 42 \quad r = 0.850 \quad s = 0.623$

2. *Oestrogenic activity of steroids in rats* [2]

$$\log A = -0.86\ \mathrm{MTD} + 1.13\pi + 5.54 \qquad (6/22)$$

$n = 20 \quad r = 0.971 \quad s = 0.39$

3. *Virostatic activity of isatin-β-isothiosemicarbazones* [67]

$$\log A = 4.17E_S^2 - 2.15E_S + 1.11 \qquad (6/23)$$

In this case, an optimal size for the substituents obviously exists.

4. *Inhibition of cholinesterase by ortho-substituted methylcarbamates* [68]

$$\log A = 3.48E_S^0 + 2.80\pi + 4.25\sigma + 2.54 \qquad (6/24)$$

5. *Interaction of haptens (substituted benzoic acids) with antibodies (prevention of the combination of anti-X$_p$-serum and X-egg albumin antigen* [11])

$$\log A = 0.864E_{S,\,ortho} + 0.084E_{S,\,meta} - 0.436E_{S,\,para} + 0.166\Sigma\pi - 0.715 \qquad (6/25)$$

$n = 22 \quad r = 0.989 \quad s = 0.120$

The interaction can be described equally well using Verloops $B\,1$ and $B\,4$ parameters [42]. Note the positional dependence of the steric substituent effect.

6. *Inhibition of xanthinoxidase by 9-phenylguanines substituted in the phenyl ring* [69]

$$\log A = 0.20(\mathrm{MR}_{meta} + \mathrm{MR}_{para}) + 1.26E_{S,\,ortho} + 0.43E_{S,\,para} + 4.33 \quad (6/26)$$

$n = 30 \quad r = 0.924 \quad s = 0.228$

The molar refractivity is primarily to be taken here as a measure of polarizability.

7. *Paralyzing activity of primary amines against American cockroaches* [70]

$$\log A = -0.54E_S^C + 4.73 \quad (6/27)$$

$n = 13 \quad r = 0.892 \quad s = 0.185$

8. *Potentiation of tryptamines in mice by 9-fluorenoximethylamines* [1]

$$\log A = -1.01\pi - 0.41B_4 + 0.32 \quad (6/28)$$

$n = 12 \quad r = 0.922 \quad s = 0.318$

Statistically, this equation is clearly better than the corresponding relation with E_S:

$$\log A = -0.80\pi + 0.35E_S - 0.75 \quad (6/29)$$

$n = 12 \quad r = 0.893 \quad s = 0.358$

9. *Activity of aromatic quaternary ammonium salts against S. aureus* [38]

$$\log A = 0.20\chi^2 + 4.58\chi + 22.24 \quad (6/30)$$

$n = 38 \quad r = 0.931 \quad s = 0.230$

In eqn. (6/30) it is anything but certain whether the relationship between biological activity and connectivity is primarily a steric or a hydrophobic one.

10. *Binding of thyroxine analogues to solubilized protein from rat liver cells* [71]

$$\log A = 1.68\pi_{3'} - 2.12\,(\mathrm{SIZE} > J)_{3'} - 0.63\pi_{5'} - 1.54I_1 - 1.35I_2 - 0.304 \quad (6/31)$$

$n = 31 \quad r = 0.946 \quad s = 0.400$

It is assumed here that those substituents in the 3-position which are larger than iodine have an unfavourable effect — to be characterized by the parameter $(\mathrm{SIZE} > J)_3'$ — on biological activity.
I_1 and I_2 denote indicator variables which take into account certain structural properties of the 2′- and 4′-positions.

11. *Binding of disubstituted* D- *and* L-N-*Acyl-α-aminoamides to chymotrypsin* [62]

$$\log 1/K = 0.72\,\mathrm{MR{-}L} + 0.230\,\mathrm{MR{-}S} + 0.323I_1 + 0.311I_2 - 1.062 \quad (6/32)$$

$n = 45 \quad r = 0.928 \quad s = 0.233$

$1/K$ = binding constant
MR—L = molar refractivity of the larger substituent

MR—S = molar refractivity of the smaller substituent
I_1 = indicator variable assigned a value of 1 for hydrazides and a value of 0 for all other cases
I_2 = indicator variable differentiating between D- ($I_2 = 1$) and L-congeners ($I_2 = 0$).

Remarkable with eqn. (6/32) is that stereoisomers are dealt with by a simple indicator variable.

12. *Inhibition of dihydrofolate reductase* (DHFR) *by phenyltriazines* (*structure XXXVa*) *and quinazolines* (*structure XXXVb*) [54a—c]

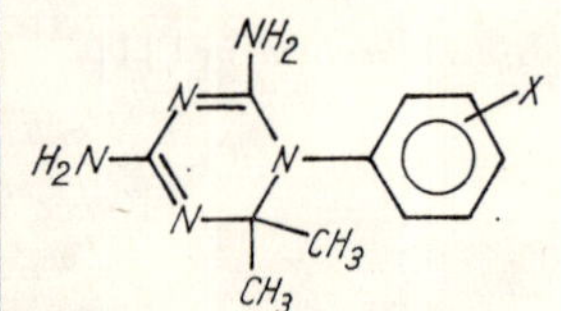

XXXV a

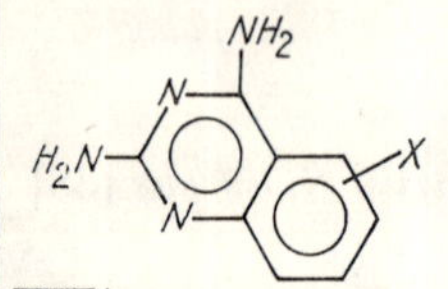

XXXV b

(i) *Phenyltriazines,* DHFR *from either Walker 256 tumours or leucaemia L 1210*

$$\log A = 1.384S_0 - 0.02127S_0^2 + 0.434\Sigma\pi - 0.574D_4 - 0.294D_4^2 - 15.66 \quad (6/33)$$

$n = 27 \quad r = 0.953 \quad s = 0.440$

reference molecule: X = 3.4 — Cl_2
assumed active conformation: $\theta = 310°$

D_4 measures a hypothetical intermolecular steric interaction involving a 4-X substituent along a vector defined by the CH bond at position 4 on the ring.

(ii) *Phenyltriazines* (*substituted only in the 3-position*), DHFR *from rat liver*

$$\log A = 1.086S_0 - 0.01606S_0^2 + 0.723\pi_3 - 0.142\pi_3^2 - 0.535D_3 - 12.17 \quad (6/34)$$

$n = 20 \quad r = 0.947 \quad s = 0.23$

reference molecule: X = $C(CH_3)_3$
assumed active conformation: $\theta = 310°$

D_3 measures the maximum distance of a nonhydrogen atom of X perpendicular to a vector defined by the CH bond at position 3 on the ring and is assumed to account for a steric interaction of 3-X substituents with a sterically restricted receptor space.

(iii) *Phenyltriazines* (*substituted only in the 3-position*), DHFR *from bovine liver*

$$\log A = 1.074 S_0 - 0.01674 S_0^2 - 0.604\,\pi_3 - 0.110 D_3^2 - 0.297 D_3 - 10.75 \quad (6/35)$$

$n = 31 \quad r = 0.926 \quad s = 0.25$

reference molecule: X = $C(CH_3)_3$

assumed active conformation: $\theta = 310°$

For the definition of D_3, see above.

(iv) *Quinazolines*, DHFR *from rat liver*

$$\log A = 0.3735 S_0 - 0.0022 S_0^2 + 0.5115(\pi_5 + \pi_6) - 0.1008\Delta\theta - 6.596 \quad (6/36)$$

$n = 35 \quad r = 0.945 \quad s = 0.451$

reference molecule: 3,4-Cl_2-2,4-diaminotriazine in its assumed active conformation

$\Delta\theta$ is defined as $(90° - \theta_{4,1})$ where $\theta_{4,1}$ represents the torsional rotation of the 4-NH_2 group such that $\theta_{4,1} = 0°$ corresponds to an NH_2 group being in the same plane as the quinazoline ring. It is supposed to reflect hydrogen-bonding properties between the 4-NH_2 group and the enzyme.

Equations (6/33)—(6/36) show high consistency. The shape descriptor S_0 is in all cases parabolically related with inhibitory potency, the optimum values of S_0 in all 4 equations being amazingly similar varying only from 79.3 to 83.1. This was interpreted to mean that the optimum inhibitor in both series of compound should occupy about 0.71 nm^3. Very remarkable is the use of 3.4-Cl_2-2,4-diaminotriazine in its postulated active conformation as reference molecule in the quinazoline study (eqn. (6/36)) which indicates the potential of molecular shape analysis to design new lead compounds. Another fact of interest is the D_3 term appearing in eqns. (6/34) and (6/35) but not in eqn. (6/33). This may indicate that this term is species specific to bovine and rat liver DHFRs. Equations (6/33) and (6/35) where shown to posses predictive value.

References

[1] Verloop, A., W. Hoogenstraaten and J. Tipker in E. J. Ariens (Ed.): Drug Design, Vol. VII, Academic Press, New York, 1976, p. 165

[2] Balaban, A. T., A. Chiriac, I. Motoc and Z. Simon: Steric Fit in Quantitative Structure-Activity Relations, Lecture Notes in Chemistry, Vol. 15, Springer-Verlag, Berlin, 1980

[3] Taft, R. W., in M. S. Newman (Ed.): Steric Effects in Organic Chemistry, Wiley, New York, 1956, p. 556

[4] Shorter, J., in N. B. Chapman and J. Shorter (Eds.): Advances in Linear Free Energy Relationships, Plenum Press, London, 1972

[5] Seydel, J. K., and K.-J. Schaper: Chemische Struktur und biologische Aktivität von Wirkstoffen, Verlag Chemie, Weinheim, 1979

[6] Martin, Y. C.: Drug Design Methods, Marcel Dekker, New York, 1978

[7] Hansch, C., and A. J. Leo: Substituent Constants for Correlation Analysis in Chemistry and Biology, Wiley, New York, 1979

[8] Charton, M.: J. Am. Chem. Soc. **91**, 615 (1969)

[8a] Mager, H., P. P. Mager and A. Barth: Tetrahedron **35**, 1953 (1979)

[8b] Berg, U., R. Gallo, G. Klatte and J. Metzger: J. Chem. Soc. Perkin II 1350 (1980)

[8c] DeTar, D. F.: J. Org. Chem. **45**, 5166 (1980)

[8d] MacPhee, J. A., A. Panaye and J. E. Dubois: Tetrahedron **34**, 3553 (1978)
[8e] Dubois, J. E., J. A. MacPhee and A. Panaye: Tetrahedron Lett. 4099 (1978)
[8f] MacPhee, J. A., A. Panaye and J. E. Dubois: J. Org. Chem. **45**, 1164 (1980)
[9] Unger, S. H., and C. Hansch: Progr. Phys. Org. Chem. **12**, 91 (1976)
[10] Kutter, E., and C. Hansch: J. Med. Chem. **12**, 647 (1969)
[11] Kutter, E., and C. Hansch: Arch. Biochem. Biophys. **135**, 126 (1969)
[12] Fujita, R., C. Takayama and M. Nakajima: J. Org. Chem. **38**, 1653 (1973)
[13] Fahmy, M. A. H., T. R. Fukuto, R. L. Metcalf and R. L. Holmstedt: J. Agr. Food Chem. **21**, 585 (1973)
[14] De Tar, D. F., and C. J. Tenpas: J. Am. Chem. Soc. **98**, 7903 (1976)
[15] Hancock, C. K., E. A. Meyers and B. J. Yager: J. Am. Chem. Soc. **83**, 4211 (1961)
[16] Hancock, C. K., and C. P. Falls: J. Am. Chem. Soc. **83**, 4214 (1961)
[17] Hancock, C. K.: J. Org. Chem. **30**, 1174 (1965)
[18] Hancock, C. K.: J. Org. Chem. **38**, 4239 (1973)
[19] Bowden, K., N. B. Chapman and J. Shorter: J. Chem. Soc. 5239 (1963)
[20] Charton, M.: J. Am. Chem. Soc. **97**, 1552 (1975)
[20a] Charton, M., in E. B. Rocke (Ed.): Design of Biopharmaceutical Properties through Prodrugs and Analogs, American Pharmaceutical Association, Washington, 1977, p. 228
[21] Fujita, T.: Pure and Appl. Chem. **50**, 987 (1978)
[22] Palm, V. A.: Grundlagen der quantitativen Theorie organischer Reaktionen, Akademie-Verlag, Berlin, 1971
[23] Charton, M.: Progr. Phys. Org. Chem. **8**, 235 (1971)
[24] Charton, M.: J. Am. Chem. Soc. **97**, 3691 (1975)
[25] Charton, M.: J. Org. Chem. **41**, 2906 (1976)
[26] Hansch, C., A. J. Leo, S. H. Unger, K. H. Kim, D. Nikaitani and E. J. Lien: J. Med. Chem. **16**, 1207 (1973)
[27] Bondi, A.: Physical Properties of Molecular Crystals, Liquids and Glasses, Wiley, New York, 1968
[27a] Pearlman, R. S., in S. H. Yalkowsky, A. A. Sinkula and S. C. Valvani (Eds.): Physical Chemical Properties of Drugs, Marcel Dekker, New York, 1980, p. 321
[28] Exner, O.: Coll. Czechoslov. Chem. Commun. **32**, 1 (1967)
[29] Tollenaere, J. P., H. Moereels and M. Protiva: Eur. J. Med. Chem. **11**, 293 (1976)
[30] Vogel, A. I.: J. Chem. Soc. 1833 (1948)
[31] Vogel, A. I.: J. Chem. Soc. 514 (1952)
[32] Quayle, O. R.: Chem. Rev. **53**, 439 (1953)
[33] Randič, M.: J. Am. Chem. Soc. **97**, 6609 (1975)
[34] Kier, L. B., L. H. Hall, W. J. Murray and M. Randič: J. Pharm. Sci. **64**, 1971 (1975)
[35] Hall, L. H., L. B. Kier and W. J. Murray: J. Pharm. Sci. **64**, 1974 (1975)
[36] Murray, W. J., L. H. Hall and L. B. Kier: J. Pharm. Sci. **64**, 1978 (1975)
[37] Kier, L. B., W. J. Murray and L. H. Hall: J. Med. Chem. **18**, 1272 (1975)
[38] Murray, W. J., L. B. Kier and L. H. Hall: J. Med. Chem. **19**, 573 (1976)
[39] Kier, L. B., and L. H. Hall: J. Pharm. Sci. **65**, 1806 (1976)
[39a] Kier, L. B., in S. H. Yalkowsky, A. A. Sinkula and S. C. Valvani (Eds.): Physical Chemical Properties of Drugs, Marcel Dekker, New York, 1980, p. 277
[40] Kier, L. B., and L. H. Hall: Molecular Connectivity in Chemistry and Drug Research, Academic Press, New York, 1976
[41] Verloop, A., and J. Tipker: Pestic. Sci. 7, 379 (1976)
[41a] Verloop, A.: Phil. Trans. R. Soc. London **B 295**, 45 (1981)
[42] Verloop, A., and J. Tipker in J. A. Keverling Buisman (Ed.): Biological Activity and Chemical Structure, Pharmacochemistry Library, Vol. 2 (Eds.: W. Th. Nauta and R. F. Rehker), Elsevier, Amsterdam, 1977, p. 63

[43] Bultsma, T., and G. J. Bijloo in J. Knoll and F. Darvas (Eds.): Chemical Structure — Biological Activity Relationships, Akadémiai Kiadó, Budapest, 1980, p. 205
[44] Silipo, C., C. Hansch, C. Grieco and A. Vittoria: Arch. Biochem. Biophys. **194**, 552 (1979)
[45] Simon, Z., and Z. Szabadai: studia biophysica **39**, 123 (1973)
[46] Simon, Z.: studia biophysica **51**, 49 (1975)
[47] Simon, Z., A. Chiriac, I. Motoc, S. Holban, D. Ciubotariu and Z. Szabadai: studia biophysica **55**, 217 (1976)
[48] Simon, Z.: Angew. Chem. **86**, 802 (1974)
[49] Simon, Z.: Quantum Biochemistry and Specific Interactions, Abacus Press, Turnbridge Wells, 1976
[50] Simon, Z., I. I. Badilescu and T. Racovitan: J. theor. Biol. **66**, 485 (1977)
[51] Simon, Z., M. Mracec, A. Maurer, S. Policec and C. Dragulescu: Rev. roum. Biochim. **14**, 117 (1977)
[52] Simon, Z.: studia biophysica **62**, 167 (1977)
[53] Simon, Z., I. I. Badilescu, A. Chiriac, D. Ciubotariu, S. Holban, F. Kerek, I. Motoc, M. Mracec, T. Szabadai and V. Popoviciu in R. Franke and P. Oehme (Eds.): Quantitative Structure-Activity Analysis, Akademie-Verlag, Berlin, 1978, p. 161
[53a] Simon, Z., N. Dragomir, M. G. Plauchithin, S. Holban, H. Glatt and F. Kerek: Eur. J. Med. Chem. **15**, 521 (1980)
[54] Simon, Z., in J. Knoll and F. Darvas (Eds.): Chemical Structure — Biological Activity Relationships, Akadémiai Kiadó, Budapest, 1980, p. 101
[54a] Hopfinger, A. J.: J. Am. Chem. Soc. **102**, 7196 (1980)
[54b] Hopfinger, A. J.: Arch. Biochem. Biophys. **206**, 153 (1981)
[54c] Battershell, C., D. Malhotra and A. J. Hopfinger: J. Med. Chem. **24**, 812 (1981)
[54d] Hopfinger, A. J.: J. Med. Chem. **24**, 818 (1981)
[54e] Testa, B., and W. P. Purcell: Eur. J. Med. Chem. **13**, 509 (1978)
[55] Amoore, J. E., G. Palmieri and E. Wanke: Nature **216**, 1084 (1967)
[56] Amoore, J. E., G. Palmieri, E. Wanke and M. S. Blum: Science **165**, 1266 (1969)
[57] Amoore, J. E.: Ann. N.Y. Acad. Sci. **116**, 457 (1964)
[58] Amoore, J. E.: Nature **214**, 1095 (1967)
[59] Lehmann, P. A., J. F. Rodrigues de Miranda and E. J. Ariens: Fortschr. Arzneimittelforsch. **20**, 101 (1976)
[60] Rodrigues de Miranda, J. F., P. A. Lehmann and E. J. Ariens: Fortschr. Arzneimittelforsch. **20**, 126 (1976)
[61] Lehmann, P. A., in J. Knoll and F. Darvas (Eds.): Chemical Structure — Biological Activity Relationships, Akadémiai Kiadó, Budapest, 1980, p. 285
[62] Yoshimoto, M., and C. Hansch: J. Org. Chem. **41**, 2269 (1976)
[63] Martin, Y. C., in E. J. Ariens (Ed.): Drug Design, Vol. VIII, Academic Press, New York, 1979, p. 1
[64] Lien, E. J., J. F. Rodrigues de Miranda and E. J. Ariens: Mol. Pharmacol. **12**, 598 (1976)
[65] Unger, S. H., K. Untch, B. Lewis, B. Berkoz, J. Edwards, A. Strosberg, R. Weissberg and R. Alvarez in J. Knoll and F. Darvas (Eds.): Chemical Structure — Biological Activity Relationships, Akadémiai Kiadó, Budapest, 1980, p. 3
[65a] Hyde, R. M., and B. Roth in J. A. Keverling Buisman (Ed.): Strategy in Drug Research, Elsevier, Amsterdam, 1982, p. 385
[66] Simon, Z.: Universitatea din Timisoara, Serie Chimie Nr. 17/1975
[67] Franke, R., M. Tonew and L. Heinisch: unpublished results
[68] Hansch, C., and E. W. Deutsch: Biochim. Biophys. Acta **126**, 117 (1966)
[69] Silipo, C., and C. Hansch: Il Farmaco **30**, 35 (1975)
[70] Tagoh, Y.: unpublished results, cited after ref. [6]
[71] Dietrich, S. W., M. B. Bolger, P. A. Kollmann and E. C. Jorgensen: J. Med. Chem. **20**, 863 (1977)

7. Interrelations of Molecular Parameters and the Collinearity Problem

As already discussed in previous chapters, there are numerous relations between the various molecular parameters; such correlated parameters are said to be *collinear*. The following categories may be distinguished:

1. Relations which can be attributed to well-known systematic features as is the case, for example, with the one between log P and CSA in the validity range of eqn. (4/5).
2. Relations which express as yet unrecognized systematics or which have validity only within a particular series (i.e., not only within the sample). A case in point may be the relation between q_n^π and E_{HOMO} (see eqn. (5/155)) in substituted piperidinoacetanilides.
3. Relations which exist solely in certain samples having a particular composition.

Relations of the first category present no problems for quantitative structure-activity analysis indicating merely that the variables involved are systematically interchangeable.

The second category is essentially more problematic as is demonstrated by some of the examples already discussed. In principle, such unpredictable or concealed collinearities may lead to a situation where instead of the relevant parameter a secondary one correlated with it enters the resultant equation (thus giving rise to misinterpretations), or where a differentiation between equations with different variables becomes impossible (so that no interpretation is possible). The simultaneous occurrence of collinear variables in a regression analysis also results in a distortion of the regression coefficients and may lead to false results. The situations reaches a crucial stage when collinearity appears between those molecular parameters which belong to different terms in eqn. (3/17), i.e., between x_h, x_e and x_s. These terms are then no longer separable so that conclusions as to the presence or absence of hydrophobic, electronic and steric substituent influences or their relative significance become impossible.

If the third category presents itself without being recognized, a quantitative structure-activity analysis can give entirely useless results. Difficulties may arise not only from a possible misinterpretation but, to make matters worse, also from the very limited predictive power of such QSARs.

The problem of collinearity is of central importance in quantatitive structure-activity analysis concerning the selection of the best equation(s) as well as mechanistic interpretability [1—18]. The problem can further be complicated by the fact that collinearities may also occur between more than two molecular parameters (so-called *multicollinearities*). It is imperative, therefore, that serious collinearities are avoided either by data preprocessing (cf., 8.4.) or, better, by an optimal selection of analogues for the training series (cf., 8.1.); another possibility is the application of special mathematical techniques such as principal component regression analysis (see e.g. [19]).

Discussed below are a few relations between molecular parameters with particular reference to the differentiation and evaluation of hydrophobic, electronic and steric molecular parameters. Relations described in preceding sections will not be considered again.

7.1. Simple Collinearities

As evidenced by the studies reported by Craig [3] and by Hansch [1, 8], no relation exists between hydrophobic and electronic substituent constants if a sufficiently large number of substituents is considered. Nevertheless, such a relation can arise if the series of substituents is limited, as emerges clearly from eqn. (4/3). Within a series of substituents which scarcely differ in CSA, Y will also show little variation. Any differences in hydrophobicity are then primarily of an electronic nature and can be attributed to dissimilar values of the term in brackets (intensity factors I_1 and I_2). If this term and σ correlate at least approximately, it follows at once that for such a series

Table 7.1. Group of substituents with collinearity between π and σ_p (from [7])

Substituent	π	σ_p
NH_2	−1.23	−0.66
OH	−0.67	−0.37
OCH_3	−0.02	−0.27
H	0.00	0.00
F	0.14	0.06
Cl	0.70	0.23
Br	0.86	0.23
SCF_3	1.44	0.50

of substituents a correlation between π and σ is to be expected. For example, a relation of this kind exists for the group of substituents presented in Table 7.1 [7]. Hydrophobic and electronic effects could not be separated for a sample with these substituents. Fortunately, however, simple collinearities between π and electronic parameters are uncommon. A relation encountered more frequently is that between π or log P and such "steric" parameters as molar refractivity, molar volume or parachor as may be expected if the validity criteria of (4/4) are satisfied. To a certain extent, this is also applicable to E_S considering its relation with the van der Waals radius for approximately top symmetric substituents (see eqn. (6/5)). As the validity criteria of (4/4) within a group of substituents are more strained the relation between π and log P and such steric quantities becomes obscured. Nevertheless, with rather a mixture of substituents Craig [3] still found statistically significant relationships between π, group polarizability, molecular refractivity, parachor and E_S. On consideration of a very large range of substituents these relations, however, disappears [1, 8]. At any rate it should be borne in mind that collinearities between π or log P and steric molecular parameters occur rather frequently (see also [20]) and in such cases it is difficult if not impossible to establish whether a given effect is primarily hydrophobic or steric.

Thus, Hansch et al. [21] derived the following equations for the inhibition of complement by disubstituted pyridinium ions (I represents an indicator variable accounting for the presence ($I = 1$) or absense ($I = 0$) of a particular structural element):

$$\log A = 0.183\pi_1 + 0.642\,\mathrm{MR}_2 + 1.024\sigma_1^+ + 0.724I + 2.122 \qquad (7/1)$$

$$n = 69 \qquad r = 0.939 \qquad s = 0.199$$

$$\log A = 0.180\pi_1 + 0.464\pi_2 + 1.008\sigma_1^+ + 0.723I + 2.500 \qquad (7/2)$$

$$n = 69 \qquad r = 0.939 \qquad s = 0.198$$

From a comparison of these two equations, it is seen that π and MR of substituents in position 2 can be freely interchanged without changing anything else. This phenomenon is due to a high collinearity between π and MR (the correlation coefficient is 0.79) rendering impossible any conclusion on the nature of substituent effects (steric or hydrophobic) in the 2-position. There is another interesting aspect of this example. The coefficients of the two π terms in (7/2) differ so that in the event of the effect being hydrophobic and not steric, it must be strongly position-dependent. Even where the π term for the 2-position represents a steric effect, a separation of π terms for the positions 1 and 2 seems to be indispensable considering the different coefficients. Surprisingly, however, the π terms can be summarized as:

$$\log A = 0.192(\pi_1 + \pi_2) + 0.131\sigma_2 + 1.112\sigma_1^+ + 0.752I + 2.468 \qquad (7/3)$$

$$n = 69 \qquad r = 0.931 \qquad s = 0.210$$

By combining the π terms, a change does occur now, namely the appearance of an additional σ term for substituents in the 2-position. What lies behind this is, in fact, a high collinearity between π_2 and σ_2. Equation (7/3) may then be interpreted as arising from a separation of the π_2 term in (7/2) into two components one of which is incorporated in the sum of the π values in (7/3) and the other (serving to correct for position-dependence) is expressed by the new σ_2 term. Equation (7/3) also illustrates clearly how collinearities can influence regression coefficients.

Had the collinearities between π_2 and MR_2 or σ_2 not been established and the position-dependence and possible connections with MR not been examined, eqn. (7/3) could have been regarded as the most appropriate equation. This would have presented a basically incorrect picture, since according to this equation the hydrophobic substituent influence from positions 1 and 2 is not position-dependent, and there is an electronic substituent influence from both positions while steric effects are entirely absent. This example once more underlines the necessity of investigating the largest meaningful number of hypotheses, while making it also clear that no equation can be interpreted unless one is aware of possible collinearities.

Direct collinearities between steric and electronic molecular parameter values are relatively rare. With a sufficient number of substituents, there is, for example, non-collinearity between electronic substituent constants and molar refractivity [3, 8]. Nevertheless, it is quite important to recognize the dualistic nature of the molar refractivity, which is associated with polarizability according to (6/13), thus representing an electronic component. Equation (7/4) provides a useful approximation to the energy of the dispersion interactions (LONDON forces) between molecules A and B:

$$E = \frac{38\,000}{r^6}\,\mathrm{MR}_A \cdot \mathrm{MR}_B = \text{constant} \cdot \mathrm{MR}_A \cdot \mathrm{MR}_B \qquad (7/4)$$

If one of the molecules is the receptor (MR = constant), it follows from (7/4) that the London energy is roughly proportional to the molar refractivity of the drug molecules. Thus, the occurrence of the molar refractivity in QSARs may also be attributed to dispersion interactions between receptor and drug. This interpretation is also considered in some of the more recent publications by Hansch and co-workers [e.g. 22—31].

Surprising and physicochemically unexplainable are the following relations presented by Koppel [32] for saturated alkyl substituents (from [33]):

$$E_S = 27.78\sigma^* - 1.90(n_H - 3) + 0.88 \qquad (7/5)$$

$$r = 0.956 \qquad s = 0.292$$

$$E_S^0 = 27.84\sigma^* - 1.71(n_H - 3) + 0.88 \qquad (7/6)$$

$$r = 0.964 \qquad s = 0.265$$

Equations (7/5) and (7/6) might be of help in the calculation of unknown E_S values of saturated alkyl substituents; n_H denotes the number of α-C-H-bonds.

7.2. Multiple Collinearities between Hydrophobic, Electronic and Steric Molecular Parameters

A very interesting relationship has recently been found among those molecular properties of organic compounds which are dependent upon non-covalent intermolecular forces, such as aqueous solvation energy, partition coefficient, boiling point, molecular refractivity, volume, vaporization energy, magnetic susceptibility, van der Waals A und B and critical temperature [34]. A principal component analysis (see 9.1.) revealed five principal components, the first two of which accounted for 96% of the variance of the data set investigated. These components can be identified with "bulk" and "cohesiveness" and were, therefore, designated as "BC" parameters by Cramer [34]. They can be estimated on the basis of an additive-constitutive model [35] and seem to provide useful new variables for characterizing non-specific non-covalent interactions in QSAR work [36].

Of special importance are multiple relationships involving π. As already pointed out in 4.1., π depends not only on substituents but also on their electronic interactions with their environment. As a consequence, π values for the same substituents from the various aromatic standard series (benzenes, phenoxyacetic acids, etc.) may be different and related through an electronic correction (for a detailed discussion of the physicochemical aspects of the aromatic π values and such electronic corrections, see 9.1.2.1.). Between the π values from two different aromatic series with the functional groups Y and Z (e.g., $-NH_2$, $-NO_2$, $-COOH$, $-OCH_2COOH$) there is usually a relationship satisfying eqn. (7/7):

$$\pi_Y = \alpha\pi_Z + \beta\sigma \qquad (7/7)$$

It appears that the coefficients α and β are connected with the Hammett constants σ_Y and σ_Z of the functional groups Y and Z (see 9.1.2.1.). From these connections the following rules emerge for meta- and para-substituents (to be considered separately):

1. In general, for the coefficient α

$$\alpha = 1, \quad \text{if} \quad \sigma_Y = \sigma_Z$$

$$\alpha \approx 1, \quad \text{if} \quad (\sigma_Y - \sigma_Z) \approx 0$$

$$\alpha > 1, \quad \text{if} \quad (\sigma_Y - \sigma_Z) < 0$$

$$\alpha < 1, \quad \text{if} \quad (\sigma_Y - \sigma_Z) > 0$$

The deviation of the coefficient α from unity becomes larger as the difference between σ_Y and σ_Z increases.

2. Usually, for the coefficient β

$$\beta = 0, \quad \text{if} \quad \sigma_Y = \sigma_Z$$

$$\beta \approx 0, \quad \text{if} \quad (\sigma_Y - \sigma_Z) \approx 0$$

$$\beta > 0, \quad \text{if} \quad (\sigma_Y - \sigma_Z) < 0$$

$$\beta < 0, \quad \text{if} \quad (\sigma_Y - \sigma_Z) > 0$$

The value of β becomes larger if the difference between σ_Z and σ_Y increases.

Tabulated aromatic π values cannot be applied in quantitative structure-activity analysis unless the condition

$$\pi_Y = \pi_Z \tag{7/8}$$

is sufficiently well fulfilled. According to the above rules this will be the case if the electronic properties of the functional groups in the standard series and the series under investigation are (almost) the same or if the electronic influence of the functional groups in both series is negligibly small.

In addition to relations of the type (7/7), relations of the following form are also possible [37]:

$$\pi_Y = \alpha\pi_Z + \beta\sigma + \gamma\pi_Z\sigma \tag{7/9}$$

$$\pi_Y = \alpha\pi_Z + \gamma\pi_Z\sigma \tag{7/10}$$

These are not typical, however, and are rare (they may, although by no means always, be met if possible position-dependences of π values are ignored).

The relations exemplified below are based on (7/7), (7/9) and (7/10) (for a detailed discussion, see 9.1.2.1. and [38]):

1. Y = $-SO_2NH_2$; Z = $-NO_2$ [39]

$$\pi_Y = 1.24\pi_Z + 0.75\sigma \tag{7/11}$$

$$n = 8 \qquad r = 0.991 \qquad s = 0.093$$

2. Y = $-SO_2NH_2$; Z = $-OH$ [39]

$$\pi_Y = 0.92\pi_Z - 0.60\sigma \tag{7/12}$$

$$n = 10 \qquad r = 0.993 \qquad s = 0.091$$

3. Y = $-OCH_2COOH$; Z = $-NH_2$ [39]

$$\pi_Y = 0.911\pi_Z - 388\pi\mathfrak{F} \tag{7/13}$$

$$n = 17 \qquad r = 0.980 \qquad s = 0.143$$

In eqn. (7/13) the field constant $\mathfrak{F}$ of SWAIN and LUPTON [40] is used instead of σ. Further examples of this kind are reported in the literature [e.g. 41—46] and in section 9.1.2.1.

Where electronic corrections based on (7/7) become necessary, it is no longer possible to separate hydrophobic and electronic substituent effects since the electronic correction term will enter the function $f_e(x_e)$ of eqn. (3/17). There may be circumstances under which an electronic substituent effect, which in reality does not exist at all, is simulated by such a correction. A case in point is eqn. (7/14) found by DRUCKREY [47] for the hypnotic activity of structure VI where $\log P$ is calculated from tabulated π values:

$$\log A = -0.53 (\log P)^2 + 1.94 \log P + 0.15\sigma^* + 1.65 \quad (7/14)$$

$$n = 6 \quad r = 0.999 \quad s = 0.024$$

As shown by experimental determination of $\log P$, the σ^* term here is exclusively a correction term since, with measured $\log P$ values, a relationship without an electronic term is obtained (eqn. (4/115)).

A relationship based on (7/9) or (7/10) is invariably associated with the occurrence of cross-products of the form $x_h x_e$. If (7/7) is valid, cross-products are to be expected in case of a non-linear relationship between $\log A$ and x_h[1]). Examples of such cross-product equations (see also (5/103) are:

1. *Synergism by 1,2-benzodioxoles* [39] (data from [48]; cf., (5/110))

$$\log A = -0.117\pi^2 - 1.833\sigma^{\cdot 2} + 0.616\pi + 3.072\sigma^{\cdot} - 0.800\pi\sigma^{\cdot} + 1.467 \quad (7/15)$$

$$n = 13 \quad r = 0.995 \quad s = 0.054$$

Statistically, eqn. (7/15) is better than (5/110), the cross-product being significant at $p < 0.01$.

2. *Virostatic activity of substituted pyrazoles* (structure XXXVI, Mengo virus [49])

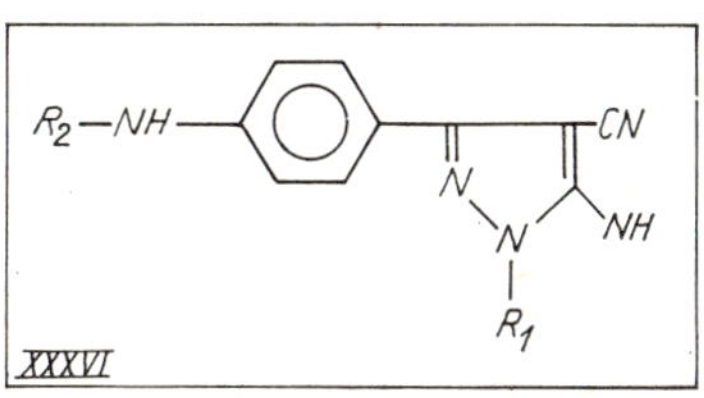

$$\log A = 0.109\pi_1 - 0.794\pi_1\sigma_1 - 2.037E_{S,2} + 0.783\sigma_2^* - 1.702 \quad (7/16)$$

$$n = 19 \quad r = 0.915 \quad s = 0.181$$

3. *Bacteriostatic activity of penicillin derivatives* [39]

$$\log A = 0.11\pi^2 - 0.69\pi - 0.27\pi\sigma + 0.42\sigma + 6.47 \quad (7/17)$$

$$n = 21 \quad r = 0.894 \quad s = 0.253$$

[1]) For the sake of completeness it should be mentioned that such cross-products may, in principle, also reflect possible differences between n-octanol and the hydrophobic biophase.

According to our experience it is important that such cross-products are allowed for in quantitative structure-activity analyses in appropriate cases although, in the literature, almost no reference is made to such terms. They can cause radical changes in the picture presented by QSARs. For example, artificial parabolic relationships with π which can arise from applying a wrong set of π values may be linearized after introducing a $\pi\sigma$ term. Unfortunately, it is always difficult to establish whether a statistically significant cross-product is also of physicochemical significance. The reason is that collinearities often occur between these cross-products and π as well as σ. In such cases additional investigations become necessary.

Equation (4/3) indicates that log P and π contain both steric as well as electronic components. It is, therefore, not surprising that multiple collinearities with varying degrees of complexity between π, electronic and steric parameters may occur for a given set of substituents as exemplified below [39].

1. *Anilines* [39]

$$\pi = -1.74E_S^2 - 1.00E_S + 2.41\sigma_I + 0.60 \tag{7/18}$$

$$n = 16 \quad r = 0.938 \quad s = 0.422$$

2. *Piperidinoacetanilides* [39]

$$r = -1.68r_v^2 + 6.20r_v - 1.52q_N^\pi - 5.13 \tag{7/19}$$

$$n = 13 \quad r = 0.893 \quad s = 0.222$$

3. *Phenols* [39]

$$\pi = -1.80E_S + 2.16E_S\sigma_I + 0.69 \tag{7/20}$$

$$n = 18 \quad r = 0.893 \quad s = 0.274$$

4. *Pyrazoles* (structure XXXVI, [49])

$$\pi_2 = -3.30E_{S,2} + 0.96\sigma_2^* + 0.81 \tag{7/21}$$

$$n = 19 \quad r = 0.827 \quad s = 0.387$$

5. *Aromatic para-substituents* [2]

$$r_v = 0.73\pi_p - 1.05\sigma_p^+ + 1.26 \tag{7/22}$$

$$n = 6 \quad r = 0.983 \quad s = 0.073$$

6. *Propynylamines* [50]

$$\mathrm{MR} = 5.49\pi - 7.03P + 1.05 \tag{7/23}$$

$$n = 22 \quad r = 0.93 \quad s = 1.35$$

7. *Carbamates* [51]

$$\pi_{carbamate} = 0.942\pi_{benzene} + 0.52\sigma^0 + 0.18E_S - 0.46\mathfrak{F} + 0.12 \tag{7/24}$$

$$n = 62 \quad r = 0.990 \quad s = 0.095$$

Equation (7/24) is also a special case of a relation based on (7/7).

Relationships of the form (7/18) up to (7/24) are not of general validity but usually only apply to a particular selection of substituents. If these relationships are not duly recognized, QSARs may lead to erroneous conclusions. Comparison of eqns. (7/21) and (7/16), for example, indicates that it should be possible to replace the linear combination of $E_{S,2}$ and σ_2^* in eqn. (7/16) by a simple π_2-term. This is indeed the case, resulting in eqn. (7/25):

$$\log A = 0.10\pi_1 - 0.51\pi_1\sigma_1 + 0.46\pi_2 - 1.88 \qquad (7/25)$$

$$n = 19 \qquad r = 0.749 \qquad s = 0.289$$

Whereas eqn. (7/16) indicates steric and electronic influences of position 2 substituents, only a hydrophobic effect is reflected by eqn. (7/25). Both equations thus lead to completely different conclusions because of the multicollinearity between π_2, σ_2^*, and $E_{S,2}$ shown by eqn. (7/21). Fortunately, eqn. (7/16) could clearly be preferred over eqn. (7/25) because of its much better statistics and of some additional criteria not discussed here. Otherwise, no decision would have been possible without including additional analogues into the analysis in order to break down the multicollinearity. It should be noted that eqn. (7/16) had high predictive power.

Another example concerns the antiadrenergic activity of β-halo-β-arylalkylamines for which the following relationship has been reported [2]:

$$\log A = 0.82 \sum \pi - 1.02 \sum \sigma^+ + 0.62 r_{v,p} + 7.06 \qquad (7/26)$$

$$n = 22 \qquad r = 0.964 \qquad s = 0.164$$

For the same series eqn. (7/27) was established by CAMMARATA [52]:

$$\log A = 0.75\pi_m - 0.91\sigma_m + 1.67 r_{v,p} + 5.77 \qquad (7/27)$$

$$n = 22 \qquad r = 0.961 \qquad s = 0.168$$

Statistically, (7/27) is equivalent to (7/26). As demonstrated by UNGER and HANSCH [2], however, eqn. (7/27) is an artefact arising from the multicollinearity embodied in (7/22). This example clearly shows that it is necessary to search for the "best equation" not only in statistical terms but also on the basis of other considerations.

An attempt was made by CAMMARATA and ROGERS [53—55] to calculate π values from quantum-chemical data. Starting from the perturbation theory reported by KLOPMAN and HUDSON [56, 57] they found the relationships

$$\log P = a_0 + a_1 \sum_r |Q_{r,N}| + a_2 \sum_r S_r^E \qquad (7/28)$$

and

$$\pi = a_0 + a_1 \sum_{r_s} |Q_{r,N}| + a_2 \sum_{r_s} S_r^E \qquad (7/29)$$

The summations are over all atoms in eqn. (7/28) and over the atoms of the substituent in eqn. (7/29). Despite some relatively crude approximations, these relationships give statistically significant descriptions of $\log P$ and π values for aromatic compounds, which follows from, for example, eqns. (7/30) and (7/31) (π values of the phenoxyacetic acid series in the octanol-water system):

$$\pi = -1.057 \sum_{r_s} |Q_{r,N}| + 0.209 \sum_{r_s} S_r^E + 0.10 \qquad (7/30)$$

$$n = 22 \qquad r = 0.810 \qquad s = 0.414$$

Equation (7/30) can be improved by omitting the substituents p-$N(CH_3)_2$, m-NH_2 and p-NH_2:

$$\pi = -0.973 \sum_{r_s} |Q_{r,N}| + 0.294 \sum_{r_s} S_r^E - 0.020 \qquad (7/31)$$

$$n = 19 \qquad r = 0.931 \qquad s = 0.205$$

This result is surprising in that hydrophobic interactions are primarily due to entropy effects, which in essence cannot be allowed for in quantum-chemical approaches. On closer inspection of the calculations it will be seen, however, that the substituents under consideration vary little in size (small entropy effect) but greatly in electronic properties. If an approximate description of hydrophobic molecular parameters by quantum-chemical indices is at all possible, it refers to such a selection of substituents. Furthermore, only a very small range of π values is covered, consisting of no more than 2π units, whereas that of the π values listed by, for example, HANSCH et al. [1] comprises 9π units, the longer alkyl chains not even being included. In view of the results obtained so far it is very doubtful whether eqns. (7/28) and (7/29) are in general suitable for the calculation of hydrophobicity parameters. A theoretical account of hydrophobic interactions is certainly of great importance; it requires, however, that changes in entropy are adequately taken into consideration, e.g., through a combination of quantum chemical and statistical mechanical approaches (e.g. [58—60]). Good results in describing or calculating π values can also be obtained with the solvent-dependent conformational analysis procedure (SCAP) [61] (see also chapter 12.). The advantage of SCAP is that the conformation is explicitly involved in the calculations, which is especially of importance in flexible molecules, where owing to intramolecular effects π may lose its additivity and eqn. (4/21) would then give rise to incorrect log P values (see also [62]).

A theoretical description of hydrophobicity within the context of a simple extra-thermodynamic approach should be confined to the calculation of hydrophobicity parameters and not lead to the replacement of π or analogous variables by more complicated expressions. Apart from possible problems with statistical degrees of freedom, it would no longer be feasible to gain information obtainable from relationships with π (e.g., the a_B rule), and the situation with a non-linear form of the function $f_h(x_h)$ would be extremely complicated. A direct use of theoretical descriptions of hydrophobic interactions cannot be dispensed with, however, in the more complex approaches to be discussed in chapter 12.

References

[1] Hansch, C., A. J. Leo, S. H. Unger, K. H. Kim, D. Nikaitani and E. J. Lien: J. Med. Chem. **16**, 1207 (1973)

[2] Unger, S. H., and C. Hansch: J. Med. Chem. **16**, 745 (1973)

[3] Craig, P. N.: J. Med. Chem. **14**, 680 (1971)

[4] Craig, P. N.: Advances Chem. Series **114**, 115 (1972)

[5] Leo, A. J., C. Hansch and C. Church: J. Med. Chem. **12**, 766 (1969)

[6] Topliss, J. G.: J. Med. Chem. **15**, 1066 (1972)

[7] Hansch, C.: Cancer Chemotherapy Reports **Part 1**, **56**, 433 (1972)

[8] Hansch, C., S. H. Unger and A. B. Forsythe: J. Med. Chem. **16**, 1217 (1973)

[9] Wootton, R., R. Cranfield, G. C. Sheppey and P. J. Goodford: J. Med. Chem. **18**, 607 (1975)

[10] Hansch, C., in J. A. Keverling Buisman (Ed.): Biological Activity and Chemical Structure, Pharmacochemistry Library (Eds.: W. Th. Nauta and R. F. Rekker), Vol. 2, Elsevier, Amsterdam, 1977, pp. 47 and 287

[11] Purcell, W. P.: Eur. J. Med. Chem. **10**, 335 (1975)

[12] Martin, Y. C.: Drug Design Methods — A Critical Introduction, Marcel Dekker, New York, 1978

[13] Martin, Y. C., in E. J. Ariens (Ed.): Drug Design, Vol. VIII, Academic Press, New York, 1980, p. 47

[14] Martin, Y. C., and H. N. Panas: J. Med. Chem. **22**, 784 (1979)

[15] Unger, S. H., in E. J. Ariens (Ed.): Drug Design, Vol. IX, Academic Press, New York, 1980, p. 47

[16] Franke, R., in A. Simkin (Ed.): Medicinal Chemistry VI, Cotswold Press, Oxford, 1979, p. 237

[17] Streich, J., S. Dove and R. Franke: J. Med. Chem. **23**, 1452 (1980)

[18] Dove, S., J. Streich and R. Franke: J. Med. Chem. **23**, 1456 (1980)

[19] Mager, P. P.: EDV in Medizin und Biologie **10**, 83 (1979)

[20] Tichý, M.: Internat. J. Quantum Chem. **26**, 509 (1979)

[21] Yoshimoto, M., C. Hansch and P. Y. C. Jow: Chem. Pharm. Bull. **23**, 437 (1975)

[22] Silipo, C., and C. Hansch: J. Am. Chem. Soc. **97**, 6849 (1975)

[23] Silipo, C., and C. Hansch: J. Med. Chem. **19**, 62 (1976)

[24] Yoshimoto, M., and C. Hansch: J. Med. Chem. **19**, 71 (1976)

[25] Hansch, C., and D. F. Calef: J. Org. Chem. **41**, 1240 (1976)

[26] Fukunaga, J. Y., C. Hansch and E. E. Steller: J. Med. Chem. **19**, 605 (1976)

[27] Hansch, C., J. Y. Fukunaga and P. Y. C. Jow: J. Med. Chem. **20**, 96 (1977)

[28] Hansch, C., R. N. Smith, A. Rockoff, D. F. Calef, P. Y. C. Jow and J. Y. Fukunaga: Arch. Biochem. Biophys. **183**, 383 (1977)

[29] Dietrich, S. W., R. N. Smith, S. Brendler and C. Hansch: Arch. Biochem. Biophys. **194**, 612 (1979)

[30] Grieco, C., C. Hansch, C. Silipo, R. N. Smith, A. Vittoria and K. Yamada: Arch. Biochem. Biophys. **194**, 542 (1979)

[31] Dietrich, S. W., J. M. Blaney, M. A. Reynolds, P. Y. C. Jow and C. Hansch: J. Med. Chem. **23**, 1205 (1980)

[32] Koppel, J. A.: Reaktionsfähigkeit organischer Verbindungen **2**, 26 (1965)

[33] Palm, V. A.: Grundlagen der quantitativen Theorie organischer Reaktionen, Akademie-Verlag, Berlin, 1971

[34] Cramer, R. D.: J. Am. Chem. Soc. **102**, 1837 (1980)

[35] Cramer, R. D.: J. Am. Chem. Soc. **102**, 1849 (1980)

[36] Cramer, R. D., in J. C. Dearden (Ed.): Quantitative Approaches to Drug Design, Pharmacochemistry Library (Eds.: W. Th. Nauta and R. F. Rekker), Vol. 6, Elsevier, Amsterdam, 1983, p. 3

[37] Franke, R., in R. Franke and P. Oehme (Eds.): Quantitative Structure — Activity Analysis, Akademie-Verlag, Berlin, 1978

[38] Franke, R., S. Dove and R. Kühne: Eur. J. Med. Chem. **14**, 363 (1979)

[39] Franke, R., and R. Kühne: unpublished results

[40] Swain, C. G., and E. C. Lupton: J. Am. Chem. Soc. **90**, 4328 (1968)

[41] Fujita, T.: Progr. Phys. Org. Chem., in press
[42] Hansch, C., in E. J. Ariens (Ed.): Drug Design, Vol. I, Academic Press, New York, 1971, p. 271
[43] Hansch, C., and E. W. Deutsch: Biochim. Biophys. Acta **112**, 381 (1966)
[44] Inonoue, S., A. Ogino, M. Kise, M. Kitano, M. Tsuchija and T. Fujita: Chem. Pharm. Bull. **22**, 2064 (1974)
[45] Lamb, D., and L. E. Harries: J. Amer. Pharm. Ass. **49**, 583 (1960)
[46] Kakemi, K., A. Arita, R. Hori and R. Konishi: Chem. Pharm. Bull. **15**, 1705 (1967)
[47] Druckrey, E., H. Schwarz and H. Leditschke: Chim. Ther. **7**, 188 (1972)
[48] Hansch, C.: J. Med. Chem. **11**, 920 (1968)
[49] Michel, H.-J., R. Franke and H. Willitzer in R. Franke, and P. Oehme (Eds.): Quantitative Structure — Activity Analysis, Akademie-Verlag, Berlin, 1978, p. 89
[50] Martin, Y. C., W. B. Martin and J. D. Taylor: J. Med. Chem. **18**, 883 (1975)
[51] Nishioka, T., T. Fujita, K. Kamoshita and M. Nakajima: Pesticide Biochem. Physiol. **7**, 107 (1977)
[52] Cammarata, A.: J. Med. Chem. **15**, 573 (1972)
[53] Rogers, K. S., and A. Cammarata: J. Med. Chem. **12**, 692 (1969)
[54] Rogers, K. S., and A. Cammarata: Biochim. Biophys. Acta **193**, 22 (1969)
[55] Cammarata, A., and K. S. Rogers: J. Med. Chem. **14**, 269 (1971)
[56] Klopman, G., and R. F. Hudson: Theor. Chim. Acta **8**, 165 (1967)
[57] Klopman, G.: J. Am. Chem. Soc. **90**, 223 (1968)
[58] Zahradnick, R., in M. Tichý (Ed.): Quantitative Structure — Activity Relationships, Akadémiai Kiadó, Budapest, 1976
[59] Zahradnick, R.: Proceedings of the 9th Annual Meeting of the Biochemical Society of the GDR, VEB Verlag Volk und Gesundheit, Berlin, 1977
[60] Zahradnick, R., P. Hobza, and S. Slanina: Collect. Czechoslov. Chem. Commun. **40**, 799 (1975)
[61] Hopfinger, A. J., and R. D. Battershell: J. Med. Chem. **19**, 569 (1976)
[62] Parker, G. R., T. L. Lemke and E. C. Moore: J. Med. Chem. **26**, 1221 (1977)

8. Practical Aspects of Quantitative Structure. – Activity Analysis by the Extrathermodynamic Approach (Hansch Analysis)

It is relatively easy to derive QSARs which yield a good description of biological potency in terms of drug properties *within* a training series. The ultimate objective of QSARs, however, is prediction, and a high descriptive power does by no means automatically guarantee predictive power. The predictive power of QSARs depends on the amount of information extractable from the data of the training series. Since even the most sophisticated QSAR cannot extract more information than is actually present the information content of the data is one of the most crucial factors for a successful QSAR analysis.

For a high information content the data must reflect the true relationship between biological potency and chemical structure completely, straightforwardly and unambiguously. Therefore, the selection of representative congeners for training series is of primary importance. These congeners must span a sufficiently large range of *all* properties governing biological potency within search space. The influence of properties not sufficiently represented cannot be detected and the resulting QSAR would consequently lead to false predictions for all compounds which differ in these properties from those in the training series. An example of this type has recently been reported by Lambrecht et al. [1] who showed that a QSAR prediction made by Lien et al. [2] of the affinity of two quaternary esters for the muscarinic receptor was not correct. The reason was that certain steric effects not varied within the training series considered by Lien et al. and, therefore, not reflected in the resulting QSAR obviously became a dominant factor in the new analogues.

It is, of course, not easy to hypothesize in an *a priori* QSAR analysis which properties will be important for biological potency. A good strategy to apply in such cases is always to start with pilot studies of small sets of compounds in an attempt to derive very simple models in a first step. These models can then aid in directing further studies during which they are refined until, eventually, a "fine tuned" QSAR is obtained and the search space exhausted. Existing QSARs for the biological effect considered may be quite helpful here. It is not the prediction of a supercompound in a dramatic overnight discovery but rather the systematic application of such stepwise strategies which will manifest the power of QSARs as a tool for the rational design of better and new drugs. Good examples demonstrating how in a process of QSAR based stepwise model building and interactive testing and refining of hypotheses the space of important properties can be systematically built up and explored may be found, for example, in the work of Zeelen et al. [3–5] (progestational lynestrenol derivatives), Unger et al. [6, 7] (cardioselective non-depressive β-blockers) and Cramer et al. [8] (pyranenamine anti-allergy compounds). The first and very important step in any rational QSAR approach is the design of an optimal training series.

8.1. Composition and Design of Training Series

Two basically different situations may be encountered in exploring a lead compound:
1. biological testing is quicker than chemical synthesis;
2. chemical synthesis is quicker than biological testing.

In the first situation the data from biological experiments make it possible to build up training series in a stepwise manner using biological information in each step. Use can be made here of certain heuristic search strategies to be discussed later (see 11.). In the second case a training series must be selected prior to biological experiments; this situation is usually referred to as a "batch situation".

The series must be designed such that a maximum of information can be obtained with the minimum of compounds. This will ensure a good basis to evaluate meaningful QSARs and, at the same time, prevent unnecessary syntheses. Therefore, the importance of a proper training series design cannot be emphasized too strongly (see also [7, 9—25]).

In an optimal training series *all* important physicochemical and structural properties governing biological activity must be varied *systematically* and *independently* from each other over a *sufficiently large range*. This means that the analogues comprising a training series must be selected in such a way that the variances (see 15.) of hydrophobic, electronic and steric molecular parameters are maximized and, at the same time, collinearities between these parameters are minimized. The analogues must, furthermore, span a sufficiently large part of the parameter space with sufficiently large and about equal distances between them within this space. This is important not only for the extrathermodynamic approach but also for other QSAR methods which can use extrathermodynamic molecular parameters as, for instance, discriminant analysis (9.2.2.).

There are various approaches to the selection of substituents for an optimal training series. Of particular simplicity is a *two-dimensional design*. If it is presumed that log A depends on not more than two molecular parameters (e.g., π and σ), all potential substituents can be represented as points in a coordinate system with the corresponding molecular parameters as coordinates (two-dimensional parameter space). Substituents are then selected in such a way that the distances between the corresponding points are about equal and that the whole space (all four quadrants) is covered. In order to avoid collinearity care must be taken, furthermore, that the points selected do not fall onto a straight line [9].

When more then two molecular parameters are to be considered, *mathematical selection methods* become necessary. All of these methods start from a presentation of all accessible substituents or analogues (*starting set*) in parameter space (cartesian coordinate system with molecular parameters as axes). Usually, the variables are used in a standardized form (see eqn. (8/40)) in order to eliminate influences due to scaling. The task now is to select substituents (points) in such a way that the distance between them is sufficiently large and that the whole space is covered in about equal-distant steps. Such substituents are then thought to fulfil sufficiently well the requirements mentioned above. As will be seen, however, the outcome of the selection procedure is dependent on the method applied. Several such methods are available.

From a purely mathematical point of view D-*optimal design* techniques (see e.g., [7, 26—28]) seem to be appropriate here. These techniques are very effective in avoiding collinearities. They tend, however, to select mainly points representing the extremes of substituents from the boundary region of the parameter space considered. As a consequence, the condition of a systematic variation of molecular parameters over the whole space may not always be sufficiently fulfilled. D-optimal design is based on maximizing the determinant of the parameter covariance matrix which may involve an enormous amount of calculations for any *ab initio* design so that this design technique cannot be recommended for this purpose. For "constrained" design problems, for example, extension of an already existing set of analogues by a limited number of additional compounds, however, stepwise procedures are available which seem to be quite effective [7].

Another possibility for series selection is to consider directly Euclidean distances in parameter space as in the methods proposed by HANSCH and co-workers [14] and by WOOTTON et al. [15]. The method applied by HANSCH is based on *cluster analysis* of substituent points. Clusters of points are obtained in such a way that the similarity of substituents with respect to all molecular parameters considered is maximal within each cluster and minimal among the clusters. Using four different parameter sets (π^2, π, $\mathfrak{F}$, $\mathfrak{R}$ and MR; π^2, π, $\mathfrak{F}$, $\mathfrak{R}$; π, $\mathfrak{F}$, $\mathfrak{R}$, MR; π, $\mathfrak{F}$, $\mathfrak{R}$) such an analysis was performed for 90 aromatic substituents [14]. An analogous investigation was carried out by MARTIN for aliphatic substituents in a parameter space with the coordinates σ^*, E_S, MR and π [18]. A good selection of substituents for a representative test series will result if substituents from different clusters are chosen.

The method of WOOTTON et al. is based on a stepwise procedure ("*multidimensional mapping*") where that substituent is selected in each step which is closest to the centre of gravity of all hitherto selected points in parameter space but further apart than a pre-set minimal Euclidian distance, D_{Min}. The first step is to chose a suitable starting substituent (e.g., hydrogen). Next, the Euclidian distances from this starting point to all other substituent points are computed, and the second substituent is selected as that closest in parameter space after deleting all substituents falling into the distance range defined by D_{Min}. The third substituent is the one closest to the centre of gravity in space of the two points already selected while ensuring that the distance to either is larger than D_{Min}. The procedure is continued systematically until the parameter space is exhausted and the desired number of substituents found; this number is adjusted by chosing an appropriate value of D_{Min}.

Both methods will yield series with high variances of molecular parameters and a well-spanned parameter space, and have proven to be of practical value [e.g., 21, 29–32]. However, collinearities are not necessarily minimized, although test series selected by these techniques are definitely better in this respect than random selections (see Table 8.1). This led us to develop what we have called the PCMM *technique* [24, 33]. PCMM is a combination of **p**rincipal **c**omponent analysis and **m**ultidimensional **m**apping and starts from the fact that a hyperplane can be fitted to substituent points in parameter space if multiple collinearities are present. The fit will be the better the stronger are the collinearities. Collinearities are mainly due to those points which are close to the hyperplane so that they could be eliminated by simply deleting such points. In order to do that without losing too much of the information contained in the corresponding region of parameter space the substituents are divided into two sets in a first step. Set 1 contains the points close to and set 2 the objects distant from the hyperplane as judged by Euclidian distances between the objects and the plane. These distances are computed with the help of principal component analysis. To each of the two sets the

Table 8.1. Values of D_S and V_S (see text) for training series[1]) selected from a starting set of 90 substituents [14] (parameter space: π, $\mathfrak{F}$, $\mathfrak{R}$, MR) by different methods (from [24])

Selection method	D_S[2])	V_S[2])
from clusters	0.370	1.668
multidimensional mapping	0.613	2.146
PCMM method	0.825	1.750
random	0.434	0.833

[1]) ten analogues
[2]) mean values from ten selections

multidimensional mapping technique of Wootton et al. [15] is now applied separately in such a way that a higher percentage of compounds is selected from set 2. In doing that the possibility must be considered that the hyperplane changes its position during the selection procedure. In order to account for this possibility an automatic stepwise iteration procedure is used where the position of the hyperplane is adjusted after each step.

Table 8.1 compares two quality criteria for training series selected from the starting set used by Hansch et al. [14] (90 substituents, parameter space: π, $\mathfrak{F}$, $\mathfrak{R}$ and MR) by four different techniques:

- stochastic selection from the clusters presented in [14],
- multidimensional mapping according to Wootton et al. [15],
- PCMM method [24],
- random selection.

The quality criteria are the determinant of the correlation matrix, D_S, as a measure of multiple collinearities and the variance coefficient, V_S, as a measure of data variance. The latter is defined as

$$V_S = \frac{1}{m} \sum_{i=1}^{m} s_{is}^2 / s_{ip}^2 \tag{8/1}$$

where m = dimensionality of parameter space (number of variables considered), s_{is}^2 = variance of the i-th variable within the training series and s_{ip}^2 = variance of the i-th variable within the starting set. Equation (8/1) can be regarded as a measure of the "information content" of a training series in terms of data variance as compared with the starting set; it becomes unity if both variances are equal. The determinant D_S converges to zero as collinearities increase and becomes unity if collinearities are completely absent. Good training series should have high values of D_S and V_S.

Table 8.1. shows that all three design techniques yield series with high data variance (V_S values), but only the PCMM technique effectively minimizes collinearities (D_S values). Randomly selected series are — as was to be expected — very far from being optimal (low data variance and high collinearities) and cannot be considered representative. Clearly, a careful selection of training series by an appropriate series design technique is indispensable.

The PCMM technique seems to be the method of choice, but for not too large starting sets (less than 50 substituents) a much simpler method turned out to have specific advantages. This method is based on the two-dimensional mapping of intra-class correlation matrices and is called the TMIC *method* [23, 25, 33]. The intra-class correlation coefficient, $r_{I(A,B)}$, for two substituents A and B is defined as

$$r_{(IA,B)} = 2 \sum_{i=1}^{m} (z_{iA} - \bar{z})(z_{iB} - \bar{z}) / \sum_{i=1}^{m} [(z_{iA} - \bar{z})^2 + (z_{iB} - z)^2] \quad (8/2)$$

with

$$\bar{z} = \frac{1}{2m} \sum_{i=1}^{m} (z_{iA} + z_{iB})$$

and

$$-1 \leqq r_{I(A,B)} \leqq 1$$

and characterizes the relatedness of the two substituents A and B with respect to m standardized (see eqn. (8/40)) variables z_i. Computation of intra-class correlation coefficients for all pairs of substituents yields an intra-class correlation matrix which can be decomposed by the principal component method (see 8.4.1.). All substituents of the starting set can then be represented in the two-dimensional cartesian space spanned by the first two components[1]). As a result a simple two-dimensional map of substituents is obtained. Such a map is shown in Fig. 8.1. It was obtained by applying TMIC to the starting set also considered by Wootton et al. [15] (parameter space: π, $\mathfrak{F}$, $\mathfrak{R}$ and MR). Substituents similar with respect to these molecular parameters are clustered together, and this clustering is chemically reasonable and in general agreement (although not strictly comparable) with the clusters obtained by Hansch and co-workers [14]. The advantage of the map in Fig. 8.1 as compared to the Hansch clusters is that the exact position of each substituent in space is known.

A good training series with high data variance and low collinearities can now be obtained by simple inspection. Substituents distant from each other are selected in such a way that the whole space is systematically covered. In addition, the inclusion of pairs of points which have a symmetrical position with respect to the origin of the coordinate system is to be avoided. The TMIC method is about as powerful as the PCMM method. It has the advantage not only of being very simple but also gives a clear representation of the full data structure in a way which is close to the usual way of thinking of organic chemists.

As already pointed out, the importance of an appropriate training series design cannot be overestimated. This has also been stressed by Hansch [16]: "Such a systematic procedure is central to the task of reducing costs in research by maximizing the information obtained from each molecular probe in a set of congeners. If QSAR accomplishes nothing more than to get chemists to take a more thoughtful and logical attitude in derivatizing a lead compound, it will have made an important contribution." Hansch [16] mentioned an example where a poor selection of substituents led to the unnecessary synthesis of a great number of substances, and Unger [34] demonstrated for a series of 104 antimalarias that the same information could have been obtained with a series of only ten properly selected analogues. This means that synthesis and testing amounting to at least 300.000 dollars has simply been wasted. According to an estimate made by Martin [21], the use of training series design strategies decreases the average number of analogues required to investigate one physical property from eleven to four; this corresponds to a 2.75-fold increase in the information gained per compound synthesized.

---

1) Provided that these two components account for a sufficiently large part of data variance (not less than 70%). This, however, will usually be the case.

Although a good series design is indispensable and can indeed save hundreds of syntheses, it must not be forgotten that all series design methods have one critical point: the parameter space to be considered must be defined *a priori*. As already discussed, stepwise strategies starting with a small pilot series may be very helpful here. The pilot series can be designed using a small standard parameter space. A preliminary QSAR is then evaluated (see, e.g., [29]) which can aid in the design of the final training series in two ways:

1. The parameter space can be modified or extended, if necessary.
2. The synthesis of inactive compounds can be avoided.

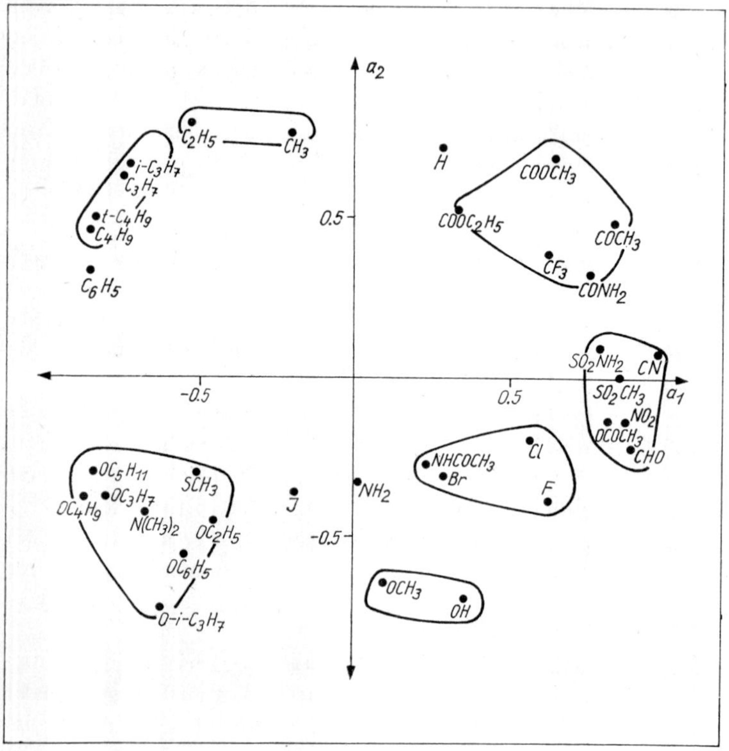

Fig. 8.1. Plot of 35 aromatic substituents in the space spanned by the first two principal components a_1 and a_2 extracted from the intra-class correlation matrix. Substituents and parameter space (π, $\mathfrak{F}$, $\mathfrak{R}$, MR) are the same as in [15]

Such an approach is always to be recommended but it is not strictly necessary. Fortunately, the space spanned by the usual hydrophobic, electronic and steric molecular parameters (for example, π, $\mathfrak{F}$, $\mathfrak{R}$ and MR) will lead to acceptable training series in most cases.

If substituents in more than one position are to be varied and positional dependencies of substituent effects are to be expected a good first step is a FREE-WILSON analysis (see 11.1.). This can be done with a first small sample of compounds in which three or four substituents are varied for each position of interest. Two of these substituents should be of average hydrophobicity and of limited size but vary greatly in their electronic properties, and the third substituent should be large and strongly hydrophobic. With the result of the FREE-WILSON analysis the most important position(s) can be identified; a selection of eight to ten additional substituents for this (these) position(s) is then made by means of one of the series design methods discussed in this chapter. Substituents in not so important positions are held constant and are selected as the most active according to the FREE-WILSON result.

Most important in series design is to account for synthetic feasibility. In TMIC alternative test series can easily be selected from the map, and the same is true for the HANSCH clusters. With WOOTTONS multidimensional mapping and the PCMM method it is always advisable to produce a set of alternative training series by simply varying the starting substituent; this is no problem since one computer run of these programs requires only a few seconds. Since synthetic feasibility may require quite different selections of substituents for different classes of chemical compounds, each training series usually poses a new design problem. This is also true because of the possibly different parameter spaces to be considered in different problems. Attempts to propose general sets of substituents for training series (see e.g., [35]) are, therefore, of only limited value.

8.2. Formulation of Equations, Search for the "Best" Equation(s) and Interpretation

A great many different types of interactions between drugs and biosystems are possible, and changes in biological potency with structural variations may be related to a variety of different mechanisms. Just as numerous are the possible hypotheses to explain these interactions and the resultant approaches. The situation may be further complicated if the training series to be considered was not properly designed. A catalogue of hypotheses may be derived from:

- already existing QSARs,
- knowledge and ideas of properties of the biosystem under investigation,
- assumptions on possible reaction mechanisms,
- knowledge and ideas of the properties of the compounds,
- type of the structural variations in the training series.

Special attention should be paid to the question whether metabolic processes may play such an important rôle that they determine decisively biological activity. If metabolic inactivation is to be expected, one should search for a function that expresses the dependence of biological activity on the rate of metabolism and the dependence of both on molecular properties. Experience in this area is scarce. It seems likely that in certain cases the QSAR approaches described here will be able to cope with such a situation since both the rate of metabolism and biological activity are functions of molecular parameters. It is, on the other hand, also possible that drugs must become metabolically activated (*bioactivation*) before they can produce a biological effect. Occurrence of bioactivation may be anticipated to a certain extent by chemical reasoning and experience in the field of biology. If it is, for example, suspected that a molecule A may be metabolically converted into a structure B, all of the following variants must be considered and included in the catalogue of hypotheses for a quantitative structure-activity analysis if more detailed information is not available:

1. Molecule A is the biologically active form (biological potency depends on the properties of A).
2. Molecule B is the biologically active form, and the bioactivation step is not rate limiting (biological activity depends on the properties of B).
3. Molecule B is biologically active but the bioactivation step becomes rate limiting (biological potency depends on the equilibrium or on the rate of conversion of A into B, and, hence, on the properties of A).

Variants 1 and 3 would require a quantitative structure-activity analysis with molecular parameters for A, whilst with variant 2 molecular parameters for B should be employed.

As already discussed (see 5.1.), an example of this type is provided by biologically active phenylsydnones where QSARs led to the conclusion that the inhibition of multifunctional microsomal oxidase is probably due to the intact compounds (case 1) whereas a toxic effect also observed with these compounds requires bioactivation to give the toxic nitrosoamino acids as cleavage products [35a] (case 2, see eqn. (5/106)). An example of case 3 is provided by the work of Hanzlik et al. [35b] who showed that the hepatotoxicity of substituted thiobenzamides follows a strict Hammett-type relationship describing a critical S-oxidative bioactivation. Another case in point are QSARs evaluated for the carcinogenic and enzyme (aryl hydrocarbon hydroxylase: AHH) inducing potency of polycyclic aromatic hydrocarbons [35c—g]. In agreement with biochemical evidence, the final results clearly showed that the hydrocarbons have to become bioactivated in a first step and that their potency as carcinogens as well as AHH inducers critically depends on their ability to undergo this bioactivation. It became evident, furthermore, that the critical bioactivation step, depending on the chemical reactivity and hydrophobicity of the hydrocarbons, is basically the same but different in some details for both processes. This led to the hypothesis that bioactivation is due to a reaction with constitutive AHH in the case of AHH induction and with induced AHH in the case of carcinogenesis, thus indicating a close connection between these two processes. The QSAR work was based on the assumption that the critical regions in the hydrocarbons for chemical reactions to occur are the most reactive double bond (K region) and the most reactive pair of para-positions (L region) according to the K-L-region theory of the Pullmans (e.g., [35h, i]). Later evidence then showed that the ultimate carcinogen may be produced through metabolic conversion not at the K region but at the so-called bay region [35j, k]. It seems, however, that the reactivities of the K and the bay regions are closely interrelated [35i] so that the results obtained are also compatible with the bay region theory.

From what has been said above, it follows that approaches to quantitative structure-activity analysis may be extremely complex and thus may require a great many equations to be calculated. If there is access to a large computer, this will not be a problem. All possible equations (possible combinations of molecular parameters) can be generated automatically through special computer programs such as the automatic quantitative structure-activity relationships finder (AQSARF-program), which has been utilized by Tollenaere et al. [36] and permits approximately 17 equations to be calculated per second on an IBM 370/135 computer. It is a matter of efficiency to compute regression coefficients solely for statistically significant correlations. These can be filtered out by a simple and rapid statistical test (see, e.g., [37]); with a modern high speed computer 10^5 correlations can be screened in a few minutes. The search for and the selection of the "best" equation(s) from the possibly very large computer outprint generated in this way may, however, present problems and be very time consuming. To circumvent this difficulty and, if necessary, to reduce computing time when a slower computer is employed, one can choose from several possible procedures.

To begin with, the catalogue of hypotheses is not worked through completely but by planned phases. Care should be taken that this mode of operation does not end in a random curtialment of the catalogue. Several of the examples discussed (see, e.g., eqns. (5/135), (5/153)—(5/155), (7/1)—(7/3)) clearly indicate how hazardous this can be. The knowledge acquired at one state is then utilized for the formulation of the approach to the subsequent stage. Such a stepwise procedure, which is particularly suitable for a dialogue with the computer, corresponds to a decision-making process involving a series of "if-then" decisions and permits an essential reduction in the number of equations to be calculated. A very nice example of how a well designed QSAR-based hypothesis testing may lead to valid conclusions after investigating only a very small number of cleverly selected analogues is provided by the work of Zeelen and colleagues [3—5] on lynestrenol derivatives. In trying to improve progestational activity, substituents were varied in the 11-β position starting with a very small pilot series comprising only four substituents (H, F, Cl, CH_3). A simple correlation with E_S was obtained indicating a steric effect:

$$\log A = -0.94E_S + 1.25 \qquad (8/3)$$

$$n = 4 \qquad r = 0.97 \qquad s = 0.32$$

Next the question was raised whether this steric effect reflects substituent-receptor interactions or whether it operates indirectly via a distortion of the steroid skleleton leading to a change in shape. Synthesis and testing of only one carefully selected analogue was sufficient to indicate that the latter was the case. In the next step the influence of hydrophobicity and of substituent shape was examined by including four additional derivatives into the series (substituents: C_2H_5, CH_3O, n-C_3H_7, n-C_4H_9) resulting in the following equation (E_S^+: modified E_S scale with E_S for hydrogen equal to zero):

$$\log A = -1.46E_S^+ - 0.14\,\mathrm{MR} + 1.97 \qquad (8/4)$$

$$n = 8 \qquad r = 0.91 \qquad s = 0.34$$

Hydrophobicity showed no effect, but the substituent bulkiness (MR term) turned out to be of importance in that substituents which stick out too far at the 11-β-position interfere with receptor binding. Thus, quite a clear picture of the factors governing activity was obtained after studying a very small set of cleverly selected compounds. It was concluded that potent derivatives of lynestrenol will result when the substituents induce a certain amount of bowing of the steroid skeleton without increasing too much the bulk of the molecules. This prediction could be verified experimentally and led to a very promising compound as a new contraceptive agent.

There exists no generally valid concept for defining the single steps of such stepwise strategies. Experience plays a major rôle here, and allowance must be made for the particular features of the problem under investigation. Fundamentally, one should always ascertain through chemical and biological reasoning which of the many possible molecular parameter combinations are most likely connected with biological potency. Less likely candidates are then tested throughout the whole process at appropriate stages by computing specially selected equations.

Especially if the training series has not been selected according to the principles dealt with in 8.1., a *factor analysis*, to be performed before the virtual regression analysis is to be recommended [38]. With this approach it is possible to single out promising equations and to avoid collinearities. As this is a practicable and relatively easy method, it will be discussed in somewhat greater detail elsewhere (see 8.4.).

A third possibility to simplify matters consists in the application of *stepwise regression techniques* (see, e.g., [18]) during which statistically non-significant variables are automatically eliminated. These techniques may work in a step-up (significant variables included successively in the computation) or step-down (non-significant variables eliminated successively) manner; both principles may also be combined in a process called forward elimination. It should be noted that the equation thus obtained is not the only possible, that is to say, objectively correct result, as variants on the procedure adopted may lead to differences in outcome. A finishing touch by calculating selected equations on the basis of fixed statements is, therefore, recommended. This limitation does not apply if step-up and step-down procedures afford the same equation.

Efficiency can also be improved markedly by breaking down the whole problem into subproblems, each referring to a given subgroup of compounds which share a structural feature, such as the variation of substituents in only one position, the cis- or trans-position of a certain group, substitution or non-substitution, mono- or polysubstitution in a certain position, etc. These subgroups are essentially less complex than the series as a whole so that it is possible to formulate simpler approaches and to obtain more exact information on the effects of the substituents at different position of substitution. With this information a more rational approach to the analysis of the entire series becomes possible, thereby reducing the complexity of the overall problem. This is particularly true if the substituent effects strongly depend on position. In this case, FREE-WILSON analysis can also be applied as a preprocessing step resulting in position-related *de novo* contributions of the substituents to biological activity in the case of polysubstituted molecules. As explained in 11.1.3., such contributions can in turn be correlated with molecular parameters.

If QSARs for variations at each separate site of substitution in the molecule are known, it is easy to recognize additivity or position-dependence for each molecular parameter and thus to combine individual equations obtained from the subproblems into more general relationships. In so doing it is often possible to account for differences among subgroups through so-called *indicator variables* some examples of which have already been presented in preceding sections. If irrespective of any other variations differences between two subgroups I and II would lead to a constant difference in $\log A$ and if $\log A$ in the two subgroups can be described by a simple linear dependence on, for example, π, two parallel straight lines with different intercepts will result according to:

$$\log A_{\mathrm{I}} = a\pi + b_{\mathrm{I}} \tag{8/5}$$

$$\log A_{\mathrm{II}} = a\pi + b_{\mathrm{II}} \tag{8/6}$$

These can be combined into one relationship with the help of an indicator variable, I, according to the following equation:

$$\log A = a\pi + \alpha I + b \tag{8/7}$$

where:

$$I = \begin{cases} 1 \text{ for compounds of subgroup I} \\ 0 \text{ for compounds of subgroup II} \end{cases} \tag{8/8}$$

The coefficient α in eqn. (8/7) can be fitted by regression analysis to give exactly the difference in the intercepts

$$\alpha = b_{\mathrm{I}} - b_{\mathrm{II}} \tag{8/9}$$

and according to the definition of the indicator variable this difference is then added to all points belonging to (8/5). In this way these points are shifted to the straight line represented by (8/6) so that both lines are united. This principle is, of course, also applicable to n-dimensional coordinate systems (equations with n variables). Furthermore, it is also possible to combine through indicator variables more than two subgroups.

A case in point is eqn. (8/10), which describe the antibacterial activity of lyndomycin derivatives against *S. lutea* [39]:

$$\log A = -0.24\pi^2 + 1.39\pi + 0.23 I_1 - 0.20 I_2 - 0.41 \tag{8/10}$$

$$n = 25 \qquad r = 0.960 \qquad s = 0.162$$

The indicator variables I_1 and I_2 distinguish, respectively, between cis- ($I_1 = 0$) and trans-substituted ($I_1 = 1$) and between N-methyl ($I_2 = 0$) and N-ethyl ($I_2 = 1$) derivatives. It follows from eqn. (8/10) that trans-compounds are about 1.7 times more active than the corresponding cis-compounds, while N-ethyl derivatives are about 1.6 times less active than the corresponding N-methyl derivatives. Another example of interest is to be found in a QSAR for the inhibition of dihydrofolate reductase from two different tumours by structurally quite different phenyltriazines (structure XXXVa, [40]):

$$\log A = 0.68\pi_3 - 0.12\pi_3{}^2 + 0.23\,\mathrm{MR}_4 - 0.02\,\mathrm{MR}_4{}^2 + 0.24 I_1$$
$$- 2.53 I_2 - 1.99 I_3 + 0.88 I_4 + 0.69 I_5 + 0.70 I_6 + 6.49 \tag{8/11}$$

$$n = 244 \qquad r = 0.923 \qquad s = 0.377$$

(the subscripts on the molecular parameters π and MR refer to the corresponding positions of substitution). In this case, as much as 76% of the variance of $\log A$ is explained by the indicator variables. While I_2—I_6 indicate the presence or absence of certain structural elements, a novel aspect is associated with I_1, namely the distinction between enzymes isolated from different sources (Walker tumours and murine leucaemia L 1210). It is thus possible to incorporate data on the inhibition by either enzyme into one equation. In a similar way, Martin [18] was able to combine QSARs for five different biological activities of barbiturates into a single equation.

As will be discussed later (see 11.), the use of indicator variables in a Hansch-type analysis amounts to a mixture of the extrathermodynamic approach and Free-Wilson analysis. Although indicator variables have proved to be very useful they should always be applied with care in order not to violate statistics or to end up with an equation of doubtful validity.

Indicator variables can also be linked with other variables in a multiplicative manner, as in eqn. (8/12), which was developed by HANSCH et al. for the inhibition of dihydrofolate reductase by quinazolines (structure XXXV b) [37]:

$$\log A = 0.810\,\mathrm{MR}_6 - 0.064\,\mathrm{MR}_6^2 + 0.775\pi_5 - 0.734 I_1 - 2.145 I_2 - 0.544 I_3 - 1.395 I_4 + 0.776 I_6 - 0.197 I_1\,\mathrm{MR}_6 + 4.924 \qquad (8/12)$$

$$n = 101 \qquad r = 0.961 \qquad s = 0.441$$

The indices refer to different positions of substitution, and the indicator variables I_1—I_6 characterize certain structural features. I_1 is defined as:

$$I_1 = \begin{cases} 1, \text{ if OH or SH is present} \\ 0, \text{ if not} \end{cases} \qquad (8/13)$$

It follows from the negative sign of the I_1 term that the presence of OH or SH has an unfavourable influence on biological activity. The negative cross-product $I_1\,\mathrm{MR}_6$ should be interpreted as implying that this influence becomes stronger as the substituents in the 6-position increase in bulk.

The first step in a HANSCH type QSAR analysis is to collect the values of the molecular parameters x_i needed to calculate all the equations. To facilitate a routine application it is recommended that the major molecular parameters such as π, f, $\log P$, E_S, MR, L, B_1, B_4, σ, σ^-, σ^+, σ_I, σ^*, $\mathfrak{F}$ and $\mathfrak{R}$ for the largest possible number of substituents be stored in a computer. It is essential that only fully reliable and compatible values should be used. The required x_i values are simply ordered from the computer, thereby saving a good deal of time and expense. Subsequently, the x_i values along with $\log A$ are processed by rows for each compounds of the training series to yield what may be called a *master file*. Activity data from different biological tests can be simultaneously included. Fed into the computer, the master file is a table of values in the form of a matrix with n rows and m columns, n being the number of compounds in the training series and m the total number of variables (inclusive of $\log A$). The formulation of equations to be calculated is achieved by selecting the columns to be included via variable selection vectors. In addition, the functional connections between the molecular parameters accounted for by these columns and $\log A$ are also defined. Subgroups can be formed through a selection of rows from the master file using row selection vectors. Variable and row selection vectors can be combined to problem vectors, each defining an equation. The computer then computes the regression coefficients and statistical data for all equations.

At least the following information should appear in the computer output for each problem vector:

1. regression coefficients with confidence intervals at an adjustable significance level (usually $P = 0.95$),
2. for each regression coefficient the significance level at which it differs from zero,
3. F value and significance level for the overall equation,

4. multiple correlation coefficient r as well as r^2,
5. s (residual error),
6. a tabulation of the log A values (with confidence intervals) — calculated with the aid of the respective regression equations — versus the input values. It is desirable that for each compound the difference log A (calculated) minus log A (input) as well as the deviation in percent of the input value should also be indicated,
7. number of degrees of freedom,
8. correlation matrix,
9. for equations with a non-linear relationship between log A and any given parameter x_i, the x_i value with confidence interval belonging to the extremum.

In order to limit the printout to a manageable size it is advisable to suppress all equations which are statistically not significant at an adjustable significance level.

The selection of the "best" equation(s) is based on statistical criteria and biological as well as physicochemical considerations. From a statistical point of view, one should choose that equation which at a sufficient number of degrees of freedom has the lowest residual error, provided, of course, that all terms are significant. The question of how many degrees of freedom are needed is not so easy to answer. There are two entirely different aspects to be considered here, namely the number of variables *included* in a regression equation and the total number of variables *considered* in evaluating the equation as compared with the number of observations. The first aspect is adequately dealt with by the usual F- and t-statistics (see appendix). These criteria, however, only relate to variables in the final equation and do not take into account how many variables were actually screened for possible inclusion in the equation. The larger this number the greater is the possibility that a significant equation as judged by F- and t-statistics will occur purely by chance. For this reason some correlations will be less significant than their standard p-values indicate. This problem has been extensively investigated by TOPLISS et al. [41—43] who analysed the probability of obtaining a statistically significant "chance correlation" as a function of the number of observations and screened variables.

For example, the probability of encountering a chance correlation for five screened variables is about 22% for six observations, 10% for eight observations, 3% for ten observations and 1% for twelve observations [42]. The number of observations per screened variable necessary to avoid chance correlation at a certain level of probability decreases as the number of variables increases. The results presented in [42] provide guidelines for planning correlation studies in such a way that an unacceptable risk of chance correlations will not be present (note that the data presented in [41] are somewhat overexaggerated and have been corrected in [42]).

The work of TOPLISS has been misunderstood by many workers who did not fully realize the difference between "*variables screened for*" and "*variables included into*" a regression equation. As a result it was considered almost a dogma by many investigators that a meaningful QSAR should be based on at least five observations per variable included. This is, of course, not correct. The ratio "number of observations per variable included" will simply be reflected in F- and t-statistics and in the confidence intervals of regression coefficients and predicted values which increase as this ratio decreases. Therefore, this ratio has simply to be adjusted in such a way that the confidence intervals do not become too large and are acceptable with regard to the objective of the QSAR investigation. For practical purposes and at the beginning of an investigation, three onservations per variable included may be completely acceptable (see also [15]). The danger of running into chance correlations by too low a ratio of "observations per variable screened" is a completely different matter and has to be considered separately on the basis of Topliss' result.

In selecting the best equation(s), chemical and biological common sense are at least as important as statistical considerations. Even when statistically highly significant, equations not in line with well established experience should always be considered with suspicion. If, for example, an electronic σ term with a ϱ value of 1000 appeared in a QSAR this would be a clear indication that σ is either not the correct parameter in this case or that the relationship found is artificial since such high ϱ values are completely incompatible with what is known from physical organic chemistry. Caution is also in order if a QSAR seems to be in contrast with knowledge about the biological mechanism of action involved in the type of activity considered. In this case, however, one should always consider the possibility that the views held on this mechanism may not be completely right and that the QSAR does in fact provide a clue to the true mechanism or additional information. All other things being equal, finally, the most simple equation is to be accepted as a working model.

Compounds which do not fit the QSAR obtained and thus deviate from the behaviour of the other compounds of the training series are of special interest. There are many possible reasons for such deviations, for example, error in measurements or inadequate data handling; they may, however, be also indicative of a special mechanism of action (for a detailed discussion, see, e.g., [44]). It is the latter point which is of special importance since the investigation of outliers may lead to a deeper insight into drug action and may even allow one to arrive at new lead compounds [44—47]. Thus, outliers may provide very valuable information (Hansch called them "a blessing in disguise" [45]) so that the detection and follow up of outliers is another important aspect of the QSAR methodology.

If outliers are present the reason for their deviating behaviour should be explored and the analysis repeated with the outliers omitted. If the outliers are simply due to an inadequate parameter space it may be helpful to plot the deviations from the regression line versus several molecular parameters. If such plots show regularities, the outliers may then be fitted by appropriate changes of parameters; care is in order here, however, to allow only for such changes which are physically meaningful. It is, for example, always possible to bring any outlier onto the regression line by including an indicator variable. This is a highly questionable procedure and should be avoided unless there is a good reason to rationalize the indicator variable. An indicator variable accounting for the behaviour of, for example, only one substance has no meaning whatever and should never be used. If a larger percentage of the training series does not fit one can no longer speak of outliers. In such cases the QSAR analysis obviously was a failure and has to be repeated. Under no circumstances can a practice be accepted where a larger portion of compounds is omitted without any good reason in order to make the equation fit the data. This does not refer to dividing a series into subgroups as discussed above.

When the best equation(s) have been selected, certain mechanistic conclusions can be drawn from the molecular parameters present and from their relation with log A. It is always worthwhile then to consider not only the best equation(s) but also the general trend in their development. By this means, it is possible to find out which properties of the molecules or the substituents are of primary importance for biological activity and in what manner drug action is influenced. In many cases, this also furnishes much information on the mechanism of drug-receptor interactions, receptor properties and the molecular mechanisms of the biological reaction. If this is what is primarily aimed at, conclusions may often be refined by some additional computations with selected quantum-chemical molecular parameters. Needless to say, with such attempts at interpretation any collinearities between molecular parameters must be carefully taken into consideration. As stated above, they can limit or even entirely prevent interpretations. As a way-out one has to extend the sample in such a way that collinearities disappear. In general, this is rather easy, requiring no more than a few compounds, provided that their selection is strictly based on the outlines provided in 8.1. The compounds so added are tested as well and the analysis is repeated for the enlarged sample.

According to the ultimate objective of QSAR work, the best equation(s) are finally used to predict biological potencies of yet uninvestigated compounds in order to guide further syntheses and testing. Predictions can be made in a quantitative way by simply inserting the values of molecular parameters of the compounds of interest into the corresponding QSAR. Sometimes, however, such quantitative predictions may lead to an overestimation of the true power of QSARs. For practical purposes it is usually sufficient to reach at more or less qualitative conclusions as to which substituent should be introduced in order to enhance potency and whether the magnitude of potency increase to be expected is worth the experimental effort. Reliable predictions can only be made within or near the "*spanned substituent* (*or parameter*) *space*" (SSS) [45]. This means that predictions from Hansch type QSARs are mainly interpolations. At first glance this might be considered a severe limitation, but one must not forget that interpolation in a multi-parameter space is a very complicated matter and can result in a substantial increase in biological potency. Within a small range outside SSS (un-SSS) predictions are, however, also possible to a certain extent. Hansch [45] has compared a QSAR with a contour map of a certain area (SSS). Conclusions as to the contours outside this map (un-SSS) will be possible for the immediate surroundings but impossible for distant areas.

An example of a successful prediction in near un-SSS is provided by the work of Hansch [45, 48, 49] on the hydrolysis of esters of the types $R-C_6H_4-OCOCH_2NHCO-C_6H_5$ (A) and $R-C_6H_4-OCOCH_2NHSO_2CH_3$ (B) by papain. The following QSAR was obtained (K_m: Michaelis-Menten constant):

$$\log 1/K_m = 0.57\,\mathrm{MR} + 0.56\sigma - 1.92I + 3.74 \tag{8/14}$$

$$n = 20 \qquad r = 0.990 \qquad s = 0.148$$

with

$$I = \begin{cases} 1 \text{ for type A compounds} \\ 0 \text{ for type B compounds} \end{cases} \tag{8/15}$$

X-ray data of papain led to the hypothesis that the amide moiety of both sets of congeners would fall into a hydrophobic crevice. If so the difference between the two sets expressed by the indicator variable term in eqn. (8/14) should reflect the difference in hydrophobic binding which must then be related to the difference in π values of the two amide moieties. From this difference amounting to

$$\Delta\pi = \pi\,(NHCOC_6H_5) - \pi\,(NHSO_3CH_3) = 0.49 - 1.92 = -1.67 \qquad (8/16)$$

and the coefficient of the I term in eqn. (8/14) a slope of about 1.15 can be estimated from

$$-1.92/-1.67 = 1.15 \qquad (8/17)$$

for a π term describing hydrophobic binding of the amide moiety to the crevice of the enzyme. The predicted slope was confirmed after synthesizing and analyzing a set of esters in which the amide moiety was varied ($CH_3OCOCH_2NHCOC_6H_4{-}R'$):

$$\log 1/K_m = 1.01\pi + 1.46 \qquad (8/18)$$

$$n = 16 \qquad r = 0.981 \qquad s = 0.165$$

This example shows nicely how predictions in un-SSS should be combined with a subsequent extension of SSS. The further away one gets from SSS the less reliable predictions become. They may still, however, be useful if they are regarded as hypotheses which can be put to test.

If collinearities are present one may end up with more than one "best" equation leading to different conclusions and predictions with no means of deciding between them. In this case predictions must be carried out with all equations keeping in mind that different results can be obtained for one and the same compound. Two decisions are then possible. Synthetic work may be confined to compounds for which, using all equations, similar activities have been predicted. This course, although most probably correct, leads to loss of information and, in addition, there is the risk that the most active compounds remain undiscovered. It is more appropriate to propose such compounds for synthesis which, on the one hand, are likely to be active and, on the other hand, break down the collinearities. The compounds proposed are synthesized and tested, and the quantitative structure-activity analysis is repeated while including all data. The knowledge available from the first QSAR makes it possible to continue with a considerably restricted set of hypotheses or fewer theoretical approaches. The new analysis provides additional or more pertinent information (e.g., by eliminating collinearities or because of higher variances of molecular parameters or log A) which can be employed for further predictions. The interplay between quantitative structure-activity analysis, prediction and experiment is continued until the search space represented by the training series has been sufficiently covered or, in other words, until all possible information from that part of space has been obtained and the most active compounds have been found with sufficiently high probability. In certain cases the most active compounds may already be present in the training series so that no further enhancement of biological potency can be achieved. This will be quickly indicated by the resulting QSARs so that unnecessary syntheses can be avoided.

The above considerations refer to cases where only a single biological effect is under investigation. In practice, however, one frequently has to contend with several biological activities, which are investigated together, and as a result optimization of drug structures tends to become a multidimensional problem. This aspect will be discussed in more detail in chapter 13.

Computer storage of QSARs is recommended. As compared to test results obtained with individual compounds, QSARs represent extremely condensed information so that computer search in a QSAR data base can result in information of a higher quality and a more generalizing capacity. Especially HANSCH and co-workers [50—52] have been actively engaged in this field and obtained interesting results (as early as 1972 they had built up a computer-based collection of approximately 1000 QSARs describing the behaviour of some 15,000 compounds in various biological systems).

Numerous searches from a large variety of angles can be carried out in the context of stored QSARs. Particularly important aspects of this kind of work include:

1. comparison of QSARs of different series acting on the same biosystem.
2. comparison of QSARs of the same or several series acting on different biosystems,
3. comparison of QSARs for different stages of biological integration (e.g., enzyme/cell/organ/organism),
4. connection of structural elements or combinations of properties with biological response profiles.

All this results in the recognition of properties which are necessary or favourable for a certain biological activity and by condensing many QSARs a first stage of structure-activity-quality relationships can be reached (see also [7, 53]). Thus, compounds with a new structure may be designed which have exactly those properties that are indicated as important by the respective QSARs (first stage of lead generation). A simple example of what can be achieved provides the rule mentioned above that many CNS drugs have an optimal log P value of about 2 as far as their transport to the site of action is concerned. It is pertinent to ask if this rule, which emerged from QSARs of a fairly large number of different series, could also have been found without computer storage of QSARs. This would, of course, have been possible if the corresponding QSARs had been established at about the same time. It would, however, no longer be possible where thousands of QSARs are involved, those of interest being randomly dispersed in the (ever-increasing) total so that a computer cannot be dispensed with. Another example of this kind is eqn. (4/58), which is to be considered as a model equation for membrane perturbation.

Finally, one can detect empirically certain systematic features or rules through such searches, cf., the a_B rule theoretically derived in 4.2. could also be derived from computer stored information about all linear relationships between log A and π or log P. This example not only demonstrates how helpful this work is but also implies a satisfactory confirmation of the theoretical derivation.

The comparison of QSARs for various biosystems can provide information regarding selectivity as well as the choice of the most meaningful combinations of different biological tests. When various stages of biological integration are compared, it should furthermore be possible to differentiate structural influences on pharmacokinetic and pharmacodynamic processes.

The significance and utility of the storage of QSAR data cannot be overemphasized. With the acquisition of knowledge and the advent of new problems in drug research, viewpoints change all the time and the QSARs can thus yield decisive information. Showing an explosive growth, these relationships need re-sorting and re-selection whenever a new standpoint presents itself, and this cannot be done with the aid of manual methods.

The considerations outlined above are represented for a one-dimensional case (= only one biological activity) in Fig. 8.2.

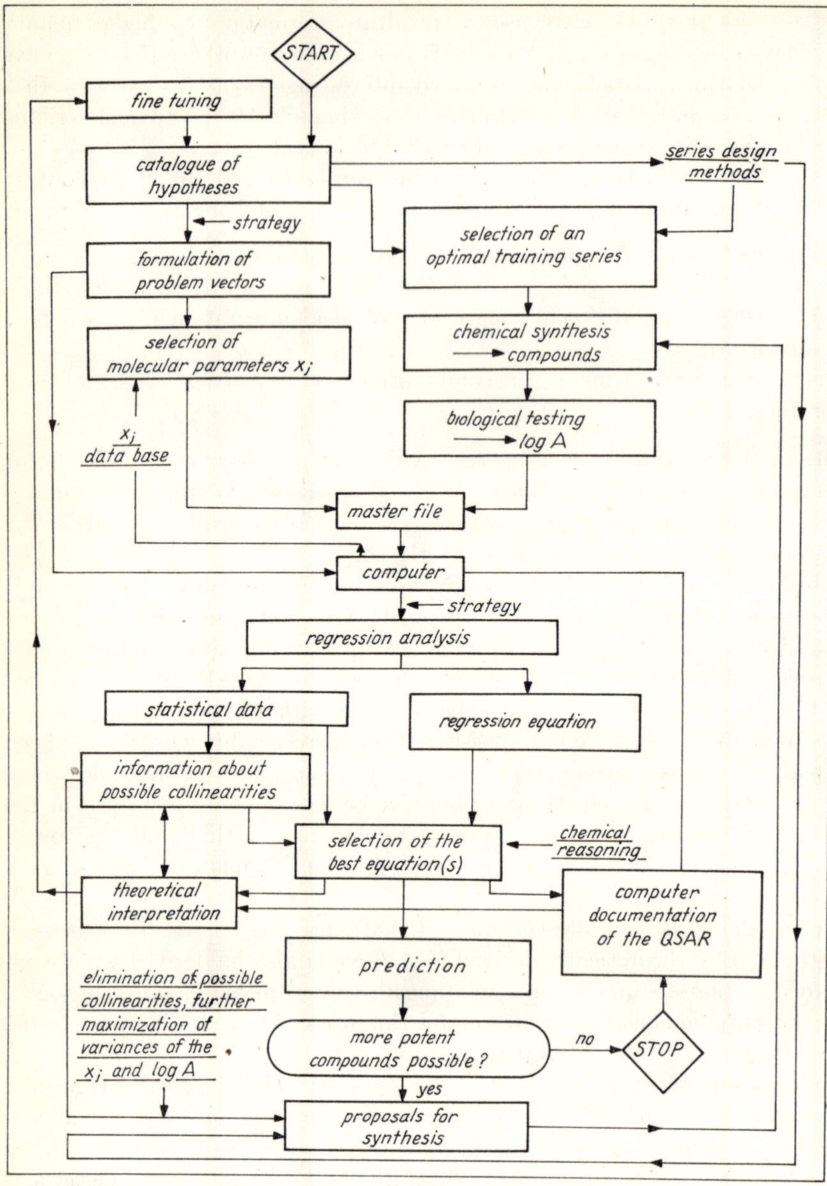

Fig. 8.2. Scheme of the quantitative structure-activity analysis following the extrathermodynamic approach (Hansch analysis)

8.3. Examples

8.3.1. Virostatic Isatin-β-Thiosemicarbazones

The reason for chosing this example [54] is that it allows a simple illustration of the procedure behind the formulation of hypotheses, their stepwise screening and the breaking down of a more complex problem into subproblems. It must be stressed that this example serves here as a *model* to demonstrate a basic strategy and that it has *many unsatisfactory features concerning the degrees of freedom and the substituent choice.*

Isatin-β-thiosemicarbazones of structure XXXVII are known for their antiviral activity [55, 56], thus providing a starting point that offers promise for the development of potential virostatics through carefully planned variations in structure. Data on the activity of a series of isatin-β-thiosemicarbazones against vaccinia virus were reported by BAUER and SADLER [55] and a quantitative structure-activity analysis was carried out in an attempt to find out whether further variations of R_1 and R_2 may lead to compounds more active than those already tested.

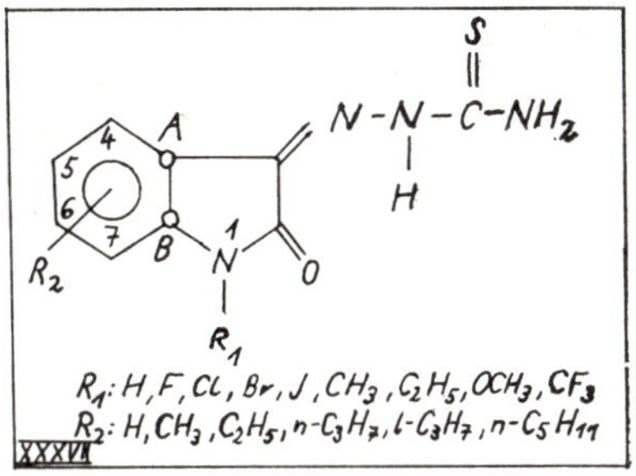

XXXVII

The first problem is that substituents are varied in several positions (1, 5, 6 and 7) while nothing is known about any position-dependence of substituent effects. In the event of all terms in the fundamental equation (3/17) being position-dependent, a relationship according to (8/19) will result (the indices refer to the position of substitution):

$$\log A = [f_h(x_h) + f_e(x_e) + f_s(x_s)]_1 + [f_h(x_h) + f_e(x_e) + f_s(x_s)]_5 + [f_h(x_h) + f_e(x_e) + f_s(x_s)]_6 + [f_h(x_h) + f_e(x_e) + f_s(x_s)]_7 + \text{constant} \quad (8/19)$$

In the case of complete additivity of the substituent influence in the various positions, on the other hand, the much simpler relationship (8/20) holds:

$$\log A = f_h(\sum x_h) + f_e(\sum x_e) + f_s(\sum x_s) + \text{constant} \quad (8/20)$$

All sorts of intermediate situations can be conceived. If, for example, position-dependence were restricted to the steric effect, eqn. (8/21) would be applicable

$$\log A = f_h(\sum x_h) + f_e(\sum x_e) + [f_s(x_s)]_1 + [f_s(x_s)]_5 + [f_s(x_s)]_6 + f_s(x_s)_7 + \text{constant} \quad (8/21)$$

and eqn. (8/22) would be valid in the case where additivity involves all ring positions:

$$\log A = f_h(x_{h,5} + x_{h,6} + x_{h,7}) + f_e(x_{e,5} + x_{e,6} + x_{e,7}) + f_s(x_{s,5} + x_{s,6} + x_{s,7}) + [f_e(x_e)]_1 + [f_h(x_h)]_1 + [f_s(x_s)]_1 + \text{constant} \quad (8/22)$$

On consideration of all conceivable position-dependences, the fundamental equation (3/17) has as many as 80 possible forms and yet any information that might help to choose the correct one *a priori* is lacking. In addition, the functions $f_h(x_h)$, $f_e(x_e)$ and

$f_s(x_s)$ can be formulated in many ways so that when all imaginable possibilities are considered the calculation of a very large number of equations becomes necessary.

The first step to reduce the number of possible equations is to divide the overall problem into subproblems and to investigate 1-, 5-, 6- and 7-substituted compounds separately considering only monosubstituted compounds in a first step. In this way the issue of position-dependence is fully eliminated. The next step comprises the formulation of hypotheses for the subgroups. Strictly, a catalogue of questions is formulated first, and an attempt is then made to find the answers formulated as hypotheses which then lead directly to the formulation of equations to be calculated. For the subgroups of ring-substituted compounds, this strategy is exemplified in Table 8.2.

The following conclusion can then be arrived at through the hypotheses:

1. The electronic substituent influences can be described by means of the simple HAMMETT constant σ.
2. Uncertainty as to whether the electronic substituent influence is directed towards A or B requires either possibility to be checked and under certain circumstances a special behaviour of substituents in the 7-position is to be expected (both σ_m and σ_p are to be applied for all positions).
3. Equations with x_e^2 or with σ_I and σ_R (or with $\mathfrak{F}$ and $\mathfrak{R}$) are not tested unless the simple HAMMETT equation will not yield a good result.
4. Hydrophobic substituent influences can be described by π values from the phenoxyacetic acid system. Cross-products are not to be expected. Any relationship with π is likely to be linear; hence, a π^2 term is only tested in one or two selected equations.
5. Steric substituent influences can be described by E_S. They are probably linear so that an $E^2{}_S$ term is tested in not more than one or two selected equations.

As already explained, the starting point is a simple one-parameter approach, which is extended stepwise to give the following results:

1. *for all three groups of ring-substituted compounds*

$$\log A = a_0 + a_1\pi \quad \text{non-significant}$$

$$= a_0 + a_1\pi^2 + a_2\pi \quad \text{non-significant}$$

$$= a_0 + a_1E_. \quad \text{non-significant}$$

$$= a_0 + a_1E_S{}^2 + a_2E_S \quad \text{non-significant} \qquad (8/23)$$

2. *for 5-substituted compounds* ($n = 5$)

$$\log A = 8.90\sigma_m - 2.43 \qquad r = 0.861 \qquad s = 0.405 \qquad (8/24)$$

$$= 14.06\sigma_m - 2.17\pi - 2.95 \qquad r = 1.000 \qquad s = 0.028 \qquad (8/25)$$

$$= 12.90\sigma_m + 2.47E_S - 4.77 \qquad r = 1.000 \qquad s = 0.059 \qquad (8/26)$$

3. *for 6-substituted compounds* ($n = 6$)

$$\log A = 3.61\sigma_m - 0.24 \qquad r = 0.971 \qquad s = 0.456 \qquad (8/27)$$

$$= 4.27\sigma_m - 1.05\pi + 0.31 \qquad r = 1.000 \qquad s = 0.028 \qquad (8/28)$$

$$= 3.07\sigma_m + 1.12E_S - 0.31 \qquad r = 0.999 \qquad s = 0.054 \qquad (8/29)$$

Table 8.2. Catalogue of questions and hypotheses for the subgroups of ring-substituted compounds

Question	Hypothesis
1. *General questions*	
1.1. Is special knowledge available on the reaction mechanism, which would require special approaches?	No
1.2. Are special metabolic reactions to be expected, which need special consideration?	No
2. *Questions on electronic substituent influences*	
2.1. To be expected?	Yes
2.2. Directed towards A or B?	No hypothesis is possible
2.3. Are coupling effects to be expected?	Principly conceivable in position 5 when the influence of the substituent is directed towards B. In any case — due to the nature of the substituents neglectible
2.4. $f_e(x_e)$ linear or non-linear?	linear, with great probability
2.5. Is separation of inductive and mesomeric effects necessary?	Unlikely, except perhaps for position 7
3. *Questions on hydrophobic substituent influences*	
3.1. To be expected?	Likely
3.2. Special intramolecular interactions to be expected — as compared with the standard series phenoxyacetic acids?	No
3.3. $f_h(x_h)$ linear or non-linear?	Likely to be linear, because only a small range of π is covered
4. *Questions on steric substituent influences*	
4.1. To be expected?	Likely
4.2. Is E_S suitable steric molecular parameter?	Yes
4.3. $f_s(x_s)$ linear or non-linear?	Likely to be linear (substituents are not so much different in bulk)

4. *for 7-substituted compounds* ($n = 7$)

$$\log A = 66.21\sigma_I^2 + 99.66\sigma_p^2 + 141.5\sigma_I\sigma_p + 0.55 \qquad (8/30)$$

$$r = 0.959 \qquad s = 0.137$$

It follows from (8/23), (8.24) and (8/27) that electronic substituent effects play a dominating role in positions 5 and 6, as illustrated by the fact that it is only with x_e that statistically significant one-parameter equations can be obtained. It is somewhat surprising that for both positions equations with σ_m occur because, whether the substituent effect be directed towards A or B, one of them must be a para-position. The electronic substituent effect shows a marked position-dependence and seems to operate more strongly from position 5 than from position 6. The resonance contribution to σ_m values, which are mainly inductive in character, is relatively small. If an inductive substituent effect is primarily directed towards point A, both the greater influence of substituents in position 5 and the occurrence of σ_m for both positions could be explained. In that event, a correlation with σ_I must afford an even better one-parameter equation, and this is, indeed, true, as indicated by a comparison of (8/31) and (8/32) with (8/24) and (8/27):

5-substituted compounds

$$\log A = 11.26\sigma_I - 0.43 \qquad r = 0.992 \qquad s = 0.195 \tag{8/31}$$

6-substituted compounds

$$\log A = 3.32\sigma_I - 0.43 \qquad r = 0.957 \qquad s = 0.269 \tag{8/32}$$

It follows from eqns. (8/24)—(8/29) and from (8/31) and (8/32) that electron-withdrawing substituents enhance virostatic activity through an inductive effect. This effect is superimposed on a position-dependent hydrophobic and/or steric effect according to (8/25), (8/26), (8/28) and (8/29) with the consequence that virostatic activity diminishes as substituents gain in hydrophobicity and/or bulk.

Unfortunately, for the substituents considered π and E_S are collinear so that the question of whether this effect is primarily hydrophobic or steric cannot be answered. Evidence for a hydrophobic effect comes from the smaller residual error of equations with π as compared to those with E_S (the difference is, however, minimal), and for a steric effect from the fact that substitution with fluorine, which, although scarcely more hydrophobic than hydrogen ($\pi_F = 0.13$, $\pi_H = 0$) exceeds it in bulk ($E_{S,H} = 1.24$, $E_{S,F} = 0.78$) markedly reduces activity when compared to that of the unsubstituted compound. If it were true that the substituent effect is primarily hydrophobic, more potent compounds could be obtained by introduction of strongly electron-withdrawing substituents with negative π values in positions 5 and 6; some of these substituents are recorded in Table 8.3. If, however, the substituents exert a steric effect, it will not be possible to find a substituent with an electron-withdrawing effect strong enough to compensate for the decrease in activity resulting from substituent bulk. Hydrogen in positions 5 and 6 would then be the most favourable substituent. A distinction between the two possibilities can easily be made by testing one or two of the substituents listed in Table 8.3.

Table 8.3. Some electron-withdrawing substituents with negative π value

Substituent	π	σ_m
CN	−0.57	0.56
JO_2	−3.46	0.68
NO_2	−0.28	0.71
$\overset{+}{N}(CH_3)_3$	−5.96	0.88
$SOCH_3$	−1.58	0.52
SO_2CH_3	−1.63	0.60

Equation (8/30) represents the non-linear form of Chartons ortho-approach (cf., eqn. (5/27)) and is the only significant relationship to be obtained for the subgroup of 7-substituted compounds. From the chemical point of view, the form of (8/30) could be interpreted to mean that substitients in position 7 undergo much steric hindrance from the adjacent N—R_1 group, as is in fact also brought out by space-filling models. Nevertheless this equation should be regarded very sceptically (note the small observations/variables ratio), and its use for predictions is, at best, hazardous (according to this equation, the OH group could be a favourable substituent).

In principle, the questions concerning the influence of ring substitution as demonstrated by the data of SADLER and BAUER have thus been answered.

The procedure with compounds substituted in position 1 on nitrogen is fully analogous to that outlined above, the questions and hypotheses corresponding to those presented in Table 8.2. An additional question to be asked at this point is whether E_S or E_S^c is more suitable to characterize the steric effect. A further point to remember is that the substituents are localized in an aliphatic environment, requiring aliphatic substituent constants to be chosen. A π^2 term is more likely to occur as a larger hydrophobicity range is covered. Again, equations only containing one molecular parameter serve as a starting point ($n = 6$):

$$\log A = -0.68\pi + 2.50 \qquad r = 0.833 \qquad s = 0.435 \qquad (8/33)$$

Adding a π^2 term does not improve this equation. The relationships with E_S and σ^* are:

$$\begin{aligned} \log A &= a_0 + a_1 E_S && \text{non-significant} \\ &= a_0 + a_1 E_S^2 + a_2 E_S && \text{non-significant} \\ &= a_0 + a_1 E_S^c && \text{non-significant} \\ &= a_0 + a_1 (E_S^c)^2 + a_2 E_S^c && \text{non-significant} \\ &= a_0 + a_1 \sigma^* && \text{non-significant} \qquad (8/34) \end{aligned}$$

It follows from (8/33) and (8/34) that the dominating influence of substituents in position 1 is hydrophobic in character, biological potency increasing as hydrophobicity decreases. Apparently, electronic and steric influences only play a secondary role. It must be kept in mind, however, that electronic properties are not sufficiently varied within the alkyl substituents considered so that conclusions concerning electronic effects are of only very limited validity.

Next, combinations of two molecular parameters are tested, always including the dominant variable π. The following relationship appears to be the best equation:

$$\log A = -1.07\pi - 1.86\sigma^* + 2.93 \qquad (8/35)$$

$$r = 0.947 \qquad s = 0.291$$

Equation (8/35) confirms the negative hydrophobicity influence, which is superimposed on an electronic effect so that electron-releasing substituents add to activity. It appears from eqn. (8/35) that the presence of electron-releasing substituents of limited size or hydrophobicity is favourable for biological activity. Obviously the favourable electronic effect overcompensates the unfavourable increase in hydrophobicity for the exchange of H for CH_3 and C_2H_5 since the latter substituents increase activity. In higher alkyl chains the latter influence predominates, causing a decrease in activity. Among the alkyl substituents the maximum is found for $R_1 = C_2H_5$ and further variations of alkyl substituents in position R_1 (including those such as CH_2X) would serve no useful purpose.

These conclusions apply to alkyl substituents only and cannot be extended to non-alkyl substituents. Considerable restrictions on conclusions to be drawn from a QSAR are, as in this case, always imposed if only alkyl substituents are varied in a given position. In such cases the hydrophobic influence is usually so overt that all other effects are obscured.

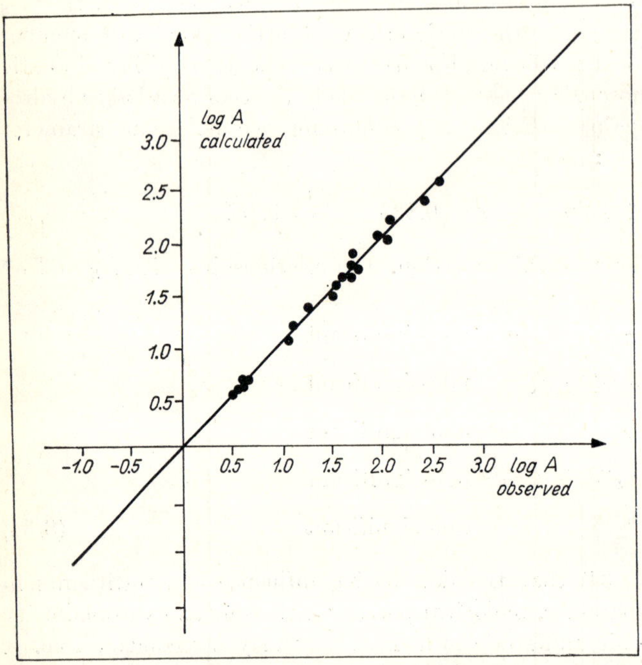

Fig. 8.3. Plot of observed versus calculated antiviral activity values of substituted isatin-β-thiosemicarbazones (from [54])

The above division into subgroups, the formulation of hypotheses and a systematic and stepwise testing of these hypotheses allowed the calculations to be restricted to a relatively few equations; for a comparison of calculated and experimental values of antiviral potency, see Fig. 8.3. Substituent influences display such a strong position-dependence that it would not be useful to reunite the subgroups in trying to derive a QSAR for the whole series. It would not be worth while anyway, since no essentially new information could be expected.

Once again, it is to be emphasized that this example was primarily chosen because it can be so easily overseen, making the procedure readily demonstrable and that its predictive value is not representative. It stands to reason that more comprehensive hypotheses and procedures are needed in the case of more complex problems. In fact, each individual problem calls for its own formulation of hypotheses and strategy in terms of quantitative structure-activity analysis.

8.3.2. Antiallergic Pyranenamines

This example from the work of the Smith Kline & French QSAR group in Philadelphia [8] was selected since it demonstrates the power of QSARs in industrial research and re-emphasizes the importance of stepwise strategies already stressed above.

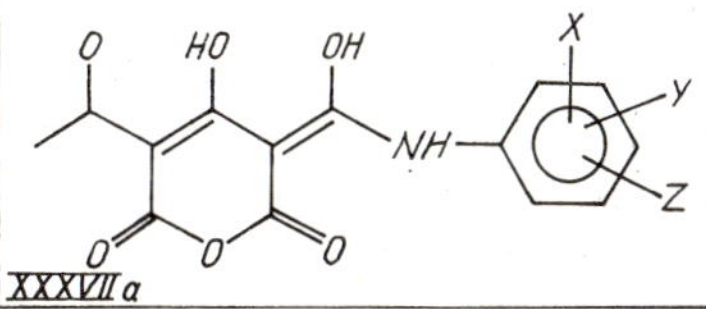

XXXVIIa

Pyranenamines (3-[arylamino)ethylidene]-5-acylpyrantriones) of the structure XXXVIIa display cromolyn sodium-like antiallergic properties in a variety of animal models [57]. The model used in this study was the passive cutaneous anaphylactic (PCA) rat. Experiments were performed in such a way that pharmacokinetic influences were minimized; the average standard error oft the response data ($A = 1/ED_{50}$) was estimated to be about ± 0.48. The task was to develop highly active compounds by varying substituents in the phenyl ring. The work proceeded through four sequential phases:

(1) a pre-QSAR phase based on the decision tree of Topliss and the concept of bioisosterism,
(2) simple QSAR-based plots resulting in the recognition of a critical structural property,
(3) synthesis of a wide variety of compounds having the desirable property and evaluation of QSARs to explore other important structural trends,
(4) refinement and confirmation of the result by synthesis of some less accessible pyranenamines expected to have maximal potency.

As was also done by Cramer et al. in their publication [8] we shall consider the sequential phases separately. For details of the substituents included in each phase the reader is referred to the original paper of these authors [8].

Phase 1: pre-QSAR Series Development

This phase started with the investigation of a first set of 19 analogues. An attempt was made to select these analogues on the basis of the decision tree according to Topliss. Based on the assumption that, in many cases, biological potency primarily depends on the hydrophobicity and electronic properties of substituents which can be characterized by π and σ, the Topliss operation scheme proceeds along sequential steps in which the π and σ values of substituents are compared with biological potency. In each step a decision can be made about which substituent should be selected next, based on the relative potencies of the preceding pair of compounds (for details, see 10.1.). The Topliss tree can be regarded as a QSAR-based heuristic technique with the ultimate objective to find the most potent compound within a series with the synthesis of the minimum number of analogues. In the present case, however, this technique was not successful since "strict adherence to the decision model would have produced nothing but derivatives less active than the starting unsubstituted compound" [8]. The reason for the failure of this basically quite efficient approach was simply that the pyranenamine problem is outside the scope of this method. This negative result with the Topliss technique seems to have somewhat discouraged the further application of QSAR techniques at this stage of development since, in the next step, a variety of close congeners (bioisosters) of the hitherto most active compound, the 4-OH derivative, were prepared and tested. As was to be expected, this "close analogue" strategy yielded only compounds which were about equipotent, but not superior to this derivative. The synthesis of these analogues could have been avoided to a large extent if a reasonable QSAR approach had been tried *prior* to synthesis. As described below, if QSAR had not been applied at all, the 4-OH derivative would probably have been regarded as optimal and the search terminated. Thus, without QSAR, the most active compounds (about 1000 times more potent) would probably have never been found.

Phase 2: Modelling by Plots

An initial analysis of the 19 compounds in the first set was carried out by plotting $\log A$ against various substituent constants. The best result was obtained with a three-dimensional plot representing $\log A$ on one axis as a joint function of π and σ on the two other axes. Since it is difficult to handle three-dimensional plots a simple two-dimensional plot with the coordinates π and σ was actually used, and biological potency was represented by contour lines. The plot immediately revealed a region of high potency corresponding to substituents with highly negative π values and σ values near zero. Consequently, it appeared possible to increase potency by introducing highly hydrophilic and, at the same time, electronically neutral substituents. Along these lines, several compounds were proposed for synthesis including multiply substituted derivatives. The proposal to include multiple substitution was at this time contrary to experience since several disubstituted analogues had turned out to be inferior to the corresponding monosubstituted derivatives. The model-based proposal, however, proved to be correct. Already the first two compounds synthesized according to the "hydrophilic—electronically neutral" concept have turned out to be highly active, one of them (3-acetamido-4-hydroxy derivative) being 2.5 times more potent than any other pyranenamine thus far synthesized.

The usefulness of this simple plot was thus confirmed and seemed worthwhile to exploring further. The same conclusion could also have been reached from a QSAR derived from the first set of 19 compounds:

$$\log A = -0.14 \sum \pi - 1.35 \left(\sum \sigma\right)^2 - 0.72 \qquad (8/36)$$

$$n = 19 \qquad r = 0.69 \qquad s = 0.47$$

$\sum \pi$ = sum of π values of all substituents (X, Y, Z)

$\sum \sigma$ = sum of σ values of all substituents (X, Y, Z)

This equation tells the same story as the plot: potency will be enhanced by hydrophilic (negative π values) and by overall electronically neutral (small sum of σ values, and, hence, $(\sum \sigma)^2 \approx 0$) substituents. The confidence intervals of the regression coefficients (not given), however, are very large so that, from a statistical point of view, eqn. (8/36) is of only dubious validity and allows, at best, a qualitative conclusion. At this stage of development, a statistical analysis of the data did not offer advantages over the simple plot, again emphasizing the importance of such plots as a starting step.

Phase 3: QSAR-*based Development of the Hydrophobicity Lead*

The breakthrough achieved on the basis of the "hydrophilic—electronically neutral" concept derived from the simple plot now offers a valuable lead to follow up. Since eqn. (8/30) only shows a poor fit it seems very likely that other structural properties in addition to hydrophilicity and overall electronic neutrality are also important. Such properties could be, for example, hydrogen bonding or substituent size. Further synthesis, therefore, not only aimed at increasing hydrophilicity but also at exploring such possible additional influences. An additional 28 compounds with a variety of hydrophilic substituents were prepared leading to the following QSAR:

$$\log A = -0.30 \sum \pi - 1.5 \left(\sum \sigma\right)^2 + 2.0\mathfrak{F}_5 + 0.78\,\mathrm{MV}_{3,5} + 0.39 I_1 - 0.63 I_2 + 0.72 I_3 - 0.75 \qquad (8/37)$$

$$n = 61 \qquad r = 0.88 \qquad s = 0.40$$

with

I_1 = number of 2,4 or 5 substituents attached to the aryl ring by —YH— where Y is not carbon,

I_2 = number of 3,4 or 5 substituents attached by $-NHSO_2-$,

I_3 = 1, if a 4-0-acyl moiety is present; otherwise zero.

In comparison with eqn. (8/36) the correlation coefficient has substantially increased, and the confidence intervals of the regression coefficients (not given) have also become much smaller so that the statistical fit of this equation has much improved. The standard deviation, however, did not change, but a lower s can not be reached since s can never become (for a meaningful equation) lower than the experimental error which was estimated to be $s = 0.48$ (see above).

The most remarkable feature of eqn. (8/37) is that it fully substantiates the concept derived in the preceding phase: potency will be enhanced by hydrophilic substituents ($\sum \pi$-term) whilst the overall electronic effect of all substituents should be close to zero ($(\sum \sigma)^2$-term). Somewhat surprising is the $\mathfrak{F}_5$-term which indicates that an inductively electron-withdrawing substituent in the 5-position may substantially enhance potency. The conclusion to be drawn from both the $(\sum \sigma)^2$- and the $\mathfrak{F}_5$-term then would be that, in multiply substituted molecules, electronic substituent effect as expressed by the respective σ values should nearly cancel each other whilst, at the same time, a directional inductive effect at the 5-position exerts a positive influence on potency. Such directional effects are very unusual and cannot be explained within the theoretical framework of classical physical organic chemistry. The explanation offered by Cramer that this term accounts for an intermolecular effect (whereas the scale of electronic substituent constants is defined by intramolecular phenomena) is a possibility but still not very convincing. It would imply that substituents in the 5-position (note the symmetry of 3- and 5-position) are always located in the same spot at the receptor site and that the $\mathfrak{F}$ value of 5-substituents somehow characterizes direct interactions between these substituents and this particular spot. In any case, the $\mathfrak{F}_5$-term needs further exploration in a next step (see phase 4), all the more so since it is only based on two analogues.

The $MV_{3,5}$-term in eqn. (8/37) seems to indicate that increasing size of substituents in the meta-positions favours high potency. Although this might well be true it is surprising that a simple volume term should be capable of describing such an effect for the highly unsymmetrical substituents considered. If steric interactions are not completely unspecific (which is unlikely for the interactions supposed to take place at a specific receptor) they require a more refined parameterization (see chapter 6.) to take into account that not simply the general bulk but rather length and width in certain directions are of importance. Thus, the $MV_{3.5}$-term certainly also requires further investigations.

One important feature in addition to hydrophilicity and electronic properties presented by eqn. (8/37) is hydrogen bonding. The I_1-term describes an increase in potency of 0.42 log units for every group of the general type —HYR attached to the 3-, 4- or 5-position, where Y may be N, O or S and R may be anything including H or a lone pair except a $—SO_2R'$ group. This may reflect hydrogen bonding with the receptor although, as CRAMER puts it, "it is not easy to understand how any number of hydrogen bond donors in any position might exert equivalent and additive effects." An exceptional behaviour of the $—NHSO_2$ group (special case of —HYR) is indicated by the negative I_2-term; obviously (but why?) this group does not have suitable properties as the other —HYR groups. In summary, hydrogen bonding clearly is important but here also more precise knowledge and a confirmation are desirable.

The I_3-term, finally, is statistically the second most important (F-test) overall to eqn. (8/37). It indicates that acyl derivatives of 4-OH are five times as potent than would be implied by the physical properties of these esters. A possible explanation of this behaviour offered by CRAMER and co-workers is that these acyl derivatives behave as prodrugs, hydrolyzing *in vivo* to produce the 4-OH analogue itself.

Phase 4: Confirmation and Refinement — the Final Phase

Several SAR questions arise from the results obtained in phase 3:

- Is there a hydrophilicity optimum?
- What substituents capable of hydrogen bonding are really potency enhancing?
- What is the importance of the $\mathfrak{F}_5$- and the $MV_{3.5}$-term in eqn. (8/37)? Are these terms real?

In order to answer these questions, to confirm the results obtained thus far and to arrive at still more potent and, eventually, an "optimal" compound some further derivatives were synthesized. The substituents were carefully selected in this final phase in order to be able to reach these objectives which required considerable synthetic effort. The regression finally obtained for all compounds was:

$$\log A = -0.33 \sum \pi - 0.034 (\sum \pi)^2 - 1.7 (\sum \sigma)^2 + 4.3\mathfrak{F}_5 + 1.3\mathfrak{R}_5 + 0.37I_1 - 0.69I_2 + 0.72I_3 - 0.86I_4 - 0.59 \quad (8/38)$$

$n = 98 \quad r = 0.87 \quad s = 0.48$

I_4 = number of substituents in 3-, 4- or 5-position ortho to another and capable of forming an intramolecular hydrogen bond.

A parabolic relationship with $\sum \pi$ is now obtained defining a hydrophilicity optimum at about $\sum \pi = -5$. Although some caution seems in order (see [8] for details), the existence of a hydrophilicity optimum can at least be accepted as a working hypothesis.

The concept of overall electronic neutrality is also again confirmed by the $(\sum \sigma)^2$ term. In addition, a directional electronic effect of substituents in the 5-position obviously does exist as indicated by the $\mathfrak{F}_5$- und $\mathfrak{R}_5$-terms, the latter indicating that resonance effects also seem to be important.

Concerning hydrogen bonding, eqn. (8/38) tells much the same story as eqn. (8/37). The potency-enhancing effect of —YHR groups (I_1-term) is even more evident (statistically, this term is the most important in eqn. (8/38)) with, again, the $—NHSO_2$ groups as an exception (potency decreasing). A new feature, however, is presented by the I_4-term constraining the I_1-term by indicating that the formation of an intramolecular hydrogen bridge between an —YHR group and another substituent attached in ortho position to it will decrease potency. There may be two reasons behind this effect. First, the intramolecular hydrogen bond may prevent the formation of a hydrogen bond with the receptor, and secondly, intramolecular hydrogen bonding increases lipophilicity (this effect was not taken into account by the π values used in the calculations) which would also result in a loss of potency.

The remaining I_3-term again indicates the potency increasing effect of acylation of the 4-OH group. The $MV_{3.5}$-term, which was probably artificial, has now disappered. It is possible that its occurrence in eqn. (8/37) was due to multicollinearities.

The most potent compound found as the final result of the investigation (the 3,5-$[NHCO(CHOH)_2H]_2$ derivative) is 1000 times more potent than any member of the original series. It shows all characteristics that eqn. (8/38) predicts for high activity with $\sum \pi = -6.2$ (near the optimum of $\sum \pi \approx -5$), two YHR groups capable of forming inter-, but not intramolecular hydrogen bonds, overall electronic neutrality $\left((\sum \sigma)^2 = 0.08\right)$ and $\mathfrak{F}_5 = 0.28$ (the latter is somewhat offset by $\mathfrak{R}_5 = -0.25$). This combination of properties yields a predicted $\log A$ of 2.3 (eqn. (8/38)) and an actual $\log A$ of 3.0.

In terms of drug-receptor interactions eqn. (8/38) could be interpreted to indicate the presence of a "hydrophilic pocket" at the receptor site which binds the aryl moiety. Increasing hydrophilicity of substituents would then favour drug-receptor interactions, and if suitable polar groups are present within this pocket capable of forming hydrogen bonds with —HYR— groups in meta and para position the potency-enhancing effect of such groups could also be easily understood.

The particular electronic effect of 5-substituents could be explained by the presence of an electropositive receptor-group (for example, a protonated lysine, arginine or histidine residue) adjacent to the 5-position. To accept this explanation, however, an additional assumption regarding the directional influence of substituent bulk for unsymmetrically 3.5-disubstituted compounds is necessary since otherwise many electron-withdrawing substituents in 3-position of such derivatives could easily be brought into the basically equivalent 5-position by flipping of the phenyl ring.

As a whole this example shows an internal consistency of results in a stepwise QSAR-based approach which finally led to a very potent compound which might not otherwise have been found.

8.4. Factor Analysis as Preprocessing Step

8.4.1. Basic Principles[1])

Factor analysis can be used to eliminate collinearities form regression equations and to reduce the number of equations to be calculated. The principal objective of factor analysis is to attain a parsimonious description of observed data, or, in other words, to simplify the structure of multidimensional data by reducing the dimensionality of the data space in order to see what basic features are behind the data.

The mathematical formalism of factor analysis will only be discussed here insofar as it is needed for an understanding of this section; extensive reviews have been published (e.g. [58—64]). When m variables x_j ($j = 1, \ldots, m$) are measured for n objects ($i = 1, \ldots, n$) the data can be arranged in the form of a matrix:

$$\boldsymbol{X} = (x_{ji})_{m,n} \tag{8/39}$$

Such a matrix is also obtained if the master file for the extrathermodynamic approach is transposed, that is if the substituents or analogues (objects) are placed in the columns and the molecular parameters as well as log A (variables) in the rows. The element x_{ji} then represents the value of the j-th variable (molecular parameter) for the i-th substituent or analogue. For the purpose of factor analysis the variables are standardized according to

$$z_{ji} = (x_{ji} - \bar{x}_j)/s_j \tag{8/40}$$

where $\bar{x}_j$ is the mean and s_j the standard deviation of the j-th variable (cf., chapter 15.). The z_{ji} have a mean of zero and unity variance and form the standardized data matrix:

$$\boldsymbol{Z} = (z_{ji})_{m,n} \tag{8/41}$$

By use of factor analysis the z_{ji}'s are now expressed by linear combinations of the smallest possible number of new variables f_{ki} ($k = 1, \ldots, p$) and q_{ji}, which are denoted as *factors:*

$$z_{ji} = \sum_{k=1}^{p} a_{jk} f_{ki} + q_{ji} \tag{8/42}$$

A distinction is to be made between *common factors* f_{ki} and *unique factors* q_{ji}. The systematic features searched for in the data space are represented by the common factors, whilst the unique factors reflect specific properties (e.g., errors) of one variable at a time. For that reason only the common factors are considered in factor analysis which span the so-called *common factor space,* i.e. the smallest space where variables can appear without loss of information. The common factors are orthogonal vectors reproducing the data matrix on the basis of a linear model within common factor space. They are to be regarded as formal mathematical quantities which, at this stage, do not allow an interpretation. The weight a_{jk} characterizes the contribution of the k-th

---

[1]) With regard to some statistical principles reference is made to chapter 15. A special knowledge of statistics is not necessary, however, for a proper understanding of this chapter.

common factor to the j-th variable and has the character of a correlation coefficient between this common factor and the corresponding variable. As a consequence, a high value of $|a_{jk}|$ points to a close relationship between the k-th common factor and the j-th variable. In other words the j-th variable is highly "loaded" in the k-th factor, and the weights a_{jk} are, therefore, also called "*factor loadings*".

In matrix notation, eqn. (8/42) can be written as:

$$\boldsymbol{Z} = \boldsymbol{AF} + \boldsymbol{Q} \tag{8/43}$$

The elements of the matrix $\boldsymbol{A}$ are the factor loadings a_{jk}. It is termed the *factor loading matrix* or *factor pattern*, and the derivation of this matrix is, in fact, the purpose of the factor analysis. The following equation serves as a starting point

$$\hat{\boldsymbol{R}} = \boldsymbol{AA}^T \tag{8/44}$$

where $\hat{\boldsymbol{R}}$ denotes the reduced correlation matrix, which according to (8/44) is the product of the factor pattern and its transpose. The only difference between this matrix and the ordinary correlation matrix is that in the former the 1's in the diagonal have been replaced by *communalities* h_j^2. As a result, the reduced correlation matrix only containes that part of the data variance which can be assigned to the common factor space. The communality for the j-th variables is defined as:

$$h_j^2 = \sum_{k=1}^{p} a_{jk}^2 \tag{8/45}$$

Like the correlation matrix, the non-diagonal elements of $\hat{\boldsymbol{R}}$ contain the correlation coefficients between the variables, the following equation pertaining to the correlation coefficient r_{jl} between the j-th and the l-th variable:

$$r_{jl} = \sum_{k=1}^{p} a_{jk} a_{lk} \tag{8/46}$$

Communalities must be estimated prior to the solution of (8/44). This can be accomplished in several manners which, however, are not discussed here. During the computations, these estimates can be improved through iteration cycles. The solution of (8/44) is achieved by use of the principal component method (not to be confused with principal component analysis to be dealt with in 9.1.). An additional condition introduced here is that the factors are determined in sequence in such a way that the first factor accounts for the largest and the last for the smallest part of the variance of $\hat{\boldsymbol{R}}$. An eigenvalue problem, then, ensues, the resulting eigenvalues λ_k corresponding to variance contributions from the factors concerned. The factor pattern $\boldsymbol{A}$ can then be obtained from the corresponding eigenvectors.

Geometrically, the roots of the eigenvalues correspond to the lengths of the principal axes of the variance ellipsoid that arises when the n objects are presented in the space of the m variables. The question of how many factors should be allowed for must be answerd from the relative length of these axes. If a principal axis is very small in comparison with the others (which means that the eigenvalue in question is low), the corresponding factor may be ignored. Only these factors are thus considered significant whose eigenvalues exceed a given borderline value (defining p in eqn. (8/42)) and which therefore account for more than a given minimum variance. The borderline value is usually taken as representing an eigenvalue of 1 or a value equal to 5% of the sum of all positive eigenvalues. It follows from the additional condition for the application of the principal component method that all large loadings occur in the first factors, thereby rendering exceedingly difficult any interpretation of the factor pattern. To eliminate this drawback and to represent the complex mass of variables and factors within the framework of common factors as simply as possible, factors are so rotated that the structure of the factor pattern becomes as simple as possible resulting in the so-called THURSTONS simple structure. This structure is characterized by the property that as many variables as possible fall on coordinate axes when presented in factor space (axes = factors) so that the largest possible number of factor loadings becomes zero; in other words, in the presence of a simple structure the variables are divided into mutually exclusive groups with, in an ideal case, non-zero loadings only in one factor (see Fig. 8.4). Rotation may be either orthogonal or oblique. Orthogonal rotation (as with the varimax method) implies that all axes of factor space are rotated about the same angle, whilst on oblique rotation the angles are different for different axes. If factor analysis is carried out as the pre-processing step for regression analysis, only orthogonal rotation is useful. This is because on oblique rotation the orthogonality of factors disappears and the implication, then, is that in the formulation of regression equations it is no longer possible to preclude collinearities. If no simple structure can be established, any interpretation is of doubtful validity.

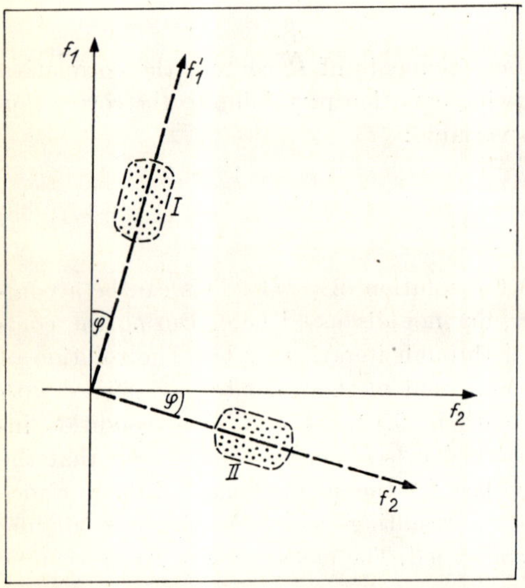

Fig. 8.4. Principle of rotation (orthogonal rotation) towards THURSTONS simple structure in the presence of two factors f_1 and f_2. The variables can be represented as points in the factor-spanned space; the coordinates of the points are the factor loadings a_{j1} and a_{j2}. In the coordinate system formed by the unrotated factors f_1 and f_2, the coordinates of the points are different from zero respective to both axes, e.g., all variables have loadings different from zero in both factors. Rotation of the coordinate axes about an angle φ, resulting in the coordinate axes f'_1 and f'_2 (rotated factors), changes the loadings of the variables: only high in group I in factor 1 and in group II in factor 2

Where following a factor analysis a simple THURSTON structure is available for a data matrix to be used in the extrathermodynamic approach, the following conclusion can be drawn from the factor pattern:

(1) Only those factors make a contribution to the variable "logarithm of biological activity (log A)" where that variable has a loading different from 0. The number

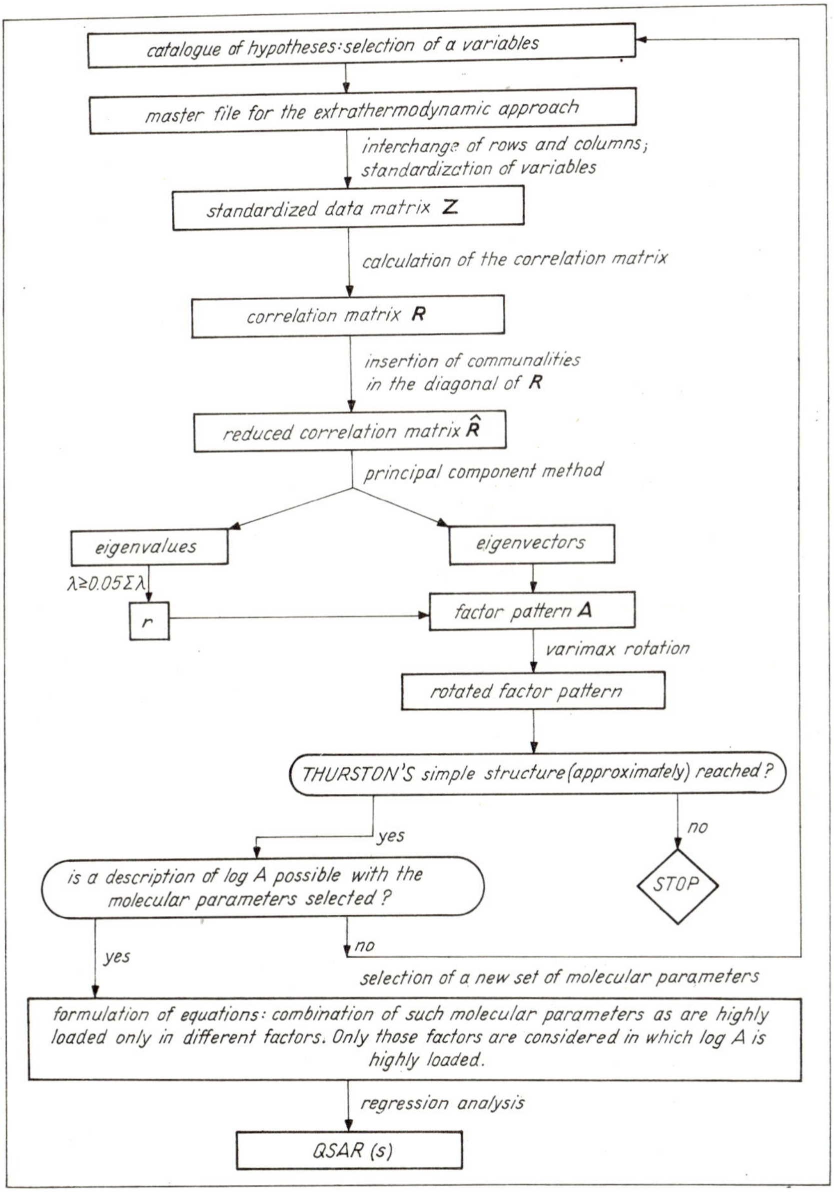

Fig. 8.5. Flow-scheme for the application of factor analysis as pre-processing step in regression analysis (number of relevant factors designated as r in this figure)

of terms in the regression equation describing log A should, therefore, be equal to that of these factors.

(2) Variables with a high loading in the same factor are interrelated and will be the more so the higher the loadings. No correlation exists between variables having non-zero loadings only in different factors.

(3) It follows from (1) and (2) that only variables with non-zero loadings in the same factors where log A also has a non-zero loading are important for the description of log A.

(4) Another consequence of (2) is that only variables with high loadings in different factors may be combined in one regression equation in order to avoid collinearities.

(5) It can be ascertained from the factor pattern whether in the variable space under consideration log A can be described in a satisfactory manner. If not, one can immediately choose a different variable space, thus preventing the calculation of — occasionally large numbers of — useless regression equations. Simple correlation coefficients can be estimated from (8/46).

The detailed information already provided by factor analysis about relationships between log A and molecular parameters allows one to select the most promising combinations of such parameters for regression analysis [38, 65—67] (see also [18]). Although collinearities can effectively be avoided it must be kept in mind that only the mathematical aspect of the collinearity problem (unstable equations) can be solved in this way. The problem of interpretability and of separating different substituent effects still remains and can only be eliminated by a proper selection of training series.

The most important steps of factor analysis are once more schematized in Fig. 8.5. It stands to reason that factor analysis needs to be applied critically. Difficulties may arise in particular when the variance contribution of the unique factors is too large compared to those of the common factors.

Factor analysis as a multivariate procedure can also be applied successfully when dealing with other questions arising from quantitative structure-activity analysis. An important problem here is the analysis of multiple biological data arising from investigations of compounds in a battery of biological tests. The objective of this kind of analyses is to disclose relations among individual test system and will be discussed under 13.2.

8.4.2. Examples

8.4.2.1. Inhibition of NADH-Oxidase by Substituted Phenoxyacetic Acids

Data about the inhibition of the NADH-oxidase system from ETP (pI_{50}; [68]) for 17 ring-substituted phenoxyacetic acids (with substituents H, 4-Br, 4-CH_3, 4-NO_2, 3-Br, 3-Cl, 3-CH_3, 3-OCH_3, 2-Br, 2-NO_2, 2-CH_3, 2,4-Cl_2, 2,3-Cl_2, 2,4,5-Cl_3 and penta-Cl) were analyzed by factor and regression analyses [65]. Substituent constants π, σ, σ^-, S, P and E_S have been employed to describe hydrophobic, electronic and steric substituent effects; for π, σ, σ^- and E_S the squares were also included. The eigenvalues of the resulting factors are shown in Table 8.4. Only the first three factors make relevant contributions to the variance in common factor space. Table 8.5. presents the pattern obtained after varimax rotation (only the high non-zero loadings are presented). The variable pI_{50} (biological activity) is loaded only in the first and third factors so that these alone are of importance for biological potency. It follows that in the space concerned two parameters are necessary and sufficient to describe the inhibition of the NADH-oxidase system by phenoxyacetic acids. Moreover, statistically significant one-parameter equations may be expected for pI_{50} with the highly-loaded substituent constants in the first and the third factor. As electronic substituent constants are highly-loaded in the first factor and E_S is highly locaded in the third factor, inhibition obviously depends on electronic and steric effects. It would appear that the electronic effect is of more importance, because pI_{50} is more highly-loaded in the first than in the third factor. Hydrophobic influences play no role, since π only has a high loading in the second factor, which is unimportant for biological activity. Another consequence of the

Table 8.4. Eigenvalues of common factors for the inhibition of the NADH-oxydase system by 17 ring-substituted phenoxyacetic acids (see text)

Factor No.	Eigenvalue
1	7.95
2	1.70
3	0.55
4	0.22
5	0.01
6	0.00
7	−0.02
8	−0.04
9	−0.05
10	−0.05
11	−0.08

Table 8.5. Factor pattern (after varimax rotation) for the inhibition of the NADH-oxydase system by 17 ring-substituted phenoxyacetic acids (see text). Only the high (significant non-zero) loadings are reported

Variable	Factor pattern		
	First factor	Second factor	Third factor
pI_{50}	0.77		0.54
π		0.76	
π^2		0.70	
σ	0.92		
σ^2	0.82		
σ^-	0.93		
σ^{-2}	0.83		
S	0.78		
P		−0.76	
E_S			−0.86
E_S^2			−0.87

loadings in the first factor is the considerable intercorrelation of the electronic substituent constants σ, σ^- and S. For the substituents considered this as well as the correlation of σ and σ^- with their squares was, of course, to be expected. E_S does not correlate with any other parameter, because it is the only substituent constant loaded in the third factor. Unexpectedly, correlations between π and π^2 and P exist, which are reflected in the high loadings of these variables in the second factor.

Starting from the factor pattern, one of the electronic substituent constants which is highly-loaded in the first factor should be combined with E_s in regression analysis, so that the following relationships result:

$$\begin{aligned} pI_{50} &= f(\sigma, E_S) \\ &= f(\sigma^-, E_S) \\ &= f(S, E_S) \end{aligned} \qquad (8/47)$$

Equations with σ^2, σ^{-2} and $E_S{}^2$ can be excluded because not more than two terms may occur and there exists a close correlation of these variables with σ, σ^- and E_S, respectively.

In order to verify these conclusions all conceivable combinations of molecular parameters have been screened by regression analysis. The results fully confirm the conclusions drawn from factor analysis:

1. Statistically significant one-parameter equations can be obtained with σ, σ^-, S and E_S, but not with π.
2. These equations are not improved by adding σ^2, σ^{-2}, π or $E_S{}^2$.
3. Relationships according to (8/47) lead to an essential improvement over the one-parameter equations.
4. No further improvement is achieved by adding more terms to (8/47). There exist no equations in which a π term is significant.

Equations in accord with (8/47) are, indeed, the best to be found in the space studied. Statistically, the best equation is:

$$pI_{50} = 0.75\sigma^- - 0.23E_S + 3.34 \qquad (8/48)$$

$$n = 17 \qquad r = 0.923 \qquad s = 0.249$$

Had equations only been calculated on the basis of (8/47), a saving of far more than 90% would have been accomplished compared to the outcome of screening all possible parameter combinations.

8.4.2.2. Inhibition of the Growth of *S. alba* Hypocotyl by Piperidinoacetanilides [65, 69]

A series of mono-substituted piperidinoacetanilides (structure XXV) with substituents H, F, Cl, Br, J, CH_3, CF_3, OCH_3, OC_2H_5 and NO_2 in ortho-, meta- and para-position were tested for inhibitory potency on the growth of *S. alba* hypocotyl (pI_{50}). A great variety of hydrophobic, electronic and steric molecular parameter (σ, σ^-, $\mathfrak{F}$, $\mathfrak{R}$, S, P, π, E_S, MR, $E_{S,ortho}$) were considered to describe inhibition. On grounds to be discussed later, subgroups of meta- and para-substituted compounds ($n = 18$) as well as ortho-substituted compounds ($n = 9$) were also investigated separately.

The eigenvalues for the three problems are listed in Table 8.6; Three factors are relevant. Table 8.7 shows those variables which have a high loading in those factors important for biological activity (high loading for pI_{50}). As regards the *overall problem*, pI_{50} is highly-loaded in all three factors so that equations with three terms are to be expected in regression analysis. The first factor represents electronic and/or steric effects. A decision either way is not possible because of the correlation of E_S with the electronic parameters. The second factor refers exclusively to special properties of ortho-substituents. I_1 is an indicator variable to be defined as follows:

$$I_1 = \begin{cases} 1 & \text{for ortho-substituents} \\ 0 & \text{for meta- and para-substituents} \end{cases} \qquad (8/49)$$

Table 8.6. Eigenvalues of common factors for the growth-inhibiting activity of substituted piperidinoacetanilides; m + p + o: all compounds (= 27), m + p: meta- and para-substituted compounds ($n = 18$), o: ortho-substituted compounds ($n = 9$)

Factor No.	Eigenvalues		
	m + p + o	m + p	o
1	4.44	4.50	5.49
2	3.29	1.56	3.30
3	1.69	1.33	1.01
4	0.53	0.21	0.30
5	0.35	0.15	0.08
6	0.10	0.00	0.06

Table 8.7. Growth inhibiting activity of piperidinoacetanilides: variables with high loadings in factors in which the biological activity (pI_{50}) is also highly loaded for the three problems meta-, para- and ortho-substututed compounds ($n = 27$), meta- and para-substituted compounds ($n = 18$) and ortho-substituted compounds ($n = 9$)

Factor No.	meta + para + ortho	meta + para	ortho
1	σ^-, $\mathfrak{R}$, E_S, P	σ^-, $\mathfrak{R}$, E_S, P	—
2	$E_{S,\text{ortho}}$, S_{ortho}, I_1	π, (MR)	—
3	π, (MR)	—	(π), MR

Hydrophobic (π) and/or steric (MR) influences are contained in the third factor, where no decision either way can be taken because of the correlation between π and MR.

These arguments taken together necessitated the combination of an electronic molecular parameter or E_S (first factor) with an indicator for the ortho-position (second

[1]) It should be remarked that E_S and MR characterize different steric properties of substituents (see 6.). This is the reason why both parameters appear in the factor pattern but in different factors.

factor) and with π or MR (third factor). Again, all possible combinations of molecular parameters were screened in regression analysis for comparative purposes. The results entirely substantiate the predictions from factor analysis, and the combinations of parameters referred to, indeed, yield the best possible relationships in the variable space considered. Three of these relations are exemplified below ($n = 27$):

$$pI_{50} = -0.64E_S + 0.78E_{S,\,ortho} + 1.15\pi + 1.08 \quad (8/50)$$

$$r = 0.872 \qquad s = 0.470$$

$$pI_{50} = 0.88\sigma^- + 0.72E_{S,\,ortho} + 1.39\pi + 0.88 \quad (8/51)$$

$$r = 0.830 \qquad s = 0.540$$

$$pI_{50} = -0.36E_S - 1.02I_1 + 1.25\pi + 1.26 \quad (8/52)$$

$$r = 0.842 \qquad s = 0.520$$

Because of the particular role of ortho-substituents as evidenced in the second factor a separate analysis of meta- and para-substituted compounds on the one and of ortho-substituted analogues on the other hand was performed. The results of the overall problem suggest two factors with a non-zero loading for pI_{50} for the group of meta- and para-substituted compounds and of one such factor for the ortho-substituted compounds. As Table 8.7 shows, this is indeed the case.

For the group of *meta- and para-substituted compounds* the first factor represents electronic or steric (substituent width) effects, whilst hydrophobic or volume effects of substituents are contained in the second factor. Therefore, regression analysis should be based on a combination of an electronic or E_S term with a π or MR term. Here, too, the best possible combinations of parameters are obtained, as illustrated below ($n = 18$):

$$pI_{50} = -0.56E_S + 1.26\pi + 1.79 \quad (8/53)$$

$$r = 0.876 \qquad s = 0.520$$

$$pI_{50} = 0.49P + 1.39\pi + 0.36 \quad (8/54)$$

$$r = 0.851 \qquad s = 0.570$$

$$pI_{50} = -0.86E_S + 0.08\,\mathrm{MR} + 2.77 \quad (8/55)$$

$$r = 0.765 \qquad s = 0.700$$

Similarly, with ortho-substituted compounds the results of factor analysis are also in agreement with the best of all possible equations ($n = 9$):

$$pI_{50} = 0.08\,\mathrm{MR} - 0.03 \quad (8/56)$$

$$r = 0.813 \qquad s = 0.270$$

The results of factor and regression analyses indicate that the first factor for the overall problem as well as for the group of meta- and para-substituted compounds may primarily be steric instead of electronic in character (eqns. (8/50) and (8/53) are statistically better than eqns. (8/51) and (8/54)), and also that the second factor for the group of meta- and para-substituted compounds (third factor for the overall problem) represents hydrophobic rather than steric effects (eqn. (8/53) is statistically better than (8/55)). It must be emphasized that these conclusions are to be considered tentative. Steric effects occur in the ortho-position.

Although all the relationships presented above are highly significant, their goodness of fit is only moderate. Most probably, the cause does not lie in the parameter space concerned but rather in the biological activity parameter pI_{50}. The reason why this conclusion can be arrived at is simply that a QSAR investigation of the same series of compounds acting as plant growth inhibitors in *B. napus* did not furnish useful results until the conventional pI_{50} value had been replaced by biological activity parameters derived from eqn. (2/10); [66]. Again, the ortho-position played a particular rôle here (associated with a changed mechanism of action), and the influence of ortho-substituents on biological activity was also purely steric in character.

References

[1] Lambrecht, G., U. Moser and E. Mutschler: Eur. J. Med. Chem. **15**, 305 (1980)
[2] Lien, E. J., E. J. Ariens and A. J. Beld: Eur. J. Pharmacol. **35**, 245 (1976)
[3] v. d. Broek, A. J., A. I. A. Broess, M. J. v. d. Heuvel, H. P. de Jongh, J. Leemhuis, K. H. Schönemann, J. Smits, J. de Visser, N. P. van Vliet and F. J. Zeelen: Steroids **30**, 481 (1980)
[4] Zeelen, F. J., in J. A. Keverling Buisman (Ed.): Biological Activity and Chemical Structure, Pharmacochemistry Library (Eds.: W. Th. Nauta and R. F. Rekker), Vol. 2, Elsevier, Amsterdam, 1977, p. 147
[5] Zeelen, F. J., in J. Knoll and F. Darvas (Eds.): Chemical Structure — Biological Activity Relationships, Akadémiai Kiadó, Budapest, 1980, p. 43
[6] Unger, S. H., K. Untch, B. Lewis, B. Berkoz, J. Edwards, A. Strosberg, R. Weissberg and R. Alvarez in J. Knoll and F. Darvas (Eds.): Chemical Structure — Biological Activity Relationships, Akadémiai Kiadó, Budapest, 1980, p. 3
[7] Unger, S. H., in E. J. Ariens (Ed.): Drug Design, Vol. IX, Academic Press, New York, 1980, p. 48
[8] Cramer, R. D., K. M. Snader, C. R. Willis, L. W. Chakrin, J. Thomas and B. M. Sutton: J. Med. Chem. **22**, 714 (1979)
[9] Craig, P. N.: J. Med. Chem. **14**, 680 (1971)
[10] Craig, P. N.: Adv. Chem. Series **114**, 115 (1972)
[11] Topliss, J. G.: J. Med. Chem. **15**, 1006 (1972)
[12] Hansch, C., A. Leo, S. H. Unger, K. H. Kim, D. Nikaitani and E. J. Lien: J. Med. Chem. **16**, 1207 (1973)
[13] Unger, S. H., and C. Hansch: J. Med. Chem. **16**, 745 (1973)
[14] Hansch, C., S. H. Unger and A. B. Forsythe: J. Med. Chem. **16**, 1217 (1973)
[15] Wootton, R., R. Cranfield, G. C. Sheppey and P. J. Goodford: J. Med. Chem. **18**, 607 (1975)
[16] Hansch, C., in K. A. Keverling Buisman (Ed.): Biological Activity and Chemical Structure, Pharmacochemistry Library (Eds.: W. Th. Nauta and R. F. Rekker), Vol. 2, Elsevier, Amsterdam, 1977, pp. 47 and 287
[17] Purcell, W. P.: Eur. J. Med. Chem. **10**, 335 (1975)
[18] Martin, Y. C.: Drug Design Methods: A Critical Introduction, Marcel Dekker, New York, 1978
[19] Martin, Y. C., in E. J. Ariens (Ed.): Drug Design, Vol. VIII, Academic Press, New York, 1979, p. 1
[20] Martin, Y. C., and H. N. Panas: J. Med. Chem. **22**, 784 (1979)

[21] Martin, Y. C.: J. Med. Chem. **24**, 229 (1981)
[22] Coats, E. A., in R. P. Spencer (Ed.): Radiopharmaceuticals — Structure-Activity Relationships, Grune & Stratton, USA, 1981, p. 4
[23] Franke, R., in A. Simkins (Ed.): Medicinal Chemistry VI, Cotswold Press, Oxford, 1979, p. 237
[24] Streich, W. J., S. Dove and R. Franke: J. Med. Chem. **23**, 1452 (1980)
[25] Dove, S., W. J. Streich and R. Franke: J. Med. Chem. **23**, 1456 (1980)
[26] Box, M. J., and N. R. Draper: Technometrics **13**, 682 (1971)
[27] Draper, N. R., and H. Smith: Applied Regression Analysis, Wiley, New York, 1966
[28] Mitchell, T. J.: Technometrics **16**, 203 (1974)
[29] Goodford, P. J., A. T. Hudson, G. C. Sheppey, R. Wootton, M. M. Blank, G. J. Sutherland and J. C. Wickham: J. Med. Chem. **19**, 1239 (1976)
[30] Dunn, W. J., M. G. Greenberg and S. S. Callojas: J. Med. Chem. **19**, 1299 (1976)
[31] Shah, K. J., and E. A. Coats: J. Med. Chem. **20**, 1001 (1977)
[32] Cranfield, R., P. J. Goodford, F. E. Norrington and W. H. G. Richards: Brit. J. Pharmac. **52**, 87 (1974)
[33] Franke, R., W. J. Streich and S. Dove in J. Knoll and F. Darvas (Eds.): Chemical Structure — Biological Activity Relationships: Quantitative Approaches, Akadémia Kiadó, Budapest, 1980, p. 153
[34] Unger, S. H.: cited in ref. [18]
[35] Woolridge, K. R. H.: Eur. J. Med. Chem. **15**, 63 (1980)
[35a] Franke, R., E. Gäbler and P. Oehme: Acta biol. med. germ. **32**, 545 (1974)
[35b] Hanzlik, R. P., J. R. Cashman and G. J. Traiger: Toxicol. Appl. Pharmacol. **55**, 260 (1980)
[35c] Franke, R.: Mol. Pharmacol. **5**, 640 (1969)
[35d] Franke, R.: Archiv Geschwulstforsch. **36**, 30 (1970)
[35e] Franke, R., and M. Büchner: Archiv Geschwulstforsch. **37**, 45 (1971)
[35f] Franke, R.: Chem. Biol. Interactions **6**, 1 (1973)
[35g] Franke, R.: Acta biol. med. germ. **30**, 151 (1973)
[35h] Pullman, A.: Biopolymers Symp. **1**, 47 (1964)
[35i] Pullman, B.: Int. J. Quantum Chem. **16**, 669 (1979)
[35j] Jerina, D. M., and J. W. Daly in D. V. Park and R. I. Smith (Eds.): Drug Metabolism, Taylor and Francis, London, 1976
[35k] Lehr, R. E., and D. M. Jerina: Toxicology Environm. Health **2**, 1259 (1977)
[36] Tollenaere, J. P., H. Mooreels and M. Protiva: Eur. J. Med. Chem. **11**, 298 (1976)
[37] Fukunaga, J. Y., C. Hansch and E. E. Steller: J. Med. Chem. **19**, 605 (1976)
[38] Laass, W., G. Eichler, S. Dove, W.-E. Vogt, R. Franke and H. Vahle in R. Franke and P. Oehme (Eds.): Quantitative Structure-Activity Analysis, Akademie-Verlag, Berlin, 1978
[39] Martin, Y. C., and K. R. Lynn: J. Med. Chem. **14**, 1162 (1971)
[40] Silipo, C., and C. Hansch: J. Am. Chem. Soc. **97**, 6849 (1975)
[41] Topliss, J. G., and R. J. Costello: J. Med. Chem. **15**, 1066 (1972)
[42] Topliss, J. G., and R. P. Edwards: J. Med. Chem. **22**, 1238 (1979)
[43] Topliss, J. G., in J. Knoll and F. Darvas (Eds.): Chemical Structure — Biological Activity Relationships, Akadémiai Kiadó, Budapest, 1980
[44] Seydel, J. K., and K.-J. Schaper in J. A. Keverling Buisman (Ed.): Strategy in Drug Research, Pharmacochemistry Library (Eds.: W. Th. Nauta and R. F. Rekker), Vol. 4, Elsevier, Amsterdam, 1982, p. 337
[45] Hansch, C., in J. A. Keverling Buisman (Ed.): Biological Activity and Chemical Structure, Pharmacochemistry Library, (Eds.: W. Th. Nanta and R. F. Rekker), Vol. 2, Elsevier, Amsterdam, 1977, p. 47
[46] Kuchař, M., in R. Franke and P. Oehme (Eds.): Quantitative Structure-Activity Analysis, Akademie-Verlag, Berlin, 1978, contribution to general discussion

[47] Zeelen, F. J., in R. Franke and P. Oehme (Eds.): Quantitative Structure-Activity Analysis, Akademie-Verlag, Berlin, 1978, contribution to general discussion
[48] Hansch, C., and D. F. Calef: J. Org. Chem. **41**, 1240 (1976)
[49] Hansch, C., R. N. Smith, A. Rockoff, D. F. Calef, P. Y. C. Jow and J. Y. Fukunaga: Arch. Biochem. Biophys. **183**, 383 (1970)
[50] Hansch, C., A. Leo and D. Elkins: J. Chem. Documentation **14**, 57 (1974)
[51] Leo, A., D. Elkins and C. Hansch: J. Chem. Documentation **14**, 1 (1974)
[52] Elkins, D., A. Leo and C. Hansch: J. Chem. Documentation **14**, 65 (1974)
[53] Cramer, R. D.: Ann. Reports Med. Chem. **2**, 301 (1976)
[54] Franke, R.: Acta biol. med. germ. **30**, 467 (1973)
[55] Bauer, D. J., and P. W. Sadler: Br. J. Pharmac. Chemother. **15**, 101 (1960)
[56] Bauer, D. J., and L. St. Vincent: Lancet 454 (1963/II)
[57] Snader, K. M., L. W. Chakrin, R. D. Cramer, Y. M. Gelernt, C. K. Miao, D. H. Shah, J. W. Venslavsky, C. R. Willis and B. M. Sutton: J. Med. Chem. **22**, 706 (1979)
[58] Überla, K.: Faktoranalyse, Springer-Verlag, Berlin (West), 1968
[59] Rummel, R. J.: Applied Factor Analysis, Northwestern University Press, Evanston, 1970
[60] Harman, H. H.: Modern Factor Analysis, 2nd edition, University of Chicago Press, 1967
[61] Malinowsky, E. R., and D. G. Howery: Factor Analysis in Chemistry, Wiley, New York, 1980
[62] Overall, J. F., and C. J. Klett: Applied Multivariate Analysis, McGraw-Hill, New York, 1972
[63] Weber, E.: Einführung in die Faktoranalyse, VEB Gustav Fischer Verlag, Jena, 1974
[64] Lewi, P. J., in E. J. Ariens (Ed.): Drug Design, Vol. VII, Academic Press, New York, 1976
[65] Franke, R.: Il Farmaco **34**, 545 (1978)
[66] Franke, R., in J. A. Keverling Buisman (Ed.): Strategy in Drug Research, Pharmacochemistry Library (Eds.: W. Th. Nauta and R. F. Rekker), Vol. 4, Elsevier, Amsterdam, 1982, p. 355
[67] Martin, Y. C.: personal communication
[68] Schewe, T., and S. M. Rapoport: personal communication
[69] Franke, R., and W. Laass: unpublished results

9. Other Approaches to Quantitative Stucture-Activity Analysis with Extrathermodynamic Molecular Parameters

Multiple regression analysis is, of course, not the only possibility to evaluate relationships between molecular parameters and biological activity. This technique is primarily to be applied when in addition to a sufficiently varied sample of structures the following conditions are fulfilled:

1. Biological activity is a continuous quantity of sufficient precision.
2. Either one or a set of uncorrelated dependent variables are taken into consideration.

Frequently, these requirements are not satisfied. This is especially true for the first at the level of mass screening, where biological activity tends to present itself in the form of an activity score (discrete quantity) or even as a yes/no judgment (logical quantity), i.e., as a classification. Classifications may also arise in connection with, for example, structure-selectivity relationships, of differentiation beween agonists, partial agonists and antagonists, and the like. *Classification procedures* such as discriminant analysis or pattern recognition methods must then be employed (the latter will only be dealt with under 11.2. along with structural molecular parameters).

Multivariate techniques are called for where several more or less interrelated biological activities (e.g., results from related or similar biological tests or from the same test but measured under different conditions) are to be analyzed. Only they make it possible to recognize unambiguously and to account adequately for basic features of data structure and to obtain results truly representative of all data in their totality (for reviews on the application of multivariate statistics in quantitative structure-activity analysis, see, e.g., [1, 2]). One multivariate technique, factor analysis, was already discussed in the preceding chapter. The present chapter will be concerned with principal component analysis as a means of determining multivariate QSARs. An alternative to this method is the classical procedure of multivariate regression, which will, however, not be dealt with here, reference being made to textbooks on statistics and, concerning applications in the QSAR field, to [3—5]. In certain cases a helpful alternative to regression analysis is provided by rank correlation analysis, which will, therefore, also be discussed briefly here.

It should be noted that in addition to the mathematical techniques to be discussed in this chapter several other possibilities also exist which will not be dealt with; most of them, however, have not widely been applied to QSAR problems so that their applicability in this area warrants further testing. The accent of the following discussions will not be on mathematical details but rather on basic principles of applicability.

9.1. Principal Component Analysis

9.1.1. Basic Principles

Principal component analysis shares many features with factor analysis. In either case, data matrices obtained by measuring a given set of variables for a given set of objects are examined. Again variables are presented as linear combinations of new variables, called *principal components* in this case. As factors, principal components also are orthogonal vectors. The only difference, although an essential one, between factor analysis and principal component analysis is that with the latter the total variance of the data matrix is considered as common variance so that the concept of unique factors is not employed. As a consequence, principal component analysis cannot be applied to unravel such basic features of multiple data which are only valid in common factor space. Rather, this analysis is basically a mathematical method of describing and reproducing variables of a data matrix by means of a new set of "abstract" variables, the principal components. The purely descriptive model thus obtained can be refined, however, by introducing the condition that the original variables are only reproduced within experimental error. In a subsequent step the abstract components can then be identified with and finally replaced by physically meaningful parameters resulting in a system of equations which describes the variables in terms of these parameters. This approach has extensively been discussed by WEINER and MALINOWSKI who applied it to a variety of problems in physical organic and analytical chemistry [6—17, 19] (for details of the method, see [6, 13, 16, 17] and also [18—20]). The first applications of principal component analysis to QSAR problems have been reported in [13, 18—22]; two examples will be discussed in 9.1.2.2. and 9.1.2.3. Principal component analysis is also particularly suitable for the investigation of complex molecular parameters as will be shown in 9.1.2.1.

The model of principal component analysis may be written as

$$x_{ij} = \sum_{k=1}^{r} u_{ik}v_{kj} + \bar{x}_j + \varepsilon_{ij} \tag{9/1}$$

or in matrix notation

$$\boldsymbol{X} = \boldsymbol{UV} + \bar{\boldsymbol{x}} + \boldsymbol{E} \tag{9/2}$$

where:

x_{ij} = value of the j-th variable for the i-th object,

r = minimum number of components necessary to reproduce the x_{ij} within ε_{ij},

u_{ik} = i-th element of the k-th so-called *object component* describing the k-th property of the i-th object (i-th row of the data matrix) or, in other words, that property of the i-th object reflected by the k-th object component,

v_{kj} = j-th element of the k-th so-called *system component* describing the k-th property of the j-th variable (or j-th system in which measurements of the objects were taken; j-th column of the data matrix) or, in other words, that property of the j-th variable (system) reflected by the k-th system component,

$\bar{x}_j$ = mean value of the j-th variable,

ε_{ij} = residual error (experimental plus model error),

$\boldsymbol{X}$ = data matrix with the objects in the rows and the variables (system) in the columns (usually standardized according to eqn. (8/40))[1]),
$\boldsymbol{U}$ = object component matrix (elements: u_{ik}),
$\boldsymbol{V}$ = system component matrix (elements: v_{kj}),
$\bar{\boldsymbol{x}}$ = vector of mean values (elements: $\bar{x}_j$),
$\boldsymbol{E}$ = error matrix (elements: ε_{ij}).

Equations (9/1) and (9/2) represent a linear model made up from a sum of products of object and system (variable) factors.

For computing the principal components the same technique as in factor analysis, the principal component method (see 8.4.1.), is applied. Since the whole data variance is considered as "common" in principal component analysis (differing from factor analysis) the computation is performed with the original and not the reduced correlation matrix. Prior to the analysis the variables are standardized according to eqn. (8/40). As already discussed in 8.4.1., the principal component method is based on solving an eigenvalue problem. Like factors, the components are also extracted in a sequence of decreasing eigenvalues, i.e., in a sequence of decreasing contributions to data variance. Thus, the first component always extracts the largest and the last the smallest part of variance. Usually, the number of extractable components is equal to the number of the columns of the data matrix (number of variables). With this number of components the data matrix is exactly reproduced. The problem, however, is to reproduce the data only within residual error according to eqns. (9/1) or (9/2), respectively, using the minimum number of components. In order to find this minimum number, r (eqn. (9/1)), the components are added step by step in order of decreasing eigenvalues to the model according to eqn. (9/1) (or (9/2)). After each step the data matrix is reproduced and the procedure continues until the following quality criteria are fulfilled:

1. The average error of the reproduced data becomes equal to the average experimental error. The average error, ε_h, of data reproduction using h principal components can be calculated from:

$$\varepsilon_h = \frac{\sum_{j=1}^{m} \sum_{i=1}^{n} \left(x_{ij} - \bar{x}_j - \sum_{k=1}^{h} u_{ik} v_{kj} \right)}{nm} \qquad (9/3)$$

n = number of objects
m = number of variables
h = number of components added

This criterion can, of course, only be applied if the average experimental error of the variables is known; it implies that the residual error ε_{ij} in eqn. (9/1) is equal to the experimental error or, in other words, that the model of principal component analysis exactly holds (no model error).

---

[1]) Note the difference to factor analysis where the objects are stored in the columns and the variables (systems) in the rows of the data matrix.

2. If the experimental error is not known the so-called ψ value according to EXNER [23] can be used

$$\psi_h = \sqrt{\frac{\sum_{j=1}^{m}\sum_{i=1}^{n} \varepsilon_{ij,h}^2 \cdot mn}{\sum_{j=1}^{m}\sum_{i=1}^{n} (x_{ij} - \bar{x})^2\, mn - h}} \tag{9/4}$$

   where $\varepsilon_{ij,h}$ is the value of ε_{ij} after adding of h components and $\bar{x}$ is the total mean. For very precise physical or chemical data as many components should be added so that ψ_h becomes smaller than 0.10. In the case of biological data which have a larger error this value would be too small; here, ψ_h should be about 0.2—0.3.

3. A further useful criterion is the multiple correlation coefficient r_h between the reproduced data after adding h components and the original data which is related to the ψ value according to:

$$r_h = \sqrt{1 - \psi_h^2 \frac{mn - h}{mn}} \tag{9/5}$$

   Sometimes it is also convenient to consider separately the correlation coefficients between h components and the variables for each variable:

$$r_{jh} = \sqrt{\sum_{k=1}^{h} r_{jk}^2} \tag{9/6}$$

   r_{jh} = correlation coefficient between h added components and the j-th column of the data matrix,
   r_{jk} = correlation coefficient between the j-th column of the data matrix and the k-th component.

4. The most important criterion is the indicator function IND introduced by MALINOWSKI [16, 17]:

$$\mathrm{IND} = \mathrm{RE}/(m - h)^2 \tag{9/7}$$

   RE is the so-called "real error":

$$\mathrm{RE} = \left\{\frac{1}{mn(n - h)}\left[\sum_{k=h+1}^{m}\sum_{i=1}^{n} u_{ik}^2\right]\left[\sum_{j=1}^{m}\sum_{i=1}^{n} (x_{ij} - \bar{x}_j)\right]\right\}^{1/2} \tag{9/7a}$$

   The indicator function passes through a minimum for the correct number of components ($h = r$). The presence of a minimum also proves that the data under investigation can be correctly expressed by the linear model of principal component analysis.

If the minimum number of principal components necessary to reproduce the data matrix within residual error has been found the principal component analysis as such is essentially complete. At this stage, however, no physical interpretation of the result is possible since the components are only abstract mathematical solutions for data reproduction and do not have any physical meaning. A very important step in the procedure of WEINER and MALINOWSKI is, therefore, a special target rotation which allows one to identify the abstract components with physically meaningful quantities. These quantities must either be known from a theoretical model, or a guess must be made as to what they might be. The components are then rotated into vectors of these quantities (e.g., π, σ, etc.) which are called *test vectors*; the elements of the test vectors are the values of the corresponding parameters for the objects of the data matrix. A least squares criterion is applied to the target rotation such that the sum of squared deviations between the rotated component and the corresponding test vector becomes a minimum according to

$$\sum_{i=1}^{n} (\hat{u}_{il} - \hat{u}_{il})^2 = \hat{\varepsilon}_l^2 = \text{Min.!} \tag{9/8}$$

or in vector notation

$$(\hat{\boldsymbol{u}}_l - \hat{\boldsymbol{u}}_l)^T (\hat{\boldsymbol{u}}_l - \hat{\boldsymbol{u}}_l) = \hat{\varepsilon}_l^1 = \text{Min.!}$$

where:

$\hat{\boldsymbol{u}}_l$ = l-th test vector,
$\hat{\boldsymbol{u}}_l$ = l-th rotated object component,
$\hat{u}_{il}$ = value of the l-th test vector for the i-th object (row) of the data matrix (i-th element of $\hat{\boldsymbol{u}}_l$),
$\hat{u}_{il}$ = value of the i-th object in the l-th rotated object component (i-th element of $\hat{\boldsymbol{u}}_l$),
$\hat{\varepsilon}_l^2$ = sum of squared deviations between the l-th object component and the l-th test vector.

The rotated object components are obtained by multiplying the object component matrix $\boldsymbol{U}$ with a rotation vector

$$\hat{\boldsymbol{u}}_l = \boldsymbol{U}\boldsymbol{t}_l \tag{9/9}$$

where $\boldsymbol{t}_l$ is defined as:

$$\boldsymbol{t}_l = \Lambda^{-1}\boldsymbol{U}^T\hat{\boldsymbol{u}}_l \tag{9/10}$$

Λ = diagonal matrix of eigenvalues

This target rotation is completely analogous to a least squares fit as used in regression analysis with the test vectors as dependent and the object components as independent variables; the elements of the corresponding rotation vectors appear as regression coefficients. In the original procedure of WEINER and MALINOWSKI the resulting regression hyperplanes are arbitrarily forced through the origin of the corresponding coordinate system (no absolute term present); this may lead to non-negligible errors. It is better, therefore, to allow adequately for the occurrence of a non-zero ordinate which can easily be done by using normalized test vectors (zero mean). According to WEINER and MALINOWSKI a test vector is accepted as being relevant for a given component if the deviation between the test vector and the corresponding component is within experimental error of the corresponding parameter. Better criteria are the correlation coefficients between test vectors and the component to be identified as well as the multiple correlation coefficient of a test vector and h principal components. The correlation coefficient between the l-th test vector and the k-th principal component is

$$r_{lk} = t_{lk} \sqrt{\lambda_k \Big/ \sum_{i=1}^{n} u_{ik}^2} \tag{9/11}$$

(λ_k = eigenvalue of the k-th component), and the multiple correlation coefficient between the k-th test vector and h principal components amounts to:

$$r_{k(h)} = \sqrt{\sum_{k=1}^{h} r_{lk}^2} \tag{9/12}$$

An advantage of the rotation procedure is that the test vectors need not be complete but may show gaps (missing values for certain objects). On rotation, the gaps are automatically filled and the missing values obtained. In this way, e.g., WEINER [12] found the relative gas phase acidities of some benzoic acids.

If the primary objective is the interpretation or identification of individual principal components with physicochemical parameters rather than their replacement by test vectors another simple approach can be used. In this case, the object components as dependent variables are correlated with molecular parameters in a standard regression procedure.

A special test vector is used in the so-called *uniqueness test* which is performed for all rows of the data matrix. This test indicates rows (objects) which show a particular behaviour. The test vector used has the element one for the row to be tested and zeros for all other rows. Rotation according to eqn. (9/9) yields the so-called *uniqueness* of the object considered and related values for all other objects. Uniqueness lies between 0 and 1, and particular behaviour is indicated for all objects having a value of $\geqq 0.3$. It is advantageous to perform the uniqueness test for each component separately and not, as WEINER and MALINOWSKI [14, 15] do, for all components simultaneously. If several objects have high uniqueness values in one component it may be concluded that this component primarily reflects the behaviour of these objects, and such knowledge may aid in selecting appropriate test vectors for the identification of this component. High uniqueness values in non-relevant components ($k > r$), on the other hand, usually indicate that the data for the corresponding objects are not compatible with the rest of the data matrix. This can be due to experimental errors, different sources of the data or simply to the fact that not all of the objects can correctly be described by the same linear model.

The uniqueness test can also be applied to the variables after repeating the principal component analysis with the transposed data matrix. The same information can, however, also be obtained in a much simpler way from the correlation coefficients r_{jk} between the columns of the data matrix and the object components; a "unique" behaviour of the j-th variable in the k-th component is indicated if the corresponding r_{jk} high.

Once all object components have been identified with test vectors they can be replaced by the latter. Equation (9/1) then transforms to:

$$x_{ij} = \sum_{k=1}^{r} \hat{u}_{ik}\hat{v}_{kj} + c_j + \varepsilon'_{ij} \tag{9/13}$$

Equation (9/13) presents a system of equations (one for each variable) with the variables x_j (columns of the data matrix) as dependent and the test vectors as independent variables. The regression coefficients $\hat{v}_{kj}$ are obtained by rotating the system component matrix with the inverse of the rotation matrix[1]) according to

$$\hat{\boldsymbol{V}} = \boldsymbol{T}^{-1}\boldsymbol{V} \qquad (9/14)$$

where $\boldsymbol{T}$ = rotation matrix with the rotation vectors $\boldsymbol{t}_l$ (see eqn. (9/9)) in the columns.

The error ε'_{ij} in eqn. (9/13) is usually somewhat larger than ε_{ij} in (9/1) since it includes the error of the target rotation; this difference is the smaller the better the test vectors match the components. Since $\hat{\varepsilon}_l^2$ and not the ε'^2_{ij} are minimized in the target rotation (see eqn. (9/8)), eqn. (9/13) does not represent a true regression equation. If, however, each test vector corresponds to a single principal component so that $\hat{\varepsilon}_l^2$ become sufficiently small, the $\hat{v}_{kj}$ in (9/13) are very close to true regression coefficients. The goodness of fit of the equations can be judged by the corresponding correlation coefficients.

Equation (9/13) is the desired result of principal component analysis, representing a multivariate system of "regression" equations. Depending on the definition of objects and systems (variables) there are many possible applications; some important ones for QSAR work are summarized in Table 9.1. The main steps of principal component analysis are summarized again below:

1. calculation of the correlation matrix,
2. evaluation of object and system components by the principal component method,
3. determination of the number (r) of relevant principal components necessary to reproduce the data matrix within experimental error,
4. uniqueness test,
5. selection of test vectors,
6. identification of the object components with test vectors (target rotation),
7. formulation of the system of "regression" equations describing the variables in terms of the parameters used as test vectors.

Table 9.1. Some possibilities for applying principal component analysis

x_{ij}	Objects ($i = 1, \ldots, n$)	Systems ($j = 1, \ldots, m$)	Result
log A	compounds	biological tests	multivariate QSARs
log A	compounds	doses	quantitative structure-activity-concentration relationships
log A	compounds	times	quantitative structure-activity-time relationships
log A	doses	times	quantitative concentration-time relationships
π, log P	substituents	series	multivariate structure-hydrophobicity relationships
π, log P	substituents	partitioning system	multivariate structure-hydrophobicity relationships

[1]) It should be noted that the number of test vectors (columns of $\boldsymbol{T}$) must be equal to the number of principal components, r. This condition is not fulfilled if, for example, object components are related to more than one molecular parameter. In this case, either weighted linear combinations of the corresponding parameters are to be used as test vectors, or a standard regression analysis is applied directly to the original data.

In addition to the work of WEINER and MALINOWSKI referred to above, principal component analysis (partly in modified form) has been applied successfully by various research teams to many problems in analytical and physical chemistry; for reviews, see, e.g. [1, 24]. Principal component analysis can also be carried out when dealing with classification problems (see 9.2.1.).

The application of this method requires data of sufficient precision and objectively existing relations among the various systems. Where such relations are absent, principal component analysis cannot be performed, as appeared to be the case in the work of WEINER and WEINER [13], where an attempt to apply this kind of analysis to the determination of multivariate QSARs in a series of diphenylaminopropanols was not successful. These compounds (objects) were tested in 11 relatively different biological tests (systems) in the mouse. Eight relevant principal components were obtained, which is a high number when taking the number of tests into consideration, and which demonstrates that the relatedness (correlations) of the individual tests is very limited. It would seem that in such an instance the overall data variance must not be regarded as being common to all variables. It then follows that the principal components can only be partially identified. Factor analysis would have been a suitable means of finding the part of commom variance represented by the communalities in a first step.

9.1.2. Examples

9.1.2.1. Principal Component Analysis of Aromatic π Values [20] (cf., [25])

As already set forth in sections 4.1. and 4.2., the values of the hydrophobic substituent constant π are dependent on the electronic environment of the substituents which is different in the various standard series of aromatic compounds. Thus, aromatic π values differ in different standard series. This must be taken into account when selecting π values for quantitative structure-activity analysis, and is reflected in electronic correction factors as in eqns. (7/11)—(7/13). The relationships of that kind thus far derived have the following disadvantages:

1. The univariate considerations, i.e., the comparison of not more than two sets of π values at a time, do not permit a complex data systematization.
2. The substituent selections underlying individual relationships as well as the contributions of meta-, para- and ortho-substituents are dissimilar, and the extent to which the result is affected by this cannot be predicted with certainty.

These two drawbacks can only be overcome by a multivariate analysis of π values for a uniform set of substituents as measured in a representative set of aromatic standard series thus considering the variation of π with the nature of substituents and functional groups simultaneously. Principal component analysis is particularly well suited to this on the following grounds:

1. π values are variables with a high and established precision, their mean error amounting to approximately 0.05π units.
2. π values from different standard series may certainly be expected to be interrelated.

3. The differences among standard series in π values can be explained by mutual perturbations of substituents and the respective functional groups. Such perturbations can usually be represented as a sum of products, which is fully in agreement with the model of principal component analysis.

The objective was to acquire more insight into the physicochemical nature of the hydrophobic substituent constant π and to arrive at pertinent conclusions for quantitative structure-activity analysis. To avoid complications due to steric effects, only π values of substituents in the meta- and para-positions of disubstituted aromatic compounds were considered (structure IX; X is the substituent and Y is the functional group). Meta- and para-substituents were treated separately. Principal component analysis was carried out with π values (variables) for the 14 substituents (objects) F, Cl, Br, I, CH_3, CF_3, OCH_3, OH, NO_2, COOH, CN, $COCH_3$, CH_2OH, H taken from the eight standard series (systems) phenoxyacetic acids (POA), phenylacetic acids (PA), benzoic acids (BA), anilines (A), nitrobenzenes (NB), piperidinoacetanilides (PAA), phenols (P) and benzenes (B) (data from the literature).

Table 9.2. Eigenvalues and quality criteria for principal components derived from π values

k[1])	λ_k		ε_h[4])		ψ[4])		r_h[4])		IND[4])	
	meta[2])	para[3])	meta[2])	para[3])	meta[2])	para[3])	meta[2])	para[3])	meta[2])	para[3])
1	7.630	7.482	0.089	0.123	0.208	0.245	0.978	0.970	0.0031	0.0038
2	0.265	0.304	0.053	0.081	0.147	0.169	0.989	0.986	0.0024	0,0036
3	0.047	0.117	0.041	0.056	0.094	0.126	0.996	0.992	0.0028	0.0037
4	0.030	0.054	0.029	0.040		0.083		0.997	0.0034	0,0044
5	0.014	0.024							0.0048	0.0060
6	0.008	0.011							0.0083	0.0113
7	0.004	0.007							0.0240	0.0310
8	0.001	0.002								

[1]) number of the principal component
[2]) values for the meta-substituent problem
[3]) values for the para-substituent problem
[4]) value after adding the k-th principal component

The eigenvalues and quality criteria for the principal components obtained are given in Table 9.2 (for explanation of symbols, see 9.1.1.). It follows from the eigenvalues that the first principal component in both problems (meta and para) already accounts for about 95% of the data variance (it should be remembered that the eigenvalues reflect the relative variance contributions of the principal components). The average error ε_h for data reproduction reaches the order of magnitude of the average experimental error (about 0.05π units) after adding the second component in the case of meta-substituents and with three components in the case of para-substituents. The implication is that for meta-values two and for para-values three principal components are needed to reproduce the data within experimental error. This is also indicated by the correlation coefficients, ψ values and the indicator function IND, the latter showing in both cases a well-defined minimum which is proof of the validity of the basic assumptions made in applying principal component analysis. The fact that the reproduction of π values of para-substituents requires an additional principal component leads to the conclusion that between the π values of para- and meta-substituents there exists a systematic difference, the former having a more complex character.

Table 9.3. Correlation coefficients r_{jk} for the relation between the π values of the individual standard series (columns of the data matrix) and the object components

Standard series[1])	para-components			meta-components		
	1	2	3	1	2	3
POA	0.982	−0.051	−0.169	0.997	−0.026	0.020
PA	0.959	0.015	0.277	0.994	−0.030	0.026
BA	0.991	0.067	0.010	0.998	0.056	0.012
A	0.974	−0.156	−0.029	0.978	−0.160	0.029
NB	0.902	0.419	−0.006	0.908	0.407	−0.095
PAA	0.985	−0.134	−0.046	0.991	−0.107	−0.030
P	0.962	−0.254	0.048	0.965	−0.215	−0.118
B	0.973	0.121	−0.079	0.977	0.104	0.147

[1]) POA phenoxyacetic acids; PA phenylacetic acids; BA benzoic acids; A anilines; NB nitrobenzenes; PAA piperidinoacetanilides; P phenols; B benzenes

Table 9.3 shows correlation coefficients r_{jk} for the correlations between the π values of individual standard series (systems, columns of the data matrix) and the relevant object components. The general picture obtained is the same for meta- and para-substituents as far as the first two components are concerned. The π values of all series are highly correlated with the first component. Obviously, this component represents that part of aromatic hydrophobicity which is independent of the type of functional group. The lowest correlations occur with the nitrobenzenes, anilines and phenols which have functional groups with relatively high $|\sigma|$ values. Just these series show the highest correlations with the second component so that a connection of this component with electronic properties is indicated. No regular pattern or connection with molecular properties can be detected in the correlations with the third component operative for the para-substituents.

The uniqueness test for the rows of the data matrix (objects, substituents X_i) was performed for each component separately. For both meta- and para-substituents, significant uniqueness values were obtained for the substituents J and CH_2OH in the first and for NO_2, CN and $COCH_3$ in the second component. This result again indicates that the first component is connected with hydrophobicity in general (J and CH_2OH have the highest and the lowest π value, respectively, of all substituents considered), whereas the second component reflects electronic properties. The third component for para-substituents showed significant uniqueness values for the substituents COOH, OH, CN and NO_2. This pattern does not allow any definite conclusions to be drawn as to the character of this component although it is not inconsistent with the view that this component may also be connected with electronic properties.

From the correlations listed in Table 9.3 and the results of the uniqueness test, the following conclusions can be drawn with respect to test vectors to identify the object components:

1. Object component 1 should be identified with quantities which describe the "normal" or "mean" hydrophobicity of aromatic substituents such as the π values from the benzene series (π_B) or REKKERS hydrophobic fragmental constant f (cf., 4.1.).
2. Object component 2 can be identified with electronic substituent constants.
3. No hints as to object component 3 (para) can be furnished.

Table 9.4. Correlation coefficients of relevant object components with substituent constants π_B (hydrophobic substituent constant of HANSCH; benzene series), f (hydrophobic fragmental constant of REKKER), σ (HAMMETT constant) and $\mathfrak{F}$ and $\mathfrak{R}$ (SWAIN-LUPTON constants); for calculation of the correlation coefficients see equation (9.11) and (9.12)

Component	Substituent constants					
	π_B	f	σ_m	σ_p	$\mathfrak{F}$	$\mathfrak{R}$
meta: 1	0.977	0.991	0.226		0.273	
2	0.104	0.042	−0.820		−0.652	
1 and 2 (multiple)	0.983	0.992	0.851		0.707	
para: 1	0.974	0.985		0.131	0.304	0.043
2	0.121	0.068		−0.915	−0.651	−0.737
3	−0.110	−0.084		0.104	0.265	−0.045
1 to 3 (multiple)	0.988	0.991		0.930	0.766	0.740

Table 9.5. Correlation coefficients of the third principal component in the para-problems with some test vectors

Test vectors							
σ_p^2	$f \cdot \sigma_p$	$\mathfrak{F}^2$	R^2	$\mathfrak{F} \cdot \mathfrak{R}$	$\pi_B \cdot \mathfrak{R}$	σ_p, σ_p^2 1)	$\mathfrak{F}^2, \mathfrak{R}^2$ 1)
0.232	−0.162	0.124	0.435	−0.112	0.576	0.434	0.440

1) multiple

Table 9.4, which shows the correlation coefficients (cf., eqns. (9/11) and (9/12)) of relevant object components with physicochemical parameters, fully substantiates the conclusions about the first two components. Therefore, test vectors suitable for the target rotation include the hydrophobicity parameters π_B or f (first component) and the HAMMETT constant σ (second component). As expected, neither $\mathfrak{F}$ or $\mathfrak{R}$ alone permits a description of electronic effects. It is, however, possible to identify the second component by a linear combination of these two quantities.

Various linear combinations of several electronic, hydrophobic and steric substituent constants (including non-linear and product terms) were tried to identify the third component of the para-problem (Table 9.5). The best correlation was obtained with the cross-product $\pi_B \Re$ as test vector with a correlation coefficient of 0.576. Although this correlation is statistically significant its poor quality does not justify an identification of the third para-component with this quantity. The correlation indicates, however, that cross-products between hydrophobic and electronic terms may come into operation when interrelating π values from different aromatic series. The failure to identify the third component is neither very serious nor surprising considering the small part of data variance accounted for by this component. In the final target rotation, therefore, only the test vectors identifiable with the first two components were included so that relationships of the same type are obtained for meta- and para-substituents. Only a slight improvement of fit would result for the para-substituent equations from a correct identification of the third component. This does not mean, however, that this component has no physical significance.

The equations obtained from the target rotation of the first two components into π_B or f and σ as test vectors are of the general form (j denotes the standard series)

$$\pi_j = a_j \pi_B + b_j \sigma + c_j \tag{9/15}$$

and

$$\pi_j = a_j' f + b_j' \sigma + c_j' \tag{9/16}$$

The coefficients of these equations are summarized in Tables 9.6 and 9.7.

Table 9.6. Coefficients a_j, b_j, c_j and correlation coefficients r for the equation $\pi_j = a_j \pi_B + b_j \sigma + c_j$ (9.15) for the calculation (reproduction) of π values from the test vectors π_B and σ (third component for para-substituents neglected)

Standard series j[1])	para π values				meta π values			
	a_j	b_j	c_j	r	a_j	b_j	c_j	r
POA	1.05	0.37	0.10	0.981	0.92	0.42	0.03	0.987
PA	0.95	0.20	0.12	0.926	0.94	0.45	0.00	0.975
BA	0.92	0.10	0.12	0.986	0.99	0.17	0.11	0.988
A	1.46	0.84	0.14	0.967	1.23	1.20	0.06	0.970
NB	0.78	−0.49	0.21	0.945	0.87	−0.91	0.39	0.924
PAA	1.00	0.53	0.17	0.975	1.04	0.79	0.05	0.984
P	1.07	0.85	0.08	0.987	0.98	1.18	0.02	0.983
B	1.00	0.00	0.00	1.000	1.00	0.00	0.00	1.000

[1]) POA phenoxyacetic acids; PA phenylacetic acids; BA benzoic acids; A anilines; NB nitrobenzenes; PAA piperidinoacetanilides; P phenols; B benzenes

It follows from these tables that within the context of the standard series and substituents under consideration π values can be described extremely well by a linear combination of π_B or f and σ. The π_B values characterize the hydrophobicity of substituents in a normal (i.e., no interference from other influences) aromatic environment, which can be regarded as being the "*normal intrinsic aromatic hydrophobicity*" of substituents. The values of the intercept c_j are 0 or not significantly different from 0, as was to be expected since c_j is equal to the π_j value of the substituent H which, by definition always is 0 $\left(\pi_B(\mathrm{H}) = \sigma(\mathrm{H}) = 0\right)$.

The situation with the corresponding f equations (Table 9.7) is similar but not identical. It is most interesting that the equations describing the benzene series in Table 9.7 have $b_j' \neq 0$. This means that an electronic correction is required if the f values are correlated with the "normal intrinsic aromatic hydrophobicity" as represented by the π_B values. The conclusion to be drawn is that f is not a "pure" hydrophobicity parameter but contains an electronic contribution which is reflected by the σ term in the π_B equations. This electronic contribution reflects an average electronic environmental effect of other substituents which is a consequence of the calculation of f values from log P values of a great number of di- and trisubstituted benzenes. Therefore, f could be regarded as representing the "*average intrinsic aromatic hydrophobicity*". The electronic differences between π_B and f result in the coefficients a_j and b_j (Table 9.6) being greater than the corresponding a_j' and b_j' (Table 9.7). The differences between the c_j and c_j' correctly reflect the value of f_H.

With the equation

$$a_j = 1 + k_j \tag{9/17}$$

eqn. (9/15) can be written as:

$$\pi_j = (1 + k_j)\,\pi_B + b_j\sigma + c_j = \pi_B + k_j\pi_B + b_j\sigma + c_j \tag{9/18}$$

With most series the constant k_j has only a low value, so that a_j in eqn. (9/15) usually is close to one.

Table 9.7. Coefficients a_j', b_j', c_j' and correlation coefficients r for the equation $\pi_j = a_j'f + b_j'\sigma + c_j'$ (9.16) for the calculation (reproduction) of π values from the test vectors f and σ (third principal component for para-substituents neglected)

Standard series j[1])	para π values				meta π values			
	a_j'	b_j'	c_j'	r	a_j'	b_j'	c_j'	r
POA	0.97	0.25	−0.15	0.972	0.86	0.23	−0.15	0.989
PA	0.88	0.10	−0.11	0.935	0.88	0.25	−0.18	0.986
BA	0.85	0.00	−0.09	0.982	0.92	−0.05	−0.08	0.993
A	1.35	0.68	−0.20	0.969	1.14	0.93	−0.30	0.970
NB	0.72	−0.58	0.03	0.961	0.80	−1.09	0.09	0.931
PAA	0.93	0.42	−0.07	0.978	0.97	0.57	−0.15	0.982
P	0.99	0.74	−0.18	0.985	0.91	0.97	−0.17	0.993
B	0.92	−0.11	−0.23	0.984	0.93	−0.22	−0.19	0.984

[1]) POA phenoxyacetic acids; PA phenylacetic acids; BA benzoic acids; A anilines; NB nitrobenzenes; PAA piperidinoacetanilides; P phenols; B benzenes

Larger deviations are only seen with nitrobenzenes and anilines. A comparison of k_j with the σ values of functional groups (see Table 9.8) shows these quantities to be related. In standard series where the functional groups are strongly electron-releasing k_j is preceded by a positive sign, and in standard series where these groups are strongly electron-attracting k_j becomes negative, the absolute values $|k_j|$ approximately paralleling the absolute value $|\sigma_j|$. The constant k_j and thus the coefficient a_j are, therefore, conditioned by the electronic properties of the functional group Y_j, a_j deviating more from unity as these properties are more pronounced. A similar relationship exists between the coefficients b_j and σ_i. These relationships are statistically highly significant according to the proportionalities (p_1, p_2 = proportionality constants):

$$k_j \sim p_1\sigma_j \quad (9/19)$$

$$b_j \sim p_2\sigma_j \quad (9/20)$$

Table 9.8. Comparison of k_j values from eqn. (9/18) with the HAMMETT constants of the functional group (σ_j) for the standard series

Standard series j	Functional group Y_j	para		meta	
		k_j	σ_j	k_j	σ_j
PAO	$-OCH_2COOH$	0.05	−0.33	−0.08	—
PA	$-CH_2COOH$	−0.05	0.18	−0.06	(0.15)
BA	$-COOH$	−0.09	0.45	−0.01	0.37
A	$-NH_2$	0.46	−0.66	0.23	−0.16
NB	$-NO_2$	−0.22	0.78	−0.13	0.71
PAA	$-NHCOCH_2NC_5H_{11}$	0.00	0.10	0.04	0.11
P	$-OH$	0.07	−0.37	−0.03	0.12
B	$-H$	0.00	00.0	0.00	0.00

The constant p_1 is practically the same for meta- and para-substituents whereas p_2 shows slight differences; these differences, however, are not significant. Equation (9/15) may now be rewritten to yield a more general relationship which if a notation analogous to eqn. (9/1) is used, reads:

$$\pi_{ij} = \pi_{iB} + p_1\sigma_j\pi_{iB} + p_2\sigma_j\sigma_i + \gamma_j \quad (9/21)$$

π_{ij} = π value of the i-th substituent in the j-th standard series containing the j-th functional group,
π_{iB} = π value of the i-th substituent in the benzene series,
σ_j = σ value of the j-th functional group,
σ_i = σ value of the i-th substituent,
γ_j = ordinate.

An analogous relationship can, of course, also be derived from eqn. (9/16). The γ_j term includes c_j (which is approximately zero) but, in addition, possibly also depends on σ_j; such a dependence, if present, would not be very important. It then follows from eqn. (9/21) (and from the corresponding relationships with f derivable from eqn. (9/16)) that π values of aromatic meta- and para-substituents can be described by a linear combination of their "*normal intrinsic aromatic hydrophobicity*" (expressed by π_B) or their "*average intrinsic aromatic hydrophobicity*" (expressed by f) and electronic corrections. These electronic corrections depend in a regular fashion on the electronic properties of both the substituents (expressed by σ_i) and the functional groups (expressed by σ_j). The first electronic correction expressed by the product $\pi_{iB}\sigma_j$ (or $f_i\sigma_j$) may be attributed to the change in π if a substituent is transferred from a normal (or average) aromatic environment to an environment disturbed by the functional group Y_j. It is logical that this effect depends both on the value of π_{iB} (or f_i) as a capacity factor and on σ_j as a measure of the degree of disturbance (intensity factor). After placement of the substituents into the new environment a mutual interaction between substituents and the functional group will take place which is reflected by the $\sigma_j\sigma_i$ term.

Equation (9/21) fully corresponds to the basic model of principal component analysis according to eqn. (9/1) since the π_{ij} are represented as a linear combination of products each comprising a substituent and a functional group factor (note that the first term in (9/21) can also be considered as such a product with a functional group factor of unity). The picture of the physical nature of aromatic π values presented by eqn. (9/21) is very reasonable, and this equation certainly reflects the most important features of aromatic hydrophobicity (see also [26]). In order to check the validity of this equation, $\log P$ values of 79 meta- or para-disubstituted benzenes were correlated with π_B and σ values of the substituents. For a disubstituted benzene with the substituents X_1 and X_2, $\log P$ is equal to:

$$\log P = \log P_{C_6H_6} + \pi_{X_1} + \pi_{X_2} \tag{9/22}$$

Since both substituents can be considered as a functional group with respect to each other the π values in (9/22) can be expressed by eqn. (9/21) according to (γ_j neglected):

$$\pi_{X_1} = \pi_1 = \pi_{1B} + p_1\sigma_2\pi_{1B} + p_2\sigma_2\sigma_1 \tag{9/23}$$

$$\pi_{X_2} = \pi_2 = \pi_{2B} + p_1\sigma_1\pi_{2B} + p_2\sigma_1\sigma_2 \tag{9/24}$$

Substituting (9/23) and (9/24) into (9/21) yields:

$$\log P = \log P_{C_6H_6} + \pi_{1B} + \pi_{2B} + p_1(\sigma_2\pi_{1B} + \sigma_1\pi_{2B}) + p_2\sigma_1\sigma_2 \tag{9/25}$$

From regression analysis, the following relationship was obtained:

$$\log P = 2.15 + 0.90\pi_{1B} + 0.84\pi_{2B} + 0.21(\sigma_2\pi_{1B} + \sigma_1\pi_{2B}) - 0.53\sigma_1\sigma_2 \tag{9/25a}$$

$$n = 79 \qquad r = 0.965 \qquad s = 0.226$$

This equation shows a good fit and is in good agreement with expectation. The ordinate exactly corresponds to the partition coefficient of benzene, and the regression coefficients of π_{1B} and π_{2B} are not significantly different from unity and from each other.

For quantitative structure-activity analysis the main conclusions from the preceding are:

1. π values of para- and meta-substituents show a clear difference in physicochemical properties but this is reflected as only a minor dissimilarity in numerical values, and can usually (but not always) be neglected. For this reason one can, in principle, accept the position-independence of aromatic fragmental constants f. In special cases, e.g., where a refinement of analysis is required, the difference between meta- and para-π values must be taken into account, and the use of the hydrophobic fragmental constant is then to be discouraged.

2. π values of substituents in mono-substituted benzenes (π_B values) and aromatic fragmental constants reflect "normal intrinsic aromatic hydrophobicity" and "average intrinsic aromatic hydrophobicity", respectively
3. π values of aromatic meta- and para-substituents can be described by their "normal intrinsic aromatic hydrophobicity" (expressed by π_B) or their "average intrinsic aromatic hydrophobicity" (expressed by f) and electronic corrections (expressed by the σ values of the substituent and the respective functional group).
4. The fundamental equation (7/7) interrelating aromatic π values from two different standard series follows directly from eqns. (9/21) and (9/22); eqns. (7/9) and (7/10) may be considered special cases. Neglecting γ_j, the following expressions can be derived from (9/21) for the constants α and β in eqn. (7/7) (σ_Y and σ_Z = Hammett constants of the functional groups Y and Z, respectively):

$$\alpha = \frac{1 + k_Y}{1 + k_Z} = \frac{1 + p_1\sigma_Y}{1 + p_1\sigma_Z} = 1 + p_1(\sigma_Y - \alpha\sigma_Z) \qquad (9/26)$$

$$\beta = -\frac{1 + k_Y}{1 + k_Z} b_Z + b_Y = p_2\sigma_Y - [(1 + p_1\sigma_Y)/(1 + p_1\sigma_Z)]\, p_2\sigma_Z$$

$$= p_2(\sigma_Y - \alpha\sigma_Z) \qquad (9/27)$$

Equations (9/26) and (9/27) can be simplified by introducing average values of p_1 ($p_1 \approx -0.3$) and p_2 ($p_2 \approx -1.1$) and neglecting the small deviations of α from unity ($\alpha \approx 1$) to yield the approximate expressions (9/28) and (9/29):

$$\alpha = 1 - 0.3(\sigma_Y - \sigma_Z) \qquad (9/28)$$

$$\beta = -1.1(\sigma_Y - \sigma_Z) \qquad (9/29)$$

All rules already discussed in connection with eqn. (7/7) immediately follow from these relationships.
5. The results of principal component analysis, the principles derived and the overall data systematization would not have been achieved by means of simple univariate analyses (= isolated pairwise comparisons of π values from various standard series using multiple regression analysis). This indicates clearly the advantage of principal component analysis as a multivariate technique. It should be noted that this technique has also been succesfully applied to other similar problems related to a real understanding of complex molecular parameters, for example, in investigations on the solvent dependence of log P [27—29] and in an analysis of σ values [30—33].

9.1.2.2. Multivariate Structure-Activity Relationships of Antibacterial Rifamycin B Amides [34]

Sensi et al. [35] have investigated the antibacterial activities (variables) of a series of rifamycin B amides (objects; structure XXXVIII) on four grampositive bacteria (systems: *M. aureus*, *S. faecalis*, *S. hemolyticus* and *B. subtilis*). These data are suitable for the application of principal component analysis to establish multivariate QSARs because an intrinsic relation between the results with the four bacterial strains and, in consequence, a sufficient covariance of the biological variables (biological activities) may be expected. A further advantage of this example is that a HANSCH analysis has already been applied to these data by QUINN et al. [36], thereby permitting a satisfactory comparison with results obtained through univariate regression analysis.

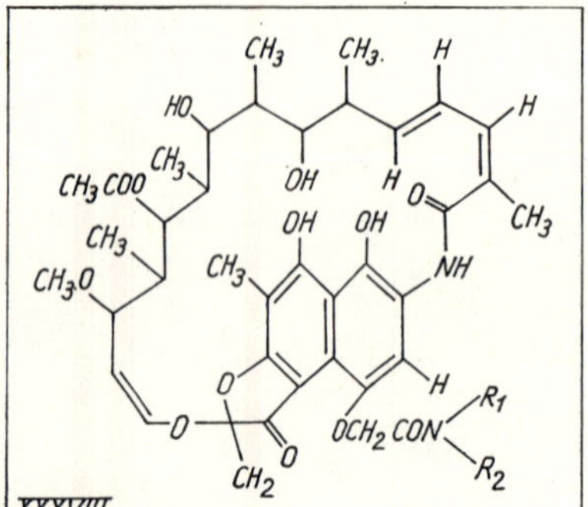

XXXVIII

The biological inhibition data for the four strains (log A) as well as the parameters log P, $\sum \sigma^*$ and $\sum E_S$ which describe, respectively, hydrophobic, electronic and steric substituent effects, were taken from [36]. The indicator variable I describes disubstitution on the amide nitrogen:

$$I = \begin{cases} 1 \text{ for N,N-disubstituted compounds} \\ 0 \text{ for non- or mono-substituted compounds} \end{cases} \qquad (9/30)$$

The compounds selected for the principal component analysis were those occurring in all regression equations presented in [36] for this homologous series for all the four bacterial test systems (compound Nos. 1, 5, 8—11, 13—18, 20—22, 25, 26, 29, 30, 32—35, 39—40) in Table I of QUINNS article [36]). Table 9.9 shows the eigenvalues and quality criteria of the extracted principal components. As no experimental error is known for the biological data concerned, the number of relevant principal components is best established with the aid of the indicator function IND. That function has a minimum at $k = 1$ (IND $= 0.042$ when $k = 0$) so that the first component should be sufficient for data reproduction within experimental error. Table 9.10, concerned with the correlations of invidual object components with the test systems (columns of the data matrix), shows this to be true for three of the four bacterial strains. Only the reproduction of inhibition data for *S. hemolyticus* by means of the first component is not satisfactory. It would appear that the second component must be added here, in which this strain shows an obvious uniqueness according to the corresponding correlation coefficient. The uniqueness test for the compounds (objects) afforded not striking value except for that of the unsubstituted rifamycin amide in the first component. The uniqueness of the primary amide is not surprising as QUINN et al. [36] have already drawn attention to the importance of the number of amide substituents.

When identifying the object components it must be borne in mind that only the first one may serve as basis for a global target rotation, the second one being specific (unique) to *S. hemolyticus*. The test vectors were determined by correlating the substituent constants mentioned above with the first component. The results of QUINNS analysis indicate that the first object component reflects linear combinations of the above mentioned molecular parameters. These combinations were evaluated by regression analysis

Table 9.9. Eigenvalues and quality criteria for principal components derived from the logarithms of antibacterial activity (log A)

k[1])	λ_k	ε_h[2])	IND[2])	ψ[2])	r_h[2])
1	3.515	0.165	0.030	0.322	0.947
2	0.370	0.089	0.039	0.181	0.984
3	0.067	0.053	0.147	0.109	0.994
4	0.049	—	—	—	—

1) number of principal component
2) value after adding the k-th principal component

Table 9.10. Correlation coefficient r_{jk} for the relation between the log A values for the four bacterial strains and the object components

Strain	Object components				
	1	2	1 and 2 (multiple)	3	1 to 3 (multiple)
M. aureus	0.976	−0.010	0.976	0.206	0.998
S. faecalis	0.962	−0.194	0.982	−0.143	0.992
S. hemolyticus	0.854	0.516	0.998	−0.057	0.999
B. subtilis	0.952	−0.257	0.986	−0.016	0.986

$$u_1 = 0.122 \log P^{(0)} - 0.510 \sum \sigma^{*(0)} - \sum E_S^{(0)} \tag{9/31}$$

$$n = 29 \qquad r = 0.867$$

$$u_1 = 0.337 \log P^{(0)} - 0.046 (\log P)^{2(0)} + 0.567 I^{(0)} \tag{9/32}$$

$$n = 29 \qquad r = 0.954$$

where the exponent "(0)" means that the parameters were normalized to a mean of zero, thereby avoiding absolute terms. By applying these two parameter combinations as test vectors (see footnote p. 202), the usual target rotation will yield multivariate "regression" equations for the four biological activities. These equations are summarized together with the corresponding univariate HANSCH equations (from [36]) in Tables 9.11 and 9.12.

As can be seen, the equations resulting from principal component analysis are in excellent agreement with the relationships ascertained through multiple regression analysis. Eqns. (9/33), (9/34) and (9/36) indicate hydrophobic, electronic and steric substituent effects in the respective bacterial test systems. In the case of *S. hemolyticus* (eqn. (9/35)) only electronic effects are demonstrable. In (9/37)—(9/40) — cf.,

Table 9.12 — the $\sum \sigma^*$ term is replaced by the highly correlated indicator variable I. Moreover, the E_S term has disappeared and the relationship between log A and log P changes from a linear into a parabolic one. No choice between the two types of equations can be made on the basis of the available data. Again, one is faced with the fact that within inexpertly composed sample, multicollinearities lead to ambiguity.

Table 9.11. Coefficients of the equation $\log A = a \log P + b \sum \sigma^* + c \sum E_S + d$ from the principal component analysis (PCA) with testvector $\hat{\hat{\boldsymbol{u}}}_1$ (equation (9/31) compared with the relevant relations from regression analysis (RA; [36]) (n number of data points; r = correlation coefficient)

Equation	Strain	Type of analysis	*a*	*b*	*c*	*d*	*r*	*n*
(9/33) a	*M. aureus*	PCA	0.284	−1.111	−0.214	7.25	0.950	29
(9/33) b		RA	0.22	−1.20	−0.25	7.41	0.915	41
(9/34) a	*S. faecalis*	PCA	0.252	−1.052	−0.190	6.47	0.927	29
(9/34) b		RA	0.31	−0.78	−0.22	6.38	0.912	41
(9/35) a	*S. hemolyticus*	PCA	0.178	−0.744	−0.134	7.41	0.811	29
(9/35) b		RA	0.00	−0.93	0.00	7.83	0.858	36
(9/36) a	*B. subtilis*	PCA	0.214	−0.895	−0.161	5.84	0.929	29
(9/36) b		RA	0.27	−0.62	−0.15	5.74	0.924	39

Table 9.12. Coefficients of the equation $\log A = a \log P + b (\log P)^2 + cI + d$ from the principal component analysis (PCA) with test vector $\hat{\hat{\boldsymbol{u}}}_2$ (equation 9/32) compared with the relevant relations from regression analysis (RA; [36]) (n number of data points; r = correlation coefficient)

Equation	Strain	Type of analysis	*a*	*b*	*c*	*d*	*r*	*n*
(9/37) a	*M. aureus*	PCA	0.807	−0.110	1.357	5.762	0.933	29
(9/37) b		RA	0.51	−0.06	1.30	6.20	0.920	42
(9/38) a	*S. faecalis*	PCA	0.714	−0.097	1.202	5.144	0.919	29
(9/38) b		RA	0.74	−0.10	0.79	5.43	0.915	42
(9/39) a	*S. hemolyticus*	PCA	0.505	−0.069	0.849	6.472	0.814	29
(9/39) b		RA	0.48	−0.10	1.18	6.40	0.866	41
(9/40) a	*B. subtilis*	PCA	0.608	−0.083	1.022	4.713	0.903	29
(9/40) b		RA	0.41	−0.03	0.76	5.04	0.909	41

As expected, the equations for *S. hemolyticus* in Tables 9.11 and 9.12 are basically poorer than those for the other strains. As already explained, it is necessary in this case to add the second component. The following relationships for the antibacterial activity against *S. hemolyticus* are then disclosed[1]).

$$\log A = -0.991 \sum \sigma^* + 7.809 \qquad (9/41)$$

$$n = 29 \qquad r = -0.881$$

$$\log A = -1.014 \sum \sigma^* + 0.072 \log P + 7.692 \qquad (9/42)$$

$$n = 29 \qquad r = 0.895$$

$$\log A = -0.088(\log P)^2 + 0.426 \log P + 1.062 I + 6.515 \qquad (9/43)$$

$$n = 29 \qquad r = 0.887$$

All three equations show an essential improvement over the corresponding relationships given in Tables 9.11 and 9.12. No significance is achieved by adding an E_S term to (9/42). The inhibitory activity on *S. hemolyticus* is in the first place governed by the electronic effects of substituents, and in addition also by a weak hydrophobic effect. Comparing (9/41) with (9/35b) (Table 9.11) again shows a good agreement.

As a whole, this example illustrates the feasibility of principal component analysis to determine multivariate QSARs where individual tests or test systems are interrelated and thus a high covariance of variables exists. In such a case, the results can be compared with those of multiple regression analysis performed for each test separately. Principal component analysis is, however, more efficient, and another major advantage of this procedure is that valuable information (e.g., about a particular behaviour of single objects or systems) is secured by data systematization. As for the present example, this is brought out clearly by the uniqueness of the unsubstituted amide group in the first component as well as of the strain. *S. hemolyticus* in the second principal component. The biological potencies in the four bacterial strains can also be directly related to the principal components resulting in multivariate activity-activity relationships [21].

9.1.2.3. Quantitative Structure-Activity-Time Relationships for Anti-Inflammatory Salicylic Acid Derivatives [22]

As remarked above (see also Table 9.1), principle component analysis may also serve for a multivariate analysis of the time-dependent biological activity of a congeneric drug series. Here, too, the compounds of the series are the objects, whilst the various times of measurement take the place of systems. A very interesting question in this context is whether principal component analysis will, in principle, make it possible to differentiate pharmacodynamic from pharmacokinetic effects. If so, time-dependent and time-independent principal components should be extractable from the data matrix.

Using the inhibition of carageenin-induced paw oedema as biological test, the anti-inflammatory activity of 14 salicylic acid derivatives (structure XXXIX) was measured in female Wistar rats 3, 4 and 5 hours after oral application of 1 mmol/kg (data

---

1) Equations (9/41)–(9/43) were obtained by applying regression analysis to log A values reproduced by the first two components.

from [37]). The data were subjected to principal component analysis. Eigenvalues and quality criteria of the resultant principal components are recorded in Table 9.13. The first principal component may in any case be looked upon as well established whilst the relvance of the second principal component is not unequivocal. The steady increase of the indicator function raises doubts as to the second principal component (the predictive usefulness of the indicator function is not invariably explicit), while the correlation coefficient and the ψ value suggest the necessity of the second principal component for data matrix reproduction (provided that the unknown error in biological data is within acceptable limits). As a test of the feasibility of principal component analysis for determining structure-activity-time relationships and especially for separating pharmacodynamic from pharmacokinetic effects, the second principal component will also be considered relevant.

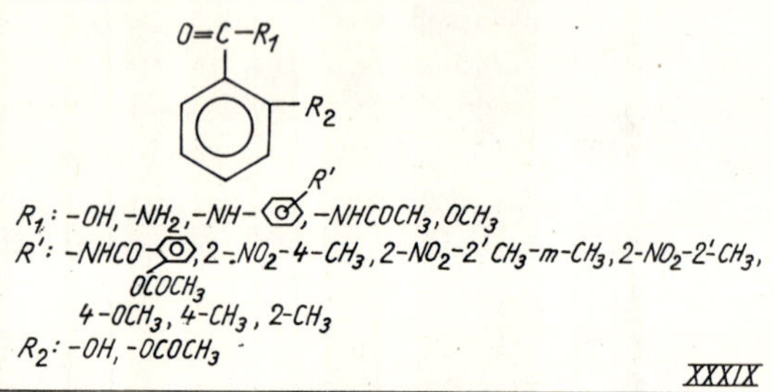

XXXIX

The correlation between the principal components and the logarithms of the inhibitory effects measured at various times are shown in Table 9.14. In view of the high correlations with the log A values of all three measuring times, the first principal component apparently embodies a time-independent (i.e., pharmacodynamic) effect. The time-dependent part is essentially contained in the second principal component, as evidenced in particular by the high correlation with the value after 5 hours.

Table 9.13. Eigenvalues and quality criteria for the principal components derived from time dependent antiinflammatory action of salicyclic acid derivatives

k[1]	λ_k	IND[2]	ψ[2]	r_h[2]
1	2.426	0.050	0.44	0.898
2	0.339	0.182	0.27	0.962
3	0.235			

[1]) number of principal component
[2]) value after adding the k-th principal component

To determine structure-pharmacodynamic relations the first principal component was correlated with a small set of selected molecular parameters (log P calculated from f values; MR and several indicator variables). In view of the complexity of the variations in R_1 resulting in complex intramolecular interactions and the relatively small number ($n = 14$) of compounds, no attempt was made to approach the problem from all angles. The only objective was to ascertain whether the discovery of quantitative relationships would be in the realm of possibility. From the few equations tested the following represents the best result for expressing the first principal component:

$$u_1 = -0.26 \sum \text{MR} + 0.33 (\sum \text{MR})^2 + 0.46 I_1 + 0.25 \qquad (9/44)$$

$$n = 14 \qquad r = 0.744$$

Indicator variable I_1 indicates the presence ($I_1 = 1$) or absence ($I_2 = 0$) of the hydroxy group in position R_1. Equation (9/44) is statistically significant ($p < 0.005$) but its descriptive power is only moderate. No doubt, a better equation could be found by considering a larger parameter space and testing all conceivable relations. What (9/44) does suggest is that steric factors may be of importance for the pharmacodynamic effect and that, moreover, in R_1 a hydroxy group tends to be more favourable than —NHR groups.

Table 9.14. Correlation coefficients r_{jk} for the relation between log A at the three times of measurement and the object components

log A after	Components			
	1	2	1 and 2 (multiple)	3
3 hours	0.914	0.189	0.933	0.360
4 hours	0.907	0.272	0.947	−0.322
5 hours	0.877	−0.479	0.999	−0.042

Identification of the second principal component was based on the *assumption* that any change in anti-inflammatory activity with time may in the first instance be described in terms of a first-order reaction

$$A_{i1} \xrightarrow{k_{i1}} A_{i2} \xrightarrow{k_{i2}} A_{i3} \qquad (9/45)$$

where A_{ij} is the measured value of the anti-inflammatory activity of the i-th compound at the j-th time ($j = 1$:3 hours; $j = 2$:4 hours; $j = 3$:5 hours) and the k_{ij}'s denote the corresponding "rate constants".[1] Assuming the A_{ij}'s to be proportional to corresponding concentrations c_{ij}'s at the receptor, it follows from the rate equation of a first-order reaction:

$$\log A_{i2} - \log A_{i1} = k_{i1}(t_2 - t_1) = k_{i1} \qquad (9/46)$$

$$\log A_{i3} - \log A_{i2} = k_{i2}(t_3 - t_2) = k_{i2} \qquad (9/47)$$

A correlation of the second object component with these "rate constants" led to a surprisingly good relationship:

$$u_2 = 0.57 k_1 + 0.29 k_2 \qquad (9/48)$$

$$n = 14 \qquad r = 0.996$$

[1]) The k_{ij} are, of course, not true rate constants. They should be regarded as apparent model parameters which are connected with the time dependence of biological activity if this dependence is of a first order.

Equation (9/48) strongly indicates that the time-dependent component of anti-inflammatory activity is, indeed, contained in the second component. Accordingly, principal component analysis would provide a means of separating pharmacodynamic and pharmacokinetic effects within a congeneric series from measured time dependences of biological activity, and, thus, of evaluating structure-pharmacodynamic and structure-pharmacokinetic relationships separately. If such is true and it is desired to identify the "pharmacokinetic" component(s), measurements performed at more than three time values are needed. Because of this restriction and the minor contribution of the second component to variance, no attempt has been made in the present case to identify this component with physicochemical parameters.

9.2. Classification Methods

Quite often objects (e.g., drugs) can be classified on the basis of an interesting property (e.g., nature or intensity of drug action). The task then is to find an algorithm (*rule for classification* or *classificator*) which describes the distribution of objects over the classes in terms of known or measurable quantities of the objects (e.g., substituent constants). The algorithm is so determined in a training series of compounds that classification is reflected as consistently as possible. The following are the points to which the determination of the algorithm is directed:

1. From the parameters appearing in the classificator one may draw conclusions as to those properties of objects which are of importance for classification.
2. With the help of the classificator it is possible to classify as yet unexamined objects, i.e., to assign them to a given class and thus to make predictions as to the property underlying the classification.
3. In a few cases the behaviour or position of objects within individual classes can be indicated beyond classification.

Which objectives are in the foreground and to what extent they can be realized are questions that depend on the type of problem, the type of data and the method of classification applied.

In drug research, the following situations can be encountered:

1. Classification according to drug activity in such cases where the biological activity cannot be represented by a continuous quantity but only as an activity score. Each score value (or possibly ranges of score values) corresponds to a class so that, for example, a score in four different levels represents classes of inactive, weakly active, strongly active and extremely active compounds. If a test affords no more than a differentiation between "active" and "inactive", there are two classes. Biological activity is frequently referred to in the form of a classification (discrete quantity) at the level of biological mass screening intended to test the largest possible number of compounds with a minimum of costs. To rationalize drug research effectively even at this level, the application of classification methods is of great importance to aid further syntheses and testing.
2. Classification according to intrinsic activity, with the result that classes of agonists, partial agonists and antagonists are obtained.

3. Classification according to the type of drug action (e.g., with respect to different actions on the central nervous system).
4. Classification according to main action and side effects. If, for example, the desired activity is A_M and the side effect is A_S the following classification may result:

   Class 1: Compounds with $A_M > A_S$ (or $A_S = 0$)

   Class 2: Compounds with $A_M \approx A_S$

   Class 3: Compounds with $A_M < A_S$ (or $A_M = 0$).

Methods of classification are diverse, and are often referred to in the literature (along with methods for entirely different purposes) as "*artificial intelligence*" or "*pattern recognition methods*". This is, however, quite an arbitrary designation, which is not necessarily adhered to because the various methods of classification differ in mathematical features. Nevertheless, a collective presentation of classification methods of importance in QSAR work in one chapter would be logical; after all, they share the same purpose, namely the discovery of rules for classification. Since, however, the organization of this monograph is such that methods of describing molecular properties rather than mathematical techniques are in the foreground and the applicability and predictive utility of methods of classification depend on the way molecules are described, a different course will be followed. In this section attention will be paid to two procedures assuming that continuous molecular parameters as in the extrathermodynamic approach are available, and in section 11.2. special "non-parametric" pattern recognition methods will be discussed, together with the use of discrete descriptors (structural parameters). Such a division is, however, not entirely free of arbitrariness, since the pattern recognition methods to be discussed in 11.2. can also be applied if the descriptors are continuous quantities.

9.2.1. Classification Using Principal Component Analysis (SIMCA Method)

Worked out and extensively used by WOLD and colleagues [38—49] this is a very elegant and efficient method, which can serve all purposes mentioned above. As principal component analysis has already been discussed, only the principle and major steps of the procedure will be dealt with; for computational details, reference is made to the original articles.

Extrathermodynamic parameters (including, for example, substituent constants) are used as features to describe molecules. The procedure is based on a search for similarities through principal component analysis, a principal component model being calculated according to eqn. (9/1) for each class separately with the molecular parameters as the x_{ij}. Geometrically, each of these models corresponds to a r-dimensional hyperplane (at r relevant principal components) in the multidimensional space spanned by the molecular parameters. The hyperplane is such that it has the closest possible fit to the objects of the respective class, and the position of the objects with respect to this plane is determined by the object components of the principal component model. In each class, the goodness of fit can be expressed by the residual standard deviation

s_q according to

$$s_q = \left[\sum_{i=1}^{n_q} \sum_{j=1}^{m} \frac{\varepsilon_{ij,q}^2}{(n_q - r_q - 1)(m - r_q)} \right]^{1/2} \tag{9/49}$$

with

$\varepsilon_{ij,q}$ = residual error of the principal component model for the q-th class,
n_q = number of compounds in the q-th class,
r_q = number of relevant principal components for the q-th class,
m = number of descriptors.

The s_q define confidence "slabs" around the class planes defined by the respective principal component models. As a result, the classes are represented as a kind of "hyper-boxes" in parameter space. The criterion for classifying a compound then is the hyper-box in which it fits best. To this end, each object is fitted to all class models by a target rotation to be performed for each class, where the system components are rotated into the standardized parameter vectors of the compounds. An object is classified into class q if the ratio of its distance to the q-th hyperplane and s_q is smaller than a critical F value. However, according to this criterion it may happen that a compound can be classified into more than one class. Such a compound may tentatively be assigned to that class for which its distance to the respective hyperplane is smallest. In certain cases, it may not be possible to classify a new compound at all; this simply means that this compound does not belong to the same data structure as the compounds of the training series. A very important feature of SIMCA is that it may also be applied to so-called asymmetric cases where only some but not all of the classes have a well defined structure in parameter space. For such cases, other linear classification procedures such as, for example, linear discriminant analysis (see 9.2.2.) may fail. A case in point is a recent SIMCA study on carcinogenic 4-nitroquinoline N-oxides [45] where only the class of active carcinogens showed a substantial structure whereas the inactive compounds did not form a homogeneous class.

If compounds classified according to one property differ *within the classes* with respect to another quantitatively measured property, it is possible with SIMCA to find a relation between the position of the objects within the individual classes and the latter. Such a situation is, for example, encountered when compounds are classified according to their intrinsic activity (classes: agonists, partial agonists and antagonists) and, at the same sime, their biological potency has been measured. The latter determines the position of compounds within the classes which can be described by the object components in terms of simple linear models. Thus, the within-class position of compounds (level of biological activity within the classes) can be quantitatively described as a function of the object components using, for example, simple plots or regression models. It should be noted that this approach has a certain similarity with the target rotation of principal components discussed in the preceding sections.

As with the extrathermodynamic approach, the definition of parameter space (selection of relevant molecular parameters as descriptors) is also a critical step with SIMCA. The importance of molecular parameters can be judged by two criteria:

1. their importance for the separation of classes (*discriminatory power*),
2. their ability to describe the relative position (e.g. gradation of activity) of objects (compounds) within classes and thus the class structure (*modelling power*).

With respect to two classes q and p, the discriminatory power, $\Phi_j^{(q,p)}$ of the j-th variable for separation of the two classes is a s follows:

$$\Phi_j^{(q,p)} = \left[\frac{(s_{i,p}^{(q)})^2 + (s_{j,q}^{(p)})^2}{(s_j^{(p)})^2 + (s_j^{(q)})^2}\right]^{1/2} - 1 \qquad (9/50)$$

where $(s_{j,p}^{(q)})^2$ $\left((s_{j,q}^{(p)})^2\right)$ is the residual variance of the j-th variable when fitting the objects from the q-th (p-th) class to the principal component model for the p-th (q-th) class and $(s_j^{(p)})^2$ and $(s_j^{(q)})^2$, respectively, are the residual variances when fitting objects in the q-th and the p-th class to the principal component model of their own class. $\Phi_j^{(q,p)}$ is $\geqq 0$ and values >1 indicate a good separation of the classes.

Modelling power ψ_j for the j-th variable can be estimated by comparing the residual variance of this variable over all principal component models (s_j^2) and its averaged within-class variance[1]) ($s_{x_j}^2$) where

$$s_{x_j}^2 = \sum_{q=1}^{Q} \sum_{i=1}^{n_q} (x_{ij}^{(q)} - \bar{x}_j^{(q)})^2/(n - Q) \qquad (9/51)$$

$x_{ij}^{(q)}$ = value of the j-th variable for the i-th compound in class q
Q = number of classes
$n = \sum_{q=1}^{Q} n_q$

$$\bar{x}_j^{(q)} = \sum_{i=1}^{n_q} x_{ij}/n_q \qquad (9/52)$$

and

$$s_j^2 = \frac{1}{Q} \sum_{q=1}^{Q} \frac{m}{(m - r_q)(n_q - r_q - 1)} \sum_{i=1}^{n_q} \varepsilon_{ij,q}^2 \qquad (9/53)$$

The smaller the quotient $s_j^2/s_{x_j}^2$, the larger is the modelling power of the j-th variable. Therefore, the expression

$$\psi_j = 1 - s_j/s_{x_j} \qquad (9/54)$$

constitutes a criterion of modelling power. If this value is approximately one the modelling power of the j-th variable is large, whilst a value of zero indicates that the j-th variable makes no contribution to the description of the class structures. Variables with low values for $\Phi_j^{q,p}$ and ψ_j should be removed from the data matrices as being non-relevant, in which case principal component analysis is repeated with the reduced data matrix. The principal steps of the SIMCA method are:

1. formulation and standardization of data matrices for each class,
2. principal component analysis within each class and determination of the number of relevant principal components (the procedure used here is different from that dealt with in 9.1.1.),

---

[1]) This differs from the original treatment of WOLD where instead of the within-class variance the total variance of the j-th variable in the training series is considered. As pointed out by DOVE [49a], however, modelling power will be overestimated with the latter.

3. elimination of non-relevant parameters on the basis of criteria $\Phi_j^{(9p)}$ and ψ_j,
4. repetition of steps 1.—3. until consistency is reached,
5. classification of unknown objects,
6. description of data structure (e.g., gradation of activity inside each class) with the aid of linear models from the object components.

In pharmacological problems, the procedure outlined above was first applied by Dunn, Wold and Martin [40] in a quantitative structure-activity analysis concerning multisubstituted phenylalkylamines acting on adrenergic β-receptors. Compounds were divided into agonists ($n = 15$) and antagonists ($n = 17$) according to intrinsic activity. Levels of activity were known for both agonists and antagonists. Agonism was characterized by stimulating the synthesis of adenylcyclase. Inhibition of isoproterenol stimulated adenylcyclase provided a measure of antagonism. The binding constants on the β-receptor (measured as the inhibition of ^{3}H-aloprenol binding), pK_a values and hydrophobic (f) as well as electronic (σ) and steric substituent constants were applied as descriptive features. Principal component models with three relevant principal components were secured for either class, permitting correct reclassification of 100% of agonists and 88% of antagonists. As remarked above, the position of objects within classes is described by object components. If the compounds are represented as points in a coordinate system spanned by the object components, both agonists and antagonists are clustered distinctly according to level of activity. Furthermore, a simple linear combination of the first two object components affords a significant relation with the level of activity in both classes.

The following are made possible by the results of this analysis:

1. classification of new compounds (i.e., prediction whether they are agonists or antagonists),
2. estimation of the level of activity of these compounds from the relation between activity and the linear combination of the first two object components,
3. inferences about molecular properties of importance for classification and activity from the features with a large discriminatory or modelling power.

Principal component analysis or, rather, simply principal component method can also be used to recognize clustering of compounds into classes by use of a technique which is called mapping (see, e.g., [1, 2]). The objects are simply plotted in the space spanned by the first two (two-dimensional plot) or three (three-dimensional plot) principal components after extracting the components from a suitable data matrix. An example of such an approach has already been presented with the TMIC procedure for series design (see 8.1.). Another typical application can be found in the work of Cammarata and Menon [50, 51] who separated 39 therapeutic compounds into their respective five therapeutic classes using special structural descriptors. This example is illustrative but the selection of descriptors is not without ambiguity.

9.2.2. Linear Discriminant Analysis

9.2.2.1. Principles

So-called *discriminant functions* serve in the discriminant analysis as classification algorithms, representing weighted linear combinations of features relevant for class separation. The same molecular parameters (substituent constants, etc.) as in the extrathermodynamic approach are used. There are several types of discriminant functions, among which the *non-elementary* ones have optimal properties that remain to be elucidated. For this reason the present section is limited to the application of these functions in quantitative structure-activity analysis. Only basic principles and the major steps will be discussed here. For mathematical details, the reader is referred to [52, 53] (see also [1, 2]).

Where Q classes occur ($q = 1, \ldots, Q$), $Q - 1$ non-elementary discriminant functions w_k ($k = 1, \ldots, Q - 1$) of the general form

$$w_k = \sum_{j=1}^{m} a_{kj} x_j \tag{9/55}$$

exist. The quantity a_{kj} denotes the weight factor (coefficient) of the j-th molecular parameter ($j = 1, \ldots, m$) in the k-th discriminant function, the w_k's also being designated as non-elementary *discriminant variables*. With this formula as a basis, individual classes are depicted as Q-1 dimensional point clouds (the points correspond to the objects) in a Q-1 dimensional space having coordinates w_k, and the a_{kj}'s are so determined that the clouds are separated as sharply as possible. This principle is schematized graphically (Fig. 9.1) for a problem with $Q = 3$ classes. If $Q = 3$ there are two discriminant functions w_1 and w_2, which span a two-dimensional space with axes w_1 and w_2. In this space the three classes constitute two-dimensional point clouds, which ideally — i.e., if classes are entirely separated — do not overlap. The distance between the centres of gravity belonging to the point clouds (class centres) is larger in the direction of coordinate w_1 than in that of coordinate w_2, as the former discriminant function contributes more to class separation on grounds to be explained later.

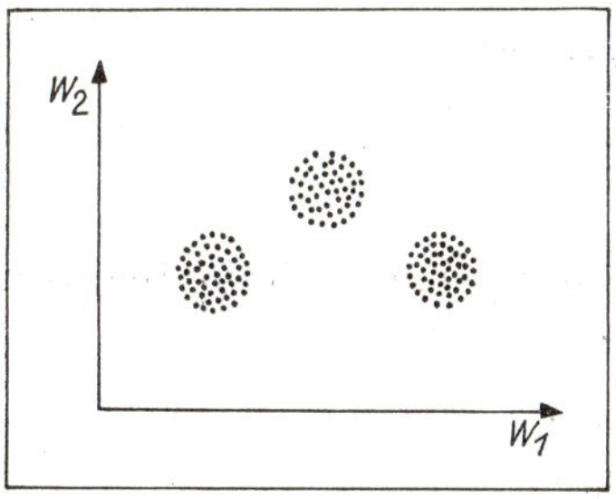

Fig. 9.1. Principle of discriminant analysis

After determination of discriminant functions from data of a training series, not yet investigated compounds can be classified and predictions made about the biological property (e.g., activity) underlying classification. As in the extrathermodynamic approach, it is possible to utilize characteristics and signs of the molecular parameters in discriminant functions for gathering hints as to molecular properties which are essential to classification and thus to the biological property of interest. It is, however, not possible to obtain information about the position of individual compounds within the classes; in this respect the SIMCA method discussed in the preceding section is superior to discriminant analysis.

The principal steps of discriminant analysis are:

1. selection of molecular parameters and formulation of approaches,

2. check whether classes can be separated using these parameters and elimination of parameters not relevant for class separation,
3. computation of non-elementary discriminant functions,
4. interpretation of discriminant functions and reclassification of the compounds from the training series as a means of testing the quality of separation,
5. classification of compounds not investigated yet so that further syntheses and tests can be planned while allowing for mechanistic conclusions from the form of the discriminant functions.

The first step is fully analogous to that in the extrathermodynamic approach, squared terms and, for example, product terms being considered in the same way in each case. Since, as shown below, non-relevant molecular parameters are automatically eliminated in the second step, one can start with relatively few or crude hypotheses, and, as demonstrated in the examples in 9.2.2.2., refine them after the first calculations. Concerning interpretation collinearities and multicollinearities of molecular parameters interfere with discriminant analysis in much the same way as with regression analysis so that a series design according to the principles outlined under 8.1. may be extremely helpful. As in regression analysis, molecular parameters can be systematized by factor analysis, as illustrated by the example in 9.2.2.2.1.

A multivariate variance analysis is performed as the second step. The test criterion is formed by HOTELLINGS T^2, a measure of the distance between classes in the space of the molecular parameters under consideration:

$$T^2 = \frac{1}{n - Q} \sum_{q=1}^{Q} n_q (\bar{\boldsymbol{x}}_q - \bar{\boldsymbol{x}})^T \boldsymbol{S}^{-1} (\bar{\boldsymbol{x}}_q - \bar{\boldsymbol{x}}) \tag{9/56}$$

where

n = number of compounds in the training series ($i = 1, \ldots, n$)

Q = number of classes ($q = 1, \ldots, Q$)

n_q = number of compounds in the q-th class

$\bar{\boldsymbol{x}}_q$ = vector of the mean values of features (molecular parameters) within the q-th class

$\bar{\boldsymbol{x}}$ = vector of the overall mean values of features

$\boldsymbol{S}$ = within-class covariance matrix, averaged over all classes

$$= \frac{1}{n - Q} \sum_{q=1}^{Q} \sum_{i=1}^{n_q} (\boldsymbol{x}_{qi} - \bar{\boldsymbol{x}}_q)(\boldsymbol{x}_{qi} - \bar{\boldsymbol{x}}_q)^T \tag{9/57}$$

The statistical test performed in variance analysis refers to the assumption (null hypothesis) that all class centres coincide in the feature space, in which case classes can no longer be separated with the aid of the selected molecular parameters. In this context, the test variable $\tilde{F}$ is calculated as

$$\tilde{F} = \left[n - Q - M + \frac{1}{(n - Q) M} \right] T^2 \tag{9/58}$$

where M = number of molecular parameters *considered* ($j = 1, \ldots, M$). The null hypothesis is rejected if the test quantity is greater than the corresponding F quantile taken from an F table (g_1, g_2 = degrees of fredom; p = critical probability of error):

$$\tilde{F} > F_{g_1, g_2; p} \tag{9/59}$$

with

$$g_1 = \begin{cases} \dfrac{(Q-1)\,M(n-Q-M)}{n-(Q-1)\,M-2} & \text{for} \quad n-(Q-1)\,M-2>0 \\ \infty & \text{for} \quad n-(Q-1)\,M-2<0 \end{cases} \tag{9/60}$$

and

$$g_2 = n - Q - M + 1 \tag{9/61}$$

Analogous tests can be done for the pairwise comparison of two classes at a time. No separation of all classes can be accomplished by means of the selected molecular parameters unless the null hypothesis has been rejected throughout.

Subsequently, such molecular features are chosen as make a significant contribution to class separation, any feature not relevant for this purpose being eliminated. This is achieved stepwise, each time one feature being added (or eliminated) and the critical probability of error p being calculated from eqns. (9/58) and (9/59). The variables are selected in such a way that p is minimized, and the resulting set of m ($m \leq M$) variables is optimal with respect to the separation of classes within the training series (*optimal set*).

The third step involves the calculation of discriminant functions according to (9/55) from the molecular parameters present in the optimal set which is done by solving an eigenvalue problem according to:

$$\frac{1}{n-Q}\,\boldsymbol{H}\boldsymbol{a}_k = \lambda_k \boldsymbol{S}\boldsymbol{a}_k \tag{9/62}$$

with

$$\boldsymbol{H} = \sum_{q=1}^{Q} n_q(\bar{\boldsymbol{x}}_q - \bar{\boldsymbol{x}})\,(\bar{\boldsymbol{x}}_q - \bar{\boldsymbol{x}})^T \tag{9/63}$$

Matrix $\boldsymbol{H}$ contains the variance of features between classes. The elements of eigenvectors $\boldsymbol{a}_k$ are the coefficients a_{kj} in (9/55); that is, the k-th eigenvector has the form

$$\boldsymbol{a}_k = \{a_{k1}, \ldots, a_{kj}, \ldots, a_{km}\} \tag{9/64}$$

where a_{kj} denotes the coefficient of the j-th feature (x_j) in the k-th discriminant function. The λ_k's are the corresponding eigenvalues which are equal to the separation factor T^2 of the discriminant functions:

$$T^2(w_k) = \lambda_k \tag{9/65}$$

As the eigenvalues decrease in the order $\lambda_1 > \lambda_2 \ldots > \lambda_k \ldots > \lambda_{Q-1}$ it follows from (9/65) that there is a similarly descending order as regards the separating power of discriminant functions. This makes it possible to eliminate those last discriminant functions which fail to contribute significantly to class separation thereby diminishing the dimensionality of the discrimination problem. Another favourable aspect of non-elementary discriminant functions is that by far the greatest contribution to the separation of classes is made by the first discriminant function so that mechanistic interpretation can usually be restricted to that. To determine the optimal number of discriminant functions the test quantity

$$\tilde{F}_t = \frac{n - Q - t + 1}{(Q - 1)\,t} \sum_{k=1}^{t} \lambda_k \tag{9/66}$$

is calculated and compared with the quantity $F_{g_1,g_2:p}$ from an F table (F test) with degree of freedom:

$$g_1 = \begin{cases} \dfrac{(Q-1)\,t(n-Q-t)}{(n-Q-1)\,t-2} & \text{for } n-(Q-k)\,t-2>0 \\ \infty & \text{for } n-(Q-1)\,t-2<0 \end{cases} \tag{9/67}$$

$$g_2 = n - Q - t + 1$$

In doing so, t as the number of relevant discriminant functions is so estimated that the probability of error p is minimized while the inequality

$$\tilde{F}_t > F_{g_1,g_2;p} \tag{9/68}$$

applies.

For the reclassification of compounds from the training series as well as for the classification of not yet investigated compounds (prediction), the values of the t relevant non-elementary discriminant variables are first calculated for all compounds. The value of the k-th discriminant variable for the i-th compound is established from eqn. (9/55) as

$$w_{ki} = \sum_{j=1}^{m} a_{kj} x_{ji} \tag{9/69}$$

where x_{ji} denotes the value of the j-th feature (molecular parameter) for the i-th compound. Subsequently, for each compound i, test quantities $F_{q/i}$ (one for each class) are calculated according to

$$\tilde{F}_{q/i} = \frac{n - Q - t + 1}{t(n - Q)} \frac{n_q}{n_q + 1} \sum_{k=1}^{t} (w_{ki} - \overline{w}_{kq})^2 \tag{9/70}$$

where $\overline{w}_{kq}$ is the mean value of the k-th discriminant variable in the q-th class:

$$\overline{w}_{kq} = \frac{1}{n_q} \sum_{i=1}^{n_q} w_{ki} \tag{9/71}$$

A compound i is classified into class q, if:

$$\tilde{F}_{q/i} \leqq F_{t,n-Q-t+1;p} \tag{9/72}$$

This criterion may be satisfied by several classes so that no unambiguous classification based on (9/72) is possible. In such cases, it is common practice to include compound i tentatively in that class for which the test quantity $\tilde{F}_{q/i}$ has its smallest value. Ideally, all compounds of the training series are reclassified correctly, which implies that the separation power of the discriminant function is optimal. Such a conclusion is, however, strictly valid only for the compounds of the training set and cannot be a priori extended to the classification of new compounds (see below).

The classification of not yet investigated compounds is fully analogous to reclassification. There may be compounds which can be assigned to no class at all because the criterion (9/72) is not properly fulfilled. Such compounds are to be regarded as belonging to a fundamentally different basis set than the compounds of the training series or to a class not represented inside the training series. As in regression analysis, such "outliers" may serve as a starting point to explore new directions in the search for active drugs.

The most suitable test for determining the quality of the discriminant functions derived is a check of their predictive power in classifying hitherto uninvestigated compound. Predictions can also be simulated. If the training series is large enough, some of the compounds can be excluded from the calculation of discriminant functions and classified as "unknowns". Another approach is to use the so-called *leave-n-out technique*. In this technique, groups of n compounds are alternatively left out of discriminant analysis and then classified with the aid of the discriminant functions obtained from the remaining compounds. The quality of discriminant functions may be viewed as proven if this procedure also reveals a good agreement between determined and real classification.

Using several modifications discriminant analysis has been widely and successfully applied in the QSAR field by several workers [54—73] (for a critical comment on [73], see [74]). In our work we have always preferred to use discriminant analysis (or another adequate classification method) for data of unknown precision rather than to force such data into a regression model. Because of its ability to make the greatest contribution to class separation, the first discriminant function can, in fact, often be interpreted analogously to a regression equation from the extrathermodynamic approach. Where for the same biological object in a crude test, activity is determined as a discrete quantity (activity score) and in a subsequent, more refined, test as a continuous quantity, the first discriminant function established using the classification corresponding to the activity score quite frequently shows a striking similarity to the regression equation for the continuous data. This occured, for example, in a structure-activity analysis for the cytostatic activity of a series of phenylthioureas [56]. The compounds were divided into two classes on the basis of data from a screening test for cytostatic activity, and the following discriminant function was obtained:

$$w = 1.56\,(\sum \pi)^2 + 0.71 E_{S,para} - 1.49 I \qquad (9/73)$$

The indicator variable I refers to a given structural feature. Test results with some of the compounds were more precise, thus allowing a regression analysis. The result so obtained for cytotoxic activity was:

$$\log A = 1.29\,(\sum \pi)^2 + 1.53 \qquad (9/74)$$

$$n = 13 \qquad r = 0.905 \qquad s = 0.153$$

The indicator variable is not needed in this equation as the structural feature which it characterizes was constant for all compounds. Accordingly, the discriminant function (9/73) and the regression equation (9/74) are practically identical, apart from the difference in E_S term. As the E_S term in (9/73) makes a basically smaller contribution to class separation than $(\sum \pi)^2$ the agreement between discriminant function and regression equation is quite close. Something similar is seen with the example dealt with in the following paragraph. Thus, discriminant analysis can be applied not only for optimization at the crude screening level but also as a means of predicting which molecular parameters may be expected in a regression approach in more sophisticated tests. This information is useful in parameter selection when one is designing an optimal sample, but in particular it may help to refine regression approaches.

A prerequisite for variance and discriminant analyses is a normal data distribution. For discrete features this need is not satisfied. In such instances pattern recognition as discussed in 11.2. is a useful procedure. As shown by experience, however, the use of an in comparison with the number of continuous variables small number of indicator variables (discrete quantities) still permits one to obtain valid discriminant functions in at least descriptive terms, even though, strictly speaking, statistical assumptions are violated. For a better understanding of discriminant analysis and some of the problems which its application entails, two examples are discussed in greater detail in the paragraphs below.

9.2.2.2. Examples

9.2.2.2.1. Fungicidal Carboxamides [60, 66]

White and Thorn [75] determined pI_{50} values for the inhibition of succinate dehydrogenase from mitochondria preparations of *Cryptococcus laurentii* by 93 carboxamide compounds of structure XL. Their inhibitory potency has been reported to correlate with their fungicidal activity [76, 77].

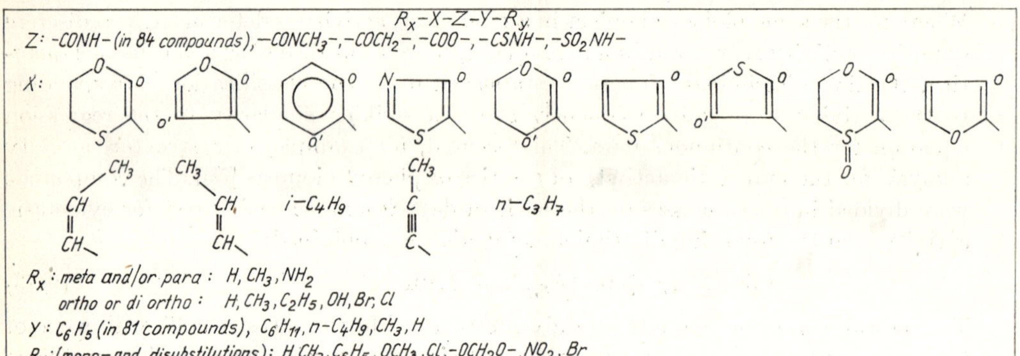

XL

Within the training series extremely large variations in structure occur so that parametrization presents difficulties where, as in the extrathermodynamic approach, LFER criteria require strict validation. In discriminant analysis, the problem is not so serious because, in contrast to regression analysis, there is no need for an exactly defined, functional relation between log A and molecular parameters to cover the entire range of values. Rather it is sufficient for the selected molecular parameters to reflect the properties of compounds in terms of classification, that is on a far coarser plane. For that reason and also to include inactive compounds in the analysis (an essential advantage of classification procedures), discriminant analysis was applied despite the continuous character of the data. Nevertheless, regression approaches have been tested in a parallel manner for comparison. This example can be regarded as a model case which can serve to clarify some essential problems and strategic aspects of discriminant analysis.

To begin with, a four-class problem with the following classes was considered:

class 1: extremely active compounds

$$pI_{50} \geqq 3.0 \qquad n_1 = 14$$

class 2: strongly active compounds

$$3.0 > pI_{50} \geqq 1.66 \qquad n_2 = 37$$

class 3: weakly active compounds

$$1{,}66 > pI_{50} \geqq 0.32 \qquad n_3 = 19$$

class 4: inactive compounds

$$0.32 > pI_{50} \qquad n_4 = 21$$

In all, 47 features served to describe the molecules. They include various hydrophobic, electronic and steric substituent constants, divided according to the positions considered in the molecule, squares of these parameters where the properties of the molecules varied sufficiently, and indicator variables for the description of certain structural features (see Table 9.15). The features are partly intercorrelated (collinear). To achieve a systematization of features and a better overview of collinearities, factor analysis was performed using the data matrix for the entire training set. As a result, seven relevant factors were obtained. Table 9.16 summarizes the variables with high loadings in these factors (factor pattern) and also some conclusions to be drawn concerning what properties are reflected by which factor. The following can then be concluded:

1. The properties of the different variable fragments in XL as well as of the ortho-, meta- and para-positions of the ring system X and Y are not interrelated.
2. The electronic molecular parameters of all fragments do not correlate with hydrophobic and steric ones.
3. Hydrophobic and steric molecular parameters are closely correlated so that hydrophobic and steric influences cannot be separated.
4. In many cases there are close correlations between a given variable and its square.

Analysis of variance afforded an optimal set of 15 features from which the three non-elementary discriminant functions w_1, w_2 and w_3 were calculated (eigenvalues: $\lambda_1 = 7.62$; $\lambda_2 = 0.48$; $\lambda_3 = 0.24$). Only the first two of these are significant at $p = 0.05$ (F test according to (9/68)). To reclassify the compounds of the training set both significant discriminant functions w_1 and w_2 are used while for interpretation it is sufficient to consider only w_1 because of the only marginal contribution of w_2 to class separation (as follows directly from the eigenvalues). The optimal set of variables and the corresponding coefficients a_{1j} belonging to them in the first discriminant function w_1

Table 9.15. Features used to describe XL

Fragment	Features
whole molecule	$\log P$, $(\log P)^2$
Z	$I_{01} = 1$, if NH is present; $= 0$, if not
	$I_{02} = 1$, if CO is present; $= 0$, if not
	$I_{03} = I_{01} + I_{02}$
X	$f, f^2, \sigma_0, \sigma_0^2, \sigma_m, \sigma_m^2, \sum \sigma, (\sum \sigma)^2$
	$I_{11} = 2$, if X is a six-ring; $= 1$, if X is a five-ring; $= 0$, otherwise
	$I_{12} = 2$, if X is aromatic; $= 1$, if X is unsaturated; $= 0$, otherwise
	$I_{13} = I_{11} + I_{12}$
R_X	$\sum \pi, (\sum \pi)^2, \pi_0, \pi_0^2, \sigma_0, \sigma_0^2, MR_0, MR_0^2$
	$I_{21} = 1$, if the cis-position with respect to Z is occupied; $= 0$, if not
	$I_{22} = 1$ for $R_X \neq H$ in meta-position to Z; $= 0$, otherwise
Y	f, f^2
	$I_{31} = 2$, if $Y = \Phi$; $= 1$, if $Y = C_6H_{11}$; $= 0$, otherwise
R_Y	$\pi_0, \pi_0^2, \pi_m, \pi_p, \sum \pi, (\sum \pi)^2, \sum \sigma, (\sum \sigma)^2, MR_0, MR_0^2, MR_m, MR_p, \sum MR, (\sum MR)^2$
	$I_{41} = 2$ for ortho-disubstitution in Y; $= 1$ for ortho-monosubstitution in Y; $= 0$, otherwise
	$I_{42} = 2$ for meta-disubstitution in Y; $= 1$ for meta-monosubstitution in Y; $= 0$, otherwise
	$I_{43} = 1$ for para-substitution in Y; $= 0$, otherwise
	$I_{44} = I_{41} + I_{42} + I_{43}$

(eqn. (9/55)) are presented in Table 9.17 systematized according to the variable fragments in XL. The mean values of w_1 for the four classes are:

	$\overline{w}_1$
class 1	24.046
class 2	23.385
class 3	21.292
class 4	16.924

Thus, $\overline{w}_1$ correlates with the activity score so that high values of w_1 are favourable for a compound being classified into the more active classes.

The complexity of the expression and particularly the numerous collinearities scarcely permit an interpretation of w_1 in chemical terms. The only remarks that can be made at this point (cfl., the results of factor analysis) are as follows:

1. The properties of individual fragments influence the biological properties of compounds independently of each other.

Table 9.16. Factor analysis for the 47 features to describe XL: features highly loaded in the 7 significant factors and assignment of factors to separate molecular porperties (listing of variables in an order of decreasing factor loading within each factor)

Factor	Features with high loadings	Molecular properties of XL, represented by this factor
1	R_Y: π_0, MR_0, $(\Sigma\ \pi)^2$, π_0^2, MR_0^2, Σ MR, I_{41}, $(\Sigma$ MR$)^2$	hydrophobic and steric properties of R_Y (mainly for the ortho-position)
	log P, $(\log P)^2$	overall hydrophobicity
2	X: f^2, f	hydrophobicity of X
	R_X: I_{22}	meta-substitution of X
3	R_X: MR_0, π_0^2, π_0, $(\Sigma\ \pi)^2$, MR_0^2, $\Sigma\ \pi$	hydrophobic and steric properties of ortho-substituents in X
4	R_Y: I_{42}, π_m, MR_m	hydrophobic and steric properties of meta-substituents in Y
5	R_Y: MR_p, I_{43}, π_p	steric and hydrophobic properties of para-substituents in Y
6	R_X: I_{21}, σ_0, σ_0^2	ortho-(cis)-substitution of X (substitution at the β-carbon atom) and electronic properties in this position
	Y: f, I_{31}	hydrophobicity of Y
	I_{03}	presence of the carboxamide group
7	X: σ_m^2, $(\Sigma\ \sigma)^2$, $\Sigma\ \sigma$, σ_0	electronic properties of X

Table 9.17. Features of the optimal set for the simultaneous separation of classes 1—4 and the accompanying coefficients a_{1j} in the first discriminant function w_1, systematized according to the variable fragments in XL. In brackets behind each variable is the number of the factor in which it is highly loaded (see Table 9.16)

Fragment of XL									
Whole molecule		X		R_X		Y		R_Y	
$+1.56 \log P$	(1)	$13.3\sigma_m^2$	(7)	$+15.0\ MR_0$	(3)	$-4.55f$	(6)	$+0.60I_{41}$	(1)
$-0.28 (\log P)^2$	(1)			$-5.67\ MR_0^2$	(3)	$+1.23f^2$	(6)	$-2.52\ (\Sigma\ \sigma)^2$	(1)
$+6.11I_{03}$	(6)			$-1.05\ \Sigma\ \pi$	(3)	$+2.79I_{31}$	(6)	$+1.56\ MR_m$	(4)
				$-2.10\sigma_0$	(6)				
				$+0.64I_{22}$	(2)				

2. In addition to the structural features revealed by the indicator variables (see Table 9.15), influences of the following properties are manifested:
   - hydrophobicity of the total molecule,
   - electronic properties of X,

— electronic (ortho-position) as well as hydrophobic and/or steric properties of R_X,
— hydrophobic properties of Y,
— electronic as well as hydrophobic and/or steric properties of R_Y.

If, in addition, the information on the indispensibility of the individual variables for class separation resulting from variance analysis (not given) is taken into consideration, the following additional conclusions can be made:

3. The three indicator variables I_{21}, I_{03} and I_{31} alone allow a significant separation of class 4 from classes 1—3 so that it would appear that the structural features described by these variables are essential to activity.
4. The term σ_m^2, which describes the electronic properties of the ring system X, is of primary importance in the separation of classes 1—3, and it thus seems that the gradation of biological potency within the group of active compounds is primarily governed by electronic properties.

Table 9.18. Statistical criteria for the separation of classes 1—4 with the features of the optimal set (see Table 9.17)

	HOTELLINGS T^2	Probability of error, p
Simultaneous separation of all classes	33.36	0
Pairwise separation of classes		
1—2	1.649	$2.6 \cdot 10^{-2}$
1—3	4.557	$2.5 \cdot 10^{-7}$
1—4	20.08	0
2—3	4.350	$1.0 \cdot 10^{-5}$
2—4	25.96	0
3—4	9.821	0

Table 9.19. Results of the reclassification of the compounds from the training series by means of discriminant functions w_1 and w_2

	Class			
	1	2	3	4
n_q	14	37	19	21
number of compounds misclassified	5	7	7	0
error of reclassification	35%	19%	36%	0%

The statistical criteria for class separation from multivariate variance analysis are presented in Table 9.18. It appears that the optimum of 15 features provides a perfect separation of class 4 from all others, whilst the separation of classes 1—3 (i.e., the classes of the active compounds) is less sharp. In particular, classes 1 and 2 are considerably more difficult to separate from each other than the others. This picture is also reflected in the result of reclassification of the training series as shown in Table 9.19. The class of inactive compounds is very sharply separated from the three classes of active compounds (reclassification error: 0%), while in three classes of active compounds a relatively large number of compounds are erroneously classified (mean reclassification error: 27%). This outcome leads to the conclusion that in the determination of whether a given compound is active or inactive other molecular properties (and thus molecular parameters) are of importance than those on which the gradation of activity within the group of active compounds depends. In other words, the pairwise separation of classes requires optimal feature sets which differ from that needed for the simultaneous separation of all classes. Such a situation is in no way uncommon in discriminant analysis. It is then helpful to divide the original problem into subproblems in such a way that the same optimal set of features is equally suitable for both pairwise and simultaneous separation of all classes involved in each subproblem. In the present case the results obtained so far suggest the following procedure:

subproblem 1: separation of inactive compounds from all the active compounds (two-class problem)
class I: active compounds (classes 1—3)
class II: inactive compounds (class 4)

subproblem 2: separation of the three classes of active compounds (description of the gradation of biological activity)

The non-elementary discriminant function presented below is obtained for *subproblem 1*:

$$w = 3.631 I_{21} + 4.291 I_{03} + 1.194 I_{31} \tag{9/75}$$

$$T^2 = 3.666 \qquad p = 0$$

$$\bar{w}_{\mathrm{I}} = 14.34 \qquad \bar{w}_{\mathrm{II}} = 11.16$$

In this way 85 of the 91 compounds from the training set can be reclassified correctly (reclassification error: 6,5%), which is a very satisfactory outcome. Three indicator variables are sufficient for the separation of active and inactive compounds. Taking into consideration $\bar{w}_{\mathrm{I}} > \bar{w}_{\mathrm{II}}$, it follows from (9/75) and the definition of the indicator variables that active compounds must have a substituent on the β-carbon atom of X in cis-position with respect to the amide group, that the NHCO group must be present and that in Y a phenyl ring (which, however, may be replaced by a cyclohexyl ring) must occur. All this is in line with some empirical conclusions reported elsewhere [75, 78] and with results obtained by different techniques to be discussed in later sections.

With *subproblem 2* a reduction of features was aimed at because the results obtained pointed to the redundancy of the original 47 features. First 10 "atypical" active compounds were eliminated to make features $I_{01} \ldots I_{03}$, $f(\mathrm{Y})$, $(f(\mathrm{Y}))^2$ as well as I_{31} vanish. The remaining features were reduced to a total number of 24 (Table 9.20) taking into consideration the outcome of factor analysis (Table 9.16), the optimal set of features for the four-class problem (Table 9.17) and the spread in individual properties in individual fragments.

Analysis of variance provides an optimal set of 10 features from which two significant discriminant functions w_1 and w_2 (eigenvalues: $\lambda_1 = 2.35$, $\lambda_2 = 0.70$) were evaluated. Although both discriminant functions are used to reclassify the training series, only

Table 9.20. Features used in subproblem 2, systematized according to variable fragments in XL

Fragment	Hydrophobic features	Electronic features	Steric features	Structural features
whole molecule	$\log P$, $(\log P)^2$	—	—	—
X	f, f^2	σ_0, σ_m, σ_m^2	—	I_{11}
R_X	$\sum \pi$, $(\sum \pi)^2$	σ_0	MR_0	I_{22}
R_Y	π_0, π_0^2, π_m, π_p, $\sum \pi$, $(\sum \pi)^2$	$\sum \sigma$, $(\sum \sigma)^2$	$\sum MR$, $(\sum MR)^2$	—

Table 9.21. Features of the optimal set for the simultaneous separation of classes 1—3 and the accompanying coefficients a_{1j} of the first discriminant function w_1, systematized according to variable fragments in XL

Fragment	Feature	Coefficient a_{1j}
X	σ_m^2	4.45
X	f	2.39
X	$\sum \sigma$	1.89
X	I_{11}	−0.73
R_X	MR_0	6.88
R_X	I_{22}	1.18
R_X	$\sum \pi$	−0.98
R_Y	$(\sum \sigma)^2$	−6.34
R_Y	π_m	2.93
R_Y	$(\sum MR)^2$	−0.41

Table 9.22. Statistical criteria for the separation of classes 1—3 with the 10 features of the optimal set (compare Table 9.21)

	HOTELLINGS T^2	Probability of error, p
Simultaneous separation of all classes	9.16	0
1—2	4.18	$3.1 \cdot 10^{-6}$
1—3	7.01	$1.5 \cdot 10^{-9}$
2—3	3.60	$2 \cdot 10^{-5}$

the first with its essentially greater separating power is of interest for interpretation. The coefficients of this discriminant function are listed, along with the optimal set of features, in Table 9.21, and Table 9.22 shows the statistical quality criteria for the separation of the three classes by the use of the optimal set. As can be seen, there is a highly significant separation of all three classes. In contrast to the four-class próblem, classes 1 and 2 are also fully separated. Eighty-eight per cent of the compounds can be correctly reclassified (reclassification error: 12%) so that, as expected, the gradation of biological activity within the biologically active compounds can be described more appropriately by solving subproblem 2 than the original four-class problem.

The mean values of w_1 for the three classes 1—3 are:

	$\overline{w}_1$
class 1	10.62
class 2	8.25
class 3	6.13

It thus follows that high positive values of the terms of the discriminant function shown in Table 9.21 are favourable for a high level of biological activity (= for the assignment to classes 1 and 2). This is fully in line with the results of the four-class problem. The stability of discriminant analysis is illustrated by the fact that the variables appearing in both the optimal set for the four-class problem (Table 9.17) and the three-class problem (Table 9.21) [$\sigma_m^2(\mathrm{X})$, $\mathrm{MR}_0(\mathrm{R}_X)$, I_{22}, $\sum \pi(\mathrm{R}_X)$, $(\sum \sigma)^2\,(\mathrm{R}_Y)$, $\pi_m(\mathrm{R}_Y)$ instead of $\mathrm{MR}_m(\mathrm{R}_Y)$] have the same sign in the respective first discriminant function.

The discriminant function (Table 9.21) for the three-class problem is not only easier to inspect than that for the four-class problem (Table 9.17) but also has the advantage that the variables occurring in it are largely uncorrelated, in accord with the results of factor analysis (Table 9.16). Thus, an interpretation in chemical terms can now be tried on more safe grounds.

To verify this conclusion, the 60 active compounds contained in the three-class problem were subjected to stepwise regression analysis (forward elimination) using their pI_{50} values and the same 24 variables (Table 9.20) as in the discriminant analysis. In all, 186 variable combinations were screened, leading to 18 significant regression equations, the best of which was:

$$pI_{50} = 0.51f(\mathrm{X}) + 17.14\sigma_m^2(\mathrm{X}) + 1.39\,\mathrm{MR}_0(\mathrm{R}_X) + 0.96\pi_m(\mathrm{R}_Y) - 2.34\,(\textstyle\sum \sigma)^2\,(\mathrm{R}_Y) - 1.11 \qquad (9/76)$$

$$n = 60 \qquad r = 0.784 \qquad s = 0.516$$

All terms in eqn. (9/76) are significant ($p < 0.05$). Although no more than ca. 62% of the data variance are "explained", this result is nonetheless quite satisfactory considering the very drastic changes in structures within the sample resulting in a relatively crude parametrization and possibly also in a violation of the rules of linear-free enthalpy relationships. A very noteworthy aspect of all this is that the variables occurring in (9/76) are exactly the same as those which contribute most to class separation in the discriminant function shown in Table 9.21. The order of features in Table 9.21 as regards importance for class separation has been found in multivariate analysis of variance to be $\sigma_m^2(\mathrm{X}) > \mathrm{MR}_0(\mathrm{R}_X) > (\sum \sigma)^2\,(\mathrm{R}_Y) > \pi_m(\mathrm{R}_Y) > f(\mathrm{X}) > I_{11} > \sum \sigma(\mathrm{X}) > (\sum \mathrm{MR})^2\,(\mathrm{R}_Y) > \sum \pi(\mathrm{R}_X) > I_{22}$. The pertinent terms in Table 9.21 and eqn. (9/76) also correspond in signs. On these grounds the major variables in the discriminant function are identical to those in the regression equation so that the results of discriminant and regression analyses may be regarded as largely running parallel. This leads automatically to the question of whether a discriminant function of significant separating power can be found using only the five variables of (9/76), i.e., with the five features of Table 9.21 which have the greatest separating power. This appears to be the case, giving rise to the non-elementary discriminant function:

$$w_1 = 1.21f(\mathrm{X}) + 43.61\sigma_m^2(\mathrm{X}) + 4.41\ \mathrm{MR}_0(\mathrm{R}_X) + 2.40\pi_m(\mathrm{R}_Y) - 5.83\,(\textstyle\sum\sigma)^2\,(\mathrm{R}_Y) \qquad (9/77)$$

$$T^2 = 4.80 \qquad p = 3.8 \cdot 10^{-8}$$

with the class means:

	$\overline{w}_1$
class 1	7.93
class 2	6.30
class 3	4.24

Taking the class means into consideration, not only are the signs of the pertinent terms of (9/77) consistent with the regression equation (9/76) but here is also agreement in the relative order of magnitude of the coefficients. The separating power of (9/77) is, of course, lower than that of the discriminant function derived from the complete optimal set (Table 9.21); this is reflected in the higher error of reclassification, 25.4%.

If only the five most important features of the optimal set which aid most in class separation are considered, Table 9.21 and eqns. (9/76) and (9/77) provide the following picture:

1. Of particular importance for the gradation of biological activity are the electronic properties of the hetero atom in the meta-position towards the carboxyl group in ring X characterized by $\sigma_m(\mathrm{X})$. According to Barlin and Perrin [79] such σ values in heterocyclic ring systems do not refer to a particular reaction centre but give a general impression of the electronic condition of the ring. The non-linear relation with $\sigma_m(\mathrm{X})$ cannot be secured because of the high correlation between $\sigma_m^2(\mathrm{X})$ and $\sigma_m(\mathrm{X})$. An indication that σ_m^2 does not artifically replace σ_m may be that when $\sigma_m^2(\mathrm{X})$ is replaced by $\sigma_m(\mathrm{X})$ the correlation coefficient for (9/76) decreases by 0.15. Even if there were unambiguous evidence of a non-linear relation a mechanistic interpretation would be prevented by the possibility of tracing such non-linearities to a variety of causes (cf., 5.1.).
2. Subproblem 1 implies that the presence of a substituent in the ortho-position in X is essential for biological activity. Additional evidence from the $\mathrm{MR}_0(\mathrm{R}_X)$ term in (9/76) and (9/77) now indicates that biological activity increases as the substituent becomes bulkier. Yet this seems to be subject to a certain maximum, as propyl substitution in this position has been reported by Snel [80] to result in a drop in fungicidal activity. In the event of such an optimum a non-linear relation with $\mathrm{MR}_0(\mathrm{R}_X)$ should result; it could not be found in the present case because of the predominance of small substituents.
3. Hydrophobic substituents in the phenyl ring Y enhance biological activity. However, since $\mathrm{MR}_m(\mathrm{R}_Y)$ and $\pi_m(\mathrm{R}_Y)$ are highly loaded in the same factor and thus correlated, it may be that steric properties of these substituents are also of importance. This explains the presence of $\mathrm{MR}_m(\mathrm{R}_Y)$ instead of $\pi_m(\mathrm{R}_Y)$ in the optimal set for the four-class problem (Table 9.17). The $(\sum\sigma)^2\,(\mathrm{R}_Y)$ term is difficult to interpret, merely

suggesting that the electronic properties of R_Y are also important for biological activity.
4. The $f(X)$ term indicates that hydrophobic rings promote biological activity. Some caution is necessary, however, because hydrophobicity among the rings under consideration varies by no more than one order of magnitude.
5. In line with the conclusions of WHITE and THORN [75], there exists no relation between the gradation of biological activity and the overall hydrophobicity of the molecules concerned.

Because of its relatively low correlation coefficients, the HANSCH equation (9/76) can only find a very limited application in the design of drugs with greater inhibitory activity. Its use is confined to assessing a certain trend and it cannot serve for the prediction of pI_{50} values. In contrast, a prediction in the sense of classification is quite possible with the help of the discriminant functions. The procedure would be as follows:

1. a list of compounds synthetically feasible or already available but not yet tested is drawn up,
2. on the basis of a classification with discriminant function (9/75) the activity and inactivity of compounds is predicted,
3. classification of the compounds classified as active in step 2 using the two discriminant functions determined for the three-class problem (Table 9.21),
4. synthesis and biological testing of those compounds assigned to class 1.

It may be that by applying the SIMCA method even further predictions can be made, e.g., about the order of compounds within a given class. Methodically, the most important conclusions from this example are as follows:

1. In such series where variations in structure are so extensive and accordingly parametrization is so crude that the extrathermodynamic approach can scarcely be followed, if at all, and thus regression analysis cannot be applied, a quantitative structure-activity analysis using discriminant analysis is still possible. Predictions from the resulting QSARs are, of course, less informative.
2. The separation of inactive from active compounds and the gradation of biological activity (separation of classes of active compounds) may be attributed to different factors, thus requiring different sets of features. In such instances, the division of the global problem into subproblems as in this example may be useful.
3. Discriminant functions can be interpreted in the same manner as regression equations. It is then necessary to consider collinearities and multicollinearities. The results of variance analysis (importance of the individual features for class separation) can be used as an additional source of information.

9.2.2.2.2. Influence of ortho-Toluenesulfonyl Ureas and Thioureas on the Blood Glucose Level in Rats [57]

In the present instance, classification is directed towards the direction of the observed effect. The blood glucose levels in rats are raised, lowered or unaffected by a series of 22 di-substituted ortho-toluenesulfonyl ureas and -thioureas of structure XLI when given as an intraperitoneal injection [81]. Accordingly, the compounds of this series fall into three different classes:

class 1: compounds raising the blood glucose level ($n_1 = 9$),

class 2: inactive compounds ($n_2 = 8$),
class 3: compounds lowering the blood glucose level ($n_3 = 5$).

The variables for discriminant analysis are presented in Table 9.23, and Table 9.24 shows the results of multivariate variance analysis (step-up procedure). MR_2 is sufficient to separate class 1 from the two others but not for the separation of classes 2 and 3. For this purpose, features I_1 and R_M must be included as well, but this does result in classes 1 and 2 being no longer separable. The optimal set for the simultaneous separation of all classes includes the variables MR_2, I_1, R_M and π_1. Again this set does not significantly separate classes 1 and 2 at the level of $p = 0.05$. The whole picture indicates that hypo- and hyperglycaemic activity are connected with different properties of the molecules.

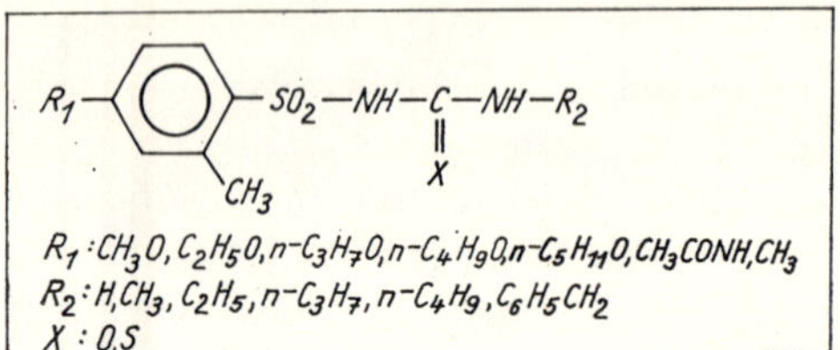

XLI

Table 9.23. Features for the molecular description of XLI

Fragement	Features
whole molecule	R_M [1])
X	$I_1 = \begin{cases} 1 & \text{for } X = S \\ 0 & \text{for } X = 0 \end{cases}$
R_1	π_1, σ_1, MR_1
R_2	π_2, MR_2 $I_2 = \begin{cases} 1 \text{ for electron attracting substituents} \\ 0 \text{ otherwise} \end{cases}$

[1]) Calculated from R_F-values (thin-layer chromatography on Siliful UV 254 with n-butanol/7 m ammonia (7:3)) [81]

Two non-elementary discriminant functions, of which only the first is statistically significant, arise from the optimum of features. The first discriminant function reads:

$$w_1 = 0.258\, MR_2 + 2.297 I_1 + 14.65\, R_M + 1.170 \pi_1 \tag{9/78}$$

	$\overline{w}_1$
class 1	8.549
class 2	9.499
class 3	11.93

Using (9/78), 19 of the 22 compounds in the training series can be reclassified correctly (reclassification error: 13%). In terms of class means of the discriminant variables it follows from (9/78) that high values for MR_2, R_M and π_1, along with the presence of the thioamide group (X = S), are favourable conditions for hypoglycaemic activity; for hyperglycaemic activity the reverse is true.

Table 9.24. Result of multivariate variance analysis for the action of XLI on the blood sugar level in rats

Feature set	Classes separated	HOTELLINGS T^2	Probability of error, p[1])
MR_2	all[2])	1.947	**0.009**
	1—2[3])	1.212	**0.012**
	1—3	1.520	**0.006**
	2—3	0.072	0.508
MR_2, I_1	all	2.823	**0.013**
	1—2	1.212	**0.047**
	1—3	2.243	**0.007**
	2—3	0.774	0.127
MR_2, I_1, R_M	all	5.175	**0.004**
	1—2	1.216	0.114
	1—3	4.126	**0.002**
	2—3	2.724	**0.010**
MR_2, I_1, R_M, π_1 (optimal set)	all	6.861	**0.004**
	1—2	1.505	0.142
	1—3	5.814	**0.001**
	2—3	3.385	**0.012**

[1]) bold values indicate a significant class-separation
[2]) simultaneous separation of all classes
[3]) pairwise separation of two classes

Since hypo- and hyperglycaemic activities obviously depend on different molecular properties it is to be concluded that also different optimal sets of variables are required to separate blood sugar increasing and blood sugar decreasing compounds from inactive compounds. It is, therefore, appropriate to consider the separation of the two classes of active compounds from class 2 as two different subproblems to be investigated separately according to:

subproblem 1: separation of classes 1 and 2
subproblem 2: separation of classes 2 and 3

As regards *subproblem 1,* the variable MR_2 is sufficient to separate these two classes ($T^2 = 0.90$; $p = 0.05$) in agreement with the results presented in Table 9.24, the non-elementary discriminant function being:

$$w = 0.143\,\mathrm{MR}_2 \tag{9/79}$$

	$\overline{w}$
class 1	1.474
class 2	2.740

With this discriminant function, 14 out of the 17 compounds considered are correctly reclassified. Three compounds cannot be unambigously classified according to the F-test (eqn. (9/72)), i.e., they fall into the region of overlap between the two classes. If the criterion of the smaller F value is used, they are assigned to the wrong class. In order to check the stability and separating power of (9/79) the leave-n-out technique (here with $n = 1$) was applied. In this technique each of the compounds is once left out from the analysis and is then classified with the discriminant function obtained from the remaining (in our case: 16) compounds. In this way a real classification in the sense of a prediction is simulated. Again, 14 compounds are correctly classified, and three fall into the region of overlap between the classes.

For *subproblem 2*, the optimal set contains the variables MR_2, I_1 and R_M ($T^2 = 4.06$; $p = 0.015$). The non-elementary discriminant function

$$w = 0.15\,\mathrm{MR}_2 + 2.82 I_1 + 8.53\,\mathrm{R}_M \tag{9/80}$$

	$\overline{w}$
class 2	5.399
class 3	8.092

affords a correct reclassification of 12 of the 13 compounds concerned. With the leave-n-out technique ($n = 1$), 10 compounds are correctly classified (three fall into the region of overlap between the two classes).

From the results, the following conclusions may be drawn:

1. The optimal sets of variables for the separation of classes 1 and 3 from class 2 are different. This leads to the occurrence of π_1 in the optimal set for the simultaneous separation of all classes as an artefact.
2. Of outstanding importance are the substituents in position R_2 which is reflected by the MR_2 term which appears in all discriminant functions. Because of a high correlation of MR_2 and π_2, no separation can, however, be achieved between hydrophobic and steric substituent effects. It follows from (9/79) and (9/80) that for a compound to raise the blood glucose level its substituents in R_2 should be small and/or hydrophilic, whilst larger and/or more hydrophobic substituents are favourable for hypoglycaemic activity (see also (9/78)). This conclusion is in agreement with the results of Ruschig et al. [82, 83], which indicate that, for N-alkyl-substituted sulfonyl ureas to be hypoglycaemic, substituents with not fewer than three C atoms are needed, and of Seydel [84] who showed that hypoglycaemic activity increases with hydrophobicity of N-substituents in another series of sulfonamides.
3. An important molecular property for hypoglycaemic activity is represented by R_M, as it is this value that leads to the separation of classes 2 and 3 (see Table 9.24).

R_M correlates negatively with the sum of π_1 and π_2 according to

$$R_M = -0.110(\pi_1 + \pi_2) + 0.502 \quad (9/81)$$

$$n = 22 \qquad r = -0.859 \qquad s = 0.006$$

and can, therefore, be regarded as a measure of the overall hydrophilicity of the molecules. The simultaneous occurrence of R_M and π_1 in (9/78) and of R_M and MR_2 in (9/80) suggests an optimum of overall hydrophobicity for hypoglycaemic activity. It may also be, however, that this simply reflects the influence of large alkoxy groups in R_2 which has been shown to be unfavourable for hypoglycaemic activity [85].

4. The amide group is not an essential part of hypoglycaemic sulfonyl ureas. Apparently, all that matters is the presence of a nitrogen-bound, sp^2-hybridizid carbon with the thioamide group promoting hypoglycaemic activity in comparison with the amide group as follows from the I_1 term in (9/80).
5. No electronic effects could be demonstrated for substituents in R_1. This is probably due to the insufficient variation of electronic properties within the R_1 substituents considered since, according to SEYDEL [84], electronic effects of such substituents are important for hypoglycaemic activity.
6. Separation of classes 1 and 3 from the class of inactive compounds cannot be accomplished unless different sets of molecular parameters are used, and, therefore, one is led to infer that hyper- and hypoglycaemic activities are regulated by two different mechanisms. This conclusion is substantiated by experimental results.

   Hypoglyceamic activity is produced by interaction with receptors in β cells [86], whereas an increase in blood glucose level is probably due to an enhanced adrenalin production [87, 88]. It would appear that the two opposite effects overlap and it depends on their relative strenght whether a given compound enhances or diminishes the blood glucose level or leaves it unaffected. As these two activities depend on different substituent effects, it is easy to understand why structurally similar compounds of the sulfonyl urea and sulfonamide types may influence the blood glucose level in totally different ways.

These conclusions are, of course, only valid for compounds belonging to that range of structural variations covered by the training series. Since these variations as well as the size of the training series are quite limited in this example the discriminant functions obtained cannot be recommended for the design of new compounds. They are, however, adequate to describe the distribution of compounds over the classes *within* the training series. This, in fact, was the primary objective of the investigation in order to understand why opposite effects on blood sugar level are present in a homologous series with only minor structural differences. The same example has recently been reinvestigated by DUNN and WOLD [49] using the SIMCA technique (see 9.2.1.) with good results. However, the conclusions of these authors, who considered SIMCA superior to discriminant analysis in this case, are invalid since they are based on the erroneous assumption that the arrangement of the compounds given in Table I presented in [57] reflects the within-class structure. This assumption is entirely wrong. In discussing their results, furthermore, these authors did not fully appreciate the importance of considering the two subproblems separately.

9.3. Rank Correlation Analysis

When applying this procedure to quantitative structure-activity analysis [89—91] it is assumed that within homologous series there exists a defined and monotonous relation between the level of biological action and molecular properties relevant to that action. This is a less strict requirement than the linear model assumed to hold in the extrathermodynamic approach which is certainly realistic expecially when dealing with quantum-chemical molecular parameters. Such relations can be examined by means of rank correlation analysis [92]. The first step comprises the transformation of the values of biological activity and the molecular parameters concerned into rank numbers. These numbers indicate the position of each value when the respective data are ranked in descending order.

With the aid of the rank numbers and eqn. (9/82)

$$r_{s,j} = 1 - 6 \sum_{i=1}^{n} d_i^2/(n^3 - n) \tag{9/82}$$

it is possible to calculate SPEARMANS rank correlation coefficient [92] which serves to characterize the connection between a given molecular property and the level of biological activity A. In this equation, d_i denotes the difference of the rank numbers of parameter x_j and biological activity of the i-th compound and n is the number of compounds in the sample. If the correlation between A and x_j is perfect, $|r_{s,j}|$ takes a value of 1.

The method developed by SKLENAR and JÄGER [89—91] permits not only the normal univariate case but also linear combinations of two and three molecular parameters p_k to be included in rank correlation analysis:

univariate case

$$x_j = x_j \tag{9/83}$$

bivariate case

$$x_j = ap_1 + bp_2 \tag{9/84}$$

trivariate case

$$x_j = ap_1 + bp_2 + cp_3 \tag{9/85}$$

The weight factors of the linear combinations (9/84) and (9/85) are so determined that the corresponding rank correlation coefficient takes a maximal value. Through a special program one can also include relations possessing a maximum or minimum which are transformed into monotonous ones by mirroring at the extreme.

The calculated rank correlation coefficients are tested using a special, distribution-free method to ascertain at what level of significance they are different from zero. Once analysis of the training series has made clear what parameters (or parameter combinations) correlate best with biological activity, corresponding values for x_j allow the inclusion of unknown compounds in the already existing rank order and thus semi-quantitative conclusions with respect to the expected level of the biological activity exerted by these compounds (optimization of structure). In addition, certain conclusions can be drawn with respect to properties of the molecules which are relevant to biological activity. The procedure in its present form is especially intended to test an extremely large number of molecular parameters for any correlation with biological activity with few, if any, hypotheses concerning possible interactions between drugs and biosystems.

Such a situation may, for example, arise when quantum-chemical parameters are considered and it is mainly this purpose for which the procedure has been designed. A specific test statistics is used in order to adequately account for the very large number of parameters involved. The procedure can be hierarchically coupled to regression analysis. It has the advantage that the values of biological activity must only be known to a precision sufficient to establish a rank order.

If a large number of quantum-chemical parameters is screened in a random fashion, collinearities and complex multicollinearities are very likely to occur. As a consequence, more than one combination of parameters may yield rank correlation coefficients of equal significance, and one is then faced with the same difficulties as already outlined in chapters 7. and 8.: a mechanistic interpretation of the result is not possible, and predictions are to be considered with caution. Therefore, a guided approach to parameter selection based on selected hypotheses and a well designed series certainly is to be preferred at some stage of the analysis. Factor analysis of the parameters may also be helpful to recognize collinearities.

References

[1] Lewi, P. J., in E. J. Ariens (Ed.): Drug Design, Vol. VII, Academic Press, New York, 1976, p. 209

[2] Lewi, P. J., in E. J. Ariens (Ed.): Drug Design, Vol. X, Academic Press, New York, 1980, p. 308

[3] Mager, H.: Thesis, Martin-Luther-Universität Halle—Wittenberg, 1977

[4] Mager, P. P., in E. J. Ariens (Ed.): Drug Design, Vol. IX, Academic Press, New York, 1980, p. 188

[5] Mager, P. P., in E. J. Ariens (Ed.): Drug Design, Vol. X, Academic Press, New York, 1980, p. 308

[6] Weiner, P. H., E. R. Malinowski and A. R. Levinstone: J. Phys. Chem. **74**, 4537 (1970)

[7] Weiner, P. H., and E. R. Malinowski: J. Phys. Chem. **75**, 1207 (1971)

[8] Weiner, P. H., and E. R. Malinowski: J. Phys. Chem. **75**, 3160 (1971)

[9] Weiner, P. H., and J. F. Parcher: J. Chromatogr. Sci. **10**, 612 (1972)

[10] Weiner, P. H., and D. G. Howery: Anal. Chem. **44**, 1189 (1972)

[11] Weiner, P. H., and D. G. Howery: Canad. J. Chem. **50**, 448 (1972)

[12] Weiner, P. H.: J. Amer. Chem. Soc. **95**, 5845 (1973)

[13] Weiner, M. L., and P. H. Weiner: J. Med. Chem. **16**, 655 (1973)

[14] Kindsvater, J. H., P. H. Weiner and T. J. Klingen: Anal. Chem. **46**, 982 (1974)

[15] Malinowski, E. R., and M. McCue: Anal. Chem. **49**, 284 (1977)

[16] Malinowski, E. R.: Anal. Chem. **49**, 606 (1977)

[17] Malinowski, E. R.: Anal. Chem. **49**, 612 (1977)

[18] Dove, S., and R. Franke in R. Franke and P. Oehme (Eds.): Quantitative Structure-Activity Analysis, Akademie-Verlag, Berlin, 1978, p. 321

[19] Malinowsky, E. R., and D. G. Howery: Factor Analysis in Chemistry, Wiley, New York, 1980

[20] Franke, R., S. Dove and R. Kühne: Eur. J. Med. Chem. **14**, 363 (1979)

[21] Lukovits, I., and A. Lopata: J. Med. Chem. **23**, 449 (1980)

[22] Dove, S., and R. Franke: Wiss. Beiträge Martin-Luther-Universität Halle—Wittenberg **42 (R 34)**, 216 (1977)

[23] Exner, O.: Coll. Czechoslov. Chem. Commun. **37**, 3222 (1966)

[24] Shoenfeld, P. S., and J. R. De Voe: Anal. Chem. **48**, 403 R (1976)

[25] Franke, R., in J. A. Keverling Buisman (Ed.): Biological Activity and Chemical Structure, Pharmacochemistry Library (Eds.: W. Th. Nauta and R. F. Rekker), Vol. 2, Elsevier, Amsterdam, 1977, p. 251

[26] Fujita, T.: Progr. Phys. Org. Chem., in press

[27] Dove, S., R. Kühne and R. Franke in F. Darvas and J. Knoll (Eds.): Chemical Structure — Biological Activity Relationships, Akadémiai Kiadó, Budapest, 1980, p. 247

[28] Dunn, W. J., and S. Wold: Acta Chem. Scand. **B 32**, 536 (1978)

[29] Kühne, R., S. Dove and R. Franke: Eur. J. Med. Chem., in press

[30] Wold, S., and M. Sjöström: Chem. Scr. **2**, 49 (1972)

[31] Wold, S., and M. Sjöström: Chem. Scr. **6**, 114 (1974)

[32] Sjöström, M., and S. Wold: Acta Chem. Scand. **B 30**, 167 (1967)

[33] Sjöström, M., and S. Wold: Chem. Scr. **9**, 200 (1976)

[34] Dove, S., and R. Franke: unpublished results

[35] Sensi, P., N. Maggi, R. Balotta, S. Furesz, R. Pallanza and V. Arioli: J. Med. Chem. **7**, 596 (1964)

[36] Quinn, F. R., J. S. Driscoll and C. Hansch: J. Med. Chem. **18**, 332 (1975)

[37] Bekemeier, H.: private communication

[38] Wold, S.: Patt. Recog. **8**, 127 (1976)

[39] Sjöström, M., and S. Wold in B. R. Kowalski (Ed.): Chemometrics: Theory and Practice, ACS Symposium Series **52**, 243 (1977)

[40] Dunn, W. J., S. Wold and Y. C. Martin: J. Med. Chem. **21**, 922 (1978)

[41] Wold, S., and M. Sjöström in N. B. Chapman and J. Shorter (Eds.): Correlation Analysis, Recent Advances, Plenum Press, London, 1978, Chapter 1

[42] Albano, C., W. J. Dunn, U. Edlund, E. Johansson, B. Nordén, M. Sjöström and S. Wold: Analyt. Chim. Acta Comp. Tech. Optim. **2**, 429 (1978)

[43] Wold, S.: Technometrics **20**, 397 (1978)

[44] Sjöström, M., and B. R. Kowalski: Analyt. Chim. Acta Comp. Tech. Optim. **112**, 11 (1979)

[45] Dunn, W. J., and S. Wold: J. Med. Chem. **21**, 1001 (1978)

[46] Dunn, W. J., and S. Wold in G. Barnett, M. Trsic and R. E. Willette (Eds.): Quantitative Structure Activity Relationships of Analgesics, Narcotic Antagonists, and Hallucinogens, NIDA Research Monograph 22, Rockville Md., 1978, p. 114

[47] Nordén, B., U. Edlund and S. Wold: Acta Chem. Scand. **B 32**, 602 (1978)

[48] Wold, S., and W. J. Dunn: Tables Rondes Roussel Uclaf **38**, 56 (1980)

[49] Dunn, W. J., and S. Wold: Bioorganic Chemistry **9**, 505 (1980)

[49a] Dove, S.: private communication

[50] Cammarata, A., and G. K. Menon: J. Med. Chem. **19**, 739 (1976)

[51] Menon, G. K., and A. Cammarata: J. Pharm. Sci. **66**, 304 (1977)

[52] Ahrens, H., and J. Läuter: Mehrdimensionale Varianzanalyse, Akademie-Verlag, Berlin, 1974

[53] Collous, T. (Ed.): Discriminant Analysis and Applications, Academic Press, New York, 1973

[54] Martin, Y. C., J. B. Holland, C. H. Jarboe and N. Plotnikoff: J. Med. Chem. **17**, 409 (1974)

[55] Franke, R., and W. Meiske: Acta biol. med. germ. **35**, 73 (1976)

[56] Franke, R., G. N. Vassiliev and S. Dove: Compt. rend. Acad. Bulg. Sci. **32**, 369 (1979)

[57] Dove, S., R. Franke, O. L. Mndshojan, W. A. Schkuljev and L. W. Chashakjan: J. Med. Chem. **22**, 90 (1978)

[58] Schönfelder, D., and R. Franke in R. Franke and P. Oehme (Eds.): Quantitative Structure-Activity Analysis, Akademie-Verlag, Berlin, 1978, p. 303

[59] Tonew, M., W. Laass, E. Tonew, R. Franke, H. Goldner and W. Zschiesche: Acta virol. **22**, 287 (1978)

[60] Dove, S., and R. Franke in R. Franke and P. Oehme (Eds.): Quantitative Structure-Activity Analysis, Akademie-Verlag, Berlin, 1978, p. 257

[61] Krause, G., R. Franke and G. N. Vassiliev: Biochem. Physiol. Plant. **174**, 128 (1979)

[62] Hagemann, R., and R. Franke: Pharmazie **31**, 130 (1976)

[63] Laass, W., W. Bercher, R. Franke and W. Grisk: Vortrag auf der 18. Jahrestagung der Gesellschaft für Pharmakologie und Toxikologie der DDR, Halle, 1976

[64] Bercher, H., W. Laass, E. Schult, A. Grisk and R. Franke: Pharmazie **34**, 336 (1979)

[65] Laass, W., H. Bercher, E. Schult, R. Franke and A. Grisk: Pharmazie **34**, 334 (1979)

[66] Franke, R., S. Dove, G. Gruska, H.-J. Michel and D. Schönfelder: unpublished results

[67] Prakash, G., and E. H. Hodnett: J. Med. Chem. **21**, 369 (1978)

[68] Dunn, W. J., and M. J. Greenberg: J. Pharm. Sci. **66**, 1416 (1977)

[69] Henry, D. R., and J. H. Block: J. Med. Chem. **22**, 465 (1979)

[70] Henry, D. R., and J. H. Block: Eur. J. Med. Chem. **15**, 133 (1980)

[71] Moriguchi, I., K. Komatsu and Y. Matsushi: J. Med. Chem. **23**, 20 (1980)

[72] Smith, C. C., C. S. Genther and E. A. Coats: Eur. J. Med. Chem. **14**, 271 (1979)

[73] Enslein, K., D. Khana and P. N. Craig: A Toxicity Estimation System. Genesee Computer Center Inc. Rochester, New York, 1978

[74] Rekker, R. F.: TIPS 383 (1980)

[75] White, G. A., and G. D. Thorn: Pesticide Biochem. Physiol. **5**, 380 (1975)

[76] Ulrich, J. T., and D. E. Mathre: J. Bacteriol. **110**, 628 (1972)

[77] White, G. A.: Biochem. Biophys. Res. Comm. **44**, 1210 (1971)

[78] Ten Haken, P., and C. L. Dunn: Proc. 6 Brit. Insectic. Fungic. Conf. **2**, 453 (1971)

[79] Barlin, G. B., and D. D. Perrin: Quart. Rev. **20**, 75 (1966)

[80] Snel, M., B. von Schmeling and L. V. Edington: Phytopathology **60**, 1164 (1970)

[81] Experimental Results by O. L. Mndshojan, W. A. Schkuljev and L. W. Chashakjan, Institut für Feinorganische Chemie der Armenischen Akademie der Wissenschaften

[82] Ruschig, H., G. Korger, W. Aumüller, H. Wagner and R. Weyer: Arzneimittel-Forschung **8**, 448 (1958)

[83] Ruschig, H., G. Korger, W. Aumüller, H. Wagner and R. Weyer: Medizin und Chemie **6**, 61 (1958)

[84] Seydel, J. K., and K.-J. Schaper: Chemische Struktur und biologische Aktivität von Wirkstoffen, Verlag Chemie, Weinheim, 1979

[85] Mhasalkar, M. Y., M. H. Shah, U. Tonse, K. G. Ananthanarayanan and C. V. Deliwala: J. Sci. Ind. Res. **21c**, 143 (1962)

[86] Gutsche, K., A. Harwart, H. Horstmann, H. Priewe, G. Raspe, E. Schraufstätter, S. Wirtz and U. Wörffel: Arzneimittel-Forschung **24**, 1028 (1974)

[87] McLamore, W. M., and G. D. Laubach: Congr. Int. Chim. Ind. **2**, 443 (1958)

[88] Bänder, A.: Arzneimittel-Forschung, **8**, 459 (1958)

[89] Sklenar, H., J. Jäger and R. Süssmilch in R. Franke and P. Oehme (Eds.): Quantitative Structure — Activity Analysis, Akademie-Verlag, Berlin, 1978, p. 239

[90] Sklenar, H., and J. Jäger: Int. J. Quant. Chem. **16**, 467 (1979)

[91] Sklenar, H., and J. Jäger: Struktur-Wirkungs-Beziehungen auf quantenchemischer Grundlage in P. Oehme, H. Löwe and E. Göres (Eds.); Beiträge zur Wirkstofforschung, No. 10, Akademie-Industrie-Komplex Arzneimittelforschung, Berlin, 1980

[92] Siegel, E.: Nonparametric Statistics for the Behavioural Sciences, McGraw Hill, New York, 1956

10. Non-Computer-Assisted Search Operations on the Basis of the Extrathermodynamic Approach

Under circumstances where compounds are difficult to synthesize it is, of course, desirable to proceed with every compound made in the most probable direction of higher biological activity. When biological testing is rapid this can be done by using the biological feedback in a stepwise decision procedure. The situation thus arising is not unlike a game of chess. The aim is to obtain a given result with the fewest possible moves, i.e., to establish the biologically active members of a family of compounds with a minimum of syntheses and tests. This has long been a usual procedure in drug design where, however, any decisions concerning each subsequent move were in general purely intuitive or at least empirical. Based on the extrathermodynamic approach the decisions can be formalized to a certain extent and are, therefore, more objective. As a result, the overall procedure becomes more effective and more rational. The reasoning underlying the extrathermodynamic approach is adopted here, implying a definite relationship between the level of biological activity and those molecular parameter which are relevant in characterizing essential molecular properties.

The consequential strategies have the advantage of being very simple and serviceable without the need for computers, and they make it possible to single out the biologically most active compounds from a limited group. Furthermore, the compounds thus selected for syntheses and biological testing usually constitute a good first move in the direction of a training series satisfying the requirements to be met for applying the extrathermodynamic QSAR approach. The strategies involved are based on the experience that biological activity can already be grossly described with fairly good results using only two or even one molecular parameters in many cases, the influence of hydrophobicity playing a major rôle here.

10.1. The Decision Tree of Topliss

The procedure presented by Topliss [1—3] rests on the assumption that the biological activity of various analogues primarily depends on hydrophobic and electronic substituent effects (that is, on π and σ). Any change in activity following the exchange of substituents is then connected with the π and σ values of the substituents in a defined and logical manner, and based on this logic a decision tree can be constructed, permitting an early discovery of active compounds (or the most favourable substituents).

The principle is illustrated in Fig. 10.1, it being assumed for convenience that an exchange of substituents will always effect biological activity. An increase in activity is indicated by a "+" sign, and a decrease in activity by a "—" sign. A fictitious example (see [4]) is considered in Fig. 10.1 to illustrate a case in which the most favourable substituent for a para-position localized in an aromatic system is to be found.

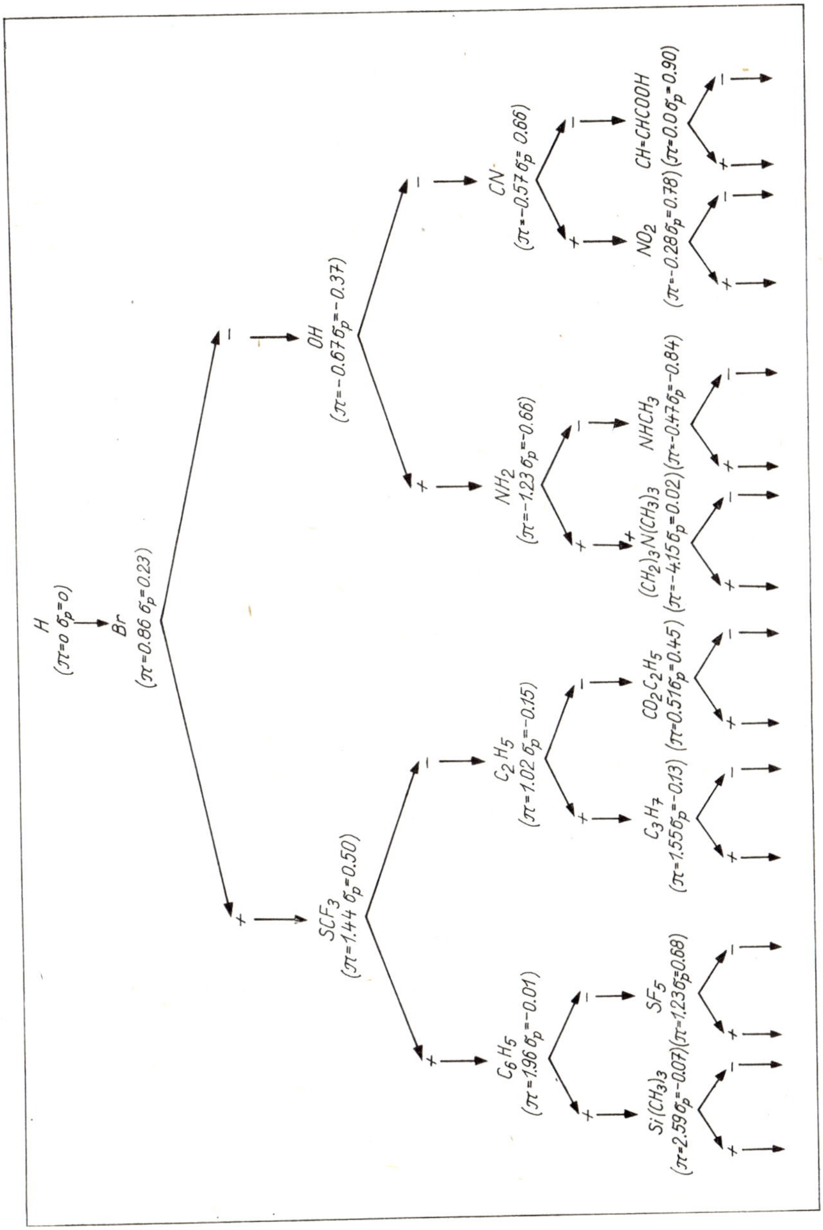

Fig. 10.1. Decision tree of Topliss

To begin with, the non-substituted compound is tested. Regardless of which substituent is selected first, it is necessary that

1. the substituent has no extremely hydrophobic or electronic properties,
2. the substituent is more hydrophobic than hydrogen, as any not too large increase in hydrophobicity often leads to an increase in biological activity,
3. the synthesis of the corresponding compound can be achieved in the simplest possible manner,
4. the substituent is not metabolized.

In the event of substituent variations in a ring system, the above conditions are best satisfied by halogens so that the preparation of the bromine derivative (which is more hydrophobic than F and Cl and less so than I and can usually be synthesized without difficulty) is recommended as the first step. If a stronger activity ensues, one moves to the *left part of the decision tree,* as will be explained first. Any increase in activity, caused by bromine, can be connected with enhanced hydrophobicity ($+\pi$ effect), with the electron-attracting effect ($+\sigma$ effect) or with both. In the last case, a substituent with higher hydrophobicity and electron-attracting power needs to be introduced; an example is the SCF_3 group. If activity continues to rise the even more hydrophobic phenyl group may be a good next move. This group has practically no electronic effect so that any further rise in activity would lead to the conclusion that biological activity is primarily dependent on hydrophobicity. Therefore, the next substituent should then be selected in such a way that hydrophobicity is further increased while electronic properties are not changed. Such a substituent is, for example, the $Si(CH_3)_3$ group, which, however, could be easily replaced by a longer alkyl chain or a hydrophobically substituted phenyl group. Activity may also be reduced by the presence of the phenyl group. The underlying cause may be that the phenyl group already exceeds the hydrophobicity optimum and/or that a $+\sigma$ effect is essential to biological activity. As the next step, therefore, it is opportune to chose a somewhat less hydrophobic substituent with a clear $+\sigma$ effect, such as the SF_5 group.

If the SCF_3 derivative is less active than the bromine compound (see right half of the left part of the decision tree), the reason may be that the group is already too hydrophobic. Another, probably better, explanation is that a $+\sigma$ effect is unfavourable for biological activity; in the bromine compound this unfavourable influence may still be overcompensated by the favourable $+\pi$ effect but this can no longer be said for the basically stronger electron-attracting SCF_3 group. This possibility is to be checked in the ethyl derivative, as the ethyl group has a $-\sigma$ effect and is also less hydrophobic. If a stronger action ensues, the $-\sigma$ character is retained with the next substituent and hydrophobicity is enhanced. A useful candidate is the propyl group. If the ethyl group, which is not essentially more hydrophobic than bromine, should lower activity, such a decrease may be interpreted to indicate that the $+\pi$ effect of the substituent must be small and that the $+\sigma$ effect is of fundamental importance. In this case bromine may already be slightly too hydrophobic and only increase activity by virtue of its $+\sigma$ effect. Subsequently, a substituent with a smaller $+\pi$ and a more pronounced $+\sigma$ effect than bromine (e.g., $CO_2C_2H_5$) needs to be chosen.

If bromine diminishes activity (see *right part of the decision tree*), hydrophobic and/or electron-attracting substituents are unfavourable. The OH group with its $-\pi$ and $-\sigma$ effects is a substituent that can be used to verify these possibilities. If the presence of the OH group results in a higher activity, such substituents are evidently favourable, thus justifying the introduction of, for example, the NH_2 group in the following step. Where activity increases further, one may try to find out whether $-\pi$ and $-\sigma$ effects are equally important or which of them dominates. Should, for example, the $(CH_2)_3 \cdot \overset{+}{N}(CH_3)_3$ group enhance biological activity the dominance of a $-\pi$ effect is indicated.

If activity is not raised by the OH group (see right half of the right part of the decision tree) it may be that, in contrast to a basically favourable $-\pi$ effect, a $-\sigma$ effect is unfavourable. Whether this is really true can be checked using, for example, the CN group which, with a $-\pi$ effect and a $+\sigma$ effect, should then be able to raise activity. If so, the choice of a hydrophilic substituent with an even more pronounced $+\sigma$ effect, like the NO_2 group, would be the subsequent step. If the opposite holds, it may be that while Br is too hydrophobic CN is already too hydrophilic. In such a case, one should decide in favour of a substituent that occupies an intermediate position between Br and CN in terms of hydrophobicity and, at the same time, exerts a strong electronic effect. Since, at this stage, no implications with regard to the possible direction of the electronic substituent influence can be made it does no matter whether a $+\sigma$ or a $-\sigma$ substituent is selected. Suitable candidates for the $+\sigma$ or the $-\sigma$ substituent to be chosen afterwards are CH=CH—COOH and the $N(CH_3)_2$ group ($\pi = 0.18$; $\sigma_p = -0.83$), respectively.

It should be noted that the choice of substituents as outlined above is in no way the only possible one. The procedure leads to certain conclusions as to properties which the substituent to be tested subsequently is required to possess. What substituent will eventually be chosen also depends, among other things, on the synthesizability of the corresponding compounds (this aspect was excluded from the proposals presented in Fig. 10.1).

The procedure does not take steric effects into account. To a certain extent, they can be recognized if biological activity only partly follows, if at all, the logic of the pure π-σ scheme, and deviations from the logic are related to steric substituent properties. As a consequence, it is possible — although within relatively narrow limits and by no means under all circumstances — to include steric substituent properties in the decision making.

The Topliss method can also be employed in the case of polysubstituted compounds, requiring, of course, assumptions to be made about the additivity of substituent influences. If the dependence on π and σ is superimposed by steric and position effects in a too complex manner, the limits of the applicability of the procedure will soon be reached. Another problem is that in general it is uncertain whether, indeed, biological activity primarily depends on π and σ, a combination of, for example, σ and E_S being also conceivable. Here, too, the Topliss procedure may find application but the possibility of using σ and E_S instead of π and σ must be checked first. On the whole, a procedure based on π and σ is more likely to be successful because that combination occurs more frequently.

By retrospective application of the Topliss scheme to examples from the literature, Martin and Dunn [5] obtained the results given in Table 10.1 which shows that an approximately 60% economy of effort can thus be achieved. Of course, the Topliss procedure implies a fairly large simplification so that it cannot always be expected to be successful. Nonetheless, it is recommended whenever testing takes less time than synthesizing, and if satisfactory results are obtained, not only the economy of effort is important but there are particularly favourable conditions for gaining much information from a subsequent quantitative structure-activity analysis insofar as the compounds selected by this method usually form a good basis for the final design of a training series. If the procedure fails (see e.g. [6]), no disadvantages will arise and there is no reason to fear larger research expenditure or a lesser chance of detecting the most active compounds.

Table 10.1. Results of a retrospective application of the TOPLISS scheme to some examples from the literature (from [5])

Substances	Biological activity	Number of compounds tested	Number of compounds which would have been necessary to find the most active derivative when applying the TOPLISS scheme
(1) 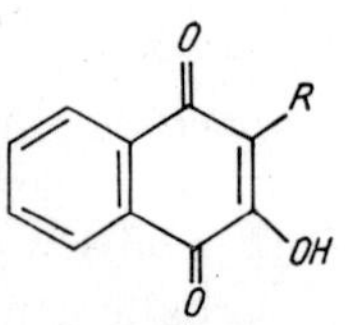	Antimalaria	295	5 (In this case, only 1 of about 26 equipotent compounds is found)
(2) 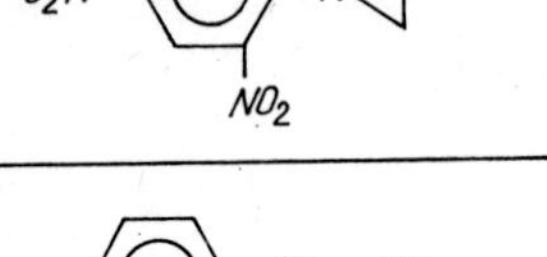	β_1-adrenergic β_2-adrenergic	9 9	3 3
(3) 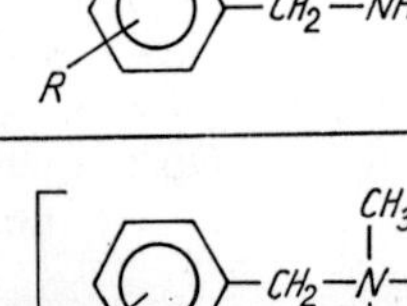	Cytostatic	11	5
(4) 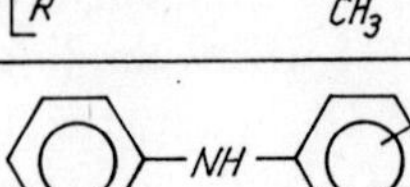	Oxydation by monoamino-oxidase	13	5
(5) 	Antibacterial, *S. aureus*	7	3
(6)	Antibacterial, *S. aureus* *E. coli*	 19 19	 4 5

10.2. Sequential Simplex Procedure

Assuming again that in many cases biological activity is sufficiently described in quantitative terms by π and σ (or any other combination of two molecular parameters), each substituent or each compound can be represented as a point in a three-dimensional coordinate system with coordinates A (biological activity), π and σ. These points lie in a plane that has a maximum in relation to A at given values of π and σ. This maximum and thus the most active compound can be found rapidly and without difficulty using the simple, geometric method of Darvas [7] (see also [8, 9]), which is based on the simplex self-directing optimization method for non-continuous fields [10].

First all compounds or substituents already available or of potential interest are shown as points in the π-σ plane. Next, three compounds are selected for experimental investigation. In general, they will include the non-substituted lead compound and two substituents, one displaying a relatively overt π effect and a limited σ effect and the other the opposite. Biological testing affords values for the third coordinate, A. The three points are then connected with one another, thus forming a triangle (called *simplex*) with a given inclination with respect to coordinate A (see Fig. 10.2).

Intuitively, one will see that more active compounds and more favourable substituents are to be found "uphill". The point for the compound with the lowest activity is connected to the midpoint of the opposite side of the triangle by a straight line and the following, presumably more active, compound is searched for in the direction of the projection of this line on the π-σ plane. The compound to be choses next is the one which lies most closely to this projection, yet sufficiently far away from the previously examined compounds. With A, determined for this new compound, one can construct a new simplex. Again, a triangle is formed by connecting the point for this compound with those two points of the first simplex which represent the two more active compounds. The second triangle is a sort of reflection of the first triangle on the side connecting the two more active compounds so that this side is a component of either triangle. The searching procedure is repeated for the second simplex, the following compound being selected in the π-σ plane in the direction of the connecting line between the point for the compound with the lowest activity and the midpoint of the opposite side of the second simplex. By means of the result for this new compound, yet another simplex can be constructed, which is the subject of the same geometrical operation. The procedure is continued until the maximum has been found, as is the case when the last simplex falls into an already existing one or when in the direction indicated no further points are found. All geometrical operations are performed in the π-σ plane, the coordinate A being viewed in such a way that the values determined for biological activity are recorded beside the corresponding points.

In Fig. 10.2 the procedure is schematized for the example of the sodiouretic activities of sulfonamides as reported by Darvas [7]. For ease of survey, not all but only those points are noted down which are, indeed, included in one of the individual simplexes. The chosen starting compounds are the non-substituted parent structure, the 4-acetyl and the 4-Cl derivatives (simplex 1). The lead compound shows the least activity (= lowest point of the simplex) so that the direction one has to search in can be gained from the direction of the line connecting point R = H and the midpoint of the opposite side of the triangle. It is in that direction that the 4-NO_2 group can be located as the subsequent substituent which, indeed, has a higher biological activity. With this, one can construct simplex 2, in which the 4-Cl compound is least active. This point can be connected to the midpoint of the opposite side of the triangle, the resultant line pointing at the 4-CN group. When tested, this compound again will show a markedly higher activity. With this compound, that is, after a total of five syntheses and five tests, the activity maximum within the sample of sixteen compounds has already been attained because in the searching direction as found by the third simplex the sample contains no further compounds.

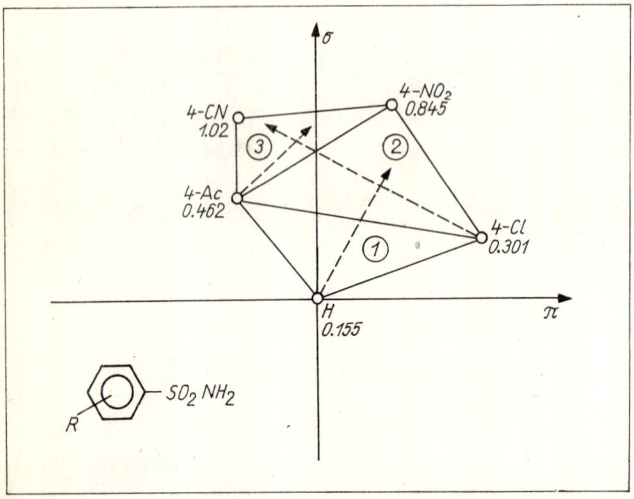

Fig. 10.2. Simplex-procedure

The simplex procedure can be applied for the same purposes and with similar results as the Topliss procedure. In either case, an about 60% economy of effort and a systematic variation in the structures of the sample can be achieved. An advantage over the Topliss procedure is the even higher degree of objectivity. Application is, of course, restricted to two molecular parameters. If more dimensions are needed, a corresponding computer variant can be used [11] (see also [8]). It is noteworthy that under certain circumstances this method may be hazardous in that it finds only a local rather than the global activity maximum.

10.3. The Fibonacci Search Technique

This technique (see e.g. [12]) can be employed whenever the biological activity within a sample of compounds primarily depends on only one molecular parameter in a mono-extremal manner. The extremum (and thus the most active compound) is found through a definite number of steps along the so-called Fibonacci frequency (numbers 1, 2, 3, 5, 8, 13, 21, 34, ...). The compounds to be synthesized are arranged in order of ascending values of the molecular parameter (for example, π) with which a monoextremal relation is presumed, and than numbered. The first compound is assigned the number 0 so that the highest number in a given sample of n compounds is equal to $n - 1$. The subsequent procedure is based on the numerical data presented in Table 10.2 and may be briefly illustrated with an example [13]. Compounds of structure XLII display antibacterial and antifungal activity. The compounds tested are arranged according to

Table 10.2. Numerical relations of the FIBONACCI search technique (from [13])

Number of internal points	Numbers of compounds to be tested	Numbers of compounds necessary to locate the maximum
2	1 and 2	2
4	2 and 3	3
7	3 and 5	4
12	5 and 8	5
20	8 and 13	6
33	13 and 21	7
54	21 and 34	8

ascending log P values as shown in Table 10.3 assuming that between log A and log P a monoextremal relation is present.

The first step serves to determine the number of what are called *internal points*, which can be expressed as $(n - 1) - 1 = (7 - 1) = 6$. This number is, however, not contained in column 1 of Table 10.2. The next following number in that table is 7 and to circumvent this problem a fictitious number 8 is added at the end of the series. The number of internal points is then $8 - 1 = 7$ and it follows from column 2 of Table 10.2 that the compound with maximal activity should be located after in all four syntheses and that compounds 3 and 5 are to be tested as the first derivatives. The test shows that compound 3 has the lower activity so that the maximum can be located between the new limits set by compounds 3 and 8. Within these limits there are four internal points, corresponding to numbers 2 and 3 in Table 10.2. These numbers are added to those for the lower limit, i.e., to 3. The numbers of the derivatives to be tested next are therefore 5 and 6, compound 5 being already tested in the previous step. This situation is typical of the FIBONACCI technique, one of two compounds involved in a given step already being dealt with by the preceding step. The new set of limits for the maxi-

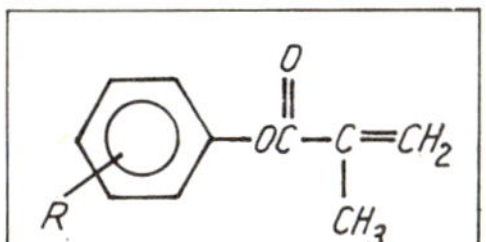

XLII

Table 10.3. Derivatives of XLII, arranged according to ascending log P values (from [13])

Compound No.	R	log P	log A
0	H	1.99	2.89
1	4-Cl	2.69	3.25
2	2-Cl	2.75	3.08
3	2.4-Cl_2	3.45	3.49
4	2.4.5-Cl_3	4.21	3.84
5	2.4.6-Cl_3	4.21	3.76
6	2.4.5.6-Cl_4	4.97	3.97
7	Br_5	6.71	3.64
8			

mum is between numbers 5 and 8, and there are two internal points. As appears from Table 10.2, numbers 1 and 2 are added to number 5 to provide items 6 and 7. The most active derivative is found as item 6 after four syntheses as predicted.

First applied to drug research by Bustard [14], the Fibonacci technique rapidly produces reliable results, if the condition that there should be a monoextremal relationship with a known molecular parameter is fully satisfied. From a given number of compounds the most active one can then be rapidly singled out by a minimum of test steps. The required presence of a monoextremal relation with only one individual molecular parameter implies, of course, a marked restriction on the applicability of the method. If more than one extremum occur, a local instead of a global maximum is apt to present itself, so that the most active compound is not found. If activity is affected by more than one molecular parameter, the procedure cannot be applied at all. Although the possibility of using the sum of different molecular parameters has been mentioned [13], many problems arise in practice. Some examples have been described [13] in which such sums as, for example ($\log P + \sigma$) have been treated as one molecular parameter. However, one has to deal here with retrospective analyses where it is always possible to play around with various parameter combinations until a successful one is found. This, however, is not possible in any true application in practice so that such an approach may lead to entirely incorrect results. A further limitation of the Fibonacci technique has recently been pointed out by Deming [15] who showed that it will fail if too much noise (e.g., from experimental errors) is present on the response surface.

The Fibonacci search provides a highly successful means of resolving specific problems (see for instance [16]), notably where one might predict with reasonable certainty a smooth monoextremal relation between biological activity and a known molecular parameter (as is the case with many CNS drugs); the maximum can then be located through the fewest possible steps of synthesis.

References

[1] Topliss, J. G.: J. Med. Chem. **15**, 1006 (1972)
[2] Topliss, J. G.: J. Med. Chem. **20**, 463 (1977)
[3] Topliss, J. G., and Y. C. Martin in E. J. Ariens (Ed.): Drug Design, Vol. V, Academic Press, New York, 1975, p. 1
[4] Hansch, C.: Cancer Chemotherapy Reports Part **1**, **56**, 433 (1972)
[5] Martin, Y. C., and W. J. Dunn: J. Med. Chem. **16**, 578 (1973)
[6] Cramer, R. D., K. M. Snader, C. R. Willis, L. W. Chakrin, J. Thomas and B. M. Sutton: J. Med. Chem. **22**, 714 (1979)
[7] Darvas, F.: J. Med. Chem. **17**, 799 (1974)
[8] Gilliom, R. D., W. P. Purcell and R. T. Bosin: Eur. J. Med. Chem. **12**, 187 (1977)
[9] Seydel, J. K., and K.-J. Schaper: Chemische Struktur und biologische Aktivität, Verlag Chemie, Weinheim, 1979
[10] Spendley, W., G. R. Hext and R. F. Himsworth: Technometrics **4**, 441 (1962)
[11] Darvas, F.: private communication
[12] Wilde, D. J.: Optimum Seeking Methods, Prentice-Hall, Englewood Cliffs, 1964
[13] Santora, N. J., and K. Auyang: J. Med. Chem. **18**, 959 (1975)
[14] Bustard, T. M.: J. Med. Chem. **17**, 777 (1974)
[15] Deming, S. N.: J. Med. Chem. **19**, 977 (1976)
[16] Zeelen, F. J., in R. Franke and P. Oehme (Eds.): Quantitative Structure-Activity Analysis. Akademie-Verlag, Berlin, 1978, p. 333

11. Procedures with Structural Parameters

There are many cases where the conditions for a meaningful application of extrathermodynamic parameters are not fulfilled or where the structural variations of the compounds to be considered are such that reliable parameters of this type are simply not available.

One possible way to deal with such situations is to use parameters derived directly from two-dimensional chemical structures as molecular descriptors; such descriptors will be called "*structural parameters*". The structures to be considered are broken down into fragments and the structural parameters then indicate the occurrence of these fragments (e.g., occurrence number) in these structures. Fragmentation and description of molecules in structural terms can be performed in many different ways, and different approaches can be used to relate structural parameters to biological activity. In the most simple case it is assumed that substituents at certain positions (fragments) make additive and constitutive contributions to biological activity which can be expressed in terms of a linear model called the FREE-WILSON model (11.1.). Essentially the same assumption is also made in the extrathermodynamic approach, and as will be shown in 11.1.3., FREE-WILSON and HANSCH analysis are, in fact, equivalent. Like HANSCH analysis, FREE-WILSON analysis can be applied to homologous series where only substituents are varied in a constant parent molecule. The selection of these substituents, however, must not meet all of the requirements of the extrathermodynamic approach. In particular, series where only a few substituents are varied in many positions can be analysed by the FREE-WILSON method, which is not possible with the HANSCH approach, and substituents constants are, of course, not needed.

When structural variations in a set of compounds become more diverse the simple assumptions of the FREE-WILSON model will no longer hold and it will usually not be possible either to define a parent molecule or to assign to molecular fragments additive increments of biological potency. With the ever increasing amount of data from large screening programs stored in large data bases this is not an unusual situation. In order still to be able to extract the information about relations between structure and activity inherent in such data, cruder approaches are then necessary. The molecules are completely broken down into fragments of, for example, atoms, atoms and their surroundings, groups of atoms (e.g., functional groups), etc., and attempts are then made to find patterns of fragments related to biological potency. This is mostly done on the basis of a classification (see 9.2.) and the patterns searched for are then found either in the form of a classificator separating the classes or as an ensemble of features typical of one particular class. The objective of such investigations is the classification of unknown compounds to guide synthesis and to increase the chance of finding active compounds in a screening program and/or to find such features which are typical and important for the production of the bilogical effect under investigation. The first aim is concerned with lead optimization whereas the second one tends to be directed towards lead generation via the evaluation of pharmacophoric groups. This division, however, is somewhat artificial and both purposes are actually two sides of the same coin; which is more prominent depends on the method applied. Since the features used in these methods consist of substructures, these methods will be discussed together under the heading "substructural approaches" in 11.2.

11.1. Free-Wilson Model

11.1.1. Basic Principles

Introduced by FREE and WILSON in 1964 [1], this procedure is based on a simple increment rule; for summaries and reviews, see [2—9]. The basic assumption is that within a homologous series of drugs *individual segments of molecules make additive and constant contributions to biological activity.* If such contributions are known, biological activity can be estimated by simple addition for all compounds obtainable by any new combination of the segments involved. In general, two kinds of segments are considered (see Fig. 11.1); a *constant segment,* which is identical to a parent structure shared by all compounds of the series, and *variable segments,* by which are understood the *substituents at the individual substitution sites.* As biological activity is affected in different manners by substituents at the various positions of substitution it follows that variable segments must be regarded as a conceptual entity of a given substituent at a fixed substitution site.

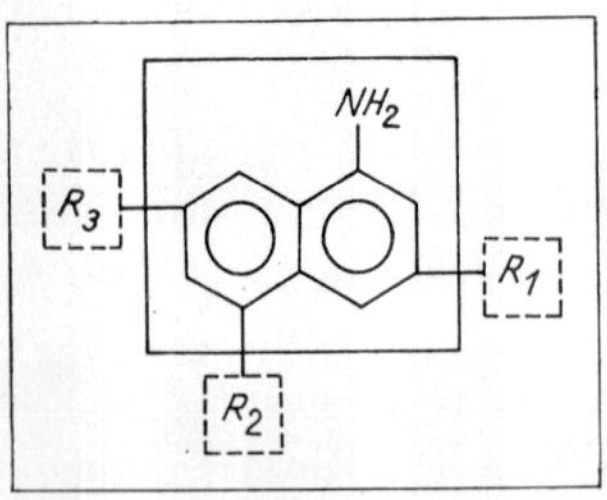

Fig. 11.1. Segments in FREE-WILSON analysis

By numbering all substitution sites and all substituents that may occur at each of them, it is possible to devise a uniform code for each variable segment on the basis of a usually two-digit number, *jk*, in which the first, *j*, identifies the substitution site and the second, *k*, the substituent. This allows the structure of any compound of the series to be described very simply by means of a vector of *structural parameters,* b_{ijk}, which have the form of a logical quantity and are assigned either a value of 0 or 1. The structural parameter b_{ijk} indicates whether in the *i*-th compound of the series the variable segment, *jk*, i.e., the *k*-th substituent at the *j*-th position, is present ($b_{ijk} = 1$) or absent ($b_{ijk} = 0$). When the contributions of the parent structure and of the variable segments to activity are designated, respectively, by μ and z_{jk} (it is often convenient to speak only of substituent contributions), it follows from the basic precept of the FREE-WILSON model that biological activity of a given compound in a series can be expressed as the sum obtained from μ and the sum of the z_{jk} for the variable segments occurring in that compound. The latter sum is equivalent to the scalar product of the vector of the structural parameters with the vector of the z_{jk} so that

$$\log A_i = \mu + \boldsymbol{b}_{ijk}^T \cdot \boldsymbol{z}_{jk} \tag{11/1}$$

where A_i = the biological activity of the i-th compound.

When the molecules of the series have p substitution sites ($j = 1, \ldots, p$) and m_j substituents may be present at the j-th substitution site ($k = 1, \ldots, m_j$), it then follows that:

$$\log A_i = \mu + \sum_{jk} b_{ijk} z_{jk} = \mu + \sum_{j=1}^{p} \sum_{k=1}^{m_j} b_{ijk} z_{jk} \tag{11/2}$$

The number of compounds obtainable from all possible combinations of the variable segments is (symmetries ignored)

$$N = \prod_{j=1}^{p} m_j \tag{11/3}$$

and the total number of all segments (including the parent structure) and, hence, of the contributions to activity to be calculated equals:

$$G = 1 + \sum_{j=1}^{p} m_j \tag{11/4}$$

Relation (11/2) constitutes a system of linear equations easily resolvable for μ and the z_{jk} through regression analysis, the number of unknowns being equal to G. To have enough degrees of freedom, one needs not fewer than about $G + 5$ equations, i.e., the test results of a sample of $n \geqq G + 5$ compounds should be available. On statistical grounds, it is desirable that the sample should be composed on a well-balanced test plan (see 11.1.4.) and that each variable segment should occur more than once.

When μ and the z_{jk} have been established, the biological activity of the remaining $N - n$ compounds can be estimated with the aid of eqn. (11/2). A comparison of (11/3) and (11/4) shows that in general $G \ll N$ so that $(N - n) \gg n$ makes the procedure very rewarding on a vast majority of cases.

The unequivocal resolvability of equation system (11/2) implies that no linear dependencies occur among the structural parameters. Such dependencies are, however, unavoidable because for each substitution site

$$\sum_{i=1}^{n} \sum_{k=1}^{m_j} b_{ijk} = n \tag{11/5}$$

(n = number of compounds in the sample = number of equations in the equation system). There are various ways of eliminating this kind of linear dependency (see e.g. [9]).

In the original procedure introduced by Free and Wilson additional restrictive equations, so-called *symmetry conditions*, are formulated so that for each position the sum of activity contributions for all substituents of the sample occurring in this position is equal to 0:

$$\sum_{i=1}^{n} \sum_{k=1}^{m_j} b_{ijk} z_{jk} = 0 \tag{11/6}$$

This implies that the activity contribution μ of the parent structure is fixed as the total mean value of all $\log A_i$:

$$\mu = \frac{1}{n} \sum_{i=1}^{n} \log A_i \tag{11/7}$$

The parent structure is to be viewed as the basic skeleton common to all compounds stripped of substituents in the variable positions (see Fig. 11.1).

Another possibility is to define the common parent structure as the non-substituted compound with hydrogen in all positions to be varied. Hydrogen is taken as a reference substituent and its contribution to activity *is equated to 0 in all positions* (instead of hydrogen, another reference substituent may, in principle, be chosen). This definition not only makes sense chemically since now μ corresponds to $\log A$ of the non-substituted compound[1]) but also provides another possibility to eliminate linear dependencies between the structural parameters. They disappear since setting $z_{j,H} = 0$ has the consequence of removing for each varied position of substitution a column from the structure matrix (see 11.1.2.). Introduced by Fujita and Ban [10], the procedure allows the calculation of the activity contributions relative to that of hydrogen.

The relation between the original solution of the Free-Wilson model (index FW) using symmetry conditions in accord with (11/6) and the results obtained with the Fujita-Ban variant (Index FB) emerges from eqns. (11/8) and (11/9)

$$[\mu]_{FB} = [\mu]_{FW} + \sum_{j=1}^{p} [z_{jH}]_{FW} \tag{11/8}$$

$$[z_{jk}]_{FB} = [z_{jk}]_{FW} - [z_{jH}]_{FW} \tag{11/9}$$

(z_{jH} = activity contribution of hydrogen in position j).

The two solutions are equivalent and can be obtained from each other through a simple linear transformation. In both cases eqn. (11/2) is valid. The following discussion chiefly refers to the original model as introduced by Free and Wilson, μ and z_{jk} being used again without indices. Solutions according to the Fujita-Ban variant will, as above, be indicated by index FB.

Another kind of linear dependence between structural parameters arises where variable segments, i.e., two given substituents in two given positions, always occur together. In such a case, the activity contributions of the two segments cannot be separated, and the system of equations described by (11/2) has no unique solution. This kind of linear dependence can be recognized simply on visual examination of the structure matrix (see 11.2.) if it had not been deliberately avoided at the time of designing the test plan. It occurs whenever the structure matrix contains two identical columns, and can be eliminated by deleting the data for those compounds which make up these columns (see [4] and [12]). Another possibility is to combine the corresponding segments to one pseudosegment and to calculate its activity contribution.

In summary, the entire Free-Wilson model (eqn. (11/2)) can be interpreted as follows. From the biological activities of the compounds forming a training series, the

---

1) Needless to say that the *estimate from the sample* is meant here. Cammarata and Yau [11] introduced the experimental value of the unsubstituted parent structure in the computations which does not take into account that this value (as all others) has an experimental error.

biological effects of individual structural elements (segments) are assessed by calculating and assigning activity contributions z_{jk} and μ on such lines that the gradation of the activity contributions quantifies the influences of the segments on biological activity.

Purcell and Clayton [13] as well as Ban and Fujita [14] have discussed the question whether, as in the work of Free and Wilson [1], the biological activity should be introduced in a linear or rather in a logarithmic manner. As the extrathermodynamic approach has shown that log A can be treated as a free enthalpy-related quantity, the logarithmic scale is basically to be preferred. It has, furthermore, the advantage that the resultant activity contributions may be treated as *biological de novo substituent constants* in extrathermodynamic terms, thus making it possible to compare these contributions with other substituent constants (e.g., π, σ, E_S; see 11.1.3.). From a purely statistical point of view, however, a decision is difficult to make. The logarithmic approach ensures a better fit but when antilogarithms are taken and the correlation coefficients between them and measured activity data A_i is determined, this correlation coefficient is, on the whole, poorer than that for the linear approach. Yet this outcome is in no way an argument for the application of the linear approach, because the fit provided by the criterion of least squares is only optimal in the applied scale. The relative sequence of z_{jk} is, however, not altered by the transformation of one scale into another [5] so that, for the reasons mentioned above, the logarithmic approach is usually employed.

The basic precept of the Free-Wilson model with respect to the additivity and stability of the z_{jk} implies that there are *no specific kinds of intramolecular interactions between the variable structure elements.* This requirement is, however, not met under all circumstances. If, for example, there are two adjacent positions 1 and 2, in which *inter alia* the two substituents OH and COOH may occur, the basic idea of the Free-Wilson model is only valid as long as the structural variants (1, COOH) and (2, OH) or (1, OH) and (2, COOH) do not appear together. As soon as OH and COOH are located in adjacent positions, a hydrogen bond is formed and this intramolecular interaction negates the constancy of the activity contributions from the two variable segments and, as a consequence, additivity is, of course, lost. The best way to avoid this problem may be to consider the two interacting substituents together as a fictitious variable segment, i.e., as one pseudosubstituent in a pseudoposition and to describe the presence or absence of this fictitious segment in terms of an additional structural parameter [6, 10, 15]. The activity contribution of this kind of segment contains those of the two substituents as well as a part resulting from their interaction.

It is also possible to account for such intramolecular interactions by means of cross-products [16—19]. Boček et al. [16—17], for example, designed the following model for disubstituted benzenes:

$$\log A_i = b_1 + b_2 + e_1 e_2 \qquad (11/10)$$

Each of the two variable segments (substituents in positions 1 and 2) has its own independent activity contribution, b_1 and b_2, as well as one which is dependent on the nature of its counterpart denoted by e_1 and e_2. For practical purposes, however, a procedure involving cross-products is not very satisfactory because the terms e_i, which are to be determined in addition to the b_i, strongly reduce the number of degrees of freedom.

11.1.2. Practical Procedure

A fictitious example (derived in a somewhat modified form from [2]) is used as an illustration. Suppose that the series shown in Fig. 11.1 is to be examined and that the substituents listed in Table 11.1 occur in positions 1—3. According to eqn. (11/3) the number of possible compounds is

$$N = \prod_{j=1}^{p} m_j = 4 \cdot 4 \cdot 4 = 64 \tag{11/11}$$

in which according to (11/4)

$$G = 1 + \sum_{j=1}^{3} m_j = 1 + 4 + 4 + 4 = 13 \tag{11/12}$$

Table 11.1. Substituents and segment codes for the fictitious example (see Fig. 11.1)

Substituent	Substituent number k	Code jk of variable segments
Position 1 (R_1)		
H	1	11
F	2	12
Cl	3	13
Br	4	14
Position 2 (R_2)		
H	1	21
NO_2	2	22
CN	3	23
$COCH_3$	4	24
Position 3 (R_3)		
H	1	31
CH_3	2	32
C_2H_5	3	33
OCH_3	4	34

segment variants in all may occur. Let us assume, furthermore, that for a series of $n = 18$ compounds biological activities are available from biological testing. The objective then is to calculate the thirteen activity contributions with the aid of this sample in order that for the remaining $N - n = 48$ compounds biological activities can be predicted.

As the first step, one draws up the so-called *structure matrix* by arranging line by line the compounds of the sample concerned and listing the structural parameters b_{ijk} and log A values in the columns (see Table 11.2). For each compound, the structure is unambiguously embodied in the structure matrix by means of the structural parameters b_{ijk}. Thus, in the case of the sixth compound ($i = 6$) in Table 11.2 the structural parameters b_{612}, b_{623} and b_{632} are equal to 1 and all others, b_{6jk}, are equal to 0. It follows immediately that this compound contains the segment variants 12, 23 and 32, i.e., sub-

Table 11.2. Structure matrix

Number of compound	Position	R_1				R_2				R_3				log A
	Substituent	H	F	Cl	Br	H	NO_2	CN	$COCH_3$	H	CH_3	C_2H_5	OCH_3	
	Segment code jk	11	12	13	14	21	22	23	24	31	32	33	34	
1	structural	1	0	0	0	1	0	0	0	1	0	0	0	3.095
2	parameter b_{ijk}	1	0	0	0	1	0	0	0	0	1	0	0	2.763
3		1	0	0	0	0	1	0	0	0	0	1	0	4.556
4		1	0	0	0	0	1	0	0	0	0	0	1	5.405
5		0	1	0	0	0	0	1	0	1	0	0	0	5.921
6		0	1	0	0	0	0	1	0	0	1	0	0	5.625
7		0	1	0	0	0	0	0	1	0	0	1	0	4.931
8		0	1	0	0	0	0	0	1	0	0	0	1	5.701
9		0	0	1	0	1	0	0	0	1	0	0	0	3.852
10		0	0	1	0	1	0	0	0	0	1	0	0	3.960
11		0	0	1	0	0	1	0	0	0	0	1	0	5.332
12		0	0	1	0	0	1	0	0	0	0	0	1	6.132
13		0	0	0	1	0	0	1	0	1	0	0	0	5.701
14		0	0	0	1	0	0	1	0	0	1	0	0	5.409
15		0	0	0	1	0	0	0	1	0	0	1	0	4.609
16		0	0	0	1	0	0	0	1	0	0	0	1	5.631
17		1	0	0	0	0	0	1	0	0	0	0	1	4.793
18		0	0	1	0	0	1	0	0	1	0	0	0	5.121

stituent F in R_1, substituent CN in R_2 and substituent CH_3 in R_3. In practice, the zeros are left out and only the ones enter into the structure matrix.

Applied to the lines of the structure matrix, eqn. (11/2) automatically affords the linear equation system (11/13):

$$\begin{aligned}
\log A_1 &= \mu + z_{11} + z_{21} + z_{31} = 3.095 \\
\log A_2 &= \mu + z_{11} + z_{21} + z_{32} = 2.763 \\
\log A_3 &= \mu + z_{11} + z_{22} + z_{33} = 4.556 \\
\log A_4 &= \mu + z_{11} + z_{22} + z_{34} = 5.405 \\
\log A_5 &= \mu + z_{12} + z_{23} + z_{31} = 5.921 \\
\log A_6 &= \mu + z_{12} + z_{23} + z_{32} = 5.625 \\
\log A_7 &= \mu + z_{12} + z_{24} + z_{33} = 4.931 \\
\log A_8 &= \mu + z_{12} + z_{24} + z_{34} = 5.701 \\
\log A_9 &= \mu + z_{13} + z_{21} + z_{31} = 3.852 \\
\log A_{10} &= \mu + z_{13} + z_{21} + z_{32} = 3.960 \\
\log A_{11} &= \mu + z_{13} + z_{22} + z_{33} = 5.332 \\
\log A_{12} &= \mu + z_{13} + z_{22} + z_{34} = 6.132 \\
\log A_{13} &= \mu + z_{14} + z_{23} + z_{31} = 5.701 \\
\log A_{14} &= \mu + z_{14} + z_{23} + z_{32} = 5.409 \\
\log A_{15} &= \mu + z_{14} + z_{24} + z_{33} = 4.609 \\
\log A_{16} &= \mu + z_{14} + z_{24} + z_{34} = 5.631 \\
\log A_{17} &= \mu + z_{11} + z_{23} + z_{34} = 4.793 \\
\log A_{18} &= \mu + z_{13} + z_{22} + z_{31} = 5.121
\end{aligned} \tag{11/13}$$

The symmetry conditions derived from (11/6) are:

$$\begin{aligned}
5z_{11} + 4z_{12} + 5z_{13} + 4z_{14} &= 0 \\
4z_{21} + 5z_{22} + 5z_{23} + 4z_{24} &= 0 \\
5z_{31} + 4z_{32} + 4z_{33} + 5z_{34} &= 0
\end{aligned} \tag{11/14}$$

The two equation systems are combined and subjected to regression analysis. An alternative is to select one of the z_{jk} at each position as a "dependent variable" and to express it as a function of the other z_{jk}. If, for example, z_{11}, z_{21} and z_{31} are so selected eqn. (11/14) can be solved to give:

$$z_{11} = -\frac{4}{5} z_{12} - z_{13} - \frac{4}{5} z_{14}$$

$$z_{12} = -\frac{4}{5} z_{22} - \frac{4}{5} z_{23} - z_{24} \qquad (11/15)$$

$$z_{31} = -\frac{4}{5} z_{32} - \frac{4}{5} z_{33} - z_{34}$$

Expressions (11/15) can then be substituted for z_{11}, z_{21} and z_{31} in the equation system (11/13). Any discrepancies between the two kinds of approach as reported by [2] and [4] disappear when by directly combining (11/13) and (11/14) the symmetry conditions are incorporated with high weighting factors [6]. On the whole, this variant is to be preferred to the procedure based on (11/15) because it is simpler and the symmetry conditions can be computed automatically after entering the structure matrix.

Regression analysis is then applied for the determination of μ, the z_{jk} values and statistical data (see p. 166 and 15.). If the solution proves significant in the F-test, it may be accepted and the Free-Wilson model may be viewed as valid. It should be noted, however, that low values of the correlation coefficient suggest caution. In such cases, a closer inspection of outliers (compounds with large differences between log A values calculated from (11/2) and experimental values) is indicated. If a rationale can be found for the deviating behaviour of such outliers it may be possible to repeat the analysis in a modified way. Thus, outliers may arise, for example, from not anticipated intramolecular interactions which can be accounted for as discussed in 11.1.1. A few compounds may also be left out from the analysis; the number of such compounds, however, must always be kept very small as compared with the size of the training series.

Results for the example discussed here are presented in Tables 11.3 and 11.4 [2]. The statistical data are extremely good, providing an excellent fit at a very high level of significance and 99.94% of the variance of the biological data being "explained" by the activity contributions. Accordingly, the differences between calculated and observed log A values are very small, and outliers are not present.

It is helpful to calculate, in addition to the data presented here, the confidence intervals of the activity contributions as well as the level of significance at which these

Table 11.3. Activity contributions and statistical data for the example presented in Table 11.2 (from [2])

$z_{11} = -1.121$	$z_{21} = -0.435$	$z_{31} = -0.253$
$z_{12} = 1.032$	$z_{22} = 0.860$	$z_{32} = -0.581$
$z_{13} = -0.382$	$z_{23} = 0.246$	$z_{33} = -0.068$
$z_{14} = 0.846$	$z_{24} = -0.948$	$z_{34} = 0.772$

$\mu = 4.895$
$r^2 = 0.9994$
$r = 0.9996$
$F = 1181.6$
$p < 0.001$

Table 11.4. Observed (index o) and from the activity contributions calculated (eqn. (11/2); index c) values of log A

i	$\log A_o$	$\log A_c$	$(\log A_o - \log A_c)$
1	3.095	3.086	0.009
2	2.763	2.759	0.004
3	4.556	4.566	−0.010
4	5.405	5.407	−0.002
5	5.921	5.921	0.000
6	5.625	5.593	0.032
7	4.931	4.912	0.019
8	5.701	5.752	−0.051
9	3.852	3.826	0.026
10	3.460	3.498	−0.038
11	5.332	5.305	0.027
12	6.132	6.146	−0.014
13	5.701	5.735	−0.034
14	5.409	5.407	0.002
15	4.690	4.725	−0.035
16	5.631	5.565	0.066
17	4.793	4.793	0.000
18	5.121	5.121	0.000

contributions are different from 0. The most favourable substituents (highest z_{jk} values) are F in R_1, NO_2 in R_2 and OCH_3 in R_3. The range, D_j, of the z_{jk} values for the j-th substitution site provides information about the sensitivity of biological activity to the variation of substituents in that position. For the present example, the ranges are:

$$D_1 = z_{12} - z_{11} = 1.032 + 1.121 = 2.153$$

$$D_2 = z_{22} - z_{24} = 0.860 + 0.948 = 1.808 \qquad (11/16)$$

$$D_3 = z_{34} - z_{32} = 0.772 + 0.581 + 1.353$$

It appears that as regards sensitivity there are no large differences among the three positions R_1, R_2 and R_3, although a $1 > 2 > 3$ order does become noticeable with R_3 differing somewhat from R_1 and from R_2.

The activities of the 46 remaining compounds in the series can be estimated on the basis of eqn. (11/2) from μ and the z_{jk} values. In general, however, only those compounds are of interest which are the most active or, if the action concerned is undesired, are the least active. A few such compounds, together with calculated log A values, are shown in the structure matrix of Table 11.5. Compound 19 is the most active one that can be obtained by a novel combination of segments because it contains the segments (substituents) with the largest activity contributions. The most active compound within the training series is No. 12 with $\log A = 6.132$ so that compound 19, with a 10 times higher activity, would display improved potency. Similarly, compounds 20 and 21 are also obviously more active than 12; hence, these three compounds may be proposed for further development when a high activity is desired. If, however, activity

Table 11.5. Structure matrix and calculated log A values for some compounds of high or low biological activity

i	R_1				R_2				R_3				log A
	11	12	13	14	21	22	23	24	31	32	33	34	
19		1				1						1	7.559
20		1					1					1	6.945
21				1		1						1	7.373
22	1							1		1			2.245
23	1							1	1				2.573
24			1					1		1			3.417

is to be minimized (undesired effect), compounds 22 and 23 are suitable candidates, their activity being less than the lowest value (compound 2) within the training series.

If it were certain that compound 19 (where maximal activity is aimed at) or compound 22 (where minimal activity is aimed at) offers the most favourable variants not only with respect to biological activity but also to synthetic feasibility, only these compounds would have to be developed further. There would be no need to explore additional analogs. In practice, such a certainty rarely exists so that usually more than one compound must be considered for further investigation. When $N - n$ is large, it would be undesirable to compute the activities of all compounds not yet tested and to make a choice of the best candidates only afterwards. It is much more effective to select these compounds automatically by means of an appropriate sub-routine incorporated into the computer program for Free-Wilson analysis. In our program [6] such a subroutine called "prediction" finds all compounds whose estimated log A values fall into the range:

$$x \cdot \log A_{max} \leqq \log A_i \leqq \log A_{max} \tag{11/17}$$

Here A_{max} is the maximum to be attained within the series after combination of segments with the largest activity contributions (in the example under discussion it is equal to 7.559 for compound 19) and $x \leqq 1$ is a factor that can be freely chosen. The compounds are arranged according to descending log A values, and it is also indicated for each compound whether log A is significantly different from log A_{max} at a preset level of statistical significance.

Precalculations must be carried out carefully as any new segment combination may imply changes in the mechanism of biological action or intramolecular interactions. In either case, the basic assumption of the Free-Wilson model would be interfered with, as would predictive power. As with all QSAR methods one should, therefore, be aware of the possibility of occasionally false predictions, although correct application of the procedure will help to minimize problems.

11.1.3. Relations between the Free-Wilson Model and the Extrathermodynamic Approach

The extrathermodynamic approach (Hansch analysis) and the Free-Wilson model are *formally equivalent* [3, 7, 10, 11, 20, 21, 22]. In both instances, the logarithm of biological activity is built up additively on the basis of a linear model from contributions of the substituents which are the z_{jk} in the case of the FREE-WILSON analysis and weighted combinations of molecular parameters in the case of HANSCH analysis. As a consequence of this equivalence there exist systematic relations in an extrathermodynamic sense between the activity contributions z_{jk} and substituent constants (hydrophobic, electronic and steric) so that the z_{jk} can be quantitatively described as functions of the appropriate parameters x_h, x_e and x_s in the same manner as log A. Such relations have, indeed, often been dealt with in the literature [3, 11, 14, 23].

In the FUJITA-BAN variant [10] of the FREE-WILSON model there is not only a formal but also a *numerical equivalence* [7] so that activity contributions $[z_{jk}]_{FB}$ can be estimated directly from the corresponding HANSCH equations[1]) whose intercept than corresponds to the activity contribution $[\mu]_{FB}$. This may be illustrated by an example from the literature [7]. Regression analysis affords inter alia the following relationship for the adrenolytic activity of ring-substituted N,N-dimethyl-2-bromophenethylamines (for substituents, see Table 11.6):

$$\log A = 0.83\pi_{meta} - 0.92\sigma^+_{meta} + 1.33\pi_{para} - 1.89\sigma^+_{para} + 7.80 \qquad (11/18)$$

$$n = 22 \qquad r = 0.966 \qquad s = 0.164$$

This equation leads to the following expressions for the FUJITA-BAN activity contributions $[z_{jk}]_{FB}$:

1. substituents in meta-position

$$[z_{meta,k}]_{FB} = 0.83\pi_{meta} - 0.92\sigma^+_{meta} \qquad (11/19)$$

2. substituents in para-position

$$[z_{para,k}]_{FB} = 1.33\pi_{para} - 1.89\sigma^+_{para} \qquad (11/20)$$

Calculated by means of (11/19) and (11/20), the respective $[z_{jk}]_{FB}$ values are in excellent agreement with those obtained by directly applying FUJITA-BAN analysis to the same data, as indicated in Table 11.6. The same is true for the intercept of (11/18) which is a very good estimate of $[\mu]_{FB}$ ($[\mu]_{FB} = 7.82$).

The equivalence between the FREE-WILSON or the FUJITA-BAN and the HANSCH model can no longer be expected for such series where the HANSCH equation contains a quadratic x_h term [18]. Consider, for example, a series in which substituents at two positions R_1 and R_2 are varied and where log A and π are interrelated according to

$$\log = a_0 + a_1(\pi_1 + \pi_2)^2 + a_2(\pi_1 + \pi_2) \qquad (11/21)$$

or

$$\log A = a_0 + a_1\pi_1^2 + 2a_1\pi_1\pi_2 + a_1\pi_2^2 + a_2(\pi_1 + \pi_2) \qquad (11/22)$$

It is because of the cross-product term that contributions of the substituents in R_1 and R_2 can no longer be separated and thus are neither independent nor constant so

---

[1]) Preconceived is that the substituent constants operating in the regression equation, just as the $[z_{jH}]_{FB}$, all have the value of 0 for substituent H. For E_S and σ^*, for example, this condition is not fulfilled, and in such cases a proper transformation is necessary by subtraction of the value of hydrogen.

that the basic assumptions of the FREE-WILSON model are not fulfilled. There may be cases, however, where the data used all lie on one wing of the parabola or where even the quadratic π contribution may additively be distributed over the positions of substitution (which would be incidental). In such cases the FREE-WILSON model would still hold so that the presence of a quadratic term in a HANSCH equation does not necessarily or always imply that the FREE-WILSON model will not also give equally good data description and predictions [24]. As a rule, however, the FREE-WILSON model will not be applicable here. The modified model according to BOČEK and KOPECKY [16, 17] (see eqn. (11/10)) can be used here which is numerically equivalent to a HANSCH equation according to (11/22) if, according to the FUJITA-BAN approach, the activity contribution of hydrogen as standard substituent is set equal to zero [7, 18].

Table 11.6. Comparison of activity contributions $[z_{jk}]_{FB}$ obtained from a FUJITA-BAN analysis and calculated from eqns. (11/19) and (11/20) for ring-substituents in adrenolytic N,N-dimethyl-2-bromophenethylamines (modified from [7])

Substituent	$[z_{jk}]_{FB}$	
	FUJITA-BAN analysis	Calculated from (11/19) and (11/20)
m-H	0.00	0.00
m-F	−0.30	−0.21
m-Cl	0.21	0.26
m-Br	0.43	0.40
m-J	0.58	0.62
m-CH_3	0.45	0.49
p-H	0.00	0.00
p-F	0.34	0.33
p-Cl	0.77	0.72
p-Br	1.02	1.07
p-J	1.43	1.41
p-CH_3	1.26	1.28

This can be illustrated by the following example [7]. For the hypnotic activity of N,N-diacylureas the regression equation is

$$\log A = -0.044n^2 + 0.760n - 0.862 \qquad (11/23)$$

$$n = 13 \qquad r = 0.918 \qquad s = 0.079$$

where n = total number of C atoms in the two acyl rests. When instead of the total number of C atoms the numbers of C atoms in the two different acyl rests R_1 and R_2 are used, it follows from (11/23):

$$\log A = -0.044(n_1^2 + n_2^2) + 0.760(n_1 + n_2) - 0.088n_1n_2 - 0.862 \quad (11/24)$$

Formally, (11/24) corresponds to (11/10) with $b_1 = -0.044n_1^2 + 0.760n_1$, $b_2 = -0.044n_2^2 + 0.760n_2$ and $e_1e_2 = -0.088n_1n_2$. Thus, the $[z_{jk}]_{FB}$ values can be calculated from (11/24) and compared with the results of a FREE-WILSON analysis in the variant of BOČEK and

KOPECKY. As shown in Table 11.7, there is again good agreement between the two sets of values.

The numerical equivalence of the FREE-WILSON model in the variants of FUJITA and BAN and of BOČEK and KOPECKY to the extrathermodynamic approach makes it possible to use the FREE-WILSON model and the HANSCH model in combination [8]. There are cases where this can be extremely helpful. If, for example, a quadratic relationship between log A and x_h is expected so that the simple FREE-WILSON model may fail, the following approach can also be applied instead of the BOČEK-KOPECKY formalism:

$$\log A_i = \left(\sum_{j=1}^{p} \sum_{k=1}^{m_j} b_{ijk}\pi_{jk}\right)^2 + [\mu]_{FB} + \sum_{j=1}^{p} \sum_{k=1}^{m_j} b_{ijk}[z_{jk}]_{FB} \qquad (11/25)$$

The square term corresponds to the $(\pi_1 + \pi_2)^2$ term in eqn. (11/21). Thus, this term contains quadratic hydrophobic terms as well as terms corresponding to the cross-product $\pi_1\pi_2$ in eqn. (11/22) or, in other words, to the interaction terms of the BOČEK-KOPECKY model. The linear π terms $\left(a_2(\pi_1 + \pi_2)\right)$ in eqns. (11/21) and (11/22)) are incorporated into the $[z_{jk}]_{FB}$. In this way, the interaction contribution which could prevent the application of the FREE-WILSON model is treated separately in the HANSCH-type part of eqn. (11/25).

Table 11.7. Comparison of activity contributions $[z_{jk}]_{FB}$ obtained from a BOČEK-KOPECKY analysis and calculated from eqn. (11/24) for acyl-substituents in hypnotic N,N'-diacylureas (from [7]). The acetyl group serves here as reference substituent whose activity contribution was set equal to zero¹)

Substituent	$[z_{jk}]_{FB}$	
	BOČEK-KOPECKY analysis	Calculated from (11/24)¹)
CH_3CO	0.00	0.00
CH_3CH_2CO	0.43	0.54
$CH_3(CH_2)_2CO$	0.91	0.99
$CH_3(CH_2)_3CO$	1.25	1.36
$CH_3(CH_2)_4CO$	1.49	1.63
$CH_3(CH_2)_5CO$	1.81	1.82
cross-product	$-0.085\ n_1n_2$	$-0.088\ n_1n_2$

¹) Since H does not occur as substituent in the present case, eqn. (11/24) transforms into: $[z_{jk}]_{FB} = -0.044n_{jk}^2 + 0.760n_{jk} - 1.344$.

For the extrathermodynamic approach to be effective in multisubstituted compounds, sufficient substituents in all positions are necessary. This is particularly true where position dependence can occur. It is, however, quite conceivable that this requirement is merely satisfied as far as some positions are concerned. In the case that substituents in positions q ($q = 1, \ldots, r$) are adequately varied whilst there are only few substituents in positions j ($j = 1, \ldots, p$), the following approach is useful:

$$\log A_i = \sum_{q=1}^{r} [f_{h,q}(x_{h,i}) + f_{e,q}(x_{e,i}) + f_{s,q}(x_{s,i})] + \sum_{j=1}^{p} \sum_{k=1}^{m_j} b_{ijk}[z_{jk}]_{FB} + \text{constant} \qquad (11/26)$$

For the functions $f_h(x_h)$, $f_e(x_e)$ and $f_s(x_s)$, the usual expressions explained in the preceding chapters can be used, the intercept in (11/26) being made up by the extrathermodynamic part of (11/26) and by $[\mu]_{FB}$. Equation (11/26) includes (11/25) as a special case. Regression equations with indicator variables (see eqn. (8/7)) to characterize the occurrence of certain structural features are likewise to be regarded as particular cases of (11/26). A simple example is that given by Kubinyi [8], who obtained the following relationship for the antibacterial activity of benzylammonium compounds substituted in the phenyl ring (R_1) and on the nitrogen atom (R_2):

$$\log A_i = -0.18(\pi_1 + \pi_2)_i^2 + 1.29\pi_{2,i} + \left[\sum_{j=1}^{p} \sum_{k=1}^{m_j} b_{jik}[z_{jk}]_{FB}\right]_{R_1} + 1.709$$

$$n = 44 \qquad r = 0.916 \qquad s = 0.281 \qquad (11/27)$$

Table 11.8. Activity contributions $[z_{jk}]_{FB}$ for aromatic substituents (eqn. (11/27)) in antibacterial benzylammonium compounds (from [8])

Substituent	$[z_{jk}]_{FB}$
2-H	0
3-H	0
4-H	0
2-Cl	0.760
4-Cl	1.004
4-NO_2	0.449
3-Cl	0.995
3,4-$(OCH_3)_2$	−0.010
3,4-OCH_2O-	0.123

The activity contributions in (11/27) refer to the substituents in the phenyl ring; their values are shown in Table 11.8. As indices in this chapter are somewhat different from those in the chapters on the extrathermodynamic approach, it may be helpful for a better understanding to re-write eqn. (11/27) in the way Hansch equations are usually presented:

$$\log A = -0.18(\pi_1 + \pi_2)^2 + 1.29\pi_2 + 0.760 I_1 + 1.004 I_2 + 0.449 I_3 + 0.995 I_4 - 0.010 I_5 + 0.123 I_6 + 1.709 \qquad (11/28)$$

$$n = 44 \qquad r = 0.916 \qquad s = 0.291$$

The coefficients of the indicator variables I_1—I_6 are identical to the $[z_{jk}]_{FB}$, and the indicator variables themselves are identical to the structural parameters b_{ijk} (see Table 11.9).

Table 11.9. Definition of indicator variables in eqn. (11/28). They have a value of 1 if substituent k is present in position j (otherwise, 0)

Indicator variable	Substituent k	in position j
I_1	Cl	2
I_2	Cl	4
I_3	NO_2	4
I_4	Cl	3
I_5	$(OCH_3)_2$	3, 4
I_6	-OCH_2O-	3, 4

11.1.4. An Approximation to Solve the Free-Wilson Model

The exact solution of the FREE-WILSON approach requires the use of computers. An approximate solution can, however, very rapidly be obtained with the aid of a simple pocket calculator [25—27].

When applying least squares (see Appendix), the following conditions must be satisfied for the solution of the linear equation system (11/2):

$$\sum_{i=1}^{n}\left[\log A_i - \left(\sum_{j=1}^{p}\sum_{k=1}^{m_j} b_{ijk} z_{jk} + \mu\right)\right]^2 = \text{Min}. \tag{11/29}$$

Differentiation of (11/29) with respect to z_{jk} and equating the first derivative to zero result in:

$$\sum_{j=1}^{p}\sum_{k=1}^{m_j} z_{jk} \sum_{i=1}^{n} b_{ijk} b_{iqr} = \sum_{i=1}^{n} (\log A_i - \mu)\, b_{iqr} \tag{11/30}$$

$$(q = 1, \ldots, p;\ r = 1, \ldots, m_q)$$

To simplify this equation system, the following abbreviations are introduced:

$$n_{jk;qr} = \sum_{i=1}^{n} b_{ijk} b_{iqr} \tag{11/31}$$

$$n_{jk} = n_{jk;jk} = \sum_{i=1}^{n} b_{ijk} \tag{11/32}$$

$$n_{qr} = n_{qr;qr} = \sum_{i=1}^{n} b_{iqr} \tag{11/33}$$

The meaning of these quantities follows from the right-hand sides of the corresponding relations. The number of compounds in which the two variable segments jk (k-th substituent in the j-th position) and qr (r-th substituent in the q-th position) occur together is expressed as $n_{jk;qr}$, and n_{jk} or n_{qr} denotes the number of compounds containing the variable segments jk or qr, respectively. From eqns. (11/30)—(11/33) and (11/7) it follows that:

$$\sum_{j=1}^{p}\sum_{k=1}^{m_j} z_{jk}(n_{jk;qr} - n_{jk}/n) = \sum_{i=1}^{n} \log A_i b_{iqr} - n_{qr}\mu \tag{11/34}$$

Within the sample, the total number of compounds which contain a given segment jk or q, is in general larger than that of compounds where both segments are present. For that reasonr the coefficients $n_{jk;jk} = n_{jk}$ which occur on the main diagonal of the equation system (11/34) are much larger than any other coefficient. When, with this in mind, only the coefficients of the main diagonal are considered and the expression n_{jk}/n, which is very small for any somewhat larger sample, is neglected, it follows from (11/34)

$$z_{jk} \approx \frac{1}{n_{jk}} \sum_{i=1}^{n} \log A_i b_{ijk} - \mu \approx \mu_{jk} - \mu \tag{11/35}$$

with

$$\mu_{jk} = \frac{1}{n_{jk}} \sum_{i=1}^{n} \log A_i b_{ijk} \tag{11/36}$$

The quantity μ_{jk} is the mean log A value for all those compounds of the sample which contain the variable segment jk. Approximate solutions for activity contributions to be denoted by

z'_{jk} can thus be obtained by use of eqn. (11/35) from:

$$z'_{jk} = \mu_{jk} - \mu \qquad (11/37)$$

At first glance, the assumptions and simplifications made in deriving (11/37) seem to be very crude. This, however, is not the case. As already explained, the size of the training series (n compounds) is in general small as related to the total number N of all possible compounds so that

$$f = \frac{N}{n} \quad \text{with} \quad f \gg 1 \qquad (11/38)$$

is usually much larger than one. The number, N_{jk}, of all conceivable compounds with the variable segment jk is:

$$N_{jk} = N/m_j \qquad (11/39)$$

By analogy, the number of all possible compounds in which the segments jk and qr occur together is:

$$N_{jk;qr} = N/m_j m_q \qquad (11/40)$$

When compounds are selected for the training series according to a well-balanced plan relation (11/41) holds

$$n_{jk;qr} = \begin{cases} N_{jk;qr}/f & \text{for } j \neq q \\ 0 & \text{for } j = q \text{ and } k \neq r \\ N_{jk}/f & \text{for } j = q \text{ and } k = r \end{cases} \qquad (11/41)$$

with

$$n_{jk} = N_{jk}/f = N/f_{mj} \qquad (11/42)$$

From eqns. (11/34), (11/41) and (11/42) it follows that:

$$\sum_{\substack{j=1\\ j \neq q}}^{p} \sum_{k=1}^{m_j} z_{jk}(N_{jk;qr}/f - 1/m_j) + \sum_{\substack{k=1\\ k \neq r}}^{m_q} z_{qk}(0 - 1/m_q)$$
$$+ z_{qr}(N_{qr}/f - 1/m_q) = \sum_{i=1}^{n} \log A_i b_{iqr} - (N_{qr}/f) \qquad (11/43)$$

Equation (11/43) can be transformed into:

$$(N - fm_q)/N \sum_{\substack{j=1\\ j \neq q}}^{p} \left(\sum_{k=1}^{m_j} z_{jk}/m_j \right) - fm_q/N \sum_{k=1}^{m_q} z_{qk}/m_q + z_{qr} = fm_q/N \sum_{i=1}^{n} \log A_i b_{iqr} - \mu \qquad (11/44)$$

The symmetry conditions for the solution of the Free-Wilson approach (eqn. (11/6)) lead to eqn. (11/45):

$$\sum_{k=1}^{m_j} z_{jk}/m_j = 0 \qquad (11/45)$$

It then follows from (11/44) that:

$$z_{qr} = fm_j/N \sum_{i=1}^{n} \log A_i b_{iqr} - \mu \qquad (11/46)$$

With indices qr and jk interchanged (11/36) and (11/39) are applied to eqn. (11/46) to give:

$$z_{jk} = 1/n_{jk} \sum_{i=1}^{n} \log A_i b_{ijk} - \mu = \mu_{kj} - \mu \tag{11/47}$$

On comparison of (11/47) with (11/37), it will be noticed that the approximation (11/37) is identical to the exact solution of the FREE-WILSON model if the substituents within the training series are selected according to a well-balanced plan. There will be closer agreement between approximate and exact solutions as the selection for the sample under discussion is more in line with a selection based on such a test plan, thereby sufficiently satisfying the synthesis chemist's requirement that substituents be properly "mixed". The determination of the z_{jk} values for position 1 of the example dealt with in 11.1.2. is shown here for illustration. From eqn. (11/36):

$$\begin{aligned}
\mu_{11} &= \frac{1}{5}(\log A_1 + \log A_2 + \log A_3 + \log A_4 + \log A_{17}) \\
\mu_{12} &= \frac{1}{4}(\log A_5 + \log A_6 + \log A_7 + \log A_8) \\
\mu_{13} &= \frac{1}{5}(\log A_9 + \log A_{10} + \log A_{11} + \log A_{12} + \log A_{18}) \\
\mu_{14} &= \frac{1}{4}(\log A_{13} + \log A_{14} + \log A_{15} + \log A_{16})
\end{aligned} \tag{11/48}$$

The total mean μ is

$$\mu = \frac{1}{18} \sum_{i=1}^{18} \log A_i = 4.895 \tag{11/49}$$

and for activity contributions it follows from (11/37):

$$\begin{aligned}
z'_{11} &= -0.773 \\
z'_{12} &= 0.649 \\
z'_{13} &= -0.201 \\
z'_{14} &= 0.398
\end{aligned}$$

The z_{1k} and z'_{1k} do not share the same absolute values but agree in sign and relative magnitude.

One may advantageously use this method of approximation for preliminary computations using only a pocket calculator. A disadvantage, however, is that the determined z'_{jk} values are no more than estimates of the real activity contributions and can thus be easily affected by error. Moreover, statistical information is not obtained, and it is no longer possible to formulate subproblems via row selection vectors since the calculations would become too laborious. Yet, as has appeared from several examples, the quality of the estimation is mostly not much below that of the exact FREE-WILSON solution (cf., Table 11.10) and there is much agreement between the z'_{jk} and the z_{jk} values on a relative scale. In addition, the sensitivity of each single position of substitution is properly indicated [26, 27]. Thus, this method affords the most important information and can very easily be applied by the experimentalist. It must be stressed, however, that it is not meant to replace the exact FREE-WILSON analysis and also, that false results will be obtained from training series which are far from being well-balanced.

Table 11.10. Comparison of the correlation coefficient, *r*, for the exact and the approximate Free-Wilson solution for some examples (from [27])

Substances	Biological activity	*r*		
		Approximate solution	Exact solution	References for the exact solution
Erythromycine derivatives	Antibacterial, *S. aureus*	0.963	0.991	[27a]
Erythromycine derivatives	Antibacterial, *K. pneumoniae*	0.958	0.991	[27a]
see Fig. 11.1	Hypothetical	0.930	1.000	[2]
N,N-dimethyl-bromophen-ethylamines	Adrenolytic	0.921	0.969	[7]
Phenanthren-aminoalkyl-carbinols	Antimalaria	0.830	0.924	[22]

11.1.5. Advantages, Disadvantages and Comparison of the Free-Wilson Analysis with the Extrathermodynamic Approach

The Free-Wilson analysis can be applied for the following purposes:

1. as an alternative to the extrathermodynamic approach with the objective to make predictions and to guide synthetic work;
2. to ascertain the most sensitive position(s) of substitution so as to compose a representative training series for use in the extrathermodynamic approach;
3. as a preprocessing step for an extrathermodynamic approach with the aim of eliminating complicated position dependencies;
4. in combination with the extrathermodynamic approach.

The Free-Wilson analysis obviously serves to supplement the extrathermodynamic approach (case 1). It is particularly suitable for samples where relatively few substituents are varied in many positions. In such instances, the extrathermodynamic approach can, in general, not be applied, simply because there are too few degrees of freedom if position dependencies occur. Conversely, the Free-Wilson analysis has limited, if any, utility where many substituents are varied in few positions because the low occurrence of individual segment variants does not permit any statistically meaningful propositions, and it is especially here that the extrathermodynamic approach gives favourable results. An advantage of the Free-Wilson analysis over the extrathermodynamic approach is that it needs no external molecular parameters to characterize substituent properties, thus allowing activity contributions to be determined also for exotic substituents for which substituent constants are not available.

A disadvantage of the Free-Wilson analysis is that in the first instance predictions must be confined to those compounds which can be composed from segment variants contained in the training series; this limitation can be overcome at least partly by additionally including external molecular parameters in the analysis (see below) or by introducing bioisosteric substituents (see [27b]) It has frequently been suggested in the literature that descriptions and predictions in terms of the FREE-WILSON model tend to be somewhat less reliable than those in the extrathermodynamic approach but as a general concept this conclusion cannot be validated.

The second case has already been discussed in 8.1. The idea is to single out from several possible positions of substitution those for which variation of substituents is most sensitive with regard to biological activity. First, a sample containing about three substituents per position is subjected to a FREE-WILSON analysis and then the position(s) with maximal D_j values (see eqn. (11/16)) are selected for further variation. It stands to reason that for any meaningful proposition the segment variants must be diverse enough from a chemical point of view.

The third case is also of great importance. It is based on the equivalence between the extrathermodynamic approach and the FREE-WILSON model (cf., 11.1.3.) allowing to correlate the z_{jk} values with hydrophobic, electronic and steric molecular parameters. This helps to solve problems due to complex position dependencies in multisubstituted molecules and the resulting intricacy of the extrathermodynamic approach in such a manner that a preprocessed FREE-WILSON analysis first determines the z_{jk} values. These values can then replace log A as dependent quantity in the extrathermodynamic approach. When the relation between z_{jk} and substituent constants is known for all positions, it is easy to check on a possible additivity of any molecular properties and positions. Such additivities may, if desired, be allowed for by combining the corresponding terms in a few selected equations, now with log A as dependent variable.

The fourth application was discussed in detail under 11.1.3. It has the advantage that where the FREE-WILSON model and the extrathermodynamic approach are combined their merits can be applied simultaneously to good effect, while also providing additional criteria of form and precision of solutions [7, 8].

11.2. Substructural Approaches

As already pointed out it is difficult if not impossible to apply HANSCH or FREE-WILSON analysis to structurally diverse data sets, which occur, for example, in large screening programmes. In order to be able to extract the information on structure-activity relationships inherent in such data, molecular parameters are needed that can yield acceptable results but can be readily obtained for any chemical structure. In principle, quantumchemical parameters are a possibility, but in addition to the problem of obtaining compatible results for very different structures by semiempirical quantum-chemical methods, the routine use of quantum chemistry for large data sets of low biological precision would not be economical. Another possibility, which has become increasingly important, is to derive molecular descriptors directly from the chemical structure. There are several ways to generate such descriptors (see e.g. [28—47]); the general principle always is to break down the two-dimensional structures into *defined substructures* (*fragments*) and then to describe the molecules in terms of the occurrence of these substructures. The resulting molecular parameters are usually called *substructural descriptors or features*. The compounds of the training series are divided into classes according to their biological activity (or other biological properties of interest), and attempts are then made to describe the distribution of the compounds over the classes and/or to find patterns of features typical of one particular class in terms of the substructural descriptors. As a result it is possible to classify not yet investigated compounds (for example, by means of a classificator) and/or to get some insight as to what pattern of features is typical of one particular class. In the first case compounds with a high probability of having (high) biological potency may be preselected for biological screening thus increasing the chance of finding chemicals with the desired activity. The directed design of novel structures, however, will usually not be possible. For that purpose the pattern of features typical of the class of interest (for example, strong agonists) must be known. These features are called *pharmacophoric groups* and their presence can be considered a necessary (but usually not sufficient) condition for a compound to evoke the particular response under consideration of the limits set by the structural information (variation) present in the training series and the approximations made by using substructural descriptors. Which of these two goals is the primary aim is dependent on the features considered and the method of analysis.

Using substructural descriptors one is, of course, asking less of the data than with, for example, extrathermodynamic parameters, but such descriptors are the only possibility for large data sets of high structural diversity, and the results can still effectively be used for guiding synthesis and biological testing. The crucial steps in all substructural QSAR methods are the generation and selection of features. If the features are in error the result will be obscured. The information obtainable with a set of substructural descriptors is highly dependent on the judgement of the person defining them. It is, therefore, generally advisable to perform substructural analysis in an interactive dialogue between chemist and computer [47a] (see also 11.2.4. and 11.2.6.).

11.2.1. Substructural Descriptors

There are several ways to code chemical structures and to define substructural features [28—47]. Consequently, there are several types of such features. Most commonly used are *topological features* which are directly derived from two-dimensional chemical structures and can be divided into the following categories (for reviews on the use of such features in QSAR work, see e.g. [43—47]):

1. non-position-coded descriptors,
2. position-coded descriptors.

For a more detailed analysis, however, the use of *geometrical descriptors* derived from molecular topography may become necessary.

11.2.1.1. Non-Position-Coded Topological Descriptors

Non-position-coded descriptors may be further divided into *atom* and *bond descriptors* which code the atom and bond types, *substructure descriptors* which code for the presence or absence of explicitly defined substructures, *environment descriptors* which code the immediate surroundings of a substructure, *pathway descriptors* which describe the distance between certain centres (e.g., heteroatoms) in the molecules and *connectivity descriptors* which are indices of the extent of branching.

Atom and bond descriptors characterize the gross composition of the molecules by indicating how many and what types of atoms (except hydrogens) and bonds are present in a given structure. A definition of such descriptors according to Stuper et al. [43] together with the corresponding values for diphenhydramin (structure II) as an example are presented in Tables 11.11 and 11.12. It stands to reason that atom and bond descriptors contain very little information about the topology of molecules, and it may be that two completely different structures have identical descriptor values. They are, therefore, of only limited utility unless additional structural information can be provided. There are certainly cases where simple parameters characterizing the global composition of molecules such as molecular weight, molar volume or partition coefficient can do the same job as these descriptors.

Table 11.11. Atom descriptors (from [43]) and the corresponding values for diphenhydramin (structure II)

Descriptor	Value for diphenhydramin
1. Total number of atoms	19
2. Number of carbon atoms	17
3. Number of oxygen atoms	1
4. Number of nitrogen atoms	1
5. Number of sulfur atoms	0
6. Number of fluorine atoms[1])	0
7. Number of chlorine atoms[1])	0
8. Number of bromine atoms[1])	0
9. Number of iodine atoms[1])	0
10. Number of phosphorus atoms	0

[1]) In many situations the total number of halogens is sufficient at this levels of description. In such cases, descriptors 6.—9. are combined into a new descriptor "total number of halogens"

Table 11.12. Bond descriptors (from [43]) and the corresponding values for diphenhydramin (structure II)

Descriptor	Value for diphenhydramin
1. Total number	14
2. Number of single bonds	8
3. Number of double bonds	0
4. Number of triple bonds	0
5. Number of aromatic bonds	6
6. Number of delocalized bonds	0
7. Number of ionic bonds	0

Substructure descriptors contain information about the presence or absence of specific substructures (substructural features) in the structures to be considered. In the most general sense such features are defined as ensembles of atoms, for example, functional groups (e.g., C=O, $-NR_2$, —OR, etc.), atoms together with the bonds and atoms connected to them (augmented atom fragments; see e.g. [41a, 48] and Table 11.15) or rings. If a substructure is found in a molecule, the descriptor is given a value equal to the number of times it appears in the structure, and if the substructure is absent the descriptor has a value of zero (see Table 11.15).

For the generation of substructure descriptors a *library of substructures* must be available. According to KIRSCHNER et al. [46] this library should include features that "(i) are thought to provide at least some information related to the biological activity, (ii) are known for the greatest majority of the compounds and (iii) if found to be related to activity, will provide the chemist with some degree of insight into the mechanism of action". There are several ways of creating a substructure library. One possibility would be systematically to combine atom and bond fragments into substructures. The number of substructures generated in this way, however, would be much too large to be manageable [43], and many of these substructures would not satisfy the conditions mentioned above. Such an approach can, therefore, not be advocated. A better alternative is to assemble a library of substructures (with the above conditions in mind) in such a way that basic chemical moieties (e.g., functional groups) are adequately represented. This can be done for each problem (training series) individually or, independent of the series under investigation, on the basis of general chemical reasoning. In the first case a series-dependent substructure library is obtained which has the advantage that it can be tailored exactly to the particular structural variations of the series under investigation; an example is provided by the work of CHU et al. [48] on anticancer compounds which will be discussed in more detail in section 11.2.5. The disadvantage of such an approach is that a new substructure library must be created for each problem, which always involves substantial work and is not a trivial task. Therefore, the second possibility of defining a series-independent substructure library once and for all and to use it for all problems is generally to be preferred. The best solution probably is to start with such a library and then to modify or extend it according to the special needs of the problem under investigation. An example is the ICI documentation and retrieval system which uses 150 defined substructures [49]. The SSFN system (substructure superposition fragment notation) used by the group in Riga [44, 50] consisting of 44 basic fragments and some additional ring and distance descriptors may also be mentioned here; this system does not represent the final library but is used as a basis to generate the library from a file of structures.

Once a substructure library is defined the descriptors can be generated for all compounds under investigation by means of substructure searching algorithms. The compounds are stored in a computer and the search algorithm then compares substructures of the compounds with the substructural features contained in the library (see e.g. [43]). All "matches" are found and counted, and the substructure descriptors are obtained for each compound as the numbers of times of occurrence of each substructural feature in its structure. Substructures may be further characterized by physicochemical parameters (e.g., π values) or theoretical indices (e.g., — electron density; see [51]).

Substructure descriptors restore part of the structural information lost in the atom and bond descriptors. A considerable part of such information, however, is still missing, and it may still be that two structurally different molecules have the same substructural descriptor values. Some of the missing information can be provided by the *environment descriptors* characterizing the environment of substructures. Chemical reasoning and intuition, in principle, offers many possibilities to define such descriptors. A very reasonable (but, of course, not the only possible) approach is that followed by JURS and colleagues [43, 43a] who derive environment descriptors by including the first and second nearest neighbours of the fragment considered and their bonds in a single parameter that reflects the atom and bond types connected to it. Three types of such descriptors are used:

1. bond environment descriptors (BED),
2. weighted environment descriptors (WED),
3. augmented environment descriptors (AED).

The BED *descriptor* is obtained by summing the non-hydrogen bonds for the first and second neighbours of the substructure to be considered. In addition to the number, the type of bonds connected to the nearest neighbours is considered in the WED *descriptors* by assigning a value for each bond type (1 for a single bond, 2 for a double bond, 3 for a triple bond, and 4 for an aromatic bond); WED simply is the sum of these values for the first and second neighbours. Finally, in the AED *descriptors*, both the type of bond and the atoms that form the bond are taken into consideration. Each atom and bond type is again arbitrarily assigned a value (a numerical code; see Table 11.13), and for each nearest neighbour the product of bond type number and the numerical value for each atom is then summed. Thus a carbon-carbon single bond would have a value of 1, a carbon-oxygen double bond a value of 4 and a carbon-oxygen single bond a value of 2. AED is finally obtained by adding together the resulting sums for the first and second nearest neighbours. If the same substructure occurs several times in a given molecule the corresponding environmental descriptors are summed; if the substructure is not present the corresponding environmental descriptors are assigned a value of 0.

Table 11.13. Numeric codes for atom and bond types (from [43])

Atom type	Numeric code	Bond type	Numeric code
C	1	Single	1
O	2	Double	2
N	3	Triple	3
S	4	Aromatic	4
F	5	Delocalized	5
Cl	6	Ionic	6
Br	7		
J	8		
P	9		

To illustrate the derivation of environmental descriptors in further detail let us consider the structures A—C presented in Fig. 11.2 as an example (from [43]). All these structures contain the fragment >C=, but the environments seen by this fragment as well as its occurrence numbers are different. In A, for example, it occurs only once with a carbon atom with a single bond, an oxygen atom with one double bond and an oxygen atom with two single bonds as first nearest neighbours. The second nearest neighbour consists of a carbon atom with one single bond. Summing of the number of bonds for all nearest neighbours gives the value for the BED descriptor which is equal to 5 in this case ($1 + 1 + 2 + 1 = 5$). A value of 6 is obtained for the WED descriptor since here the oxygen atom with the double bond has a value of two. The AED descriptor for structure A, finally, becomes 10 with the contributions

— 1 from the carbon-carbon single bond between atoms 1 and 2,
— 4 from the carbon-oxygen double bond,
— 4 from the two carbon-oxygen single bonds,
— 1 from the single bond starting at carbon 5.

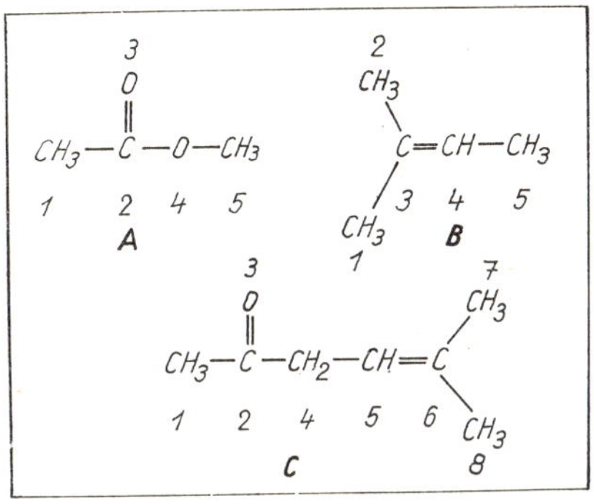

Fig. 11.2. Structures containing the substructure $\rangle$C= (from [43])

The corresponding values for B are: BED = 5, WED = 6 and AED = 6. In structure C, the fragment to be considered occurs twice (C atoms 2 and 6). The values for the environmental descriptors are as follows:

1. BED

for the fragment at C_2

from the bond starting at C_1:	1
from the C=O bond:	1
from the two single bonds starting at C_4:	2
from the two bonds starting at C_5:	2
sum:	6

for the fragment at C_6

from the two single bonds starting at C_7 and C_8:	2
from the two bonds starting at C_5:	2
from the two single bonds starting at C_4:	2
sum:	6

Total = BED = 6 + 6 = 12

2. WED

Same as BED except that the C = O bond (at C_2) now contributes a value of 2 instead of 1 and the C = C bond (connecting C_6 and C_5) a value of $2 \cdot 2 = 4$ (once for the fragment at C_2 and once for the fragment at C_6) instead of $2 \cdot 1$, so that WED = 15.

3. AED (see Table 11.13)

for the fragment at C_2

from the single bond starting at C_1:	1
for the C=O bond:	4 (= 2 · 2)
for the two single bonds starting at C_4:	2
for the single bond starting at C_5:	1
for the double bond starting at C_5:	2
sum:	10

for the fragment at C_6

from the two single bonds starting at C_7 and C_8:	2
for the C=C bond:	2
for the single bond starting at C_5:	1
for the two single bonds starting at C_4:	2
sum:	7

Total = AED = 10 + 7 = 17

The concept of environment may be extended further by using electron densities, bond distances, electronegativities or other physical parameters instead of the numerical codes assigned to the bond and atom types. In this way the information provided by the descriptors can be increased. The utility of environment descriptors depends, on the one hand, on the chemical intuition and the experience of the person defining them and, on the other hand, on the type of environment considered, the molecules under investigation and the purpose of the investigation.

Connectivity descriptors provide some basic information concerning branching and the overall composition of molecules. A very useful parameter of this kind is the *molecular connectivity* based on the work of Randić [52] and introduced into QSAR work by Kier and Hall [53, 53a], already discussed in chapter 6. Molecular connectivity has been shown to be related to many fundamental chemical properties [53] and thus obviously presents exactly the type of information wanted. The calculation of this index is straightforward (see [53]) and can be performed with the help of a computer. A disadvantage of connectivity is that its chemical meaning is not always easy to interpret.

The above mentioned descriptors can be derived automatically by means of computers using graph-theoretical methods. Each molecule can be represented as a graph with the atoms as nodes and the bonds between them as edges, and such a graph can then be described in terms of a so-called *connection table* (also called *adjacency matrix*) indicating which nodes of the graph are connected (for basic articles and reviews on graph theoretical and matrix representation and manipulation of chemical structures, see e.g. [28, 35, 36, 54—56]; an introduction to graph theory can be found in [57, 58]). The connection table is a symmetrical matrix with the atoms (nodes) in the rows (hydrogens neglected) and the columns. The elements of the main diagonal are 0 and the off-diagonal elements either 1 or 0 depending on whether the corresponding atoms (nodes) are connected (an edge is there) or not. More information can be stored if the types of atoms and the bond type are also included. This can be done by using a simple numerical code for atoms and bonds as represented in Table 11.13 [43]. The code for the atoms appears in the main diagonal, and the ones in the off-diagonal elements are replaced by the bond type code number. An example of this type is presented in Table 11.14 describing the structure of caffeine (XLIIa; from [43]) using the code from Table 11.13. Each substructure of a library can be represented as a subgraph or submatrix, and substructural descriptors are then generated by special algorithms searching for the appearance of these submatrices in the connection tables (see [43]). Adjacency matrices may also be subjected to intersection procedures for which special algorithms are available [44, 59, 60]. As a result subgraphs are obtained which are common to the molecules considered (common subgraphs). For active molecules, such subgraphs may directly represent pharmacophoric groups.

Table 11.14. Connection table for caffeine (XLIIa) using the numeric code from Table 11.13 (from [43]). Since the matrix is symmetric the lower triangle can be neglected

Atom No.	1	2	3	4	5	6	7	8	9	10	11	12	13	14
1	1	1	0	0	0	1	0	0	0	0	2	0	0	0
2		1	2	0	0	0	1	0	0	0	0	0	0	0
3			1	1	0	0	0	0	1	0	0	0	0	0
4				3	1	0	0	0	0	0	0	0	0	1
5					1	1	0	0	0	0	0	0	2	0
6						3	0	0	0	0	0	1	0	0
7							3	1	0	1	0	0	0	0
8								1	2	0	0	0	0	0
9									3	0	0	0	0	0
10										1	0	0	0	0
11											2	0	0	0
12												1	0	0
13													2	0
14														1

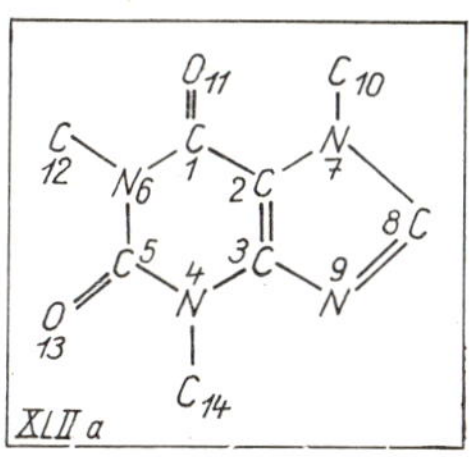

Connection tables are not the only possible matrix representation of chemical structures. Instead of including each atom it may be advantageous, for example, to consider only potentially active or important centres in the molecules which may be certain atoms and/or groups of atoms. These centres may be called *descriptor centres,* and chemical structures can then be represented in the form of a *descriptor centre matrix* [44] (see also [61—64]). In such a matrix the atoms are replaced by the descriptor centres the type of which can be coded in the main diagonal. In the off-diagonal elements information on the distance between these centres can be given.

11.2.1.2. Position-Coded Topological Descriptors

Position-coded topological descriptors indicate the presence or absence of defined fragments in defined positions of molecules. Typical descriptors of this kind are the b_{ijk} used in the FREE-WILSON analysis (see 11.1.) which have a value of 1 if in a compound i the substituent k is present in the j-th position of substitution. Position-coded descriptors contain much structural information and are thus particularly suitable if the main purpose of a substructural analysis is the evaluation of pharmacophoric groups. Unfortunately, the derivation of such descriptors becomes the more difficult the more diverse are the chemical structures to be considered so that their applicability is limited. The FREE-WILSON type of position coding is restricted to such series where only substituents are varied in fixed positions of a common parent molecule. It can, however, sometimes be extended somewhat by defining an artificial parent molecule (some chemical moiety occurring in all compounds) and then treating all fragments not belonging to this moiety as substituents. A more general procedure is the supermolecule technique first used in this connection by CAMMARATA and MENON [65, 66] and later in a modified version by us [67, 68]. The principle is very simple. In a first step all molecules to be considered are superimposed. As a result an artificial supermolecule is obtained. This supermolecule contains all information about all structures. It can be visualized as graph with atoms or groups of atoms as nodes each node representing a substructural feature. In the second step, the molecules of the series are superimposed over the supermolecule one at a time, and for all nodes which match the descriptor value will be 1 and otherwise 0. In other words a set of binary descriptors is obtained for each molecule describing its structure in terms of the features present in the supermolecule. These descriptors are defined as:

$$x_{ji} = \begin{cases} 1 & \text{if feature } j \text{ (the } j\text{-th node of the supermolecule) is present in compound } i \\ 0 & \text{if not} \end{cases} \qquad (11/50)$$

The critical and most difficult step in this procedure is the construction of the supermolecule which must fulfil two important conditions:

- It must be possible to superimpose all molecules of the training series over the supermolecule in a well defined and the same manner.
- It must be defined in such a way that it cannot be identified with itself by symmetry operations.

A more detailed discussion of this technique and an example will be presented in 11.2.6.

11.2.1.3. Geometrical Descriptors

Matrix representations of molecular structure may be extended to include information on the topography of molecules and thus also provide a simple possibility of arriving at geometrical descriptors. There are several possibilities of doing this (see also [68a]) once the geometry (bond length, etc.) of the molecules to be considered is known (a brief discussion of methods suitable for the calculation of molecular geometries will be given in chapter 12.). The general principle consists in substituting the bond type descriptors in a connection table by geometrical distances between atoms. Distances between chemically non-bonded atoms can also be included in this way. In addition, the atom type code in the main diagonal can be replaced by a physically more meaningful quantity such as, for example, electronic charges (see e.g. [36, 44, 56, 69]).

In flexible molecules, the distances between atoms depend on conformation. In such cases either a conformational choice has to be made (which may be difficult; see 12.), or ranges of bond distances corresponding to the allowed conformational space (maximal and minimal distances) are to be used instead of a single value (see e.g. [64, 70, 71]). The resulting distance matrices can be handled in the same way as simple connection tables. Matrix-based geometrical descriptors may, for example, simply be obtained as a result of general matrix intersection.

Other geometrical descriptors are used by Stuper et al. [43], namely the three principal axes of rotation and the van der Waals volume; the molecular shape introduced into QSAR work by Hopfinger [72—73] (see 6.) also constitutes such a descriptor.

Geometrical descriptors are closer to the three-dimensional reality of drug-receptor interactions than the simple topological descriptors. They contain more structural information, but their evaluation is more laborious. As Stuper et al. [43] point out, "the actual value of any geometric descriptor depends on the specific application in which it is used".

11.2.1.4. Feature Extraction, Feature Selection and Data Preprocessing

For small data sets it is possible to generate substructural descriptors manually. This however, will always be a very laborious procedure and subject to errors. Much more effective and reliable are computer-based feature generation and extraction procedures in general use now at many places and within several molecular modelling systems (see e.g. [28, 43, 49, 74]). The input of chemical structures is very simple and usually does not require knowledge of computer programming or languages so that these procedures can easily be applied by any chemist or pharmacologist. With the more sophisticated programs use can be made of the powerful possibilities of modern computer graphics (see e.g. [28, 71, 75, 76]) allowing three-dimensional representations of molecules to be viewed and manipulated at a TV screen (see also 12.).

Once the descriptors have been generated (this process is frequently referred to as "*feature generation*" or "*feature extraction*") each compound can be described by a vector of its descriptor values. This is demonstrated in Table 11.15 for three simple compounds using augmented atom fragments as substructure features (from [48]). Before applying the features in, for example, pattern recognition methods (see 11.2.5.) it is usually appropriate to improve the feature space by *data preprocessing*. The first step in preprocessing usually is scaling and normalization. This is necessary if the data are on different scales (for example, if substructure features are to be used together with molar refractivity) in order to avoid the larger descriptors dominating those of smaller values. Usually, the autoscaling technique is applied here which translates and normalizes the features so that they have a mean of zero and constant variance (see eqn. (8/40)). The descriptors may also be transformed in several ways. They may be weighted according to their usefulness such that features contributing most to, for example, a clustering of compounds in feature space get a higher weight. Another possibility is to apply principal component analysis or the so-called KARHUNEN-LOEVE transform which will result in a new feature space of lower dimensionality. New features can also be obtained by combining features (e.g., ratios or cross-products of the original features). Finally, the dimensionality of the feature space is reduced by discarding unnecessary descriptors and retaining those that are necessary for describing a clustering of compounds. This step is called *feature selection*, and it is completely analogous to the evaluation of the optimal set of variables in discriminant analysis (see 9.2.2.). Several mathematical techniques can be used here which will, however, not be discussed in any detail (see e.g. [43, 77]). Feature selection is not only important in the context of data preprocessing but may also serve its own purpose. If it is so designed that the features typical for one particular category of compounds (e.g., agonists) can be found it can be used as a tool to derive pharmacophoric groups and thus aid in lead generation. A typical example will be presented in 11.2.6. (see also 11.2.4.).

Table 11.15. Augmented atom fragments and descriptor value vectors for three simple compounds (from [48])

No.	Fragments	$CH_3-C(=O)-H$	$CH_3-C(=O)-CH_3$	$CH_3-C(=O)-OH$
1	C=O	1	1	1
2	H_3C-C	1	2	1
3	C–C(=O)–H	1	0	0
	C–C(=O)–C	0	1	0
5	C–O–H	0	0	1
6	C–C(=O)–O	0	0	1

11.2.2. Cramer's Substructural Analysis [78—80]

Developed by BERKOFF, CRAMER and REDL this method is one of the first attempts to apply substructural analysis in the QSAR field. The compounds of a training series are divided into two classes (active and inactive) and fragmented into substructures using a library of atom, bond and substructure topological features. For each feature the so-called substructure activity frequency (SAF) is then calculated according to:

$$\mathrm{SAF}_j = \frac{\text{number of active compounds containing the feature } j}{\text{total number of compounds containing the feature } j} \tag{11/51}$$

The SAF_j value embodies the probability contribution of the j-th feature to the overall probability that the compound containing that feature will be biologically active. To characterize the activity of compounds the mean substructure activity frequency (MSAF) is used. For the i-th compound this value is

$$\mathrm{MASF}_i = \frac{1}{m_i} \sum_j b_{ij}\, \mathrm{SAF}_j \tag{11/52}$$

where m_i is the number of features (fragments) occurring in the i-th compound and b_{ij} is a substructural descriptor defined as:

$$b_{ij} = \begin{cases} 1, & \text{if the } j\text{-th feature is present in the } i\text{-th compound} \\ 0, & \text{if not} \end{cases} \tag{11/53}$$

As shown by an example concerning the immunoregulatory potency of 770 compounds, the MSAF values are indeed connected with biological potency. The compounds were ordered in the sequence of decreasing MSAF values and divided into groups with either equal numbers of compounds or spanning equal ranges of MSAF. For each group, the mean MSAF value and the mean relative incidence of biologically active compounds were determined, and there appeared a clear relation between these two quantities. The relation between MSAF and biological activity will be the closer the higher is the discriminating power of the features. Compounds can be arranged in a sequence of decreasing MSAF values, and the probability of a compound being active will then be related to its place in this sequence and will be highest for compounds at the top. An unequivocal classification of compounds simply by means of MSAF values, however, is not possible. For that purpose a threshold MSAF value and a decision rule would be required.

11.2.3. Preselection of Compounds for Screening: a Statistical-Heuristic Method [41, 81, 82]

Substructural analysis as discussed in the preceding section was developed further and statistically refined by Hodes and colleagues who introduced a statistical-heuristic method for the automated selection of drugs for screening [41, 81, 82] with the objective of increasing the incidence of biologically active compounds (see also [83, 83a]). The method is based on an analysis of the probabilities that structural features present in the molecules to be considered are connected with biological activity and inactivity. For each feature a weighting for activity and inactivity is derived, and an activity and inactivity score for a compound can then simply be obtained by summing the respective weightings of all its structural features.

To evaluate the weightings a training series is used which is divided into active and inactive compounds. The active set is used to derive activity weightings and scores, and the inactivity weightings and scores are derived from the inactive set. In a first step, all compounds are broken down into fragments using a library of substructural features (ring, nucleus and augmented atom fragments). Each fragment is then tested to determine whether its incidence, p_j, in both classes is significantly different from the randomly expected incidence, p_j^0. The latter is derived from the incidence, p_j', the features have in the 280000 compounds stored in the NCI file.

Let us consider first the set of active compounds. When this set contains n_a compounds (index a for active) the randomly expected incidence, $p_{j,a}^0$, of the j-th feature is:

$$p_{j,a}^0 = n_a p_j' \tag{11/54}$$

When

$$p_{j,a}^0 = p_{j,a} \tag{11/55}$$

it is assumed that the j-th fragment is of no consequence for biological activity. This means that for biological activity (and hence assignment to the class of active compounds) only those fragments are significant for which the incidence in the test set differs from the randomly expected incidence. A particular fragment will gain in importance as this difference becomes larger. A measure of the importance of the j-th fragment is provided by the reciprocal of the probability $P_{j,a}$ that the difference between $p^0_{j,a}$ and $p_{j,a}$ can be generated by chance. Accordingly, an activity index, $I_{j,a}$, for each feature can be defined as:

$$I_{j,a} = 1/P_{j,a} \qquad (11/56)$$

The activity score for any given compound X with fragments $j = 1, \ldots, n$ can be derived as

$$I_{X,a} = \prod_{j=a}^{n} (1/P_{j,a}) \qquad (11/57)$$

from the $P_{j,a}$ values calculated for the n features in the class of active compounds. On numerical grounds, it is desirable to perform a logarithmic transformation and to define the activity score as:

$$I'_{X,a} = \log I_{X,a} = \sum_{j=1}^{n} \log (1/P_{j,a}) \qquad (11/58)$$

The activity score constitutes a criterion of the probability that compound X will belong to the class of active compounds. The probability that it should be included among the inactives is provisionally ignored. $I_{X,a}$ becomes zero when all fragments contained in the compound under consideration satisfy eqn. (11/55). On summation, it should be borne in mind that contributions $\log (1/P_{j,a})$ are preceded by a negative sign when $p_{j,a} < p^0_{j,a}$.

In a fully analogous manner, an inactivity score, $I'_{X,in}$ (index *in* for inactive), can be defined with the aid of the probabilities $P_{j,in}$, to be deduced from the class of inactive compounds:

$$I'_{X,in} = \sum_{j=1}^{n} \log (1/P_{j,in}) \qquad (11/59)$$

The inactivity score provides a measure of the probability that compound X will belong to the class of inactives.

If compounds are to be selected for a screening program with the objective of increasing the incidence of actives both the activity as well as the inactivity score have to be taken into account. These scores can be combined in various ways depending on the needs of the selection program [41]. A very simple way is to combine both scores into a single value which can be used to establish priorities. A high value would mean that the corresponding compounds would have a high probability of being active and, thus, a priority for testing. Another possibility is to use a linear combination of both scores. To this end, the compounds to be considered are plotted as points in a cartesian coordinate system with $I'_{X,a}$ and $I'_{X,in}$ as axes and their respective score values as coordinates. Then any linear combination of the two scores can be represented geometrically as a projection of each point onto a line of a given direction, and the priority can be measured along the line. It is advantageous to use a line along the so-called FISHER direction [84] since in that case an optimal separation of active and inactive compounds can be achieved.

The procedure designed by HODES et al. has already been successfully applied in the screening of cytostatics [41, 81, 82]. It has much in common with the substructural analysis described in the preceding chapter but as a predictive tool it has far broader scope and utility. Another important aspect of the procedure of HODES et al. is that redundancies of substructures (see also [39, 40]) and the novelty of compounds can be taken into account. Nevertheless, it is to be noted that the procedure is not intended as an exact classification, merely serving to enrich the incidence of actives in screening via a preselection of compounds. Compounds classified on the basis of $I'_{X,a}$ and $I'_{X,in}$ stand a significantly greater chance of turning out to be active than randomly selected compounds.

An extension of the HODES procedure has recently been presented by TINKER [83, 83a] who introduced the following modifications:

- as many as eight classes may be considered,
- confidence limits for statistically significant differences between each pair of classes are calculated,
- for each substance to be classified or reclassified various measures of the correctness of classification can be obtained,
- data can be traced through the program.

The main purpose of this extended program is its application to mutagenicity data. First results look promising [83] but it must be stressed that estimates of mutagenicity made in this way should never be allowed to replace experimental values.

11.2.4. The Logico-Structural Approach [44—45]

Developed by the Riga QSAR group this approach is a further step forward to predicting biological activities by means of substructural features. It allows one to classify compounds according to their activities using certain threshold values to be discussed below and is based on a simulation of the logical processes of a medicinal chemist who tries to find connections between particular structural features of compounds and their activities. Two techniques are used, one designed for lead optimization (STRAC) and the other for the preselection of compounds in screening programmes based on a battery of biological tests (ORACLE).

Let us first consider lead optimization (STRAC *procedure*). A training series of compounds is divided into the classes "active" and "inactive" as a first step. In the next step substructural features are defined. In the STRAC procedure these features are selected as in the FREE-WILSON approach as substituents in their positions of substitution (position-coded descriptors). Therefore, STRAC is limited to more or less homologous series. The advantage over the FREE-WILSON analysis is that the assumption on the additivity of substituent contributions is not necessary here. Next, the discriminating power of the features is investigated (feature selection). A feature is considered discriminating if the probability that a compound containing this feature belongs to one of the two classes is greater than a certain threshold value, λ. This probability can easily be computed from the occurrence numbers of features in the classes, and the threshold is found by an interactive trial and error procedure based on the leave-one-out technique (see p. 227).

In many cases the discriminating features found in this way are not sufficient to classify the compounds of the training series. For this reason the next steps of the procedure are aimed at deriving new discriminating features. This is done in the following way:

1. A non-discriminating feature is selected, and all compounds containing this feature are displayed and inspected.
2. This inspection of a (small) number of compounds will usually reveal a new feature not yet considered which has a high probability of being typical of one of the two classes.
3. A more complex feature is now generated by combining the non-discriminating and the new feature into a new complex feature using the logical operation "and"; in addition, the negation of the new feature (that it is not present) is also considered and used to derive a second complex feature in an analogous way (a more detailed discussion of such logical operations will be presented in 11.2.6.).
4. The statistical characteristics of the new complex feature are determined. If it is discriminating it is stored together with the other discriminating features. If not, the procedure is continued with step 5.
5. All compounds having the new non-discriminating feature are inspected and an additional feature is selected and added according to 3. In this way a still more complex feature is obtained.
6. With this feature step 4 is repeated.
7. The procedure is continued until sufficient new features have been added to the originally non-discriminant feature that it becomes discriminating.
8. The procedure is repeated for the other non-discriminating features.
9. As a result a set of discriminating features sufficient to separate the classes of active and inactive compounds is obtained. These features are either typical of the active ("activity features") or of the inactive ("inactivity features") compounds.
10. With this set the activity of new compounds can be predicted. This is usually done according to their predominant features. A compound is classified as active, if

$$V_a - V_{in} > \eta \tag{11/60}$$

and as inactive, if

$$V_{in} - V_a > \eta \tag{11/61}$$

where V_a and V_{in} are the occurrence numbers of activity and inactivity features, respectively, in this compound and η is a certain threshold value.

This technique has successfully been applied to several problems as, for example, to antimicrobial alkylaminosilanes [44] or to anticonvulsive indandione-1,3 derivatives [44, 45]; in both cases, the predictions could be experimentally verified. It has the advantage that feature generation and selection are performed interactively by the medicinal chemist operating the computer, making decisions in each step (for example, about which feature should be included) using his experience and intuition.

The ORACLE *procedure* was developed for the purpose of generating topological pharmacophores. These pharmacophores are then used as a criterion to guide the screening of compounds in a battery of biological tests. The basis for ORACLE is a structure and pharmacological activity file including about 6000 compounds and 55 major types of pharmacological activities [85]. Structural descriptors of the compounds are generated by means of fragmentation using the substructure superposition fragment notation (SSFN) [50] which consists of a library of substructures, rings and certain distance measures (pathways).

The compounds of the data file are now divided into 55 classes according to the type of their pharmacological activity. Each class is then separately compared with the rest of the compounds contained in the remaining 54 classes in order to find descriptors which represent the particular type of activity exhibited by the class under investigation. A descriptor is considered to represent a particular activity feature if its presence in this class is not a chance event. For a feature j this is tested after counting the number of all compounds having this feature in the data base (l^j_{total}) and in the class considered (l^j_{class}). From these numbers the probability of the chance occurrence of feature j of less than l^j_{class} in the class can be computed. If this probability is large and higher than a threshold value it can be concluded that feature j is connected with the class type of pharmacological activity. As an additional criterion the so-called coefficient of prognostic feature utility is also considered. The procedure is applied to all descriptors and classes until sets of discriminating features typical of each respective class are found.

In a way these sets constitute topological pharmacophores the presence of which can be considered a necessary (but not sufficient) condition for production of a desired type of biological effect (see 11.2.6.). Once these sets are known the type of pharmacological activity to be expected for a new compound can be predicted. These predictions can then be used to decide what compounds should be investigated with regard to which of the 55 pharmacological effects. This is, of course, extremely useful for large screening programmes since it allows one to select the most promising from a battery of pharmacological tests for all compounds and thus not only increases the incidence of actives but also may save quite a lot of biological testing. To a certain extent knowledge of the pharmacophores will also allow the design of novel structures simply by devising new combinations of discriminating features.

The method will, of course, fail if a pharmacological effect can be produced via more than one mechanism of action. In such cases, different pharmacophores for the different mechanisms of action are to be expected so that a common pharmacophore (a set of descriptors typical of the effect) does not exist. Nevertheless, ORACLE has successfully been applied. The system correctly recognized the presence of earlier established activities for the majority of compounds in the data base, and a number of unknown activities could be predicted for many compounds [44].

11.2.5. Classification by Pattern Recognition Methods

As was already pointed out in section 9.2., the evaluation of classification rules to describe the distribution of compounds over classes of different biological activities and the classification of as yet untested compounds is an important task in QSAR work which may serve several objectives. The methods outlined in 9.2. can, however, only be applied if the data are normally distributed. For substructural descriptors (discrete or logical quantities) this condition is no longer fulfilled so that other classification methods not based on this assumption are required. Suitable methods are the so-called "non-probabilistic", "non-parametric" or "heuristic" techniques which belong to the field of pattern recognition methods. Non-parametric pattern recognition methods are, therefore, the only choice for deriving decision rules or classificators if substructural descriptors are to be used as variables[1]). They are based on geometrical and not on statistical considerations, starting from a representation of the compounds of the training series as points in the space spanned by the descriptors. If there are m descriptors this space will be m-dimensional, each axis corresponding to a particular feature, and the coordinates of the points are the descriptor values of the compound. If the features selected are meaningful and somehow connected with the biological property underlying the division of compounds into classes, points belonging to the same class will be clustered together with a certain distance between the clusters belonging to the different classes. In other words, the members of different classes will be found in different regions of the feature space. Once these regions are known a new compounds can be classified by observing in which region it would fall. For a two- or three-dimensional space this could be done by simple inspection. In a higher dimensional space, however, this is not possible, and mathematical approaches become necessary. The pattern recognition methods to be discussed here actually do the same thing in an m-dimensional space as a scientist viewing a two- or three-dimensional space. They are nothing more than a mathematically formulated empirism designed to elucidate similarities within sets of data with respect to a set of features. There are two main types of decision rules which can be generated:

1. *Hypersurface seperators* which seperate the classes with hypersurfaces. Classification of a compound then is based on the determination of the regions of feature space containing the different classes partitioned by the hypersurfaces.
2. *Distance classifiers* which classify compounds by considering their distance in space to and the class membership of the nearest neighbours.

The most important method of the first category is the so-called *linear learning machine* (LLM), and the most commonly used distance classifier is the so-called *k-nearest neighbour method* (KNN). The discussion in this section will be restricted to these two methods. Note, however, that the logico-structural approach discussed in the preceding section may also be regarded as a pattern recognition method since it is non-parametric and heuristic. Furthermore, the spectrum of pattern recognition methods implies also other techniques not to be discussed in this book, and the methods discussed in 9.2. may also be considered as belonging to pattern recognition. Pattern recognition methods have been successfully applied to a variety of fields (for extensive reviews and mathematical details, see e.g. [43, 84, 86—101]), and some reviews on the application of such methods in drug design have also recently been published [43, 46, 47, 102].

Let us first consider the *linear learning machine* (LLM) [88]. The basic steps are, in principle, the same as in discriminant analysis (see 9.2.2.):

1. Division of the compounds of the training series into classes according to the biological property to be considered (e.g., biological potency).

---

[1]) It should again be stressed that continuous parameters (e.g., substituent constants) can also be applied in these methods (see also 9.2.).

2. Generation of descriptors (11.2.1.).
3. Data preprocessing including feature selection yielding an "optimal set" of features (11.2.1.).
4. Evaluation of the classificator. This is done by a process which is called supervised learning and which will not be discussed here. It starts from an initial estimate of the classificator which is then improved in such a way that the separation of classes is optimal (the computer learns how to separate the classes in a supervised manner).
5. Testing of the discriminating power of the classificator by reclassification, leave-n-out technique or classification of the compounds of a test series (see 9.2.2.).
6. Interpretation of the classificator; classification and design of new compounds.

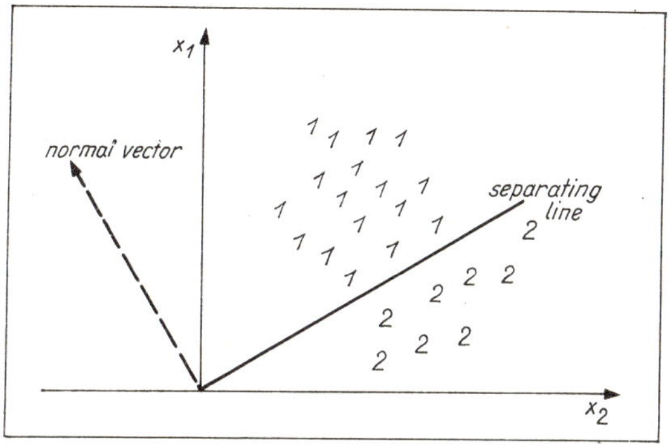

Fig. 11.3. Separating line in two-dimensional feature space

For simplicity let us start with a two-class problem (e.g., class 1 = active compounds, class 2 = inactive compounds) assuming that steps 1—3 have already been performed and that two features (descriptors), x_1 and x_2, have been found which are sufficient to separate the two classes. All compounds of the training series can then be presented as points in a two-dimensional coordinate system with coordinates x_1 and x_2 (Fig. 11.3) and the objective is to find a straight line separating the two classes from each other. In a simple case of two-dimensionality the problem can, of course, be solved graphically but this possibility does not exist in m-dimensional space (m features). In the latter case, one needs a hyper-surface to separate classes, which in Fig. 11.3 simplifies to a straight line.

In m-dimensional space each object can be denoted by a point with the descriptor values for the m features as coordinates, i.e., by a *feature vector* $\boldsymbol{x}$ of all features for this object. The elements of this vector are the m descriptor values corresponding to the m features (see e.g. Table 11.15) according to

$$\boldsymbol{x}_i = \begin{pmatrix} x_{1,i} \\ \vdots \\ x_{ji} \\ \vdots \\ x_{mi} \end{pmatrix} \qquad (11/62)$$

where x_{ji} is the value for the j-th feature of the i-th compound. The separating hyper-surface can be described by its *normal vector* which is exactly perpendicular to that plane (see Fig. 11.3), an element w_j of this vector being assigned to each feature x_j:

$$\boldsymbol{w}^T = (w_1 \ldots w_j \ldots w_m) \tag{11/63}$$

The separating hypersurface between the classes is determined in such a way as to satisfy relation (11/64) in the best possible manner that is for a maximum number or, ideally, for all objects in the training series:

$$^T\boldsymbol{x} = (w_1 \ldots w_j \ldots w_m w_{m+1}) \begin{pmatrix} x_1 \\ \vdots \\ x_j \\ \vdots \\ x_m \\ x_{m+1} \end{pmatrix} = \sum_{j=1}^{m+1} x_j w_j = \begin{cases} > 0 \text{ for compounds of class 1} \\ < 0 \text{ for compounds of class 2} \end{cases} \tag{11/64}$$

The additional element w_{m+1} of the normal vector fixes the position of the separating hypersurface in feature space; the corresponding extra element x_{m+1} of the feature vector has a value of 1. For the two-dimensional case in Fig. 11.3, (11/64) leads to:

$$(w_1 w_2 w_3) \begin{pmatrix} x_1 \\ x_2 \\ 1 \end{pmatrix} = \sum_{j=1}^{3} x_j w_j = x_1 w_1 + x_2 w_2 + 1 \cdot w_3 = \begin{cases} > 0 \text{ for compounds of cass 1} \\ < 0 \text{ for compounds of class 2} \end{cases} \tag{11/65}$$

Following the determination of normal vector $\boldsymbol{w}$, it is very easy to classify new objects by multiplication of their feature vectors by that vector. In accord with (11/64) they are to be assigned to class 1 if the product is positive, and to class 2 in the case of negative product. In two-class problems the elements w_j permit certain conclusions with respect to the importance of individual features for classification. A high positive value for a given w_j, for example, indicates that a high value for the corresponding feature x_j argues in favour of assignment of the object to class 1 and thus may be important for the biological activity considered. To a certain extent such information can be used for designing new structures in the sense of lead generation and may also be helpful in understanding certain mechanistic aspects of drug action.

A good example of the application of the LLM is provided by the work of Chu et al. [48] on the classification of antineoplastics (further examples will be presented in 11.2.6.). The training series contained 138 compounds of widely differing structures including metal complexes, antimetabolites, alkylating agents and alkaloids. These compounds were divided into two classes (class 1 = active compounds, class 2 = inactive compounds) and fragmented using a library of the following substructure types: augmented atom fragments (Table 11.16), ring fragments (Table 11.18) and heteropath fragments (number of C atoms between defined heteroatoms, see Table 11.17). A total of 421 features was obtained from which 384 were discarded as non-relevant by feature selection, leaving an "optimal set" of 37 features. These features and the corresponding weights, w_j, in the normal vector are summarized in Tables 11.16—11.18. The presence of fragments with high positive w_j values is favourable for antineoplastic activity whereas fragments with high negative w_j lead to inactive compounds. Thus, the hypothetical compound XLIV contains fragments 2 (twice), 7 (once), 29 (once) and 33 (three times). This means that the seventh and twenty-ninth elements of the feature

Table 11.16. Augmented atom fragments and the corresponding elements of the normal vector, w_j (from [48])

No.	Fragments	w_j
1	C=C–C	0.57
2	H_3C–C	–0.75
3	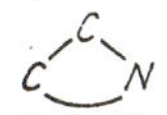	0.14
4	H_3C–N	0.53
5	N–C(=O)–N	1.76
6	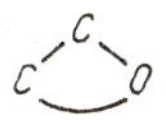	1.26
7	C–C(=O)–C	–0.01
8	Cl–C	0.29
9	Cl–Pt	0.71
10	H_2N–C	–0.05
11	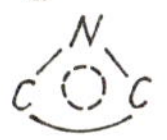	1.11
12	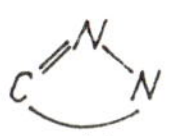	–1.52
13	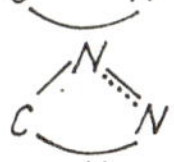	1.39
14	C–N(–N)–C	0.12
15	N–N=O	1.72
16	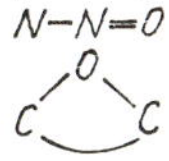	–0.59
17	C=O	–0.16
18	C⋯O	–0.74

Table 11.17. Heteropath fragments and the corresponding elements of the normal vector, w_j (from [48])

No.	Heteroatom 1	Heteroatom 2	Number of C atoms between 1 and 2	w_j
19	N	N	0	–0.38
20	N	N	2	0.45
21	N	N	6	0.35
22	O	N	6	0.39
23	O	O	2	0.22
24	O	O	4	0.54
25	O	O	6	–0.95
26	S	N	3	0.61
27	S	O	0	–1.56

Table 11.18. Ring fragments and the corresponding elements of the normal vector, w_j (from [48])

No.	Fragments	W_j
28	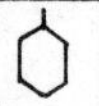	0.58
29	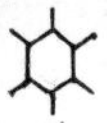	−0.26
30	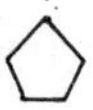	−2.15
31		−2.18
32	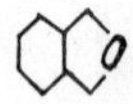	0.69
33	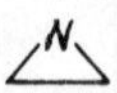	1.22
34	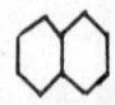	0.22
35	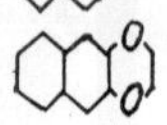	0.69
36	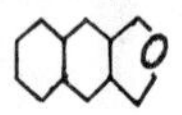	0.53
37	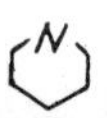	1.90
38	constant	−1.15

vector of this compound are equal to 1, the second element is equal to 2, the thirty-third element is equal to 3 and all other elements (except the additional element 38) are equal to 0. Multiplication of this feature vector by the weight vector through (11/64) affords:

$$\begin{aligned} \boldsymbol{w}^T\boldsymbol{x} &= 2w_2 + 1w_7 + 1w_{29} + 3w_{33} + w_{38} \\ &= 2 \cdot (-0.75) + 1 \cdot (-0.01) + 1 \cdot (-0.26) + 3 \cdot 1.22 - 1.15 \\ &= 0.74 > 0 \end{aligned} \qquad (11/66)$$

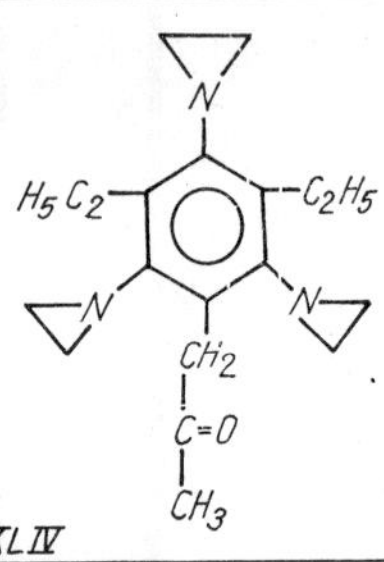

XLIV

Thus, this compound is classified in class 1 (the class of the active compounds). In this way CHU et al. [48] classified 24 new compounds according to anticipated antineoplastic activity. Predictions were experimentally found to be correct in 92% of cases.

LLM is also applicable where more than two classes occur. For a case of J classes, $J(J-1)/2$ normal vectors have to be determined. A prerequisite for its applicability is a configuration of the objects in feature space such that a good separation by hypersurfaces is possible.

The second technique, the *k-nearest-neighbours method* (KNN) [103, 104] is based on the consideration of distances between objects in feature space. The basic steps are the same as for LLM except that the classificator is not explicitly stated and remains hidden in the computer. Therefore, an interpretation of the result in structural terms is not possible. An unknown object (compound) is classified by comparing its position in feature space with that of its k nearest neighbours. For this purpose the distances between the object and all objects of the training series are calculated (usually, the Euclidian distance is employed). The k nearest neighbours receive a vote for the class they belong to, and the unknown object is then assigned to that class which has accumulated the most votes. For vote weighting, various methods are available. For a two-class case the decision can be made very easily according to

$$\sum_{i=1}^{k} \frac{V_i}{d_i^2} = \begin{cases} > 0\text{: assignment to class 1} \\ < 0\text{: assignment to class 2} \end{cases} \qquad (11/67)$$

where d_i denotes the EUCLIDEAN distance and V_i is to be defined as:

$$V_i = \begin{cases} 1 \text{ for class 1} \\ -1 \text{ for class 2} \end{cases} \qquad (11/68)$$

The KNN method has the advantage that it is applicable in cases where data are not separable by a linear decision surface and performs best on data that contain a high density of points.

Pattern recognition methods have become increasingly important in QSAR work and have been applied to a variety of problems. Table 11.19 provides a survey of applications of LLM and KNN in this field (for an extensive review, see [46]). As already pointed out, the crucial step in these methods is the generation of the feature space including data preprocessing and feature selection. If the features are in error the result of the analysis will be misleading. Chemical experience and intuition may play an important part here, and an interactive process in feature generation, preprocessing and selection is always recommended [47a] (see also 11.2.4.). In doing so, correlations between features must be adequately considered; otherwise, wrong conclusions may be drawn (see also [41, 107]). An example where the features selected led to a wrong conclusion is provided by the work of KOWALSKI and BENDER [109] on the classification of 200 purine and pyrimidine derivatives with respect to their antitumor activity (two-class problem). From these compounds 50 different structural features were derived, 16 of which were eliminated by variance weighting and 14 on account of their rare occurrence. The remaining structural features were used for classification. Among them the ratio of the number of C—S bonds to the total number of C atoms as well as the number of SH groups turned out to be of outstanding importance for activity. This led to the conclusion that an increase in the number of C—S bonds or SH groups is almost certain to give active compounds. However, on closer inspection of the compounds and the data it is seen that with only one exception the sulphur atom always occurs in position 6 of the purine molecule. The features referred to above are therefore misleading. It would rather have to be concluded that *sulphur in position 6* of a purine ring represents a substructure extremely favourable for biological activity [110]. Other problems which may arise in this example from relations among the various structural

Table 11.19. Application of the LLM and the KNN method in QSAR work (examples for the application of other pattern recognition methods not included)

Biological activity and classes	Method	Error of reclassification	Reference
Sedatives and tranquilizers	KNN	17%	[105]
	KNN	5%	[106][1])
	KNN	16%	[107][1])
	KNN	10%	[108]
	LLM	10%[2])	[43, 111]
	LLM	10%[2])	[112]
Antitumor, active and inactive compounds	KNN	6.5–10%[2])	[109][3])
	LLM		
	KNN		[48][4])
	LLM		
	LLM	0–17%	[51]
	KNN		
	LLM	10–26%	[113]
	KNN		
Carcinogens, active and inactive	LLM	4.5%	[114]
	KNN		
	LLM	0–23%	[115]
	KNN		
	LLM	20%	[121]
Duration of action of barbiturates	LLM	5–6%[2])	[116]
Analgesics, antidepressive, antihistaminic, anticholinergic and anti-Parkinson drugs	KNN	40–22%	[117]
Herbicides, active and inactive compounds	LLM	12%	[118]
Inhibitors of succinate dehydrogenase, active and inactive compounds	LLM	5%	[119]
	KNN		
Olfactory stimulants, active and inactive compounds	LLM	7%	[43]
Trigeminal compounds, active and inactive	LLM	7–21%	[43]
Analgesics and antispasmodic agents	LLM	15–18%	[120]
	KNN		

[1]) Critisize the data set used in [105] as nonrepresentative since the sedatives as well as the tranquilizers are structurally very similar; this makes the separation of the two classes a more or less trivial task.

[2]) Leave — 1 — out technique.

[3]) The weighting of features in this work was critisized by MATHEWS [47a] who argued that several features with a high weight are, in fact, not important. This work was also critisized by UNGER [110] who showed that some of the features selected lead to erreneous conclusions.

[4]) See text.

features have been pointed out be MATHEWS [47a], who stressed that the chemist should be consulted at all stages of pattern recognition.

The validity of pattern recognition results is highly dependent on how representative are the training series and the biological data. If the structural variations within the training series are too narrow the predictive power of the resulting classificator is, of course, limited. The result is also not independent of the specific methods used for data preprocessing, feature selection and derivation of the classificator. It is recommended that the result be verified by applying leave-n-out techniques. The result can be trusted only if the classificator remains stable during such procedures. In some cases it may be advantageous to apply molecular parameters characterizing certain physical properties of the molecules or parts of them along with substructural descriptors.

The possibility to arrive at conclusions as to which substructures are of special importances for the biological eff ectconsidered has already been mentioned. Such conclusions may allow one, to a certain extent, to arrive at hypotheses on which processes are involved in the production of the biological effect and which substructures might be considered of having the character of topological pharmacophoric groups. The knowledge of such groups should, in principle, allow the design of novel structures expected to exert the type of response under investigation (lead generation). Such approaches are certainly useful (see also 11.2.4.) but, as will be shown in more detail in 11.2.6. and 12., the information presented by such topological pharmacophores on the complex events taking place at a receptor is, of course, very limited.

For the sake of completeness two other approaches useful in visualizing a classification or clustering of compounds should be mentioned. The first concerns *cluster analysis* [122—124] briefly discussed already in section 8.1. This method finds clusters of similar objects in a given feature space but does not result in a classificator. Another possibility is provided by the so-called *display methods* (see e.g. [43, 46]. In essence, these methods project an m-dimensional feature space into a two- or three-dimensional space in such a way that as much information as possible is retained. The latter can then be simply inspected by eye. A typical example is the map presented in Fig. 8.1. Some more examples will be briefly discussed in section 13.2. (see also [65, 66, 125]).

11.2.6. Heuristic Approach to Topological Pharmacophores [67, 68]

This approach is based on

— position coding,
— division of the compounds of a training series into classes according to a biological property of interest, such as the strength of a response (e.g., differentiation between active and inactive compounds), the quality of an effect (differentiation between agonists, partial agonists and antagonists) or the type of an effect (differentiation with respect to specificity),
— stepwise and iterative generation of complex from simple features using logical operations (similar to the logico-structural approach, 11.2.4.),
— analysis of the relative frequencies of occurrence of features within different classes of biological activity using, as a criterion, SHANNONS entropy in multiclass cases.

As a result features are found which are typical of one particular class which means that they are present in this but not in the other classes. These features are believed to constitute a topological pharmacophore so that their presence in a compound is considered necessary (but not sufficient) for this compound to possess the biological property characteristic of the class considered. As will follow from a more detailed discussion on pharmacophores presented in chapter 12., results of such simple topological considerations cannot be expected to be truly representative of the complex three-dimensional events taking place at the receptor. Since, however, the evaluation of true three-dimensional pharmacophores of general validity is still an extremely difficult task, approximate approaches at different levels of sophistication are justified and, in fact, necessary. The concept of topological pharmacophores goes far back into the history of medicinal chemistry and pharmacology, and in spite of the limited validity and predictive power of such pharmacophores they have been used quite successfully in the stepwise development of drugs and systematization of drug actions (see, e.g., [126]). In the past the evaluation of pharmacophores has mainly been by simple inspection and intuitive reasoning using principles of analogy and similarity. The approach to be discussed in this section uses the same principles on a somewhat higher level, namely with a computer-based and thus more efficient and objective method. Since this method works along the same lines as the medicinal chemist is used to think and is interactively guided by him, he can make full use of his experience and intuition.

Let us first consider the generation of the basic feature set. The procedure used here is similar to that of CAMMARATA and MENON [65, 66]. An *artificial supermolecule* (*reference diagram*) is constructed in a first step by superposing all compounds of the training series. This supermolecule represents the basic structure common to all compounds as well as the structural variations possible. For the examples considered in this chapter the supermolecule could be evaluated by simple inspection. For larger series with more complicated structures, however, this will usually not be possible; in such cases the supermolecule should be generated by computer.

In the next step all molecules of the training series are superposed one at a time over the supermolecule, and substructural descriptors are generated by comparing the features present. Thus, the descriptor vector obtained for each compound has as many elements as the number of variable features present in the supermolecule, each descriptor indicating whether a given feature of the supermolecule is present or absent in a given molecule. The value of the j-th descriptor (corresponding to the j-th feature of the supermolecule) of the i-th compound is thus defined as:

$$x_{ji} = \begin{cases} 1, \text{ if feature } j \text{ is present in compound } i \\ 0, \text{ if not} \end{cases} \qquad (11/69)$$

The descriptor space can be extended by the logical operators "not" (*negation*, symbolized by a "$\sim$" sign) and "or" (*disjunction*, symbolized by a "$\vee$" sign). A negation means that the absence of the j-th feature is considered important and is used as a new feature. The corresponding descriptor for the i-th compound is then defined by:

$$\sim x_{ji} = \begin{cases} 1, \text{ if feature } j \text{ is } \textit{not} \text{ present in compound } i \\ 0, \text{ if it is present} \end{cases} \qquad (11/70)$$

The operator "*or*" combines several single features into one new feature. If, for example, F, Cl, Br and J in a certain position of the supermolecule are originally considered as four different features it may often be convenient to combine them into a common feature for halogens. The corresponding descriptor for the i-th compound would then be defined as:

$$x_{halogen,i} = \begin{cases} 1, \text{ if F } or \text{ Cl } or \text{ Br } or \text{ J (if halogen) is present in compound } i \\ 0, \text{ if not} \end{cases} \quad (11/71)$$

In the next step the following quantities are calculated for each feature:

— a_{kj} = number of occurrence of feature j in class k

$$(k = 1, \ldots, m) \quad (11/72)$$

— $p_{kj} = a_{kj}/n_k$
n_k = number of compounds in class k
p_{kj} = relative frequency of occurrence of feature j in class k

— $$P_{kj} = p_{kj} \Big/ \sum_{k=1}^{m} p_{kj} \quad (11/73)$$

P_{kj} = probability of occurrence of feature j in class k defined as the relative frequency of occurrence normalized to 1

— $$H_j' = -\left(\sum_{k=1}^{m} P_{kj} \log P_{kj}\right) (1/\log m) \quad (11/74)$$

H_j' = entropy according to Shannon [127—129], normalized to 1[1]). The entropy is only needed in multi-class problems. In two-class problems the same information can be obtained directly from the P_{kj}'s (see below).

The task now is to construct *conjunctions of features* for the classes of interest by the logical operation "and" which is indicated by a "$\wedge$" sign in a stepwise process. A conjunction of two features, say j and r, means that the two are combined into one new and more complex feature indicating the presence of both of them according to:

$$x_{ji} \wedge x_{ri} = \begin{cases} 1, \text{ if features } j \text{ } and \text{ } r \text{ are present in compound } i \\ 0, \text{ if not} \end{cases} \quad (11/75)$$

More features can be added to the conjunction by the same operation. Adding a third feature s to the above conjunction, for example, would result in:

$$x_{ji} \wedge x_{ri} \wedge x_{si} = \begin{cases} 1, \text{ if features } j \text{ } and \text{ } r \text{ } and \text{ } s \text{ are present in compound } i \\ 0, \text{ if not} \end{cases} \quad (11/76)$$

---

1) Shannons entropy, H, is a measure of information and should not be mixed up with the thermodynamic entropy, S.

The single features are added step by step to the conjunctions in an iterative process so that more and more complex features are generated resembling larger substructures of the supermolecule. For each new feature all the above quantities are calculated. The process is continued until, in the ideal case, a conjunction (a complex substructure of the supermolecule) is found which is typical of only one class (the corresponding P_{kj} becomes 1). This substructure is then regarded as the topological pharmacophore.

As guiding criteria in this procedure the p_{kj} and P_{kj} or, in multi-class problems, the normalized entropy H_j' are used. The entropy is a measure of the distribution of features over the classes. It will be maximal if a feature is equally distributed ($P_{1j} = P_{2j} = \cdots = P_{mj}$) and equal to 0, if a feature occurs in one class only (one of the probabilities P_{kj} becomes unity). Because of the normalization by multiplying with ($1/\log m$) according to eqn. (11/74), the maximal value of H_j' is always 1 independent of the number of classes.

The stepwise development of conjunctions requires a decision of the operator in each step. Let us consider first the most simple case of two classes of biological activity, where only one class (class 1) represents a specific biological effect. This is true, for instance, if compounds active with respect to an interesting biological activity (specific effect) are to be compared with inactive ones (no specific effect). It is obvious that the existence of a pharmacophore can only be expected in the class of active compounds (class 1). The search of a pharmacophore for inactivity would be meaningless. The pharmacophore for activity must then meet the condition that it is present in all of the active and in none of the inactive compounds. In other words for the final conjunction of features p_{1j} and P_{1j} must be 1 in the ideal case. The construction of this conjunction is performed in the following steps (index 1 refers to the class of active compounds and index 2 to inactive compounds):

— Poorly represented features with

$$p_{ij} < 1/m = 1/2$$

and equally distributed features with

$$P_{1j} = P_{2j} = 0.5$$

are eliminated.

— Features with $P_{1j} < P_{2j}$ are also eliminated because they cannot be considered as typical of class 1 (active compounds).

— All features with $p_{1j} = 1$ are selected, and from these features the first conjunction is constructed using those two features which have the highest values of P_{1j}.

— p_{1j} and P_{1j} are calculated for this conjunction, and from the remaining features that with the highest P_{1j} is added.

— This procedure is continued until P_{1j} becomes unity. The corresponding conjunction has the desired property: it is present in the active compounds and absent from all inactive compounds. In other words, the features contained in this conjunction are essential for a compound to belong to class 1, and this set of features will therefore be called "*essential pharmacophore*". Sometimes it is not possible to increase P_{1j} to 1 with only those features having $p_{1j} = 1$. In such cases conjunctions with $p_{1j} = 1$ and $P_{1j} \gg P_{2j}$ or with $P_{1j} = 1$ and $p_{1j} \approx 0.8$ may be accepted as a good approximation of the essential pharmacophore.

— Some of the features with $p_{1j} < 1$ may also be important for the specific effect considered. They are added to such conjunctions which already have a high P_{1j} to see whether they increase P_{1j} (in the ideal case, to a value of one). These features are not present in all compounds of class 1, but they are nevertheless to be considered as pharmacophoric groups in the sense that they support the production of the effect investigated. These features will therefore be called "*supporting pharmacophore*".

It may be that several different conjunctions fulfil the conditions mentioned above. In this case it may be concluded that different pharmacophores exist (corresponding to different mechanisms of action). It is an advantage of this procedure that it can account for the existence of more than one pharmacophore to a certain extent. For such cases, however, its limits will soon be reached. Extended and modified versions were therefore, developed which can adequately handle such situations [130, 131].

In multi-class problems, the entropy H_j' is used as a criterion for the stepwise construction of conjunctions. Features are selected in the order of entropy and the conjunction is complete if the entropy becomes 0 or close to 0; P_{kj} for the class considered is then 1 or approximately equal to 1. The same procedure as outlined above is also used here.

The approach is very flexible and makes full use of the intuition and experience of medicinal chemists. In spite of this, it is, however, not possible to violate the algorithm according to preformed ideas or wishes. In the examples considered in the next sections attempts were made to force the algorithm into routes different from those resulting from the criteria presented above, but without success. Either no acceptable result at all was obtained or the different routes led to exactly the same result.

The definition of the reference diagram is a very critical step. If it is poorly designed the resulting pharmacophore (if any) will also contain only poor information and may be grossly misleading. The procedure may also be applied to non-position coded substructural features which extends its applicability to large series with wide variations in chemical structure. Since such features bear less information than position-coded ones the result will also be less informative.

In two-class cases the method may also be regarded as a feature selection technique since a pharmacophore by its very definition constitutes a set of features typical of one and atypical of the other classes. Such a set will, of course, have optimal discriminating power and can be used directly to derive a good separating hypersurface in the linear learning machine (see 11.2.5.). In multiclass cases, however, this is no longer true. Here, the optimal set for a classificator will comprise those features which have the highest power for the simultaneous separation of all classes which may thus be regarded as representing typical "between-classes" properties. The topological pharmacophore, on the other hand, represents the typical "within-classes" properties and thus yields a different type of information.

Once topological pharmacophores are known they can be used to design new structures (lead generation). Their scope is, of course, limited to those features actually appearing in them but can be extended by introducing bioisosteric features. As already pointed out, they are only a rather crude approximation and valid only insofar as the complex three-dimensional events of drug-receptor interactions can at least approximately be reflected by simple topological considerations. Furthermore, the result of an analysis will depend heavily on the structural variations in the training series since the pharmacophore can only reflect such substructures adequately presented in the compounds investigated. In spite of these limitations, the information contained in such pharmacophores may still be very useful for guiding practical work or as starting hypotheses for more sophisticated approaches (see 12.). The method outlined here is rapid and straightforward and certainly more powerful than a simple inspection of data. No large computer is needed, and it may even be implemented on a small desk-top-calculator. In the following sections two examples will be discussed. The results are not thought or meant to represent new pharmacological knowledge. Rather, the examples were selected to be as simple as possible in order to illustrate the main steps of the procedure in some detail.

11.2.6.1. Example 1: Intrinsic and Affinity Pharmacophore for Phenethylamine Adrenergic Agonists and Antagonists [68]

A series of 15β-agonists and 17β-antagonists of the general structure XLIII was investigated by Mukherjee et al. [132] using racemic mixtures. Structure-activity relationships in this series have recently been investigated by Dunn, Wold and Martin [133] by using SIMCA classification (see 9.2.1.) and the data of intrinsic activity α (relative to isoprenaline) as well as the potency log A to stimulate (agonists) or to inhibit agonist stimulation (antagonists) of the β-adrenergic coupled adenylate cyclase have been taken directly from their paper.

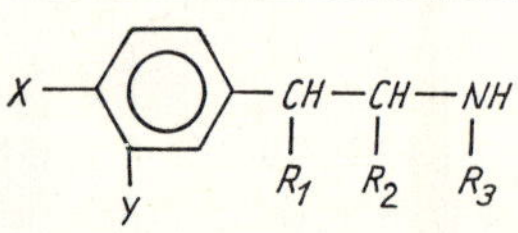

X : OH, H, Cl, $NHSO_2CH_3$, $CH_2SO_2NH_2$

Y: OH, H, Cl, $NHSO_2CH_3$, $CH_2SO_2N(CH_3)_2$, OCH_3

R_1: OH, H

R_2: H, CH_3, C_2H_5, $C(CH_3)_3$

R_3: H, CH_3, C_2H_5, $CH(C_2H_4)_2$, $CHCH_3O_2$, $C(CH_3)_2CH_2C_6H_5$
$CH(CH_3)CH_2C_6H_4$-4-OH, $CH(CH_3)CH_2C_6H_3$-3,4-OCH_2O-
$CH_2CH_2C_6H_4$-4-OH, $CH(CH_3)(CH_2)_2C_6H_4$-4-OH,
$C(CH_3)_2CH_2C_6H_4$-4-OH, $(CH_2)_3C_6H_4$-4-OH

XLIII

The compounds were classified into four classes according to:

class 1: strong agonists ($\alpha > 0$)

$\log A > 5.2$ $(n_1 = 7)$

class 2: weak agonists ($\alpha > 0$)

$\log A < 5.2$ $(n_2 = 8)$

class 3: weak antagonists ($\alpha = 0$)

$\log A < 5.2$ $(n_3 = 8)$

class 4: strong antagonists ($\alpha = 0$)

$\log A > 5.2$ $(n_4 = 9)$

The same classification also results from data on the affinity of the compounds for the β-receptor in vitro. The supermolecule (reference diagram) obtained from superimposing all molecules is presented in Fig. 11.4, and the descriptors are summarized and defined in Table 11.20.

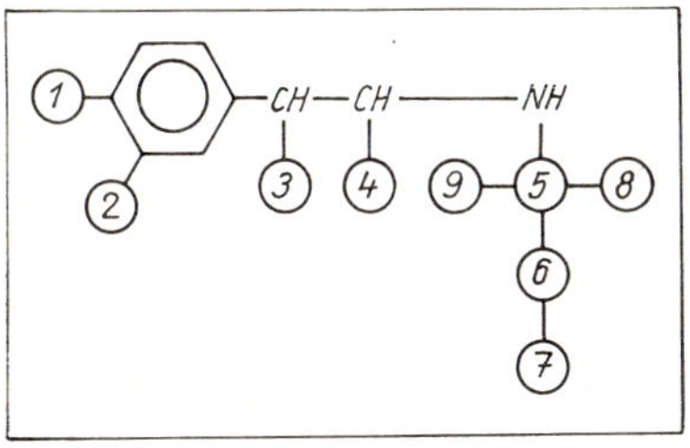

Fig. 11.4. Reference diagram for the phenethanolamines

Table 11.20. Descriptors defined by the supermolecule in Fig. 11.4

Descriptor	equal to 1	equal to 0
x_1	if OH is present in position 1	if not
x_2	if OH or NH— is present in position 2	if not
x_3	if OH is present in position 3	if not
x_4	if a substituent other than hydrogen is present in position 4	if not
x_5	if —C—C— is present in position 5	if not
x_6	if $—CH_2—$ is present in position 6	if not
x_7	if a phenyl ring is attached to the side chain at the nitrogen	if not
x_8	if C_2H_5 is present at position 8 (at the α-C-atom of a —C—C-group in position 5)	if not
x_9	if $—CH_3$ is present in position 9	if not

In a first analysis it was atempted to evaluate pharmacophores for the classes 1, 2, and 4 simultaneously by treating the complete four-class problem. It was not expected to find a pharmacophore in class 3 since the weak antagonists interact much less specifically with the receptor than agonists and strong antagonists. Since more than two classes are to be considered the entropy was used here as indicator for the distribution of the features over the classes. The relative frequencies of occurrence p_1—p_4, the probabilities P_1—P_4 and the entropies of all important features (underrepresented features already eliminated) are summarized in Table 11.21. The conjunctions derived with the entropy as first and p_{kj} as second criterion are summarized in Tables 11.22—11.24. For class 1, features 1, 2, 3, ∼ 4, 5, ∼ 6, and 8 have $p_1 = 1$. Since 8 has the lowest entropy the generation of conjunctions for class 1 starts with this feature (see Table 11.22). By adding features 2, 1 and ∼ 4 the entropy is drastically decreased, and it becomes zero if either feature 3 or ∼ 6 is finally included into the pharmacophore. The resulting two conjunctions can be extended by feature 5 without decreasing p_1, and Table 11.22 shows that the conjunction $8 \wedge 2 \wedge 1 \wedge (\sim 4) \wedge 5$ also has quite a low entropy, a high value of P_1, a low value of P_2 and $P_3 = P_4 = 0$. It is to be concluded, therefore, that this feature is also important for strong agonist activity and has to be included into the pharmacophore for these compounds (class 1). This pharmacophore is presented in Fig. 11.5. The phenyl ring was added in brackets since feature 7 also decreases the entropy but has only quite a low p_1 value (0.571).

The results for class 2 are summarized in Table 11.23. A very simple pharmacophore results which is shown in Fig. 11.6. This pharmacophore which is also present in class 1 (Fig. 11.5) is probably essential for intrinsic activity.

Table 11.21. Relative frequencies of occurrence (p_1—p_4), probabilities (P_1—P_4), and the entropy H' of single features in classes 1—4 (indices refer to class numbers); non-relevant features already eliminated

Feature	p_1	p_2	p_3	p_4	P_1	P_2	P_3	P_4	H'
1	1.000	1.000	0.125	0.556	0.373	0.373	0.047	0.207	0.859
2	1.000	1.000	0.500	0.222	0.367	0.367	0.184	0.082	0.903
3	1.000	0.625	1.000	1.000	0.276	0.172	0.276	0.276	0.987
4	0.000	0.500	0.375	0.667	0.000	0.324	0.243	0.433	0.773
∼4	1.000	0.500	0.625	0.333	0.407	0.203	0.253	0.135	0.942
5	1.000	0.625	0.250	1.000	0.348	0.217	0.087	0.348	0.922
∼6	1.000	0.625	1.000	0.889	0.285	0.178	0.285	0.253	0.996
7	0.571	0.375	0.000	0.444	0.395	0.259	0.000	0.346	0.782
8	1.000	0.375	0.125	0.889	0.419	0.157	0.052	0.372	0.849

Table 11.22. Stepwise development of conjunctions for class 1 versus classes 2—4: relative frequencies of occurrence (p_1—p_4), probabilities (P_1—P_4), and entropy (H'); the indices refer to class numbers

Features in conjunction	p_1	p_2	p_3	p_4	P_1	P_2	P_3	P_4	H'
8	1.000	0.375	0.125	0.889	0.419	0.157	0.052	0.372	0.849
8 ∧ 2	1.000	0.375	0.000	0.222	0.626	0.235	0.000	0.139	0.655
8 ∧ 2 ∧ 1	1.000	0.375	0.000	0.000	0.727	0.273	0.000	0.000	0.423
8 ∧ 2 ∧ 1 ∧ (∼4)	1.000	0.125	0.000	0.000	0.889	0.111	0.000	0.000	0.251
8 ∧ 2 ∧ 1 ∧ (∼4) ∧ 3	1.000	0.000	0.000	0.000	1.000	0.000	0.000	0.000	0.000
8 ∧ 2 ∧ 1 ∧ (∼4) ∧ 3 ∧ 5	1.000	0.000	0.000	0.000	1.000	0.000	0.000	0.000	0.000
8 ∧ 2 ∧ 1 ∧ (∼4) ∧ 5	1.000	0.125	0.000	0.000	0.889	0.111	0.000	0.000	0.251

Table 11.23. Stepwise development of conjunctions for class 2 versus classes 1, 3, and 4: relative frequencies of occurrence (p_1—p_4), probabilities (P_1—P_4), and entropy (H'); the indices refer to class numbers

Features in conjunction	p_1	p_2	p_3	p_4	P_1	P_2	P_3	P_4	H'
1	1.000	1.000	0.125	0.556	0.373	0.373	0.047	0.207	0.859
1 ∧ 2	1.000	1.000	0.000	0.000	0.500	0.500	0.000	0.000	0.500

Table 11.24 shows the results for class 4. It is very interesting that the probabilities for the conjunctions 5 ∧ 3 are the same for the two classes with high affinity (classes 1 and 4) and also for the two classes with low affinity. This indicates that these features are probably connected with affinity. The conjunction 5 ∧ 3 ∧ ~ 2 decreases the entropy to a reasonable value but is only present in 77.8% of the compounds in this class. Addition of feature 4 brings the entropy to zero, but at the same time, p_4 decreases to 55.5%. If feature 8 is added instead of 4 the entropy is still reasonable low, and p_4 amounts to 0.666. The probabilities of feature 8 indicate that it is probably also involved in strong antagonist activity so that the pharmacophore presented in Fig. 11.7 is revealed for class 4.

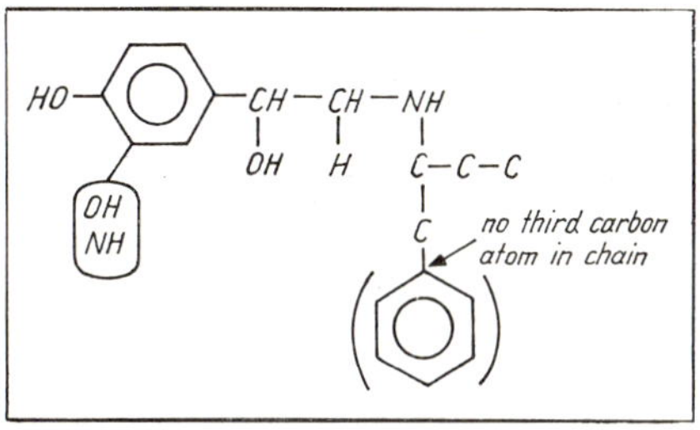

Fig. 11.5. Pharmacophore for strong β-agonists (class 1)

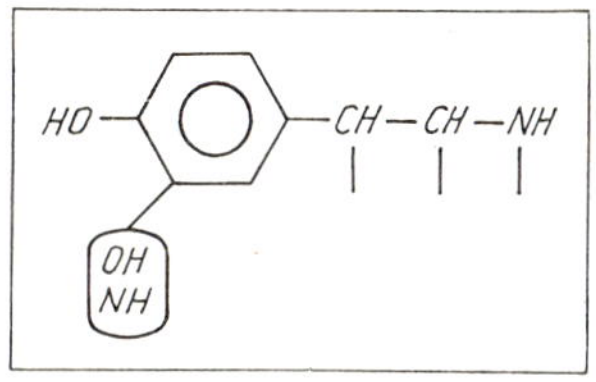

Fig. 11.6. Pharmacophore for weak β-agonists (class 2)

Table 11.24. Stepwise development of conjunctions for class 4 versus classes 1—3: relative frequencies of occurence (p_1—p_4), probabilities (P_1—P_4), and entropy (H'); the indices refer to class numbers

Features in conjunction	p_1	p_2	p_3	p_4	P_1	P_2	P_3	P_4	H'
5	1.000	0.675	0.250	1.000	0.348	0.217	0.087	0.348	0.922
5 ∧ 3	1.000	0.250	0.250	1.000	0.400	0.100	0.100	0.400	0.861
5 ∧ 3 ∧ (~ 2)	0.000	0.000	0.125	0.778	0.000	0.000	0.138	0.862	0.289
5 ∧ 3 ∧ (~ 2) ∧ 4	0.000	0.000	0.000	0.555	0.000	0.000	0.000	1.000	0.000
5 ∧ 3 ∧ (~ 2) ∧ 8	0.000	0.000	0.125	0.666	0.000	0.000	0.158	0.842	0.315

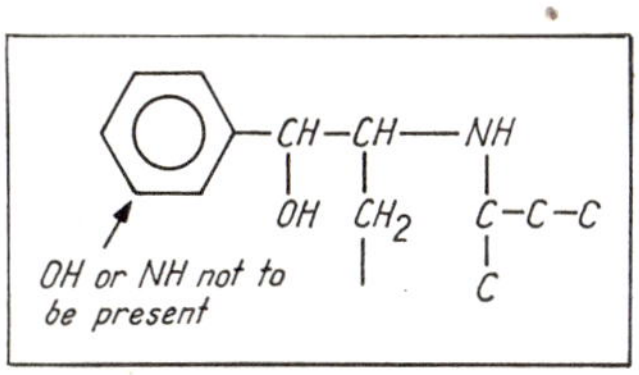

Fig. 11.7. Pharmacophore for strong β-antagonists (class 4)

By comparing the pharmacophores for classes 1, 2 and 4 some further conclusions are possible. The branched carbon chain at the nitrogen as well as the hydroxy group at the β-C-atom appear in both the pharmacophore of the strong agonists and that of the strong antagonists (Figs. 11.5 and 11.7). This can only be explained by assuming that these groups are involved in receptor binding and constitute the *affinity pharmacophore*. The parmacophore for weak agonists (Fig. 11.6) also contained in the pharmacophore for strong agonists (Fig. 11.5) probably reflects the basic requirements for agonist activity and may thus be referred to as the *essential intrinsic pharmacophore*. The differences between the pharmacophore in Fig. 11.5 and those in Figs. 11.6 and 11.7 lead to the conclusion that an unsubstituted α-C-atom and the presence of the phenyl ring in the side chain at the nitrogen support intrinsic activity. These features may therefore be regarded as the *supporting intrinsic pharmacophore*. All these conclusions which could be verified in [68] through some additional analyses are summarized in Fig. 11.8. This result is in agreement with well-known facts on the structural requirements for β-adrenergic compounds. Since only phenethylamines were present in the training series the pharmacophore is only valid for this group of compounds and only insofar as the compounds included in the training series are truly representative of this family. No conclusions on, for example, the effect of replacing the phenyl by a heterocyclic ring, are possible. Thus, this example clearly demonstrates that the result cannot be more representative than is the training series.

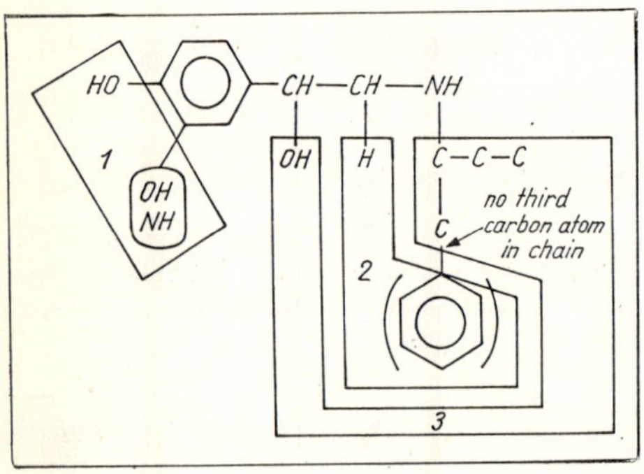

Fig. 11.8. Suggested pharmacophore for β-agonists from the phenethenolamine series. 1 = essential intrinsic pharmacophore; 2 = supporting intrinsic pharmacophore; 3 = affinity pharmacophore

11.2.6.2. Example 2: Carboxamides as Inhibitors of Succinate Dehydrogenase [68]

These compounds have already been dealt with in 9.2.2.2.1. where the results of a discriminant analysis were presented, together with details on the structures and biological activity. In applying the topological pharmacophore approach to this training series two questions were investigated:

1. What is the essential topological pharmacophore for active compounds?
2. Is it possible to find a supporting pharmacophore for very active compounds?

For the first problem, the compounds were divided into two classes according to:

class 1: active compounds

$$pI_{50} \geqq 0.40 \qquad n_1 = 64$$

class 2: inactive compounds

$$pI_{50} < 0.40 \qquad n_2 = 25$$

The second problem requires another classification since it is connected with the gradation of activity within the class of active compounds. In the search for the supporting pharmacophore, therefore, very active compounds were compared with weakly active ones using the following classification:

class 3: very active compounds

$$pI_{50} \geqq 3.00 \qquad n_3 = 14$$

class 4: weakly active compounds

$$0.40 \leqq pI_{50} < 1.6 \qquad n_4 = 14$$

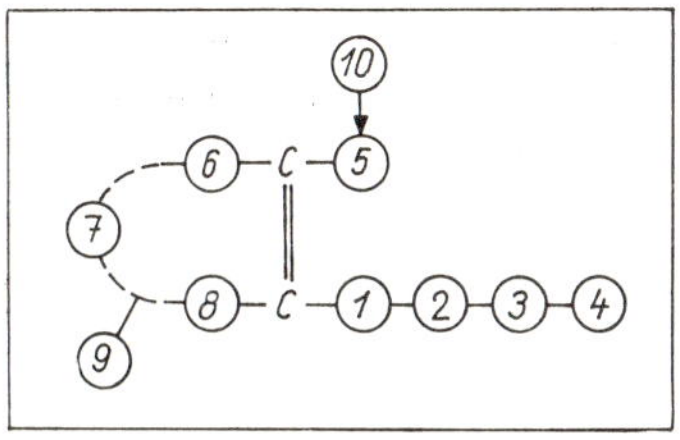

Fig. 11.9. Reference diagram for the carboxamides

The reference diagram used is presented in Fig. 11.9, and the descriptors are summarized in Table 11.25. The variables x_4 and x_6 are already disjunctions from single features which are only poorly represented alone. These disjunctions are:

$$x_4 = \begin{cases} 1, \text{ if a substituent with } \pi > 0 \text{ is present in ortho- or meta- or para-position} \\ 0, \text{ if not} \end{cases} \tag{11/77}$$

$$x_6 = \begin{cases} 1, \text{ if N or S or O is present in position 6} \\ 0, \text{ if not} \end{cases} \tag{11/78}$$

Since only two-class problems are treated in this example, it is not necessary to calculate entropies; the same information can be obtained directly from the probabilities P_1 and P_2.

The relative frequencies of occurrence and the probabilities of all relevant features for the first problem (active versus inactive compounds) are summarized in Table 11.26. Features 9 and 10 had to be eliminated because they are underrepresented. Table 11.27 shows the stepwise development of conjunctions using p_1 as primary and P_1 as secondary criterion. In the fourth step a conjunction with the features 5, 3, 1 and 2 is found which appears in practically all (98.4%) of the active compounds with a very high probability (0.925) for class 1 and a very low probability for class 2 (0.075). There is only one active compound which does not contain the complete set of these features and only one inactive compound in which this set is present. These exceptions might well be due to errors of measurement so that features 5, 3, 1 and 2 together with the C=C-group already included into the reference diagram (see Fig. 11.9) obviously constitute the *essential pharmacophore* for enzyme inhibiting potency (see Fig. 11.10).

Table 11.25. Descriptors defined by the supermolecule in Fig. 11.9

Descriptor	equal to 1	equal to 0
x_1	if CO in position 1	if not
x_2	if NH or NCH_3 in position 2	if not
x_3	if phenyl or cyclohexyl in position 3	if not
x_4	if substituents with π[1]) > 0 are present in *o*-, *m*-, or *p*-position of a phenyl ring in position 3	if not
x_5	if a substituent other than H or F is present in position 5	if not
x_6	if N, S, or O are in position 6	if not
x_7	if a six-membered ring is present in X (structure XL)	if not
x_8	if S is present in position 8	if not
x_9	if a methyl-substituent is present in m-position to position 1	if not
x_{10}	if a substituent with size greater than methyl is present in position 5	if not

[1]) hydrophobic substituent constant

Table 11.26. Relative frequencies of occurence (p_1, p_2) and probabilities (P_1, P_2) of relevant single features in class 1 (index 1: active compounds) and class 2 (index 2: inactive compounds)

Feature	p_1	p_2	P_1	P_2
1	1.000	0.880	0.532	0.468
2	1.000	0.920	0.521	0.479
3	1.000	0.800	0.556	0.444
4	0.609	0.080	0.884	0.116
5	0.984	0.440	0.691	0.309
6	0.641	0.240	0.727	0.273
7	0.609	0.440	0.581	0.419
8	0.453	0.320	0.586	0.414

Table 11.27. Stepwise development of conjunctions for class 1 versus class 2: relative frequencies of occurence (p_1, p_2) and probabilities (P_1, P_2); the indices refer to class numbers

Features in conjunction	p_1	p_2	P_1	P_2
5	0.984	0.800	0.691	0.309
$5 \wedge 3$	0.984	0.240	0.804	0.196
$5 \wedge 3 \wedge 1$	0.984	0.120	0.891	0.109
$5 \wedge 3 \wedge 1 \wedge 2$	0.984	0.080	0.925	0.075
$(5 \wedge 3 \wedge 1 \wedge 2) \wedge 6$	0.641	0.040	0.941	0.059
$(5 \wedge 3 \wedge 1 \wedge 2) \wedge 4$	0.594	0.000	1.000	0.000
$(5 \wedge 3 \wedge 1 \wedge 2) \wedge 4 \wedge 6$	0.406	0.000	1.000	0.000

If features 4 or 6 are added to the conjunction representing the essential pharmacophore P_1 eventually increases to 1 and P_2 becomes zero. These extended sets of features are still present in a reasonably high percentage of the active compounds. Since as follows from Table 11.26, features 4 and 6 already alone have $P_1 \ll P_2$ it is to be concluded that both are typical of active compounds and form part of the supporting pharmacophore (see Fig. 11.10). This view is fully supported by the results of the second two-class problem (with the features already present in the essential pharmacophore discarded) which are summarized in Tables 11.28 and 11.29. After eliminating poorly represented and equally distributed ($P_3 = P_4 = 0.500$) features, only the features 4, 6 and 8 remain to be considered. All three of them are fairly well represented in class 3 and have $P_3 > P_4$. The most important feature is 6 which is present in 85.7% of the very active compounds with $P_3 = 0.706$. Adding 4 or 8 increases P_3 to 0.818, and the combination of all three features has a very high P_3 and is still present in 50% of the very active compounds, but only in 7% of the weakly active compounds. It thus follows that these three features are important for activity and form the *supporting pharmacophore.*

Table 11.28. Relative frequencies of occurence (p_3, p_4) and probabilities (P_3, P_4) of single features in class 3 (index 3: very active compounds) and class 4 (index 4: weakly active compounds)

Feature	p_3	p_4	P_3	P_4
4	0.714	0.429	0.625	0.375
6	0.857	0.357	0.706	0.294
7	0.643	0.643	0.500	0.500
8	0.643	0.286	0.692	0.308
9	0.357	0.214	0.625	0.375

Table 11.29. Stepwise development of conjunctions for class 3 versus class 4: relative frequencies of occurence (p_3, p_4) and probabilities (P_3, P_4); the indices refer to class numbers

Features in conjunction	p_3	p_4	P_3	P_4
6	0.857	0.357	0.706	0.294
$6 \wedge 4$	0.643	0.143	0.818	0.182
$6 \wedge 8$	0.643	0.143	0.818	0.182
$6 \wedge 4 \wedge 8$	0.500	0.071	0.875	0.125

The whole pharmacophore is represented in Fig. 11.10. Essential for enzyme inhibiting activity is the intact carboxamide group, the presence of a substituent larger than hydrogen or fluorine in position 5 and the presence of a ring in position 3 (see Fig. 11.9). Activity is enhanced by hydrophobic substituents in the ring, by the presence of heteroatoms in position 6 and by the presence of sulphur in position 8. As far as variation goes in the series, no importance of the features 7, 9 and 10 can be detected by the method used. This pharmacophore is in good accord with the results of discriminant analysis presented in 9.2.2.2.1. Apart from slight differences in the definition of indicator variables used there, the discriminant function (9/75) separating active from inactive compounds tells the same story as the essential pharmacophore.

If a separating hypersurface for the classes 1 and 2 is evaluated by means of the linear learning machine using the same features but a different feature selection procedure the result of the essential pharmacophore is confirmed [134]. The feature selection step finds the features 1, 2, 3 and 4 as optimal set, and the classificator (see eqn. (11/64) has the form:

$$\boldsymbol{w}^T\boldsymbol{x} = 0.360x_1 + 0.162x_2 + 0.408x_3 + 0.367x_4 + 0.316 \qquad (11/79)$$

This classificator correctly reclassifies 97% of the compounds of the training series.

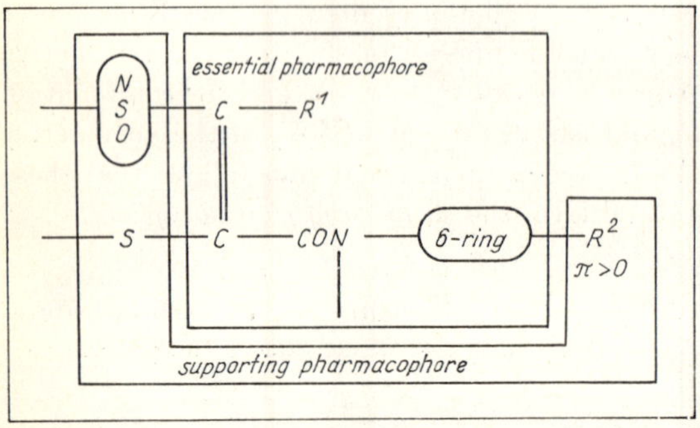

Fig. 11.10. Essential and supporting pharmacophore for the inhibition of succinate dehydrogenase by carboxamides and related compounds

Finally, the results of discriminant analysis for the separation of the classes of active compounds (eqn. (9/77) and Table 9.21) nicely resemble the supporting pharmacophore. If, for the sake of simplicity, only the first five most important variables (discriminant function (9/77)) are considered, the following picture is obtained. The first term depends on the features 6, 7 and 8, and the second term reflects feature 6. All of these features except 7, which is underrepresented and thus was eliminated, are also present in the supporting pharmacophore (Fig. 11.10). It was not clear why $\sigma_m{}^2(X)$ does a better job than $\sigma_m(X)$ in the discriminant function. With the knowledge of the supporting pharmacophore the reason becomes evident: like x_6, $\sigma_m{}^2(X)$ discriminates between heteroatoms in position 6 (Fig. 11.9) and carbon whereas $\sigma_m(X)$ does not. The $MR_0(R_X)$ term indicates that activity increases with increasing size of substituents in position 5 corresponding to feature 10. This information could not be obtained in the present study since feature 10 was only poorly represented and had to be eliminated.

Finally, the importance of substituents in position 4 for activity expressed by the supporting pharmacophore is reflected by the last two terms of the discriminant function.

As a whole, the agreement between the results from discriminant analysis, the linear learning machine and from the present investigation is very acceptable. The present method, however, is certainly more rapid and efficient than discriminant analysis if complex structural modifications as those in this example occur which are mostly difficult to describe in terms of continuous physical-chemical parameters. It has the further advantage that the result is directly obtained in structural terms whereas a discriminant function has to be translated back to structure; this is not always easy because of collinearities which may occur between different parameters.

References

[1] Free, S. M., and J. W. Wilson: J. Med. Chem. **7**, 395 (1964)
[2] Purcell, W. P., G. E. Bass and J. M. Clayton: Strategy of Drug Design, Wiley, New York, 1973
[3] Cammarata, A.: J. Med. Chem. **15**, 573 (1972)
[4] Craig, P. N.: Adv. in Chemistry Series **114**, 115 (1972)
[5] Gäbler, E., R. Franke and P. Oehme: Pharmazie **31**, 1 (1976)
[6] Meiske, W., E. Gäbler and R. Franke: Pharmazie **31**, 741 (1976)
[7] Kubinyi, H., and O.-H. Kehrhahn: J. Med. Chem. **19**, 578 (1976)
[8] Kubinyi, H.: J. Med. Chem. **19**, 587 (1976)
[9] Kubinyi, H., and O.-H. Kehrhahn: J. Med. Chem. **19**, 1040 (1976)
[10] Fujita, T., and T. Ban: J. Med. Chem. **14**, 148 (1971)
[11] Cammarata, A., and S. J. Yau: J. Med. Chem. **13**, 93 (1970)
[12] Hudson, D. R., G. E. Bass and W. P. Purcell: J. Med. Chem. **13**, 1184 (1970)
[13] Purcell, W. P., and J. M. Clayton: J. Med. Chem. **11**, 199 (1968)
[14] Ban, T., and T. Fujita: J. Med. Chem. **12**, 353 (1969)
[15] Cammarata, A., and T. M. Bustard: J. Med. Chem. **17**, 981 (1974)
[16] Boček, K., J. Kopecky, M. Krivucova and D. Vlachová: Experientia **20**, 667 (1964)
[17] Kopecky, J., K. Boček and D. Vlachová: Nature **207**, 981 (1965)
[18] Singer, J. A., and W. P. Purcell: J. Med. Chem. **10**, 1000 (1967)
[19] Schwarz, G., A. Barth and R. Franke: unpublished results
[20] Cammarata, A., and K. S. Rogers in N. B. Chapman and J. Shorter (Eds.): Advances in Linear Free Energy Relationships, Plenum Press, London, 1972, p. 369
[21] Craig, P. N.: J. Med. Chem. **15**, 144 (1972)
[22] Craig, P. N., and C. Hansch: J. Med. Chem. **16**, 661 (1973)
[23] Franke, R., D. Labes, M. Tonew, W. Zschiesche and L. Heinisch: Acta biol. med. germ. **34**, 491 (1975)
[24] Schaad, L. J., B. A. Hess Jr., W. P. Purcell, A. Cammarata, R. Franke and H. Kubinyi: J. Med. Chem. **24**, 900 (1981)
[25] Rösner, R., R. Kühne and R. Franke: Paper presented at the 17. Jahrestagung der Gesellschaft für Pharmakologie und Toxikologie der DDR, Berlin, 1975
[26] Rösner, T., R. Franke and R. Kühne in R. Franke and P. Oehme (Eds.): Quantitative Structure-Activity Analysis, Akademie-Verlag, Berlin, 1978, p. 317
[27] Rösner, R., R. Franke and R. Kühne: Pharmazie **33**, 226 (1978)
[27a] Martin, Y. C., P. H. Jones, T. J. Perun, W. E. Grundy, S. Bell, P. R. Bower and N. L. Shipkowitz: J. Med. Chem. **15**, 635 (1972)
[27b] Magee, P. S., in E. C. Olson and R. E. Christoffersen (Eds.): Computer-Assisted Drug Design, ACS Symp. Ser. **112**, 319 (1979)
[28] Wipke, W. T., S. R. Heller, R. J. Feldmann and E. Hyde (Eds.): Computer Representation and Manipulation of Chemical Information, Wiley, New York, 1974
[29] Feldmann, R. J., W. A. Milne, S. R. Heller, A. Fein, J. A. Miller and B. Koch: J. Chem. Inf. Comput. Sci. **17**, 157 (1977)
[30] Christofferson, R. E.: ACS Symp. Series **46**, (1977)
[31] Friedrich, J., and I. Ugi: Inf. Commun. Math. Chem. **6**, 201 (1979)
[32] Friedrich, J., and I. Ugi: Tables Rondes Roussel Uclaf **38**, 44 (1980)
[33] Friedrich, J., and I. Ugi: J. Chem. Res. (S) **70** (1980)
[34] Friedrich, J., and I. Ugi: J. Chem. Res. (M), 1301, 1401, 1501 (1980)
[35] Schubert, W., and I. Ugi: Chimica **33**, 183 (1979)
[36] Ugi, I., J. Bauer, J. Brandt, J. Friedrich, J. Gasteiger, C. Jochum and W. Schubert: Angew. Chem. (Internat. Ed.) **18**, 111 (1979)

[37] Lynch, M. F., J. M. Harrison, W. G. Town and J. E. Ash: Computer Handling of Chemical Structural Information, Mac Donald, London, 1971

[38] Balaban, A. T.: Chemical Application of Graph Theory, Academic Press, New York, 1976

[39] Feldman, A., and L. Hodes: J. Chem. Inf. Comput. Sci. **15**, 147 (1975)

[40] Hodes, L.: J. Chem. Inf. Comput. Sci. **16**, 88 (1976)

[41] Hodes, L., G. F. Hazard, R. F. Geran and S. Richman: J. Med. Chem. **20**, 469 (1977)

[41a] Hodes, L.: J. Chem. Inf. Comput. Sci. **21**, 132 (1981)

[42] Smith, E. G.: The Wiswesser Line-Formula Chemical Notation, McGraw-Hill, New York, 1968

[42a] Milne, M., D. Lefkovitz and H. Hill: J. Chem. Doc. **12**, 183 (1972)

[43] Stuper, A. J., W. E. Brugger and P. C. Jurs: Computer Assisted Studies of Chemical Structure and Biological Function, Wiley-Interscience, New York, 1979

[43a] Brugger, W. E., A. J. Stuper and P. C. Jurs: J. Chem. Inf. Comput. Sci. **16**, 105 (1976)

[44] Golender, V. E., and A. B. Rozenblit in E. J. Ariens (Ed.): Drug Design, Vol. IX, Academic Press, New York, 1980, p. 300

[44a] Rozenblit, A. B., in J. A. Keverling Buisman (Ed.): Strategy in Drug Research, Pharmacochemistry Library (Eds.: W. Th. Nauta and R. F. Rekker), Vol. 4, Elsevier, Amsterdam, 1982, p. 287

[45] Golender, V. E., and A. B. Rozenblit: Computer Assisted Methods of Drug Design, Zinatne, Riga, 1978 (in Russian)

[46] Kirschner, G. L., and B. R. Kowalski in E. J. Ariens (Ed.): Drug Design, Vol. VIII, Academic Press, New York, 1979, p. 73

[47] Jurs, P. C., J. T. Chou and M. Yuan in E. C. Olson and R. E. Christoffersen (Eds.): Computer-Assisted Drug Design, ACS Symp. Series **112**, 103 (1979)

[47a] Mathews, R. J.: J. Am. Chem. Soc. **97**, 935 (1975)

[48] Chu, K. C., R. J. Feldman, M. B. Shapiro, G. F. Hazard and R. I. Geran: J. Med. Chem. **18**, 539 (1975)

[49] Eakin, D. R. and E. Hyde in W. T. Wipke, S. R. Heller, R. J. Feldmann and E. Hyde (Eds.): Computer Representation and Manipulation of Chemical Information, Wiley, New York, 1974, p. 1

[50] Avidon, V. V.: Khim.-Farm. Zh. **8**, 22 (1974)

[51] Chou, J. T., and P. C. Jurs: J. Med. Chem. **22**, 792 (1979)

[52] Randić, M.: J. Am. Chem. Soc. **97**, 6609 (1975)

[53] Kier, L. B., and L. H. Hall: Molecular Connectivity in Chemistry and Drug Research, Academic Press, New York, 1976

[53a] Kier, L. B., in S. H. Yalkowsky, A. A. Sinkula and S. C. Valvani (Eds.): Physical Chemical Properties of Drugs, Marcel Dekker, New York, 1980, p. 277

[54] Balaban, A. T., A. Chiriac, I. Motoc and Z. Simon: Steric Fit in Quantitative Structure-Activity Relations, Springer-Verlag, Berlin, 1980

[55] Sussenguth, E. H.: J. Chem. Doc. **5**, 36 (1965)

[56] Dugundji, I., and I. Ugi: Topics Curr. Chem. **39**, 19 (1973)

[57] Harris, B.: Graph Theory and Its Application, Academic Press, New York, 1970

[58] Knödel, W.: Graphentheoretische Methoden und ihre Anwendung, Springer-Verlag, Heidelberg, 1969

[59] Gitlina, V. S., V. E. Golender and A. B. Rosenblit: IV. Int. Conf. on Comp. in Chem. Res. and Educ. Abstracts, Novosibirsk, 2—17 (1978)

[60] Cone, M. M., R. Venkataraghavan and F. W. McLaferty: J. Am. Chem. Soc. **98**, 7668 (1977)

[61] Crippen, G. M.: J. Med. Chem. **22**, 988 (1979)

[62] Crippen, G. M.: Tables Rondes Roussel Uclaf, **38**, 28 (1980)

[63] Crippen, G. M.: J. Med. Chem. **23**, 599 (1980)

[64] Crippen, G. M.: Distance Geometry and Conformational Calculations, Research Studies Press, Chichester, 1981
[65] Cammarata, A., and G. K. Menon: J. Med. Chem. **19**, 739 (1976)
[66] Menon, G. K., and A. Cammarata: J. Pharm. Sci. **66**, 304 (1977)
[67] Franke, R.: Tables Rondes Roussel Uclaf **38**, 20 (1980)
[68] Hübel, S., T. Rösner and R. Franke: Pharmazie **35**, 424 (1980)
[68a] Stoltzberg, L. J., and C. L. Wilkins: J. Am. Chem. Soc. **99**, 439 (1977)
[69] Blair, J., J. Gasteiger, C. Gillespie, P. D. Gillespie and I. Ugi: Tetrahedron **30**, 1845 (1974)
[70] Marshall, G. R., in M. A. Simkins (Ed.): Medicinal Chemistry VI, Cotswold Press, Oxford, 1979, p. 225
[71] Marshall, G. R., C. D. Barry, H. E. Bosshard, R. A. Dammkoehler and D. A. Dunn in E. C. Olson and R. E. Christoffersen (Eds.): Computer-Assisted Drug Design, ACS Symp. Ser. **112**, 205 (1979)
[72] Hopfinger, A. J.: J. Am. Chem. Soc. **102**, 7196 (1980)
[72a] Hopfinger, A. J.: Arch. Biochem. Biophys. **206**, 153 (1981)
[72b] Battershell, C., D. Malhotra and A. J. Hopfinger: J. Med. Chem. **24**, 812 (1981)
[73] Hopfinger, A. J.: J. Med. Chem. **24**, 818 (1981)
[74] Dyott, T. M., A. J. Stuper and G. S. Zander: J. Chem. Inf. Comput. Sci. **20**, 28 (1980)
[75] Meyer, Jr., E. F., in E. J. Ariens (Ed.): Drug Design, Vol. IX, Academic Press, New York, 1980, p. 267
[76] Langridge, R., T. E. Ferrin, I. D. Kuntz and M. L. Conolly: Science **211**, 661 (1981)
[77] Mucciardi, A. N., and E. E. Gose: IEEE Trans. Comp. **C-20**, 1023 (1971)
[78] Cramer, R. D., in M. Tichy (Ed.): Quantitative Structure-Activity Relationships, Akadémiai Kiadó, Budapest, 1978
[79] Cramer, R. D., G. Redl and C. E. Berkoff: J. Med. Chem. **17**, 533 (1974)
[80] Redl, G., R. D. Cramer and C. E. Berkoff: Chem.-Soc. Rev. **3**, 273 (1974)
[81] Hodes, L., in E. C. Olson and R. E. Christofferson (Eds.): Computer-Assisted Drug Design, ACS Symp. Series **112**, 583 (1979)
[82] Hodes, L.: J. Chem. Inf. Comput. Sci. **21**, 128 (1981)
[83] Tinker, J.: J. Chem. Inf. Comput. Sci. **21**, 3 (1981)
[83a] Tinker, J. F.: J. Comput. Chem. **2**, 231 (1981)
[84] Duda, R. O., and P. E. Hart: Pattern Classification and Game Analysis, Wiley, New York, 1973
[85] Piruzjan, L. A., V. V. Avidon, A. B. Rozenblit, V. S. Arolovich, V. E. Golender, S. P. Kozlova, E. M. Michailovsky and E. G. Gavrischuk: Khim.- Farm. Zh. **11**, 35 (1977)
[86] Lewi, P. J., in E. J. Ariens (Ed.): Drug Design, Vol. VII, Academic Press, New York, 1976
[87] Shoenfeld, P. S., and J. R. De Voe: Anal. Chem. **48**, 403 R (1976)
[88] Nilsson, N. J.: Learning Machines, McGraw-Hill, New York, 1965
[89] Meisel, W. S.: Computer-Oriented Approaches to Pattern Recognition, Academic Press, New York, 1972
[90] Mendel, J. M., and K. S. Fu (Eds.): Adaptive, Learning and Pattern Recognition Systems: Theory and Applications, Academic Press, New York, 1970
[91] Kowalski, B. R., and C. F. Bender: J. Am. Chem. Soc. **94**, 5632 (1972)
[92] Kowalski, B. R., and C. F. Bender: J. Am. Chem. Soc. **95**, 686 (1973)
[93] Kowalski, B. R., in C. E. Klopfenstein and C. L. Wilkins (Eds.): Computers in Chemical and Biochemical Research, Vol. 2, New York, Academic Press, 1974, p. 1
[94] Kowalski, B. R., and C. F. Bender: Naturwissenschaften **62**, 10 (1975)
[95] Batchelor, B. G.: Practical Approach to Pattern Classification, Plenum Press, New York, 1974
[96] Fu, K. S. (Ed.): Digital Pattern Recognition, Springer-Verlag, New York, 1976

[97] Fukunaga, K.: Introduction to Statistical Pattern Recognition, Academic Press, New York, 1972
[98] Fu, K. S.: IEEE Transactions on Computers **C-25**, 1336 (1976)
[99] Jurs, P. C., and T. L. Isenhour: Chemical Applications of Pattern Recognition, Interscience, New York, 1975
[100] Andrews, H. C.: Introduction to Mathematical Techniques in Pattern Recognition, Wiley, New York, 1972
[101] Watanabe, S. (Ed.): Methodologies of Pattern Recognition, Academic Press, New York, 1969
[102] Streich, J.: Kongreß- und Tagungsberichte der Martin-Luther-Universität Halle-Wittenberg **N 10**, 97 (1981)
[103] Cover, T. M., and P. E. Hart: IEEE Trans. Inf. Theory **IT-13**, 21 (1967)
[104] Hart, P. E.: IEEE Trans. Inf. Theory **IT-14**, 515 (1968)
[105] Ting, K.-L. H., R. C. T. Lee, G. W. A. Milne, M. Shapiro and A. M. Guarino: Science **180**, 417 (1973)
[106] Clerc, J. T., P. Naegeli and J. Seibl: Chimia **27**, 639 (1973)
[107] Perrin, C. L.: Science **183**, 551 (1974)
[108] Chu, K.: Anal. Chem. **46**, 1181 (1974)
[109] Kowalski, B. R., and C. F. Bender: J. Am. Chem. Soc. **96**, 916 (1974)
[110] Unger, S. H.: Cancer Chemotherapy Reports Part 2 4, 45 (1974)
[111] Stuper, A. J., and P. C. Jurs: J. Am. Chem. Soc. **97**, 182 (1975)
[112] Soltzberg, C. J., and C. L. Wilkins: J. Am. Chem. Soc. **99**, 439 (1977)
[113] Jurs, P. C., J. T. Chou and M. Yuan: J. Med. Chem. **22**, 476 (1979)
[114] Yuan, M., and P. C. Jurs: Toxicol. Appl. Pharmacol. **52**, 294 (1980)
[115] Yuta, K., and P. C. Jurs: J. Med. Chem. **24**, 241 (1981)
[116] Stuper, A. J., W. E. Brugger and P. C. Jurs in B. R. Kowalski (Ed.): Chemometrics: Theory and Application, ACS Symp. Series **52**, 165 (1977)
[117] Henry, D. R., and J. H. Block: J. Med. Chem. **22**, 465 (1979)
[118] Schönfelder, D., and R. Franke in R. Franke and P. Oehme (Eds.): Quantitative Structure-Activity Analysis, Akademie-Verlag, Berlin 1978, p. 303
[119] Streich, W. J., and R. Franke: unpublished results
[120] Abe, H., S. Kumazawa, T. Taju and S. Sasaki: Biomed. Mass. Spectrom. **3**, 151 (1976)
[121] Dierdorf, D. S., and B. R. Kowalski: cited in Ref. [46]
[122] Duran, B. S., and P. L. Odell: Cluster Analysis — A Survey, Springer-Verlag, New York, 1974
[123] Everitt, B.: Cluster Analysis, Wiley, New York, 1974
[124] Hartigan, J. A.: Clustering Algorithms, Wiley, New York, 1975
[125] Lewi, P. J., in E. J. Ariens (Ed.): Drug Design, Vol. X, Academic Press, New York, 1980, p. 308
[126] Korokovas, A.: Essentials of Molecular Pharmacology, Wiley, New York, 1970
[127] Shannon, C. E., and W. Weaver: Mathematische Grundlagen der Informationstheorie, Oldenburg-Verlag, München, 1976
[128] Shannon, C. E., and W. Weaver: The Mathematical Theory of Communication, University of Illinois Press, Urbana, 1949
[129] Brillouin, L.: Science and Information Theory, Academic Press, New York, 1962
[130] Franke, R., W. J, Streich and S. Hübel: studia biophysica **97**, 11 (1983)
[131] Streich, W. J., and R. Franke: paper to be submitted
[132] Mukherjee, C., M. C. Caron, D. Mulliken and R. J. Lefkowitz: Mol. Pharmacol. **12**, 16 (1976)
[133] Dunn, W. J., S. Wold and Y. C. Martin: J. Med. Chem. **21**, 922 (1978)
[134] Streich, W. J., and R. Franke: unpublished results

12. Receptor Mapping and Pharmacophores

The most straightforward approach to a real understanding of structure-activity relationships at the receptor level would be a direct study of the forces and properties involved in drug-receptor interactions. In the case of some enzymes of known structure or where a reasonable guess as to the nature of the binding site could be made such studies have indeed led to very promising results (e.g., [1—10]; see also 12.7.). For example, a novel antihypertensive compound acting as an inhibitor of the angiotensin-converting enzyme (ACE) could be designed by taking the structure of the active site of carboxypeptidase as a model of the ACE site [4]. Another simple example concerns the work of the Wellcome group on compounds releasing oxygen from oxygenated hemoglobin [11—13]. Compounds with a high 2,3-diphosphoglycerate(DPG)-like activity not resembling DPG (the natural oxygen releaser) could theoretically be designed by starting from the known architecture of the DPG binding site in hemoglobin.

Unfortunately, for pharmacological receptors the time where such studies can be applied is yet to come since the structure of most receptors is not known. This is the reason why the concepts of receptor mapping and pharmacophores have been introduced. The term receptor mapping refers to a variety of methods employed to attempt to evaluate the structure of a receptor binding site by regarding it as complementary to drugs which fit the receptor. A pharmacophore is frequently defined as an arrangement of atoms appearing in the structures of all these drugs necessary for a specific interaction with that receptor. Once the receptor thought to be complementary to the corresponding pharmacophore or the pharmacophore itself are known or can be guessed at the design of compounds fitting the receptor becomes possible. The structure of such compounds may be novel and it is, thus, lead generation which is aimed at here. The principle seems to be very easy: a compound is expected to be capable of interacting with a given receptor and, hence, of producing the biological effect connected with such interactions when it contains the pharmacophore in its structure. As we shall see it is not as simple as that although the principle as such is valid.

Although the term "pharmacophore" seems to have a clear meaning and is very frequently used in pharmacology and medicinal chemistry, a generally valid definition of pharmacophores does, in fact, not exist. As we shall see it can only be defined in the context of the method used for its evaluation. In order to get a better understanding of what one is really talking about if this term is used a short discussion on drug-receptor interactions is necessary before proceeding to the methods of pharmacophore evaluation and receptor mapping.

12.1. Some Basic Aspects of Drug-Receptor Interactions and the Definition of Pharmacophores

A variety of hypotheses on possible molecular mechanisms of drug-receptor interactions can be found in the literature (for recent reviews, see e.g. [14, 15]; see also chapters 2. and 3.). Although none of them can be considered definitely and unambiguously proven it seems that most pharmacologists and medicinal chemists tend to believe in the concept that the production of a stimulus (see chapter 2.) is somehow related to a specific conformational change in the corresponding receptor (see e.g. [16—18]). This conformational change was referred to in chapters 2. and 3. as a "specific perturbation (SP)" of the receptor and considered to be the final result of agonist-receptor interactions subsequent to the formation of the drug-receptor complex. Quite a lot of evidence supporting such a view can be found in the literature. Investigations on the interaction of several agonists and antagonists with the acetylcholine receptor using rapid-reaction kinetics [19], for example, indicated the presence of two reaction steps, the first probably referring to the formation of a drug-receptor complex and the second related to a conformational change in the receptor. There seems to be a parallelism between such changes and the intrinsic activity as may be concluded from the results of DAMLE and KARLIN [20] on the protection of the acetylcholine receptor by various compounds against the reduction of a disulphide bridge which is related to a change in receptor conformation. The concept of relating the production of a stimulus to conformational changes of the receptor is also supported by several thermodynamic investigations [e.g. 21—30]. WEILAND et al. [21], for example, found that the binding of agonists to β-adrenergic receptors is enthalpy driven whereas antagonist binding primarily depends on entropy. This may be explained by assuming that agonist binding is followed by a conformational change of the receptor such that its state of order increases. This would result in a decrease of entropy compensating the entropy increase typical of many protein-ligand interactions. The latter is observed only in the case of antagonists, that is they are not able to produce the same type of conformational change in the receptor as can the agonists. It should be mentioned, finally, that changes in shape or size of isolated receptors after drug binding could also be directly observed [e.g. 31, 31a].

Theoretical evidence for the conformational concept of drug-receptor interactions is provided by the work of KIER and co-workers [32—36] who considered in more detail the chain of events taking place as a drug approaches a receptor. Using very simple models of receptors (benzene, acetamide, acetate ion, n-propylguanidinium ion) and drugs (phenyl ring, carbinol group, various onium groups, methanol, aniline, ethylbenzene) they analysed the interaction energy as well as the mutual perturbation of drugs and receptors (conformation, electron distribution) as a function of drug-receptor distance. The most important results of these studies may be summarized as follows:

1. There is a significant degree of drug-receptor interaction *before* any perturbation of the drug structure occurs. The separation distance marking the onset of such interactions in the approach of the drug to the receptor was termed *recognition point.* This led KIER to his hypothesis on the "remote recognition of preferred conformation" stating that the "recognition" of a drug by a receptor depends on the preferred conformation of the isolated drug molecule.

2. As the approach of the drug to the receptor continues there is an increase of interaction energy leading to the perturbation of both drug and receptor. This perturbation starts *before* the equilibrium distance corresponding to the formation of the drug-receptor complex is reached. From that KIER concluded that the formation of this complex may actually not be necessary and that weak long-range interactions when producing a certain amount of receptor perturbation are sufficient to evoke a stimulus [35, 37]. This view would be in keeping with PATONS [38] rate theory (see chapter 2.), but it is incompatible with, for example, results from receptor binding studies as KIER himself realized [37]. Many such studies have demonstrated that the affinity of drugs for receptor preparations is usually (but not always) closely related to biological potency *in vivo* if transport to the site of action is adequately accounted for [e.g. 18, 39—52a], and some evidence that the thermodynamics of binding (enthalpy, entropy) may be related to intrinsic activity has already been presented above. In this book, therefore, the formation of a drug-receptor complex will be considered a necessary event for evoking a biological stimulus.

3. At equilibrium distance, finally, the drug molecule may be in a high energy conformation, the low energy conformer not participating in the equilibrium to any extent. That means, in other words, that an originally unpreferred conformation of the drug molecule predominates and interacts with the receptor.

Summarizing all evidence and the above discussion one may schematically picture the events of drug-receptor interactions to proceed through the following three steps:

1. Recognition:

   Recognition occurs at the recognition point due to weak long-range interactions between drug and receptor. At this point the receptor recognizes such structures which appear to have the right features to match its own structure. The drug is in its ground state. Recognition is a necessary but not sufficient condition for the next step (binding) to occur.

2. Binding:

   At equilibrium distance the drug-receptor complex is formed provided that this process is not sterically hindered and results in a decrease in energy. The former condition may imply that the drug molecule is capable of changing its conformation so that an optimal fit can be achieved in a cooperative process according, for example, to the "zipper mechanism" proposed by BURGEN et al. [53]. Usually, both drug and receptor will be perturbed at this stage. This means that the drug usually is no longer in its ground but in an "excited" state in which a high-energy conformation may predominate.

3. Final specific perturbation (SP) of the receptor:

   Binding is a necessary but still not sufficient condition for the production of a biological stimulus. For that, a very specific perturbation of the three-dimensional receptor structure is obviously necessary (see also chapter 2.) which can only be brought about by agonists, not by antagonists. This perturbation will be assumed here to occur after the formation of an initial drug-receptor complex. This assumption cannot be proven directly but it is supported to some extent by, for example, results of kinetic investigations of protein-ligand or drug-receptor interactions (see also above). The initial drug-receptor complex would then be regarded as resembling a transition state.

This scheme is, of course, an oversimplification. In particular, the distinction made between binding and the final specific receptor perturbation, although physically reasonable, appears to be somewhat artificial. It is of interest to note in this connection, that reasoning along very similar lines recently led KAETHNER [54] to advance his conformational change theory for auxin[1]) structure-activity relationships. According to this theory auxins are first recognized and then bound by the auxin receptor in what is called the "recognition conformation"; this would correspond to steps 1 and 2 of the above scheme. Subsequent to the binding a conformational change of both the bound auxin molecule as well as the receptor occurs (corresponding to step 3). The new conformation of the auxin triggering the effect is termed the "modulation conformation". Thus, auxin activity requires adoption of the recognition conformation and the ability to change into the modulation conformation. Molecules which possess the recognition conformation but are unable to move to the modulation conformation will be bound to the receptor but will behave as antagonists. This theory represented a rationalization and extension of previous concepts and could explain all basic features of the complicated auxin structure-activity relationships including such subleties as different activities of enantiomers (but see also [54a]). A similar concept was also used by KHROMOV-BORISOV [55] to explain agonist and antagonist activity in bis-ammonium compounds acting on the cholinergic receptor. The receptor is viewed as a tetrameric protein consisting of four subunits each bearing a negatively charged centre. In the free state of the receptor the distances between these centres are believed to be 1.4 and 2 nm, respectively. In order to produce a stimulus the conformation of the receptor must be changed to that of an activated state in which the distances between the negative centres are much shorter, namely 0.85 and 1.2 nm, respectively. A bis-ammonium compound will be an agonist if its N-N distance in the ground state is approximately equal to either 1.4 or 2 nm (prerequisite for binding; corresponds to steps 1 and 2) and if it has enough flexibility to change its conformation subsequent to binding so that the receptor is able to move to its activated state while maintaining the contact with the drug (corresponds to step 3). Compounds which are not capable to undergo this conformational change (rigid compounds) will behave as antagonists. Although this model has been arrived at only indirectly through analyses of structure-activity relationships and cannot be considered proven is has turned out to be useful in the directed design of new cholinergic compounds.

Thus, the above scheme adopted to describe drug-receptor interactions can obviously be considered as biologically reasonable. It leads to the following *pharmacophore definition for agonists*: a pharmacophore is a certain pattern of elements (e.g., atoms) the presence of which in a drug is a necessary and sufficient condition for the production of a stimulus at the receptor under consideration. This implies that:

— this pattern must be recognized by the receptor at the recognition point (step 1),
— it is capable of binding to the receptor which means that it may be necessary to change its conformation (step 2),

---

[1]) Auxins are plant growth hormones related to indol-3-yl-acetic acid.

— it can induce the specific perturbation of the receptor subsequent to binding (step 3) which is usually accompanied by a further change in its own conformation.

The agonist pharmacophore will change into that for a competitive antagonist if the last condition is not fulfilled. Thus, an agonist pharmacophore in the general sense not only implies a certain three-dimensional pattern but also the ability of that pattern to change its structure during drug-receptor interactions.

A straightforward evaluation of such a pharmacophore would actually require knowledge of the receptor and details of the molecular mechanisms of drug-receptor interactions. Since such knowledge usually is not available approximations become necessary. All these approximations have in common that the pharmacophore is elucidated in an indirect way by comparing drug structures and biological data in an attempt to find patterns which are common and typical of compounds specifically interacting with a given receptor. This is always a difficult task and it is not surprising, therefore, that many different attempts at quite different levels are being used which may lead to different results. It is because of this fact that it is always necessary to specify the approach used when defining a pharmacophore and to state what it actually describes and what it can predict.

There are three main types of approximations usually implied concerning:

— the definition of the elements constituting the pharmacophore,
— the step(s) of drug-receptor interactions considered,
— the informational content of biological data.

Let us start with the first point. If one looks at drugs the way a receptor "senses" them they must be viewed as a more or less flexible three-dimensional arrangement of perturbable fields and forces capable of interacting with comparable fields at the receptor (see e.g. [33, 34, 37]). Thus, the most straightforward and physically meaningful way to define the elements constituting a pharmacophore would be to identify them with such fields and forces. A pharmacophore in terms of such elements would be of general validity and include a variety of quite different possible chemical structures. The problem is that it is difficult to evaluate such pharmacophores by comparing drug structures since it is not obvious which fields and forces in which spatial regions are to be considered. First attempts in this direction will be outlined in sections 12.4. and 12.6.

One may also look at the drug structures as an organic chemist usually does. In that case, the elements will be identified with atoms and the pharmacophore ist then viewed as a (flexible) three-dimensional arrangement of specified atoms in specified positions. Clearly, such a pharmacophore is of less general validity and does not allow one to make as far reaching predictions on novel structures as the pharmacophore in terms of fields and forces.

The second point is related to the scheme presented above which leads to an operational distinction between three types of pharmacophores:

1. Recognition pharmacophore
   Pattern of elements which can be recognized by the receptor at the recognition point as being complementary to its own structure.
2. Binding or affinity pharmacophores
   (Flexible) pattern of elements the presence of which is necessary and sufficient for

the binding of a drug at the active site of the receptor resulting in the formation of the (initial) drug-receptor complex.

3. Intrinsic pharmacophore
   Pattern of elements necessary and sufficient to induce specific perturbations in the receptor subsequent to the binding step including, if necessary, its ability to change its arrangement.

This distinction is, of course, somewhat philosophical but it is certainly helpful for a better systematization which is commonly lacking in the literature and for a clearer understanding of prerequisites and limits of the different methods used in the evaluation of pharmacophores.

Following Kiers concept of the remote recognition of preferred conformation, the *recognition pharmacophore* can be evaluated from an analysis of drug molecules in their ground state corresponding to their minimum energy conformation. Since this is relatively simple it is this approach which is most frequently applied. In many cases, however, the fact that the resulting pharmacophore is not a sufficient condition for either binding or specific receptor pertubations to occur is simply overlooked. In other words, the presence of a recognition pharmacophore in a compound does not guarantee that this compound will actually bind to the receptor or will have intrinsic activity. This will be the case only insofar as the recognition pharmacophore also contains features of the binding or the intrinsic pharmacophore, which is, of course, possible.

To evaluate *binding* and *intrinsic pharmacophores, dynamic considerations* of drug structures become necessary. This means that the whole accessible conformational space must be considered and not only the preferred conformation in the ground state in order adequately to sample the possible receptor-bound conformation induced on binding to the receptor. The same is, of course, true for the intrinsic pharmacophore. The binding pharmacophore will usually imply the recognition pharmacophore, and its presence in a structure is a necessary and sufficient condition for the formation of the drug-receptor complex. Since the binding pharmacophore may be shared by agonists and antagonists, conclusions concerning intrinsic activity can usually not safely be drawn from the presence of this pharmacophore. This is only possible with the help of the intrinsic pharmacophore as far as this is really separable from the binding pharmacophore.

This, of course, is not a dogma. Rather, these three types of pharmacophores are to be considered as borderline cases. What type is actually obtained in an analysis and what a resulting pharmacophore really can describe and predict not only depends on the way the molecules are considered but also on the type of data available and the manner the data are handled (third point). First of all the general validity of a pharmacophore heavily depends on the extent of structural variation inherent in the compounds analysed. If this range is too small the validity of the resulting pharmacophore will be limited. Secondly, there are two ways of approach to evaluating pharmacophores by comparing drug structure:

1. Only drugs showing the same type (quality) of action at a given receptor (e.g., only agonists) are compared.
2. Drugs with different or opposite effects (e.g., agonists and antagonists) are compared.

In the first case an attempt is made to find a pattern which is common to all compounds. This pattern is then regarded as being typical of that type or quality of action and is identified with the pharmacophore. The disadvantage of this approach is that parts of this pattern may also be typical of compounds not showing the particular quality of biological effect considered. For example, if only agonists are considered the resulting pharmacophore will usually contain both the pattern for binding and those for intrinsic activity. The former, however, is also shared by competetive antagonists which bind to the same site as the agonists. As a consequence it is not possible to conclude what parts of the pharmacophore are connected with binding in general and which are related to intrinsic activity, and new compounds designed after this pharmacophore are not with certainty agonists but may also be antagonists.

This disadvantage can at least partly be avoided if the second strategy is used by, for example, comparing agonists and antagonists. In this case it should, in principle, be possible to separate the binding pharmacophore (which is present in both, agonists and antagonists) from the intrinsic pharmacophore typical of the agonists only. It should be noted in this context that a pharmacophore is not necessarily to be defined only in terms of elements supposed to be present but may also contain elements characterizing the absence of certain features (compare 11.). The problem here is that a comparison of agonists and antagonists will only lead to meaningful results when both bind to the same site with a comparable degree of specificity. This, however, is not necessarily true. It seems that some receptors have accessory binding areas outside or in addition to the specific agonist binding site with which antagonists, but not agonists, can interact (see e.g. [17, 56, 57a, b]; a similar situation may be encountered in enzymes [58]). This seems to be the case, for example, for certain antihistimines, antiserotonines and anticholinergics which show a greater similarity among each other than with the respective agonists and also show cross-reactivity [17]. Another aspect to be taken into account here is a possible heterogeneity of receptors which may result not only in binding differences between agonist and antagonists but also among agonists themselves (see e.g. [59, 59a]).

For a full characterization of agonists both the binding constant as well as a suitable measure of intrinsic activity (factor F in eqn. (2/7)) should be available. The pD_2 value ($-\log ED_{50}$) which can be derived from dose-response curves (see chapter 2.) is only then a true measure of binding if the relationship between receptor occupancy (or stimulus) and the observable biological effect is linear. With many receptors, however, the maximum response can already be obtained when only a small fraction of the receptors is occupied (see chapters 2. and 3.) so that this is more an exception than a rule. In such cases the pD_2 value is not related to the binding constant. Furthermore, the commonly used quantity

$$\alpha = \frac{E_M}{E_{\max}} \qquad (12/1)$$

$E_{\max}$ = maximum possible effect
E_M = maximum effect of the drug under investigation

called intrinsic activity is also not a reliable measure of the true intrinsic activity of an agonist since agonists which all have the same value of $\alpha = 1$ may still appreciably differ in their ability to induce specific perturbations at the receptor. In order to get reliable binding constants and measures of intrinsic activity it is then necessary to apply the well known technique of irreversible receptor blocking (see e.g. [60—61]) which, however, requires that an irreversible blocker is available. Another possibility is to study drug-receptor interaction *in vitro* using isolated or membrane-bound receptors. Such studies have become increasingly important (see e.g. [14, 15, 21, 52a, 59, 59a, 62—69]) and have several advantages:

— the assay is usually rapid once the problems of receptor isolation and the evaluation of its biological relevance have been solved,
— the data are of high precision and well defined in a physicochemical sense,
— pharmacokinetic processes are eliminated.

Although primarily designed to estimate binding constants such receptor assays may also yield information about intrinsic activity. There are several possibilities:

1. For membrane-bound receptors the cyclic nucleotide synthesis can be measured which should be directly related to the stimulus [57, 63, 64, 65, 69].
2. Detailed analysis of enthalpy and entropy (see e.g. [21]).
3. Application of kinetics (see e.g. [19]).
4. Analysis of special effects as, for example, the so-called sodium shift typical of the opiate receptor [70]. There, the addition of sodium ions to the incubation medium decreases the affinities of agonists but not of antagonists.

It stands to reason that pharmacokinetic processes must always be adequately accounted for if *in vivo* data are to be used for analysing drug-receptor interactions. Another problem which may become important with such data is that not only antagonists but also agonists may interact with more than one receptor (see e.g. [57]). It may then become necessary to separate a global observable biological effect into its components (see 13.2.).

In this chapter we have always considered a pharmacophore as a three-dimensional (topographical) pattern. This is certainly true but does not completely rule out the possibility of topological considerations as, for example, in section 11.2.6. From the above discussion, however, it clearly follows that a topological pharmacophore can only be valid insofar as it codes essential features of the actual topographical pattern (see also [71—74]). For more rigid molecules this condition will often be fulfilled since the geometrical structure of such compounds is often inherent in the two-dimensional structural diagram.

12.2. Some Basic Aspects of Deriving Drug Molecule Geometry

For deriving pharmacophores as three-dimensional patterns it is necessary to know and to manipulate the three-dimensional structures of the drug molecules to be compared. This structure is determined by the conformation which presents itself as a set of coordinates describing the spatial position of all atoms or as a set of bond lengths, bond angles and torsion angles. Most biologically active molecules are, at least to a certain extent, flexible and can change their conformation by distortion of bonds or rotation about single bonds. These changes are accompanied by an energy change. In other words, different conformations of a flexible molecule have different energies, and the preferred conformation will be that with minimum energy. The investigation of the different geometries of flexible molecules and the energies connected with them is the subject of *conformational analysis*. A variety of techniques can be applied here which will, however, not be discussed in detail. Only some of the basic aspects will be considered.

Molecular structures can be derived from experimental and theoretical studies. The most important experimental techniques are:

1. For molecules in the solid state (crystals):
   X-ray [75] and neutron diffraction [75a].
2. For molecules in solution:
   NMR spectroscopy [76, 76a].
3. For molecules in the gas phase:
   Electron diffraction [77] and microwave spectroscopy [78].

The *gas-phase methods* require that the molecules to be investigated can be transferred into the gas phase by evaporation *in vacuo* without destruction. This condition automatically limits these techniques to small molecules so that they usually cannot be directly applied to drug structures. Using suitable small model compounds mimicking parts of such structures which are of special interest, valid information may still be obtained. NMR *spectroscopy* refers to the conformation of molecules in solution which is more relevant to the biological situation than the solid state or *in vacuo* conformations in the context of recognition pharmacophores. If a molecule has more than one relatively stable conformation all of them will be detected, and the results will also show their relative population. The first category of methods, finally, gives precise information about the *conformation in crystals*. This conformation may appreciably differ from that in solution if the crystal packing forces are strong. Since, furthermore, only one conformation is usually present in the crystal other possible low-energy conformations which may be present in solution would go undetected. However, the information obtainable from crystals is still very valuable as the solid state conformation represents in a very precise way at least one of the many possibly minimum energy conformations a molecule can adopt. The solid state conformation can be used for comparison with the conformation in solution and as a primary input for theoretical calculations (see below). Over 24000 crystal structures are available from the Cambridge Crystallographic Data File [79] (see also [80, 81]), and a number of macromolecular structures is stored in the Protein Data Bank [82]. Recently, a very useful compilation of drug structures became available in book form [83].

The principle of *theoretical* (*computational*) *methods* of conformational analysis is to vary the position of different parts of a molecule with respect to each other and then to calculate and compare the energies for each variation. The standard geometry operation applied here is the clock-wise rotation about bonds. If only one rotatable bond exists the result may be represented as plot of the calculated energy versus the torsion angle which is usually symbolized by the letters τ or θ. An example is provided in Fig. 12.1 (from [84]) which shows the variation of conformational potential energy of the benzamidinium cation with the variation of the torsion angle, indicating the orientation of the plane of the amidinium part with respect to the plane of the phenyl ring. The energy minimum indicating the stable conformation corresponds to an angle of 37.5°, and this value could also be verified experimentally [85]. In drug molecules commonly two (or even more) rotable bonds exist. This would result in a three-dimensional plot with both angles and, again, the energy as axes. Since such a plot is difficult

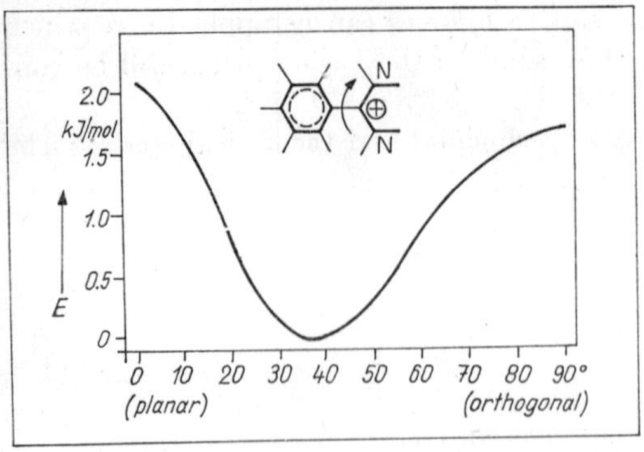

Abb. 12.1. Energy of the benzamidinium cation as function of the torsion angle (from [84])

to handle, it is common practice to project the three-dimensional picture onto a plane so that again a two-dimensional picture is obtained. The axes in this projection are the torsion angles, and the energies appear as contour lines. An example of such an energy map is presented in Fig. 12.2 (from [86]) for structure XLV. On such maps, minima represent stable conformations with the relative depths being indicative of their stability. The maps also give the heights and shapes of energy barriers between conformational isomers from which it is possible to calculate rates of interconversion. The population of different conformations (the percentages of molecules being in these conformations) can be calculated via the BOLTZMAN distribution function [87, 88], and via probability functions maps can be derived which emphasize how flexible a molecule is [87] (see also 12.5.).

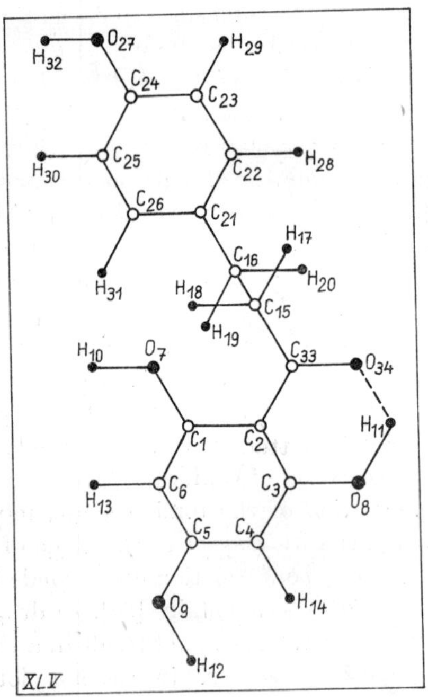

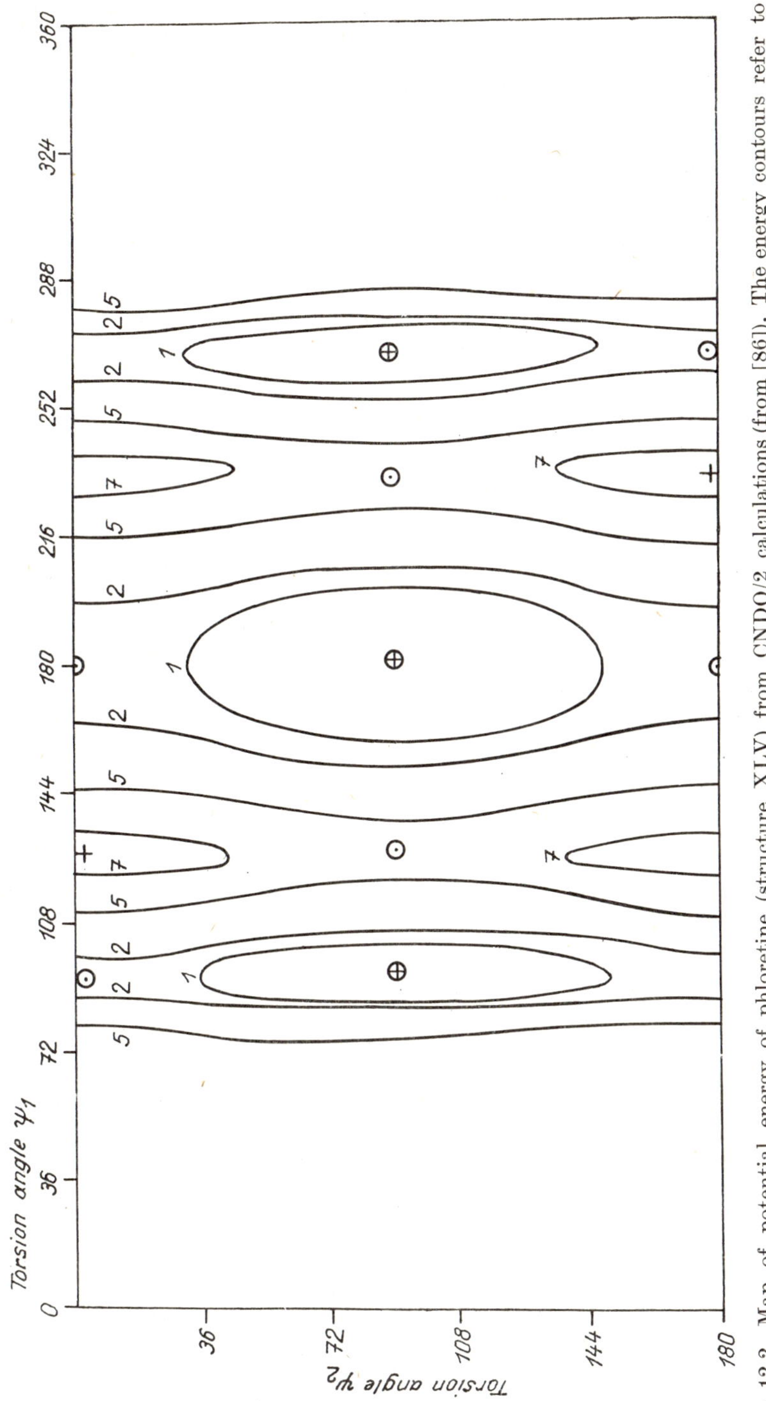

Fig. 12.2. Map of potential energy of phloretine (structure XLV) from CNDO/2 calculations (from [86]). The energy contours refer to 4.2, 8.4, 21 and 29.3 kJ/mol relative to the global minimum; ⊕ = minima, ⊙ = saddle points, + = maxima

Theoretical techniques for conformational analysis start either from *quantum* or from *classical mechanics*. *Quantum mechanical methods* have already been referred to in section 5.3. in the context of calculating electronic indices of molecules. They have become more and more important in the QSAR field (for some recent reviews, see e.g. [72—74, 87—101]) and have been developed into a powerful tool to analyse conformations (e.g. [87, 95, 98, 102—104]. Considering molecules as a unit, quantum mechanical methods are based on the analysis and description of *wavefunctions* and their energies using various levels of approximation. The most rigorous treatment is provided by the so-called *ab initio* approaches which do not use empirical parameters [105]. These approaches involve quite complicated calculations and need a lot of computer time. Therefore, a variety of so-called semi-empirical methods (for reviews, see e.g. [103, 106]) have been developed and also extensively applied in the field of drug research. These methods are based on several simplifying assumptions and usually apply empirical parameters obtained from experimental data. Methods of this type are the Extended Hückel Theory (EHT) [107], the Interacted Extended Hückel Theory [IEHT) [108], various methods based on neglect of diatomic differential overlap (CNDO/2, INDO, PRDDO and MINDO) [109—112], and the Perturbative Configuration Interactions using Localized Orbitals [PCILO) [113]. Each of these methods has its own set of idiosyncracies [102], and any attempt to discuss their relative merits, their reliability and specific applications would be far beyond the scope of this chapter. Today, the most commonly used methods for the analysis of drug conformations probably are CNDO/2 and PCILO. Standard computer programs are available through the Quantum Chemistry Program Exchange (QCPE) run from the Department of Chemistry at the University of Indiana (USA) which can, in principle, be used without detailed knowledge of the methods involved. This is an advantage but at the same time a danger. It should be emphasized that a potential user of any of these methods must become familiar with them in order to avoid serious pitfalls.

Quantum mechanical methods have the advantage of providing, in addition to conformation, information about electronic properties (see also section 5.3.) of the molecules investigated, which classical mechanics cannot. They have been applied to a large variety of biologically active molecules with, as a whole, satisfactory results. It must be noted, however, that the results may largely depend not only on the type but also on the details of the method applied (e.g., the input geometry used). A weak point of these methods is the principle of rigid rotation: if there are several rotatable bonds in a molecule only two of them are varied at one time taking the rest of the structure as rigid. Although such an approach provides at least a good approximation in most cases it may lead to failures in certain instances. Depending on the method used quantum mechanical calculations occasionally tend to either under or overestimate rotational barriers and the strength of intramolecular interactions. For all these reasons, quantum mechanical methods (especially the semi-empirical ones) may sometimes lead to unrealistic conformational predictions (see e.g. [2, 114—118]). Another problem with even the simplified semi-empirical methods is that they still need too much computer time to be applicable to larger numbers of highly flexible drugs. Conformational analysis presents a combinatorial problem. An analysis involving 360° rotations in D degree increments about N different bonds requires the examination of $(360/D)^N$ conformations. Thus, the number of conformations increases exponentially with the number of bonds being rotated and may easily become as large as 10^5—10^6 if a small D is selected and

$N > 2$ [119]. If only local minima (corresponding to minimum energy conformations) are of interest it is not necessary to consider all of these conformations since such minima can be directly detected by special geometry optimization algorithms (see e.g. [120—122] and the references given there). In the dynamic approaches aiming at the elucidation of binding and intrinsic pharmacophores, however, the exploration of the whole conformational space besomes necessary, and the sheer magnitude of such a problem then rules out even the fastest quantum mechanical technique. Classical mechanical methods are then the only practical means of examining such large number of conformations.

In *classical mechanics* a molecule is viewed as a collection of particles held together by simple harmonic or elastic forces. These forces can be defined by an *empirical potential function* and the conformational energy can then be computed by summing the non-bonded interactions over all atoms whose distances can change relative to each other [123—129]. The potential function is made up from various individual potentials describing different types of interactions. The most important contributions are from non-bonded repulsive and attractive interactions, bond deformations, hydrogen bonding, torsional strain and electrostatic interactions. A rough qualitative picture about the permissible conformational space may already be obtained by considering only repulsive forces.

Methods using empirical potentials have the advantage of being much faster (by several orders of magnitude) than quantum mechanical methods (see e.g. [119]) thus allowing the full exploration of conformational spaces and an easy manipulation of structures. A critical point is the correct parametrization of the potential functions, and a need for developing a consistent set of potentials that includes both intra- and intermolecular interactions over a broad range of molecules, still exists. Potentials derived from quantum mechanical *ab initio* calculations have been very helpful here (e.g. [130—132]).

If correctly applied and parametrized, empirical potentials will yield reliable results. Therefore, such methods have been implemented in many *molecular modelling system* [2] as, for example, the Merck modelling system (MMMS, Merck, Sharp & Dohme, USA) [2, 133—134], the CAMSEQ conformational analysis system [135—137] which is part of the CIS system (National Institute of Health, USA) [80, 138], the MMS-X system (Washington University, USA) [139], the SCRIPT molecular modelling program (Roussel Uclaf, France) [140], the MOLOCH-2 system (Searle, USA) [141], the system MOLY (Rohm & Haas, USA) [119, 142], the TRIBBLE system (Du Pont, USA) [143] and the video vector dynamics chemical graphics system [143a] which is in use at Pfizer Central Research [143b][1]). Since classical mechanics cannot provide information on electronic properties, some of these systems also contain quantum mechanical methods.

Classical and quantum mechanical methods may also supplement each other in conformational analysis. For example, it is possible to evaluate a rough picture of the energy hypersurface by using simple empirical potentials (may be considering only attractive and repulsive interactions) and then to refine the result by applying quantum mechanical calculations to points of special interest (minima, maxima, saddle points). Vice versa, such points may also be evaluated first by quantum chemical calculations

---

[1]) The following empirical energy function programs should also be mentioned: QCFF/PI [143c], UNICEPP [143d), MMI [143e] and AMBER [143f]; for a recent review of Molecular Modelling Systems applied to drug design, see e.g. [143g].

using rigid rotations and then be refined by potential methods allowing for a full flexibility of the molecule.

Even with empirical potentials some problems need further simplification in order to reduce computer time. Several strategies can be followed here. In many cases it is sufficient to eliminate all conformations which are not permissible and to find all sterically allowed conformations. This can be done by considering only the repulsive interactions between nonbonded atoms neglecting all other contributions. High energies will be assigned to all conformations in which there is significant atomic overlap, and a clear picture of the permissible conformational space is revealed [114, 115, 139]. Other possibilities are to detect and eliminate high energy conformations without having to calculate them, to eliminate the calculation of interactions which are unaffected by the various rotational changes or to couple stepwise pharmacophore search strategies directly with the conformational analysis [119, 139, 142, 144].

A very important strategy to be applied in connection with conformational analysis and pharmacophoric pattern searching is the "*restricted* (*or rigid*) *analogue approach*" [e.g. 145, 146] which makes use of specially designed rigid or semi-rigid conformationally restricted analogues. An attempt is made to constrain molecules into a hypothesized receptor-preferred conformation by, for example, the addition of an extra ring system to replace a flexible side-chain. When such an analogue exhibits biological activity, the conformational possibilities responsible for that activity are well defined. Unfortunately, the opposite is not true: a lack of activity does not necessarily indicate a wrong conformation but may be due to a number of other reasons. The extra number of atoms added to make a molecule less flexible may sterically interfere with drug-receptor interactions, and the loss of flexibility itself may prevent the final specific receptor perturbation and, thus, the generation of a biological stimulus. In addition, absorption, distribution, metabolism and other cellular processes may also be altered. In spite of these limitations the rigid analogue approach has already proven to be very useful and can effectively rationalize the search for pharmacophores. Some recent examples can be found in the work of GRUNEWALD et al. [145] on sympathomimetic amines, of HORN and ROGERS [146], GOLDBERG at al. [147], RANDALL et al. [147a], OLSON et al. [147b] and of HUMBER et al. [148] on dopamine analogues, of NICHOLS et al. on hallucinogens [149] and of VEBER et al. [150—155] and SEPRODI et al. [156] on peptide hormones (for some possibilities to constrain peptides, see also [157, 158]).

Basically, molecular modelling methods describe isolated molecules in the gaseous state. Although the results usually provide valid information it must be emphasized that conformation and other properties may appreciably differ in solution. It is, therefore, important to extend and modify methods for conformational analysis to account for solvation where necessary. This can be done with both quantum mechanical methods [159—163] as well as empirical potential functions [126, 131, 132, 135, 164—169]. For the purpose of pharmacophoric pattern searching the modifications based on empirical potentials seem to be more appropriate.

Most of the molecular modelling systems mentioned above make use of highly advanced *interactive computer graphics* (for recent reviews on computer graphics, see e.g. [1, 3, 170—174]). In the first step a geometrical model of the molecules to be analyzed is generated in the computer. There are two ways of molecular input:

— batch mode: input via coordinates,
— interactive mode: graphical input.

For the *batch mode*, three different types of coordinates can be used. When a crystal structure is available the input consists of unit cell coordinates which are converted by common subroutines into cartesian coordinates. The latter can, of course, also be used directly if known. A structure may also be generated from internal atomic coordinates using standard bond lengths, bond angles and torsion angles from available compilations [175, 176]. The structure generated can then be displayed on a screen and the pictorial view thus provided can very easily be checked for input errors.

More convenient than the batch mode and very easy to use for any chemist is the *graphical input* via a graphical input program module. The two-dimensional structure of the molecule to be considered is simply drawn on the display screen by means of a light-pen. The computer will then generate a crude geometrical model which is subsequently refined by strain energy minimization procedures based on empirical potentials.

The stereochemical model created in the input routine serves as starting geometry for conformational analysis. An analysis is defined by specifying the bonds to rotate, the increments of rotation and the total number of degrees to rotate. In addition, details of the method to be used for conformational analysis (e.g., the types of potentials) and the way in which the results are to be presented have also to be specified. With respect to the latter aspect the molecular modelling systems mentioned above differ somewhat but, in general, the following results may be obtained (see e.g. [119, 137, 142]):

- lists of the energy of all conformations examined,
- lists of all conformations within a specified number of kJ/mol of the minimum,
- graphs of energy as a function of rotation about a specified bond,
- contour maps of energy and populations as a function of rotation about two specified bonds,
- lists of atomic coordinates, bond angles and interatomic distances in specified conformations.

The great power of interactive computer graphics is its ability to display molecules so that a visual inspection becomes possible. At any stage of conformational analysis stereochemical pictures can be generated which may be three-dimensional and coloured. The molecules can be rotated in space and thus viewed from different angles. It is also possible to observe the rotation about bonds selecting and manipulating only the interesting parts of a molecule at various degrees of structural details. Several types of structural representations can be selected as, for example, simple stick figures, space-filling models, surface models and space-filling or surface models with imbedded stick figures. Molecules can be moved relative to one another, compared, superimposed (see 12.5.) and parameters of their interaction calculated. All these operations are performed interactively so that the user, at any given moment, can decide and specify what and how to look at. Thus, interactive computer graphics provides a powerful means of comparing molecules, understanding the spatial arrangement of atoms, functional groups or electron distributions (which would require quantum mechanical methods) and properties derived therefrom (as, e.g., electrostatic potential maps, see 12.4.) and developing an understanding of the features required for the interaction with the receptor. This may be emphasized by a quotation from a recent review written by Langridge and colleagues [1]: "It is said that one picture is worth 10,000 words, but by altering the image interactively one can procedure thousands of different pictures in a single session with the graphics system."

Access to interactive computer graphics is not indispensable for pharmacophore searching but it will always be very helpful. Some of the approaches to be discussed in the following sections (e.g., active analogue approach, see 12.6.) would be extremely difficult if not impossible to realize without this technique.

12.3. Kier's Work: Static Pharmacophores and Receptor Mapping by Model Interaction Calculations

Based on his pioneering concept of "remote recognition of preferred conformation" [33, 34] KIER suggested that the initial contact between drug and receptor (recognition) is dependent on the placement of essential atoms in the preferred conformation of the isolated drug molecule. The spatial arrangement of these essential atoms (which may also be replaced by charges) is then regarded as the pharmacophore and has been investigated by KIER and colleagues for a variety of biologically active compounds [90—92, 177—193]. Clearly, this pharmacophore is a typical recognition pharmacophore with all its limitations. Its evaluation usually proceeds through the following steps:

1. Selection of some compounds specifically interacting with a particular receptor.
2. Conformational analysis of these compounds and evaluation of their minimum energy (preferred) conformation(s). In addition, some electronic indices (e.g., charges) may also be calculated.
3. Assumptions are made as to which atoms (mostly heteroatoms) should be regarded as "essential" for drug-receptor interactions.
4. The spatial arrangement of these atoms in the molecules considered is compared and related to biological activity, until, eventually, the pharmacophore emerges. The assumption(s) made in step 3 may change during this comparison.

The last two steps are based on an intuitive trial-and-error approach leaving much space for subjective decisions, and a more efficient decision making procedure based on objective criteria would certainly be more appropriate. The practice of identifying essential centres for drug-receptor interactions with heteroatoms is also somewhat questionable since the receptor does not "see" atoms but rather centres of force fields. The position of these centres must not be identical with the position of the heteroatoms (see 12.4.). Furthermore, the EHT method used in most of KIERS calculations has several limitations although it frequently yields better results for the conformation of molecules in solution than more sophisticated semi-empirical quantum mechanical methods (this effect may simply be due to a cancellation of errors, see e.g. [194—196]).

For these reasons and because of its very nature as the recognition pharmacophore, the static pharmacophore is of only limited descriptive and predictive power and usually restricted to relatively similar compounds. In particular, it does not allow one to draw conclusions on intrinsic activity. For a first rationalization and understanding of the potential ability of drugs to interact with a given receptor as well as a starting point for the evaluation of more sophisticated models it is, however, useful, and KIERS work can in fact be regarded as an important step in exploring the field of pharmacophores.

As an example the static pharmacophore proposed by KIER [92, 177, 184] for the muscarinic receptor is presented in Fig. 12.3. This pharmacophore is in fact present in several important muscarinic agents but it cannot explain all experimental facts. In some rigid compounds with muscarinic activity, for example, the $N—O_1$ distance does not fit the range of 0.32 ± 0.02 nm predicted in Fig. 12.3 [197]. Not all muscarinic agonists contain three heteroatoms and it must then be assumed that heteroatoms may be replaced by other structural features. For oxotremorine which mimics the muscarinic pharmacophore in its preferred conformation but does not have the ether oxygen, for example, KIER had to assume that the electronic character of the triple bond is the receptor equivalent of the ether oxygen atom in acetylcholine. As will be shown in 12.4. this is not an unreasonable assumption.

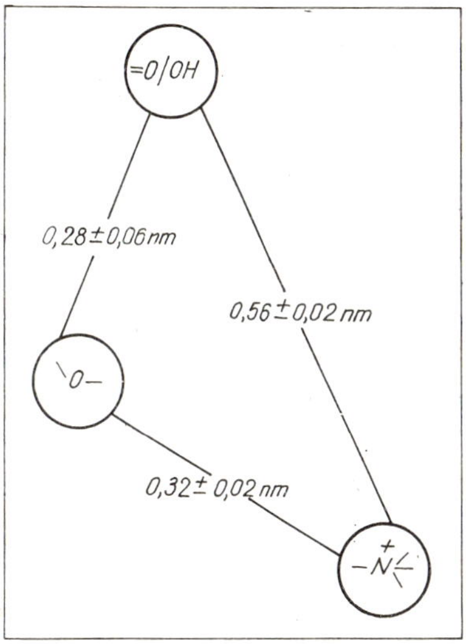

Abb. 12.3. Static pharmacophore for the muscarinic receptor [92, 177, 184]

Another interesting example concerns the histamine pharmacophores. The dual nature of the activity of histamine at H_1- and H_2-receptors was presumed to be connected with the existence of two distinctly different histamine conformations (gauche and trans) which are of equal preference [92, 178] assuming that the gauche-conformation is responsible for H_2- and the trans-conformation for H_1-activity (for a recent review on the conformation of histamine derivatives, see e.g. [166]). Based on this hypothesis a static H_2-pharmacophore was proposed by BUSTARD and MARTIN as follows [198]:

- presence of two heteroatoms with,
- a distance of about 0.36 nm between them,
- one of them must have a free electron pair,
- the other must belong to an aromatic system or be in conjugation with double bonds.

It was shown that various compounds of widely differing structures acting upon the H_2-receptor indeed possess these features so that the fact that compounds bearing, at a first glance, no obvious structural resemblance are capable of interacting with the same receptor could be rationalized to a certain extent. Because of the limitations inherent in a recognition pharmacophore this pattern does not allow one to differentiate between agonists and antagonists. Furthermore, it cannot explain the H_1/H_2 activity ratios observed in methylhistamines (see Table 12.1). Detailed conformational analyses were performed by GANELLIN and co-workers [196, 199—201]. If different conformations are required at the two receptors as proposed by KIER and if activity depends on the concentration of the relevant conformer, then the ratio of H_1 and H_2 activities should parallel the population ratio of the two conformations concerned. This however, is not the case since the population ratio of trans/gauche conformers appears to be unrelated with the H_1/H_2 activity ratio (Table 12.1). This does not disprove KIERS idea but clearly shows the limits of recognition pharmacophores. It may well be that histamine arrives at the recognition point in the conformations proposed by KIER but the receptor-bound conformations are different. The results of GANELLIN and colleagues [87, 196, 201] in fact indicate that the bioactive conformation at the H_1-receptor is not a minimum energy conformation. In order to understand the selective interactions of histamine compounds with the two histamine receptors dynamic considerations are required (see 12.5.). In addition, further effects such as tautomeric equilibria must also to be taken into account [202—206].

Table 12.1. Agonist activity of methylhistamines[1]) at the H_1- and the H_2-receptor relative to histamine (histamine = 100) and trans/gauche population ratio (from [200])

Position of Me substituent	H_1 (ileum)	H_2 (atrium)	Activity ratio H_1/H_2	Conformer ratio trans/gauche
2	16.5	4.4	4	1.2
3	0.42	<0.1		1.2
4	0.23	43	0.005	3
N	72	74	1	1.2
N, N	44	51	1	3.5
β	0.83	0.89	1	0.02
α	0.36	0.74	0.5[2])	0.1

[1]) for the histamine structure, see Fig. 12.9
[2]) not significantly different from 1

KIER realized the limitations inherent in any approach considering only static molecules isolated from each other or from the receptor. In an effort to create a more dynamic model of interacting species and an attempt to predict the energies of such interactions, he and HÖLTJE developed their method of "receptor mapping by model interaction calculations" and applied it to a variety of problems [207—215]. The method consists of the calculation of the interaction energy between pharmacophoric groups of drugs and a model compound simulating a possible receptor feature. If the interaction energies evaluated at some constant distance and orientation of the drugs with respect to the receptor model correlate with biological activity it can be concluded that this model is isomorphic with reality. Although this does not necessarily mean that it really constitutes the actual receptor feature interacting with the drugs the results can aid in a better understanding of the nature of drug-receptor interactions and of possible receptor characteristics. A study of trimethylammonium group interaction, for example, revealed that it is probably not the classic candidate, the carboxylate ion, but rather an aromatic amino acid side-chain which is the essential receptor feature for interactions with onium groups in drugs [208], and a similar result was also obtained for the α-binding site of acetylcholinesterase [211]. The value of such models, furthermore, lies in their ability to predict the activity of other untested modifications of a drug molecule and to create a rationale for further compound design.

The active site model is taken as an amino acid side-chain assuming that a single side-chain is dominant in drug-receptor interactions. This is, of course, an oversimplification, but it keeps the complexity of calculations to a reasonable limit. The monopole polarizabilities method of CLAVERIE and REIN [216, 217] is used for the numerical calculations of the interaction energies. Within this approximation, the interaction energy between a receptor model and a drug is described in terms of the charge distributions of the two molecules approximated by point charges centred at the nuclei and the polarizabilities of the bonds, together with an algorithm for computing the repulsive energy component. The calculations are performed for a variety of amino acid side-chains and for various modes of approach of the drugs as a function of distance, and that model is finally accepted which gives the best correlation between the interaction energies and log A. As a rule, side-chains of aromatic amino acids like toluene (surrogate for phenylalanine) or methylindole (surrogate for tryptophan) turned out to be the best models. In order further to reduce the complexity of calculations, assumptions on anchoring of the drug molecules at the receptor through certain groups, e.g., onium groups, are usually made which limits the freedom in the alignment of the pharmacophoric groups considered to the receptor model. Some of the results summarized in Table 12.2 show that this approach works surprisingly well.

The examples investigated refer to homologous series with very limited structural variations, and the pharmacophoric groups considered were defined *a priori*. In order to get useful information about pharmacophores it would be necessary to consider more diverse structures and systematically to vary those parts of them involved in interactions in addition to the receptor models, allowing for appropriate conformational and/or orientational changes with distance. In addition, it may also be necessary to consider more complex receptor models consisting of more than one amino acid side-chain as, for example, in the work of HÖLTJE and VOGELSANG [215] (see Table 12.2). This, however, would enormously increase the complexity of calculations. Maybe a strategy starting with the simplest possible model which is then refined in a stepwise procedure could help here. For example, different homologous series acting upon the same receptor could be used to arrive at simple receptor models which may be different for these series. These models could then be combined to construct a more complex model with which it may then be possible to investigate more diverse structures. The importance of the "receptor mapping by interaction calculations" approach lies in its potential to characterize drugs with respect to their "ability to interact" in a certain manner and to provide information on how the real situation at the receptor can be simulated.

Table 12.2. Examples for the application of the concept of "receptor mapping using model interaction calculations"

Compounds	Pharmacophoric group[1])	Biological activity	Side chain model	Surrogate for	Distance[2]) (in nm)	r[3])	References
R—CH—CO—OCH_3 \ NH—CO—CH_3	R	Hydrolysis by amino acid acylase	Toluene	Phenylalanine	0.45	0.974	[207]
Chloramphenicol congeners	Substituent at the carbonyl group	Antibacterial	Indole	Tryptophan	0.45	0.914	[209]
Nitroanilines	para-Substituent	Sweet Taste	3-Methylindole	Tryptophan	0.425	0.887	[210]
Phenoxy-cyclopropyl-amines	Substituents at the phenyl ring	Inhibition of monoaminooxydase	N-Propylguanidin	Arginin	0.475	0.938	[212]
Amphetamines	Phenyl ring substituents	Hallucinogenic	3-Methylindole	Tryptophan	0.45	0.73[4])	[213]
Phenethylamines	Phenyl ring[5]) Side chain	Re-uptake of norepinephrin	N-Methylguanidin, Benzene	Arginin[5]) Phenylalanin		−0.814	[215]

[1]) Group whose interaction with the receptor model is considered assuming that this group is responsible for the gradation of biological potency.
[2]) Distance between drugs and the receptor model for which the interaction energy gives the optimal correlation with log A.
[3]) Correlation coefficient of the correlation between interaction energy and log A.
[4]) The correlation coefficient can be improved to $r = 0.88$ by adding an indicator variable accounting for the occurrence of methoxy groups in meta- and para-position and log P.
[5]) The model here consists of two amino acid side chains in a fixed spatial position.

12.4. Molecular Electrostatic Potentials: the Interaction Pharmacophore

The molecular electrostatic potential (MESP) is the global potential created by a molecule in the surrounding space by its nuclear charges and electron distribution and can straight-forwardly be calculated via standard quantum mechanical procedures [218 to 221] (for a recent review on MESPs, see [221a]). It represents the electrostatic interaction energy for each point in this space which is equal to the work needed to bring a unit positive charge from infinity to that point assuming that the unit charge has no perturbing effect on the molecule. It may be visualized as a "cloud" around a molecule with varying density (amount of interaction energy) and colour (sign of interaction energy) which is "seen" by an approaching charged reagent. The contours of this "cloud" determine the electrostatic interactions with this reagent and its orientation since the electrostatic energy of interaction of a point charge, q, placed in a potential, V, is qV. In a series of drugs interacting with the same receptor the reagent (the receptor) is constant so that the recognition of the drugs by the receptor will depend on their MESPs as far as electrostatic interactions are dominant in the recognition step. This led Weinstein and co-workers [222, 223] to the concept of the *interaction pharmacophore* which may be defined as a certain MESP pattern necessary and sufficient for the recognition step to occur. In the evaluation of such interaction pharmacophores it is not the complete three dimensional MESP that is considered but only a two-dimensional picture in a plane intersecting the three-dimensional MESP at a defined distance and orientation to the molecule. The MESP then appears as a contour diagram (map) of isoenergy lines (see Fig. 12.4) allowing one to visualize the path of the easiest approach of positive charges (negative potential minima) or of negative ones (positive maxima).

Although sometimes claimed to be dynamic, interaction pharmacophores derivable from such MESP maps are, in fact, static and have all the limitations of a recognition pharmacophore. This follows from the fact that only electrostatic interactions are considered and other interactions including possible conformational changes are neglected. This is basically only correct at a drug-receptor distance corresponding to the recognition point. Such pharmacophores are true interaction pharmacophores only insofar as a unit charge placed at different positions around drug molecules can be considered to be a receptor model. In comparison with the static pharmacophore of Kier it has the advantage that one interaction pharmacophore may comprise many arrangements of atoms or static pharmacophores, respectively. It is, thus, possible to arrive at entirely new structures (new lead compounds) with the help of such interaction pharmacophores. Another advantage is that the interaction pharmacophores reflect the true centres of electrostatic interactions which must not coincide with the position of atoms.

Applied to a variety of biologically active compounds MESPs and the concept of interaction pharmacophores have been useful in understanding drug-receptor interactions and drug activity in molecular terms (4c, 94a, 222—243]. MESPs were even calculated for a few enzymes in attempts better to understand enzyme activity [4e, 244—249] and for DNA [249a]. A short discussion of a few examples may serve to illustrate this point.

Cholinergic agonists and antagonists were investigated by Weinstein and co-workers

[222—225]. First, the MESP of acetylcholine was analysed assuming that the positively charged trimethylammonium group may play a leading role in directing the molecule towards the receptor and that its interaction with an anionic site might be a first step in the recognition process. To simulate this step and to account for its influence, an arbitrary anionic model group (NH_2^-) was placed in the vicinity of the cationic head of acetylcholine at a configuration and distance which would attain an energy minimum for the entire complex. The resulting MESP is presented in Fig. 12.4. It shows regions of negative potential around the two oxygens and a positive region at the cationic head. By comparing the MESP for acetylcholine with that of other compounds it was concluded that the essential MESP pattern for the recognition step at the cholinergic receptor constists of a negative potential region at the ester oxygen and a positive region at the nitrogen. This pattern was, in fact, found in other cholinergic agonists and antagonists as demonstrated in Fig. 12.5 which shows a schematic representation of the interaction pharmacophore in acetylcholine (agonist), 3-acetoxyquinuclidine (agonist) and phencylidine (antagonist). In the last compound the environment of the ether oxygen in the two agonists is simulated by a negative potential surrounding the phenyl ring. The degree to which various compounds investigated by Weinstein et al. generate the MESP pattern constituting the cholinergic interaction pharmacophore determines their interaction with the cholinergic receptor, and compounds devoid of this pattern show no cholinergic or anticholinergic activity. If, for example, 3-acetoxyquinuclidine (see Fig. 12.5) is methylated at the nitrogen, the cholinergic activity is drastically decreased. With classical considerations this is difficult to explain since both molecules have the same minimum energy conformation corresponding to the presumed active configuration of acetylcholine, and the charge distribution is also practically identical. Comparison of the MESPs of the two compounds, however, reveals two important differences for the N-methyl derivative:

— the negative region near the ester oxygen is less developed,
— the shortest distance achievable to the simulated anionic receptor site supposed to interact with the cationic head is greater by $\approx$ 0,075 nm.

These differences may well lead to a much weaker interaction with the cholinergic receptor.

If in phencyclidine the phenyl ring is substituted or replaced by other groups the following observations can be made:

1. p-nitro derivative: inactive
   MESP: the negative potential is shifted away from the required region,
2. p-amino derivative: higher activity
   MESP: the negative potential in the required region is enhanced,
3. replacement of the phenylring by an ethynyl group: active
   MESP: the negative potential of the ester oxygen in acetylcholine is mimicked by the triple bond and situated in the required region,
4. replacement of the phenyl ring by a nitrile group: inactive
   MESP: the negative potential is shifted away from the required region.

Thus, as a whole, there is a good agreement between the predictions from MESP and the observed biological activity demonstrating the power of the MESP approach, although the number of compounds and the structural variations investigated are still too limited

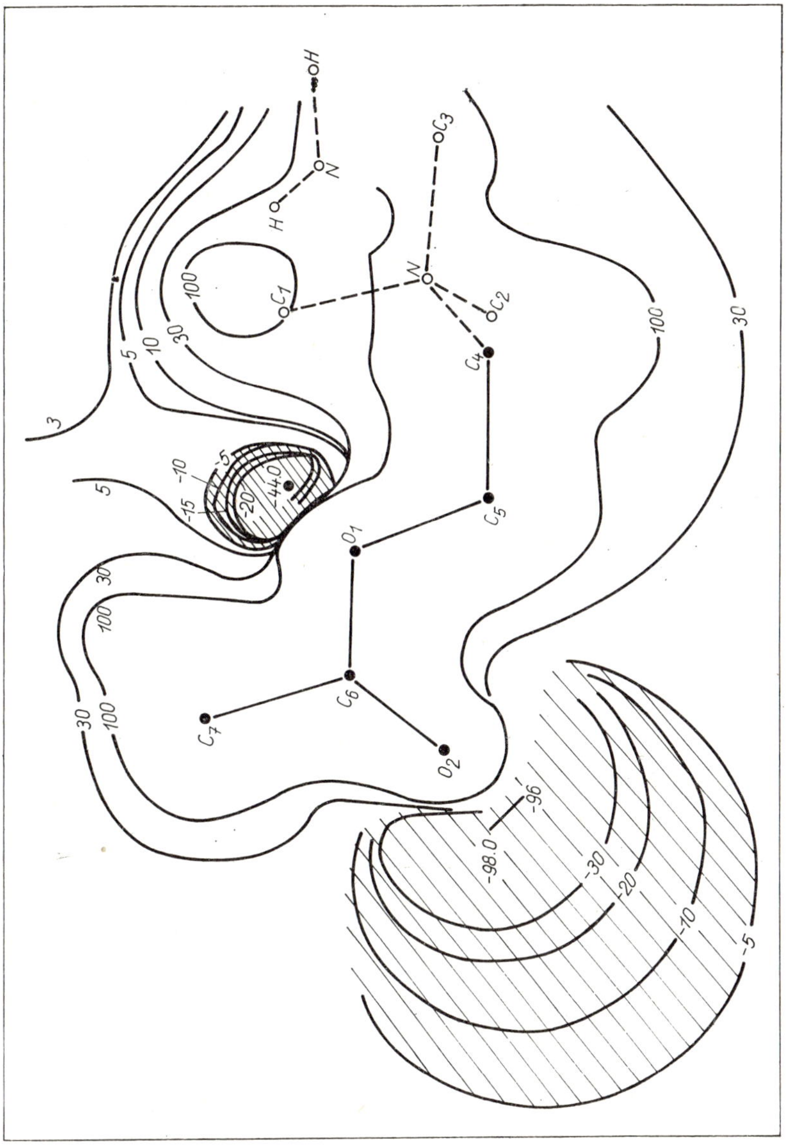

Fig. 12.4. Molecular electrostatic potential for acetylcholine interacting with a negative group (see text). Regions of negative potentials are represented by shaded areas (from [223])

in order to accept the cholinergic interaction pharmacophore as of general validity. Being of the recognition pharmacophore type, the cholinergic interaction pharmacophore can only globally characterize the ability of compounds to interact with the receptor and cannot differentiate between agonists and antagonists.

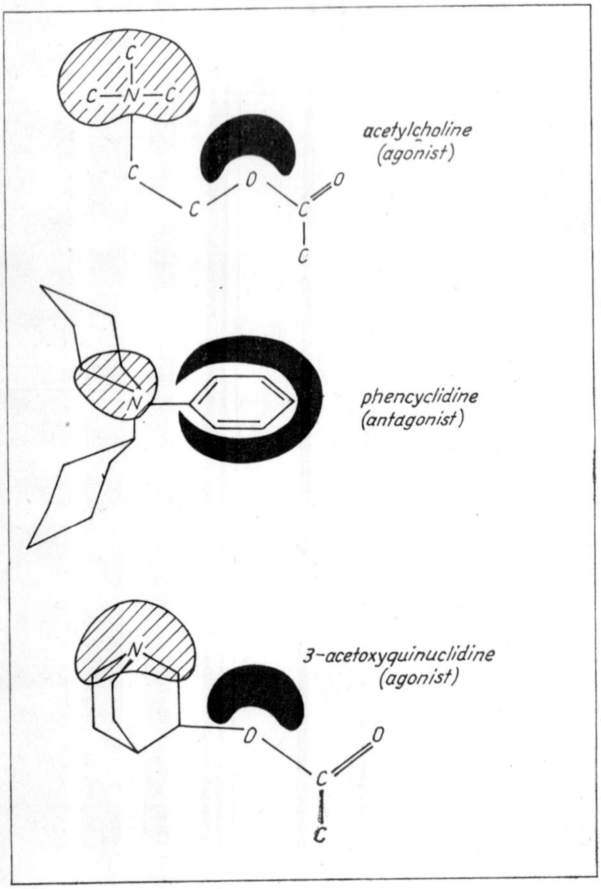

Fig. 12.5. Schematic representation of the cholinergic interaction pharmacophore in two cholinergic agonists and one antagonist. Shaded areas represent regions of negative electrostatic potential and straited areas positive regions (after [223])

There are, however, situations where the interaction pharmacophore is capable of yielding information about affinity or even intrinsic activity. This will be the case when the dynamic events of drug-receptor interactions leading to the production of a biological stimulus are already sufficiently well reflected by the MESPs. An example of this kind seems to be provided, to a certain extent, by investigations on β-adrenergic drugs of the phenethanolamine (I) and phenoxypropanolamine (II) type [234—238]. Petrongolo and colleagues [234—238] investigated the MESP pattern of the phenyl part of the former and of the aryl-OCH_2 moiety of the latter compounds in relation to their activity at β-adrenergic receptors using model compounds. Two regions of negative electrostatic potential could be identified in the agonists, and following a suggestion by MACCHIA et al. [238] on a possible interaction pattern at the β-adrenergic receptor site these regions will be called S- and Φ-regions, respectively. In type I compounds the S-region is located at the aromatic substituents and the Φ-region above the phenyl ring, while the S-region in type II compounds is at the phenyl ring and the Φ-region shifted towards the $-OCH_2-$ group. In other words, the potential generated at the aromatic substituents in type I compounds must be compared with that at the phenyl ring in type II compounds and that at the phenyl ring in the former with that in the vicinity of the OCH_2 group in the latter in order to give a coherent picture. Antagonists differ from agonists in that the potential in the Φ-region is positive while they still have a negative potential in the S-region. The authors, therefore, concluded that the negative potential in the S-region (common to both, agonists and antagonists) may be connected with affinity while that in the Φ-region (different for agonists and antagonists) may relate to intrinsic activity. If testing dipoles are placed in the vicinity of the S- and Φ-regions (positive charges pointing towards the drug molecules), the interaction of the Φ dipole is attractive only for the β-agonist drugs while the interaction with the S-dipole is attractive for both agonists and antagonist with, however, more negative values of interaction energy for the former. This simple model is attractive but needs verification by extending the analysis to a greater number of compounds. It has the further advantage that assumptions about a special conformation of type II compounds proposed in the literature to make these compounds superimposable over type I compounds (see e.g. [249b]) are not needed (for a discussion of this point, see [238, 249b]). For a full understanding of adrenergic drug action, the reactivity of the side-chain has, of course, also to be taken into account [238] (see also 11.). It is interesting to note, however, that from this model it may implicitly be derived that type I and type II compounds should have very similar distances between the hydroxylic oxygen and the amino N atom, and this has in fact been found in a recent quantum-chemical investigation [249c]. The model is further supported by a recent MESP analysis of adrenergic phenethanolamines performed by HADŽI et al. [240] which also demonstrated the importance of the negative potential region at the aromatic substituents for adrenergic activity. When the depth of the negative electrostatic potential minimum in the region of 3,4-aromatic ring substitution is plotted against adenylate cyclase stimulating potency (measure for β-adrenergic activity) a good relationship is obtained for a series of eleven β-adrenergic agonists (Fig. 12.6). The selectivity of adrenergic compounds for α- and β-receptors may also be connected with MESPs [240].

Judging from recent experience the analysis of MESPs can be regarded as a promising approach to a better understanding of drug action at the molecular level and to pharmacophoric pattern searching. As long as MESPs are considered to characterize the recognition step, the usual choice of minimum energy conformations as a basis for the calculations is reasonable since the interactions at the recognition point are still so weak that a conformational perturbation of the approaching drug is unlikely to occur. At this point, furthermore, long-range electrostatic interactions will usually dominate so that it is justified to neglect other interaction energies and also polarization effects due to the approaching charge (at least to a first approximation). Beyond the recognition point, however, this is no longer true, and if results directly concerning the formation of the drug-receptor complex are aimed at through an analysis of MESPs it will become necessary to allow for conformational flexibility, to include other types of interactions (e.g., dispersion forces) and to account for polarization effects. In such cases the calculation of MESPs should be based on the biologically active conformation likely to be present at the receptor which can, for example, be obtained from molecular matching techniques (see 12.5.).

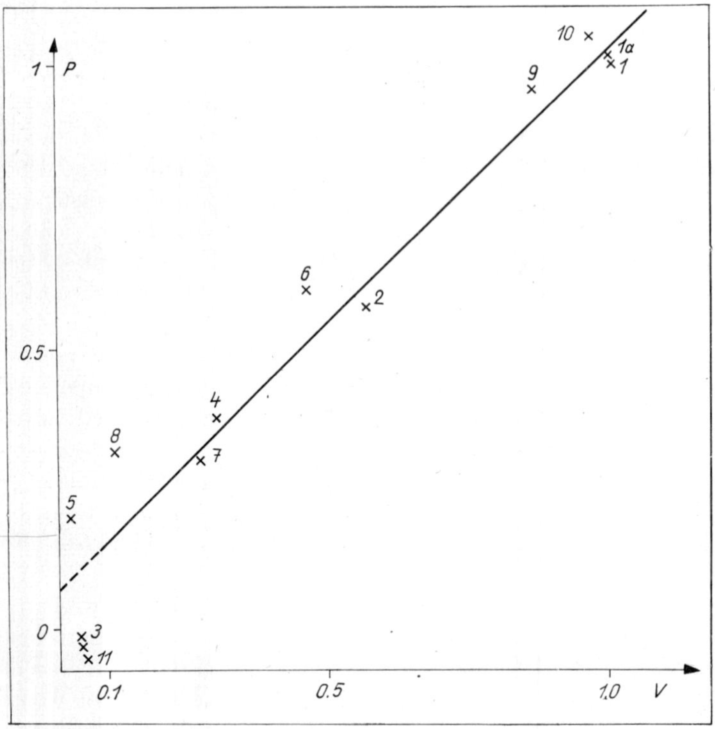

Fig. 12.6. Correlation of adenylate cyclase stimulating potency (P) of some β-adrenergic agonists with the depth of the negative potential minimum in the region of 3,4-aromatic ring substitution (V). 1 = Noradrenaline, 2 = Isoproterenol, 3 = Sotatol, 4 = Octopamine, 5 = Normetanephrine, 6 = Salbutamol, 7 = Metaraminol, 8 = Metaproterenol, 9 = Pirbuterol, 10 = 2-fluoronoradrenaline, 11 = 6-fluoronoradrenaline (from [240])

The two-dimensional analysis of MESPs via isoenergy contour maps may sometimes be difficult and arbitrary since the result may depend on the position and orientation of the plane selected, especially in non-symmetrical molecules. Furthermore, the evaluation of interaction pharmacophores from MESPs by simple inspection should be replaced by more objective and efficient procedures as, for example, pattern recognition methods. Such methods would, in principle, allow one to analyse the whole spatial MESP distribution around a molecule which should yield more information than a simple map referring to only a plane through that space; procedures based on gradients to describe the shape of MESPs in space may also be helpful here (see e.g. [299]). An interesting alternative is to consider the MESP on the surface of the molecular envelope [250].

12.5. Molecular Matching and Superimposition

The biologically active conformation of drugs may be evaluated to a certain extent by a systematic comparison of the molecular geometries of different compounds interacting with the same receptor. Usually, a drug of particularly high and specific activity (e.g., morphine in the case of the opiate receptor) is selected as a kind of standard with which the other molecules to be considered are then compared one at a time. At the beginning of this comparison an initial position and conformation is chosen for each molecule. They are then considered as free to move and to modify their geometries within a pre-established limit of the total molecular energy. In this way the comparison includes not only minimum energy conformations but a large part of the accessible conformational space and is thus truly dynamic. If a match between the molecules within this space can be found there is good reason to assume that the corresponding spatial arrangement of atoms corresponds to the biologically active conformation and represents the geometry of the pharmacophore. Other molecules may then be designed which conform to the desired geometric requirements.

A critical point is the selection of a reasonable limit for the increase in total energy resulting from the deformation of the molecules during the matching procedure. In a biological situation these energy costs would be provided from the energy of drug-receptor interactions which may, however, be quite different in different cases. Since, furthermore, the flexibility of molecules also varies over a broad range, no clear or general rule for establishing an amount of allowed energy costs can be given, and quite different views have been presented in the literature [94, 250—252]. As a rule of thumb an upper limit of 42—63 kJ/mol seems to be reasonable (see e.g. [250, 253]) but it may be necessary to vary this amount according to specific features of the problems considered.

Several techniques are available for the matching of molecules (e.g. [2, 71, 75, 119, 142, 250, 254—259]) most of them based on interactive computer graphics. Usually, a stepwise procedure is applied to optimize the extent of fit between the pair of molecules considered with respect to intermolecular rotation and translation as well as conformational changes. The simplest criteria of fit are the sum of squares of the distances between corresponding atoms in the two molecules (see e.g. [254]) or the root mean square deviation of all interatomic distances [71]. Another possibility is to use the total exposed molecular area of the overlapping molecules [250], and some modification of the molecular shape parameter introduced by Hopfinger [260—261] might also be applicable. During the optimization these criteria are minimized while limiting the total increase in molecular energy resulting from deformations of the molecules to the pre-established amount. A different approach can be based on the superposition of energy maps (or, rather, probability contours obtainable from such maps) of different molecules resulting from conformational analysis [87, 196] which will be discussed below.

The technique of molecular matching or superimposition has recently been successfully applied to a variety of problems (see also 12.6. and 12.7.; e.g. [2, 71, 134, 250, 253, 256, 259, 262—280]). Some example are summarized in Table 12.3. A few details should suffice to give an idea of what can be achieved.

Green et al. [264, 265, 271] showed that LSD is a competitive antagonist of histamine H_2-receptors in the brain. They compared the structure of LSD with those of the well

Table 12.3. Some recent examples for the application of molecular matching and similar techniques to derive pharmacophoric pattern

Type of drugs	References
Atileukemics	[71]
Histamine analogs	[87, 196]
Catecholamines	[122]
Somatostatine derivatives	[151, 154, 155]
LHRH derivatives	[155]
Cyclic hexapeptide analogs of cyclo-(Ala-Sar)$_3$	[155]
Opiates, Analgesics	[71, 253, 267–269, 272–277]
Substrate for transpeptidase	[256]
Digitoxines	[259, 266]
Antiinflammatory Arylacetic acids	[262]
Chloramphenicol	[263]
H_2-Antagonists	[264, 265, 271]
Penicillins	[270]
GABA analogs	[278–280]

known selective H_2-antagonists cimetidine and metiamide (Fig. 12.7) which, at a first glance, show no obvious similarities. However, sterically the molecules neatly superimpose, the oxygen of the amide group of LSD being congruent with the nitrogen of the cyano group of cimetidine or the sulphur atom of the thiourea group in metiamide. The moiety in D-LSD which is sterically congruent with metiamide or cimetidine is hexanoic acid-4-aza-4-methyl-6-(3-pyrrolyl)-N,N-diethylamide (Fig. 12.7), and it was proposed that this structure as well as its indolyl and imidazole analogues and their derivatives have H_2-antagonist activity. Available was hexanoic acid-4-aza-4,5-dimethyl-6-(3-indolyl)-N,N-diethylamide (SK & F 10,856; see Fig. 12.7), and biological testing proved it to be a potent competitive antagonist of histamine at the H_2-receptor. Thus, a new biologically active structure could be predicted by simple matching of three known compounds.

Intensive studies have been performed on the biologically active conformation of analgesics and the opiate pharmacophore (see e.g. [101]). Using molecular mechanics Cheney et al. [253] investigated and compared the geometries of several analgesics and related compounds starting with morphine (see Fig. 12.8). They found that morphine has a considerable amount of flexibility and concluded that, when compared to other molecules, its geometry must also be varied and should not be assumed to be rigid. With this in mind morphine was matched with fentanyl and meperidine (Fig. 12.8) using a four-point model including the following atoms:

morphine: quaternary nitrogen, C_3, C_1, C_{12};
fentanyl: quaternary nitrogen, para- and the two meta-positions of the F ring;
meperidine: quaternary nitrogen, para- and the two meta positions of the phenyl ring.

A good match could be obtained in both cases at energy costs that might be expected to be covered in a drug-receptor interaction (Table 12.4) indicating a common bioactive conformation for all three molecules. This conformation is not a minimum energy con-

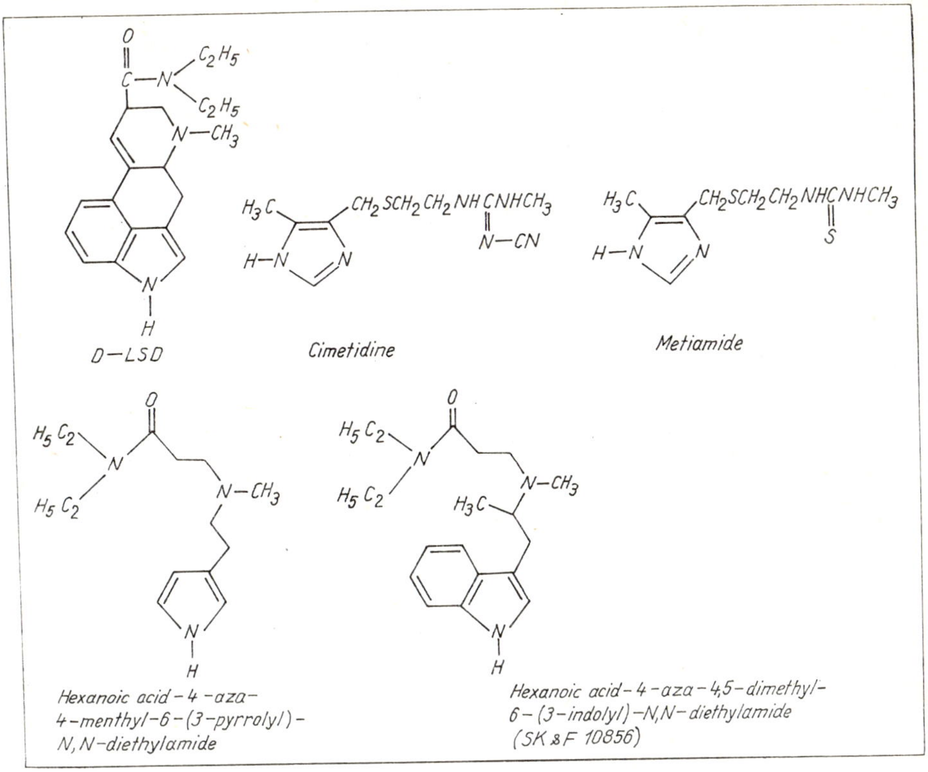

Fig. 12.7. Structural formulas of D-LSD, Cimetidine, Metiamide and of two new compounds with H_2-antagonistic activity derived from molecular superimposition [265]

Table 12.4. Results of the matching of Fentanyl and Meperidine with Morphine: energy costs and distances between the 4 selected points (from [253])

Point	Distances between corresponding points (in nm)		
	Morphine/ Fentanyl	Morphine/ Meperidine[1])	Morphine/ Meperidine[2])
(1)	0.05	0.03	0.04
(2)	0.01	0	0
(3)	0.02	0	0
(4)	0.02	0	0
energy costs[3]) (in kJ/mol)	10.9/21.8	8.8/15.1	11.3/28.9

[1]) axial form

[2]) equatorial form

[3]) increase in energy of the "matching" conformation compared to the minimum energy of the isolated molecule

formation. The same was true of the two antagonists nalorphine and naloxane which can also be closely matched.

These and some additional results led Cheney et al. [253] to conclude that "for several of the important classes of analgesic agonist and antagonists, quite similar geometric environments for atoms believed to be important to the drug-receptor interaction can be attained at only modest energy cost". In other words, a well defined bioactive conformation (pharmacophore) exists for the interaction with the opiate receptor and compounds capable of interacting with that receptor must be able to match the required spatial arrangements. In addition to these geometric demands (which are still under investigation, see e.g. [143g, 268—269]) electronic factors seem also to be important [241a, 242, 253]. Of particular interest is the question whether opiates and enkephalins have a similar active conformation. A number of conformational comparisons with rigid opiates considering overlaps of different assumed critical regions have been made [253, 272—277]. Gorin and Marshall [267] used the tetrapeptide Tyr-Ala-Gly-Phe as enkephalin model and tried to fit it to morphine starting from the following two conditions:

1. The amino terminus and phenolic ring of Tyr[1] must spatially correspond to the phenolic A ring and the nitrogen atom of morphine (see Fig. 12.8).
2. The para and meta positions of Phe[4] should spatially correspond to the C 5 and C 6 atoms of morphine which were assumed to make an important contribution to the opiate pharmacophore.

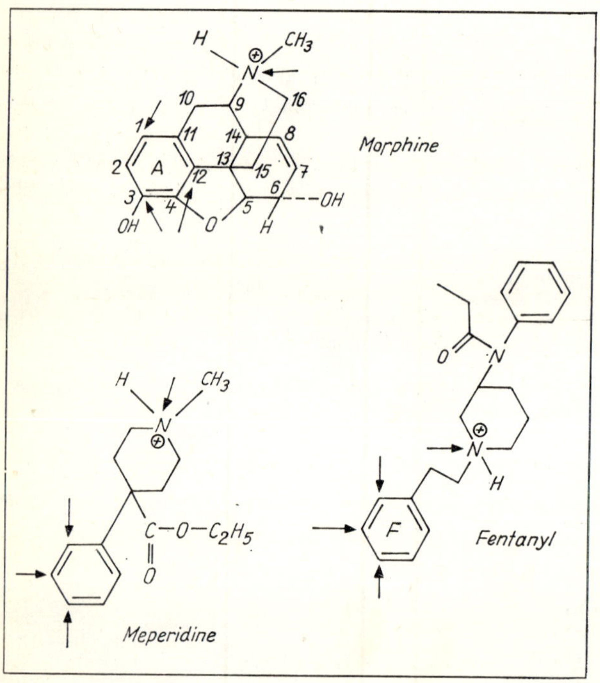

Fig. 12.8. Structural formulas of Morphine, Fentanyl and Meperidine. The 4 points selected for matching [253] are arrowed (see text)

The first condition could easily be fulfilled by fixing the side-chain torsion angles of Tyr[1] at $\tau_1 = 197°$ and $\tau_2 = 106°$ which gives an aromatic ring centre — to — nitrogen distance of 0.45 nm (morphine: 0.45 nm; naloxone: 0.448 nm). In order to check the second condition two target points were placed relative to the phenolic ring and amino terminus of Tyr[1] so as to correspond spatially to C 5 and C 6 of morphine, and the torsion angle space of the eight remaining rotatable bonds of the peptide backbone and the side-chains of Phe[4] was then explored systematically. As a result a single conformer was found in which the distances between the para and meta positions of Phe[4] and the target points were within 0.04 nm the latter being as small as 0.022 nm. Gorin and Marshall proposed this conformation as the one bound to the analgesic receptor. It is satisfactory that predictions made on this basis regarding the activity of enkephalin analogues in which modifications affect backbone conformational possibilities turned out to be correct [267, 267a—c]. Work along similar lines was done by Loew et al. [276, 277] who investigated the overlap of met-enkephalin conformers over rigid opiates using the following criteria:

- modest energy costs,
- significant overlap involving at least the tyramine moieties of enkephalin and the opiates,
- accommodation of D-Ala[2] but not L-Ala[2] in place of the Gly[2] residue.

They found a low energy conformer (12.56 kJ/mol above the minimum energy) with significant rigid opiate overlap beyond the imposed tyramine matching and concluded that enkephalin binds to the receptor by an induced fit initiated at the crucial tyramine region, followed by the binding of the C-terminal residues. From all these studies it follows that enkephalins may in fact sterically resemble opiate molecules and that the biologically active conformation at the opiate receptor is not a minimum energy conformation. With a static approach considering only the properties of isolated molecules in their minimum energy states, this information could not have been obtained.

It is very satisfactory that not only small molecules but also peptides can successfully be handled in such approaches. In this connection the work done by Veber and colleagues [150—155] on analogues of cyclo-(Ala-Sar)$_3$, LHRH and somatostatin should be mentioned. Using the Merck Molecular Modeling System [2, 133, 134] and a strategy of narrowing the conformational possibilities of the peptides through selective conformational constraint, they were able to derive detailed conclusions on the bioactive conformations. In the somatostatin case a bridged analogue was found which had only four of the original fourteen amino acid residues, yet had three times the insulin inhibiting activity but only 5% of the gastric secretion inhibition of somatostatin. In addition, it also exhibited increased duration of action and even some activity when given orally. Detailed analyses of this and other analogues led to a refined picture of the bioactive conformation which may now aid in the design of further therapeutically useful analogues.

Instead of directly matching molecular structures, conformational energy maps containing the information on the whole conformational space (at least as far as rotation about two bonds in concerned) may also be superimposed. A direct comparison of energy contours has, however, two disadvantages: the result heavily depends on the scaling of the energy contours, and the entropy factor is completely neglected. For this reason it is more appropriate to compare probability contours in conformational space which can easily be obtained from the energy maps. Such contours may either represent the probability of the occurrence of certain conformations or the possible range of conformations for a pre-established probability. For the comparison of molecules in order to find regions of bioactive conformations the latter variant is more convenient. The conformations which can be adopted at the pre-set probability occur as certain regions in the same coordinate system used for representing the energy contours with angles of rotation as axes. Such probability maps directly show how flexible a molecule may be and which regions of conformational space are favoured, and comparison of such maps for a series of analogues will show whether there are conformational requirements for activity. An interesting example of this type of analysis is provided by the work of GANELLIN and colleagues on the conformation of histamine derivatives in relation to their dual receptor activity [87, 196] at H_1- and H_2-receptors. As already pointed out, the potency of histamine (Fig. 12.9) at these two receptors is extremely sensitive to methylation (see Table 12.1). Figures 12.10—12.13 show probability maps for histamine, 4-methylhistamine, N,N-dimethylhistamine and α-methylhistamine. The smallest H_1/H_2 activity ratio (highest selectivity for the H_2-receptor) is that of 4-methylhistamine. If it is assumed that this selectivity is related to conformational properties, the inability of 4-methylhistamine to function properly as an H_1-receptor stimulant can be viewed as a consequence of its inability to assume a necessary bioactive conformation. Since this conformation must be accessible for histamine it may be found by superimposing the maps for histamine and 4-methylhistamine as that region available to histamine but not to 4-methylhistamine. The result is shown in Fig. 12.14. If all H_1 agonists are considered this region may further be narrowed as shown by the dark

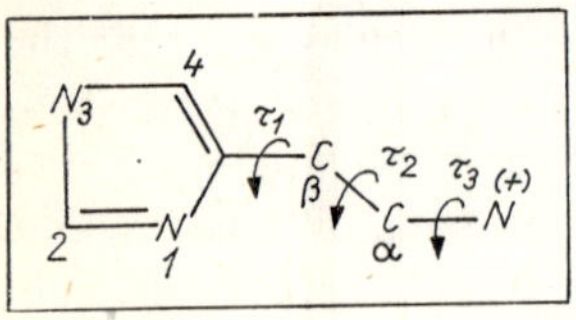

Fig. 12.9. Histamine structure and angles for rotation

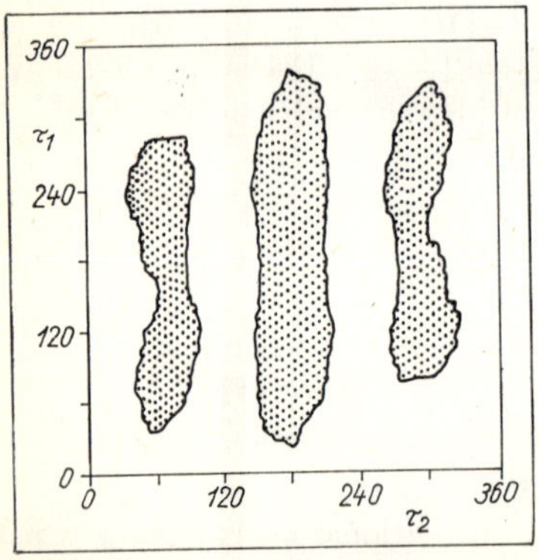

Fig. 12.10

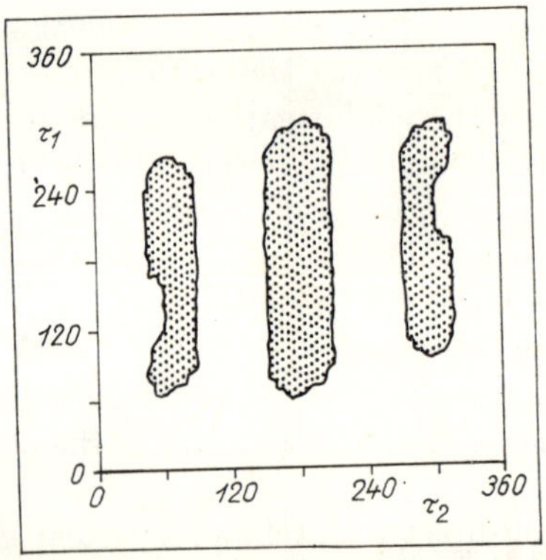

Fig. 12.11

Fig. 12.10. Probability map for histamine. The shaded area indicates the range of conformation which would encompass 99% of the molecules at 310.3 K (from [87])

Fig. 12.11. Probability map for 4-methylhistamine. The shaded area indicates the range of conformation that would encompass 99% of the molecules at 310.3 K (from [87])

areas in Fig. 12.14. These areas may be regarded as representing the H_1 essential conformation. As in the preceding examples this conformation is not a minimum energy conformation and could thus not have been found by static considerations (see 12.3.). A similar approach was used by KUMBAR [169] in a study on the hallucinogenic and antiserotonin activity of lysergic acid derivatives.

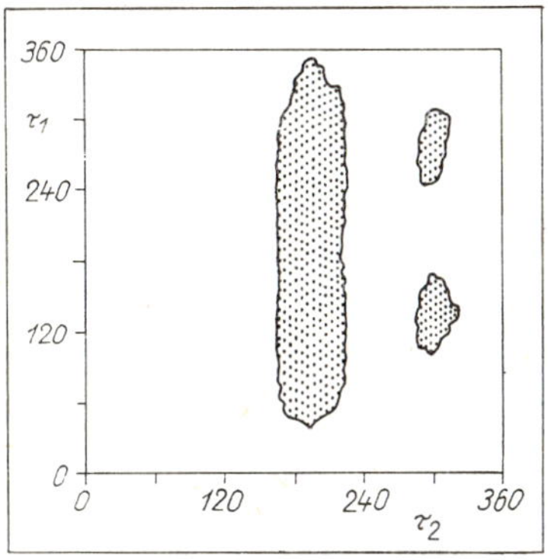

Fig. 12.12. Probability map for N,N-dimethylhistamine. The shaded area indicates the range of conformation which would encampass 99% of the molecules at 310.3 K (from [87])

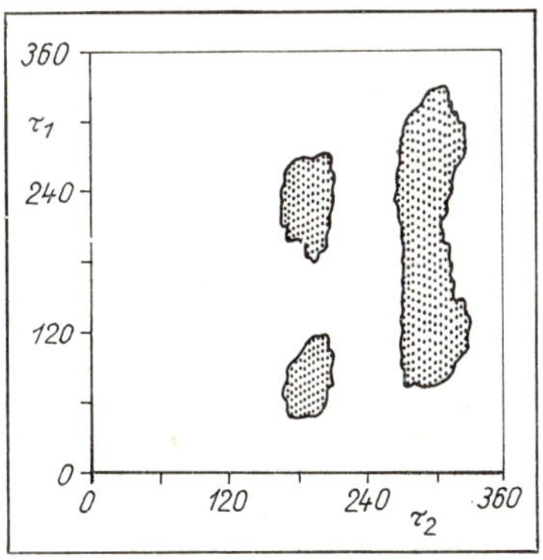

Fig. 12.13. Probability map for α-methylhistamine. The shaded area indicates the range of conformation which would encompass 99% of the molecules at 310.3 K (from [87])

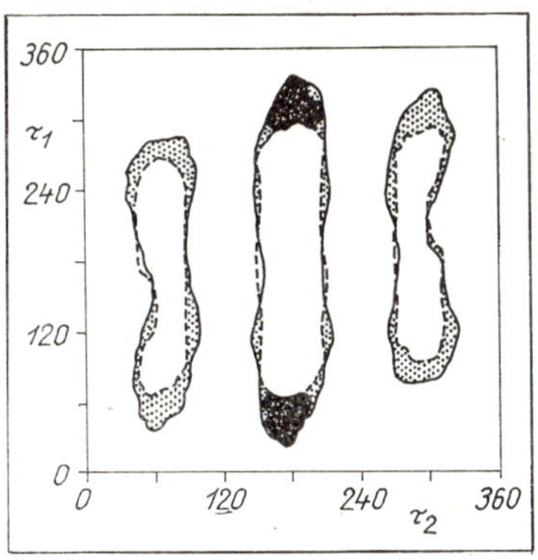

Fig. 12.14. Comparison of probability maps for histamine and its methyl derivatives. The dotted area indicates regions available to histamine but not to the 4-methyl derivative. The dark area is within the 99% contour for all H_1 active agonists and represents the conformation "essential" for H_1 activity

The advantages of dynamic approaches over static considerations are obvious. The resulting information on bioactive conformations represents affinity or even intrinsic pharmacophores (depending on the types of compounds included in an analysis) as far as spatial properties are concerned. Such pharmacophores may, of course, involve additional properties as, for example, certain charge distributions, etc. Activity, intrinsic activity and selectivity of histamine compounds for the H_1- and H_2-receptors, for example, are not only related to conformational properties but heavily depend also on electronic properties and tautomeric equilibria [204—206]. A tremendous advantage of knowing the bioactive conformation in a dynamic sense is that such additional properties may now be calculated for that molecular geometry presumed to be involved in the binding to the receptor. This was done, for instances, in the above mentioned work of Cheney et al. [253] on opiates. Another example is provided by an investigation of Cohen [250] on hypolipidemic agents. After matching the compounds, the energy contours of the electrostatic potentials were drawn on the surface of their molecular envelopes (defined from the van der Waals radii of the atoms). The result showed that the similarities between the compounds in question were not only geometrical but also electronic.

Difficulties may sometimes arise if molecules can be matched in more than one way. In such cases *a priori* assumptions may become necessary about essential centres and the mutual orientation of the molecules which may, of course, turn out to be wrong. Information from topological analyses (see chapter 11.) may sometimes be helpful in making the correct decisions.

12.6. The Active Analogue Approach (AAA)

Developed on the basis of the MMS-X molecular modelling and graphic display system by Marshall and colleagues [139, 144, 281, 282] and successfully applied to a variety of problems [143g, 267—267c, 268a, 269, 281—287) the AAA is a dynamic approach which has essential parts in common with the matching techniques discussed in the preceding section. It is based on the following propositions:

1. Compounds active at a given receptor have in common a spatial arrangement of certain atoms (for example, heteroatoms) or groups (pharmacophoric groups) which is essential for the recognition by and the activation of the receptor. This arrangement is called the pharmacophore in the context of the AAA. Its presence is a necessary but not sufficient condition for biological activity.
2. Only a limited volume is available at the receptor for the binding of agonists which is called "*receptor excluded volume*".
3. A necessary and sufficient condition for a compound to be active is that is possesses the pharmacophore and does not occupy any extra volume outside the "receptor excluded volume" at the receptor.
4. Even when correctly representing the pharmacophore, a compound will be inactive if it requires volume at the receptor binding site which is occupied by the receptor itself (extra volume outside the receptor excluded volume). Such extra volume is termed "*receptor essential volume*".

The pharmacophore and receptor excluded volume are evaluated by a systematic comparison of active analogues taking into account that the biologically active conformation induced on binding to the receptor is probably not a minimum energy conformation. Therefore, all possible conformations of all analogues have to be examined which is a tremendous task even with sophisticated programs and high-speed computers. In order to limit the computations to a manageable size a very effective strategy is applied based mainly on the following principles:

1. conformational analyses are performed on the basis of molecular mechanics considering only VAN DER WAALS interactions,
2. systematic use of conformationally restricted analogues in order to narrow the search space (see also 12.1.),
3. interactive and stepwise performance where information from preceding steps can be used to reduce computational complexity in subsequent steps,
4. decomposition of complex searches into tractable sub-problems,
5. application of special constrained search techniques.

The initial task is the evaluation of the pharmacophore. This requires that a hypophesis can be derived from existing structure-activity relationships and known facts as to which centres or atoms of the molecules are to be regarded as pharmacophoric groups. All allowed conformations are now evaluated for each active analogue, and for each conformation the relative position of the proposed pharmacophoric groups is determined. This can be expressed as an *orientation map* in which each point represents one possible arrangement of these groups, i.e., a possible pharmacophoric pattern. The coordinates of the orientation map are the pairwise distances between all groups. For three pharmacophoric groups A, B and C, for example, the orientation map has three dimensions with the distances $\overline{AB}$, $\overline{AC}$ and $\overline{BC}$ as axes where each point represents a specific triangle. The intersection of the orientation maps of all compounds yields the possible pharmacophoric pattern available to the entire set of active analogues. Philosophically, this approach is very similar to that of RICHARDS and colleagues applied to histaminic compounds (see Fig. 12.10—12.14). If the set of compounds is large enough and shows sufficient structural variation, a unique definition of the pharmacophore will usually be possible.

The determination of the pharmacophoric groups can be assisted by the use of distance range matrices (see chapter 11.). Constructed for each active analogue to be compared, such a matrix contains the maximum and minimum pairwise distances between atoms in the accessible conformation space. Additional information such as the elevation of atoms above the plane of an aromatic ring can also be included. Any hypothesis on possible pharmacophoric groups can now easily be checked by comparing such matrices The very definition of the pharmacophore implies that it is common to all active analogues. Hence, the minimum condition for accepting a pair of centres as pharmacophoric groups is that the distance ranges between these centres overlap for all molecules. On the other hand, only the overlapping ranges between possible pharmacophoric groups are of biological importance so that conformations corresponding to distances not within the overlap need not be considered. The intersection of the distance ranges of the active analogues thus leads to a limitation of the original space to be searched creating a subspace designated as *target space*. As a result much of the computation may be eliminated. This is especially true if sterically constrained molecules are available which, as a consequence of their smaller possible distance ranges, place narrower limits on the possible pharmacophore which translate into distance constraints for subsequent molecules.

Once the pharmacophore has been defined, the steric demands for activity at the receptor are investigated using the concept of receptor excluded volume. Using the pharmacophore as a common frame of reference for orienting the molecules, a pseudo-electron density map contured according to space-filling physical models is constructed for each compound in its presumed receptor-bound conformation. These three-dimensional maps represent the volumes of the analogues when correctly representing the pharmacophore, and the receptor excluded volume is then simply obtained as the union of these maps for all active analogues. The activity of new compounds can now be predicted by determining whether they can both represent the pharmacophore and fit within the excluded volume map.

In the last step inactive analogues possessing the pharmacophore are included in the analysis in order to evaluate the receptor essential volume. The assumption made here is that the inactivity of such compounds is due to their requirement of extra volumes outside the receptor excluded volume which is occupied by the receptor itself, so that they cannot bind or do not bind in the correct way. This assumption is reasonable if the inactives considered are physically similar to the active analogues. The receptor essential volume can be evaluated as follows:

1. volume union of all inactives, again using the pharmacophore as a frame of reference,
2. intersection of this volume union with the receptor excluded volume,
3. subtraction of the volume resulting from the intersection from the volume union of inactives = receptor essential volume.

Unfortunately, one cannot presume which part of the receptor essential volume is responsible for inactivity unless a unique area can be found for all inactive. One possibility of overcoming this problem which is being investigated by MARSHALLS group is to score each segment of this volume by considering the number of inactives in which it is present. In this way a probabilistic value could be given to possible inactivity of novel compounds requiring volume outside the receptor excluded volume.

The active analogue approach provides a powerful and logical technique for pharmacophore identification and exploration. It should be noted that the definition of a pharmacophore used here is different from that given in section 12.1. According to the latter the true pharmacophore should include the whole information obtainable from the AAA, namely:

- the pharmacophore as defined in the context of the AAA (spatial arrangement of essential groups),
- the receptor excluded volume,
- the receptor essential volume which may be regarded as an "antipharmacophoric" feature.

Depending on the type of analogues considered, this information will resemble:

- an affinity pharmacophore, if all analogues have the same intrinsic activity,
- an intrinsic pharmacophore, if all compounds have the same affinity,
- a mixture of both, if affinity and intrinsic activity both vary.

The way in which the volumes are compared is conceptionally similar to SIMONS MTD concept (e.g. [288]) and to the molecular shape analysis introduced by HOPFINGER

[260—261] (see chapter 6.) with the important difference that these approaches are not dynamic.

A volume representation as a basic feature of the AAA was selected instead of an electrostatic potential field since van der Waals forces show a much sharper dependence on distance (proportional to r^{-6}) than coulombic forces (proportional to r^{-2}) and it was felt that this is required to explain the high discriminating power of receptors. This is certainly a reasonable argument for drug-receptor interactions beyond the recognition point, but even there an analysis of MESPs (see 12.4.) instead of or in addition to volumes using similar techniques could be a promising alternative. A spatial comparison of MESPs would, of course, be much more complicated since the magnitude and sign of the potential at each point in space would appear as additional dimensions.

Problems may sometimes arise in formulating a valid proposal on the nature of the pharmacophoric groups. Topological approaches as outlined in chapter 11. may be of some help here and capable of providing a reasonable hypothesis to start with.

12.7. Transition State Analogues

Inhibitors resembling the transition state geometry of an enzymatically catalyzed reaction are some orders of magnitude more potent than substrate analogues since the transition state is bound much more tightly than the substrate itself [289—291]; in addition, they are also more specific. This has led to the use of the structure of transition states as templates for the design of powerful and highly selective enzyme inhibitors which are called *transition state analogues* (for reviews, see [292—300]).

Since only an extremely small number of molecules will exist in the transition state at any given time it is impossible to study transition state structures directly. These structures have, therefore, to be derived from an interpolation between substrate(s) and product(s) along the reaction coordinate with the help of quantum chemical methods Of the alternative molecular orbital methods available, especially the MINDO/3 method. [301] has been recommended for this purpose [297, 302]. As the reaction coordinate, an internal coordinate is chosen which changes continuously on the way from the substrate(s) to the product(s). If details of the enzymatically catalyzed reaction are not known the corresponding non-enzymatic chemical reaction is taken as a model which can be expected to be similar with regard to bond breaking and bond making processes [303]. The energies at various points along the reaction coordinate are computed, and the transition state is located at the point with the energy maximum. The corresponding molecular geometry can then serve as a template for the design of transition state analogue inhibitors. Because of the complexity of many reaction surfaces it may become necessary to calculate reaction pathways for several starting geometries of the substrate(s) and different reaction coordinates. As a result a number of alternative transition state structures may be obtained. The most likely candidate of the true transition state is that corresponding to the minimum energy pathway. If, however, the different pathways do not differ much in their energy a decision on the basis of the computations alone will be impossible. It may then become necessary to design structural analogues for each of the alternative transition state geometries and to test their inhibitory potency against the enzyme in question; the inhibitor resembling the true transition state will then produce the strongest inhibition.

Once the transition state structure has been elucidated, analogues resembling it as closely as possible are to be designed. This is not an easy task since the long partial bonds and abnormal hybridization of transition state structures are difficult to mimic in stable compounds, but a number of plausible analogues can usually be derived by inspection and chemical reasoning. To facilitate comparison of these analogues with the transition state structure, interactive computer graphics and molecular superimposition techniques (see 12.5.) can be used. Those analogues which optimally match the transition state structure are then selected for synthesis and biological testing.

Table 12.5. Some examples of transition state analogue inhibitors [296, 299]

Enzyme	Substrate	Transition state analogue inhibitor
Dihydrofolate reductase	Folate	Methotrexate
Aspartate transcarbamylase	Carbamylphosphate	N-Phosphonoacetyl-L-Aspartate
Adenosine deaminase	Adenosine	Conformycin
Acetoacetate decarboxylase	Acetoacetate	Acetopyruvate
Proline racemase	L-Proline	Pyrrole-2-Carboxylate
t-RNA-Ligases	L-Alanine	DL-Alaninol-AMP-ester

The transition state analogue concept is becoming more and more important and has already led to potentially valuable drugs (see e.g. [304—306]). Brodbeck [299] estimates that about 70 enzymes are recognized targets for inhibition by transition state analogues. Some selected examples are presented in Table 12.5. Transition state analogue inhibitors are of special importance in the field of chemotherapy since they can be specifically designed to inhibit enzymes which are vital to microorganisms or abnormal cells, but of no importance for the host. Most interestingly, β-lactam antibiotics (penicillins, cephalosporins), for example, seem to belong to this class resembling the structure of the possible transition state for the scission of the peptide bond in D-Ala-D-Ala, a reaction specific for bacterial cell wall biosynthesis [307—314]. The antibiotics and the proposed transition state can match almost exactly, and a quantitative relationship exists between the transition state energy for a model gas-phase reaction of β-lactam structures with an approaching nucleophile (OH^-) and antibacterial potency. Another enzyme of interest as a potential target for compounds with antibacterial activity is chorismate mutase which catalyzes the rearrangement of chorismate to prephenate (first step in the biosynthetic pathway leading to tyrosine and phenylalanine in bacteria [315] which is absent in man). Intensive theoretical studies of Andrews and colleagues [297, 298, 316—318] using the transition state analogue concept in fact led to potent inhibitiors.

References

[1] Langridge, R., T. E. Ferrin, I. D. Kuntz and M. L. Conolly: Science **211**, 661 (1981)
[2] Gund, P., J. D. Andose, J. B. Rhodes and G. M. Smith: Science **208**, 1425 (1980)
[3] Meyer, E. F., in E. J. Ariens (Ed.): Drug Design, Vol. X, Academic Press, New York, 1980, p. 267
[4] Cushman, D. W., H. S. Cheung, E. F. Sabo and M. A. Ondetti: Biochemistry **16**, 5484 (1977)

[4a] Lipscomb, W. N., in H. Weinstein and J. P. Green (Eds.): Quantum Chemistry in Biomedical Sciences, Ann. N. Y. Acad. Sci. **367**, 326 (1981)

[4b] Pullman, A., in H. Weinstein and J. P. Green (Eds.): Quantum Chemistry in Biomedical Sciences, Ann. N. Y. Acad. Sci. **367**, 340 (1981)

[4c] Osman, R., H. Weinstein and S. Topiol in H. Weinstein and J. P. Green (Eds.): Quantum Chemistry in Biomedical Sciences, Ann. N. Y. Acad. Sci. **367**, 356 (1981)

[4d] Warshel, A., and R. M. Weiss in H. Weinstein and J. P. Green (Eds.): Quantum Chemistry in Biomedical Sciences, Ann. N. Y. Acad. Sci. **367**, 370 (1981)

[4e] Allen, L. C., in H. Weinstein and J. P. Green (Eds.): Quantum Chemistry in Biomedical Sciences, Ann. N. Y. Acad. Sci. **367**, 383 (1981)

[5] Mathews, D. A., R. A. Alden, J. T. Bolin, D. J. Filman, S. T. Freer, R. Hamlin, W. G. J. Hol, R. L. Kislink, E. J. Postore, L. T. Plante, N. Xuong and J. Kraut: J. Biol. Chem. **253**, 6946 (1978)

[6] Platzer, K. E. B., F. A. Momany and H. A. Scheraga: Int. J. Peptide Protein Res. **4**, 201 (1972)

[6a] Pincus, M. R. and H. A. Scheraga: Biochemistry **20**, 3960 (1981)

[7] Bolis, G., M. Ragazzi, D. Salvaderi, D. R. Ferro and E. Clementi: Gazz. Chim. Ital. **108**, 425 (1978)

[8] Scheiner, S., D. A. Kleier and W. N. Lipscomb: Proc. Natl. Acad. Sci. (USA) **72**, 2606 (1975)

[9] Sheridan, R. P., and L. C. Allen: J. Am. Chem. Soc. **103**, 1544 (1981)

[10] Levitt, M.: J. Mol. Biol. **82**, 393 (1974)

[11] Bedell, C. R., P. J. Goodford, F. E. Norrington, S. Wilkinson and R. Wootton: Brit. J. Pharmac. **57**, 201 (1976)

[12] Norrington, F. E., in R. Franke and P. Oehme (Eds.): Quantitative Structure-Activity Analysis, Akademie-Verlag, Berlin, 1978, p. 69

[13] Brown, F. E., and P. J. Goodford: Brit. J. Pharmac. **60**, 337 (1977)

[14] Gualtieri, F., M. Gianella and C. Melchiorre (Eds.): Recent Advances in Receptor Chemistry, Elsevier, Amsterdam, 1979

[15] O'Brien, R. D.: The Receptors: A Comprehensive Treatise, Plenum Press, New York, 1980

[16] Belleau, B.: J. Med. Chem. **7**, 776 (1964)

[17] Ariens, E. J., and A. M. Simonis in P. R. Saxena and R. P. Forsythe (Eds.): Beta-adrenoreceptor Blocking Agents, North-Holland, Amsterdam, 1976, p. 3

[17a] Burgen, A. S. V.: Fed. Proc. **40**, 2723 (1981)

[18] Ariens, E. J., and R. DeMiranda in F. Gualtieri, M. Gianella and C. Melchiorre (Eds.): Recent Advances in Receptor Chemistry, Elsevier, Amsterdam, 1979

[19] Grünhagen, H. H., M. Iwatsubo and J. P. Changeux: Eur. J. Biochem. **80**, 225 (1977)

[20] Damle, V. N., and A. Karlin: Biochemistry **19**, 3924 (1980)

[21] Weiland, G. A., K. P. Minnemann and P. B. Molinoff: Nature **281**, 114 (1979)

[22] Pike, L. J., and R. J. Lefkowitz: Mol Pharmacol. **14**, 370 (1978)

[23] Insel, P. A., and M. J. Sanda: J. Biol. Chem. **254**, 6554 (1979)

[24] Reinhardt, D., J. Wagner and H. J. Schumann: Naunyn-Schmiedebergs Arch. Pharmak. **275**, 95 (1972)

[25] Harri, M. E.: Acta pharmac. tox. **33**, 273 (1973)

[26] Woppel, W., and U. Trendelenburg: Eur. J. Pharmacol. **23**, 302 (1973)

[27] Downing, D., R. C. Kolbeck, J. E. Holl, W. A. Bransome Jr. and J. Speir: Life Sci. **24**, 603 (1979)

[28] Levitzki, A., in R. M. Featherstone (Ed.): A Guide to Molecular Pharmacology — Toxicology, Marcel Dekker, New York, 1973, part I, p. 305

[29] Maelicke, A., B. W. Fulpius, R. P. Klett and E. Reich: J. Biol. Chem. **252**, 4811 (1977)

[30] Repke, K. R. H., and F. Dittrich: TIPS **1** (1980)

[31] Limbird, L. L., and R. J. Lefkowitz: Proc. Natl. Acad. Sci. (USA) **75**, 228 (1978)

[31a] Harmon, J. T., E. S. Kempner and C. R. Kahn: J. Biol. Chem. **256**, 7719 (1981)
[32] Kier, L. B.: Pure appl. Chem. **35**, 509 (1973)
[33] Kier, L. B., and H.-D. Höltje: J. theor. Biol. **49**, 401 (1975)
[34] Hall, L. H., and L. B. Kier: J. theor. Biol. **58**, 177 (1976)
[35] Kier, L. B.: TIBS N 80 (1976)
[36] Höltje, H.-D.: Int. J. Quant. Chem. QBS **4**, 245 (1977)
[37] Kier, L. B.: personal communication, 1981
[38] Paton, W. D. M.: Proc. Roy. Soc. Ser. B. **154**, 21 (1961)
[39] Beld, A. J., and E. J. Ariens: Eur. J. Pharmacol. **25**, 203 (1974)
[40] Raynaud, J. P., T. Ojasoo, M. M. Bouton and D. Philbert in E. J. Ariens (Ed.): Drug Design, Vol. VIII, Academic Press, New York, 1979, p. 170
[41] Jacobson, A. E., W. A. Klee and W. J. Dunn: Eur. J. Med. Chem. **12**, 49 (1977)
[42] Seeman, P.: Fed. Proc. **37**, 130 (1978)
[43] Seeman, P.: Pharmac. Rev. **32**, 229 (1980)
[44] Möhler, H., and T. Okada: Science **198**, 849 (1977)
[45] Creese, I., D. R. Burt and S. H. Snyder: Science **192**, 481 (1976)
[46] Jacobson, A. E., in G. Barnett, M. Trsic and R. E. Wilette (Eds.): Quantitative Structure Activity Relationships of Analgesics, Narcotic Antagonists and Hallucinogens, NIDA Research Monograph 22, Rockville, 1978, p. 129
[47] Iorio, M. A., and W. A. Klee: J. Med. Chem. **20**, 309 (1977)
[48] Rogers, M. E., H. H. Ong and E. L. May: J. Med. Chem. **18**, 1036 (1975)
[49] Creese, I., and S. H. Snyder: J. Pharmac. Exptl. Therap. **194**, 205 (1975)
[50] Pert, C. B., S. H. Snyder and P. S. Portoghese: J. Med. Chem. **19**, 1248 (1976)
[51] Wilson, R. S., M. E. Rogers, C. B. Pert and S. H. Snyder: J. Med. Chem. **18**, 240 (1975)
[52] Glennon, R. A., and P. K. Gessner: J. Med. Chem. **22**, 428 (1979)
[52a] Titeler, M., in M. A. Simkins (Ed.): Medicinal Chemistry VI, Cotswold Press, Oxford, 1979, p. 437
[53] Burgen, A. S. V., G. C. Robert and J. Feeney: Nature **253**, 753 (1975)
[54] Kaethner, T. M.: Nature **267**, 19 (1977)
[54a] Raghunathan, S., and V. Pattabhi: Int. J. Quant. Chem. **20**, 151 (1981)
[55] Khromov-Borisov, N. V., in R. Franke and P. Oehme (Eds.): Quantitative Structure-Activity Analysis, Akademie-Verlag, Berlin, 1978, p. 149
[56] Ariens, E. J., and M. Simonis: Arch. Int. Pharmacodyn. **127**, 479 (1960)
[57] Ariens, E. J., and M. Simonis: Ann. N.Y. Acad. Sci. **114**, 842 (1967)
[57a] Ariens, E. J., in J. A. Keverling Buisman (Ed.): Biological Activity and Chemical Structure, Pharmacochemistry Library (Eds.: W. Th. Nauta and R. F. Rekker), Vol. 2, Elsevier, Amsterdam 1977, p. 1
[57b] Ariens, E. J., in E. J. Ariens (Ed.): Drug Design, Vol. I, Academic Press, New York, 1971, p. 1
[58] Baker, B. R.: Design of Active-Site Directed Irreversible Enzyme Inhibitors, Wiley, New York, 1967
[59] Terenius, L., in J. A. Keverling Buisman (Ed.): Biological Activity and Chemical Structure, Pharmacochemistry Library (Eds.: W. Th. Nauta and R. F. Rekker), Vol. 2, Elsevier, Amsterdam, 1977, p. 161
[59a] Burgen, A. S. V., N. J. M. Birdsall and E. C. Hulme in M. A. Simkins (Ed.): Medicinal Chemistry VI, Cotswold Press, Oxford, 1979, p. 25
[60] Furchgott, R. F.: Adv. Drug. Res. **3**, 21 (1966)
[60a] Stephenson, R. P.: Brit. J. Pharmacol. Chemother. **11**, 379 (1956)
[61] Furchgott, R. F., and P. Bursztyn: Ann. N.Y. Acad. Sci. **144**, 882 (1967)
[62] Jorgensen, E. C., in E. B. Roche (Ed.): Design of Biopharmaceutical Properties through Prodrugs and Analogs, American Pharmaceutical Association, Washington, 1977, p. 18

[63] Robinson, G. A., F. R. W. Butcher and E. W. Sutherland: Cyclic AMP, Academic Press, New York, 1971
[64] Greengard, P.: Nature **260**, 101 (1976)
[65] Mukherjee, C., M. C. Caron, D. Mulliken and R. J. Lefkowitz: Mol. Pharmacol. **12**, 16 (1976)
[66] Feinberg, A. P., I. Creese and S. H. Snyder: Proc. Natl. Acad. Sci. (USA) **73**, 4215 (1976)
[67] Harden, T. K., B. B. Wolfe and P. B. Molinoff: Mol. Pharmacol. **12**, 1 (1976)
[68] Kolata, G. B.: Science **197**, 36 (1977)
[69] Seelig, S., and G. Sayers: Arch. Biochem. Biophys. **154**, 230 (1973)
[70] Pert, C. B., and S. H. Snyder: Mol. Pharmacol. **10**, 868 (1974)
[71] Gund, P., in F. Hahn, H. Kersten, W. Kersten and W. Szybalski (Eds.): Progress in Molecular and Subcellular Biology, Springer-Verlag, Berlin, 1977, p. 117
[72] Kaufmann, J. J., and E. Kerman in I. S. Forrest, C. J. Carr and E. Usdin (Eds.): The Phenothiazines and Structurally Related Compounds, Raven Press, New York, 1974, p. 55
[73] Kaufmann, J. J., and W. S. Koski: Int. J. Quant. Chem. QBS **2**, 35 (1975)
[74] Kaufmann, J. J., and W. S. Koski in E. J. Ariens (Ed.): Drug Design, Vol. V, Academic Press, New York, 1975, p. 252
[75] Duchamp, D., in R. E. Christoffersen (Ed.): Algorithms for Chemical Computation, ACS, Washington, 1977, p. 98
[75a] Chen, S. H., B. Chu and R. Nossal (Eds.): Scattering Techniques Applied to Supramolecular and Nonequilibrium Systems, NATO Advanced Study Institutes Series, Ser. B: Physics, Vol. 73, Plenum Publishing Corporation, London, 1981
[76] Bovey, I. A.: Nuclear Magnetic Resonance Spectroscopy, Academic Press, New York, 1969
[76a] Pullmann, B. (Ed.): Nuclear Magnetic Resonance Spectroscopy in Molecular Biology, D. Reidl Publishing Company, Dordrecht, 1978
[77] Hargittai, I.: Topics Current Chem. **96**, 43 (1981)
[78] Gordy, W., and R. L. Cook: Microwave Molecular Spectra, Interscience, New York, 1970
[79] Allen, F. H., O. Kennard, W. D. S. Motherwell, W. G. Town and D. G. Watson: J. Chem. Doc. **13**, 119 (1973)
[80] Milne, G. W. A., S. R. Heller, A. E. Fein, E. F. Frees, R. G. Marquardt, J. A. McGill, J. A. Miller and D. S. Spiers: J. Chem. Inf. Comp. Sci. **18**, 181 (1978)
[81] Motherwell, S., and P. Murray-Rost: Acta Cryst. **B 34**, 2518 (1978)
[82] Bernstein, F. C., T. F. Koetzle, G. J. B. Williams, E. F. Meyer Jr., M. D. Brice, J. R. Rogers, O. Kennard, T. Shimanouchi and M. Tasumi: J. Mol. Biol. **112**, 535 (1977)
[83] Tollenaere, J. P., H. Moereels and L. A. Raymaekers: Atlas of the Three-Dimensional Structure of Drugs, Janssen Research Foundation Series, Vol. 1, Elsevier, Amsterdam, 1979
[84] Scharfenberg, P.: Z. Chem. **21**, 328 (1981)
[85] Reck, G.: personal communication
[86] Hache, A., and A. Sklenar: personal communication
[87] Richards, W. G.: Quantum Pharmacology, Butterworth, London, 1977
[87a] Weinstein, H., and J.-P. Green (Eds.): Quantum Chemistry in Biomedical Sciences, Ann. N.Y. Acad. Sci. **367** (1981)
[88] Scharfenberg, P., and J. Sauer: Int. J. Quant. Chem. **18**, 1309 (1980)
[89] Pullman, B., and A. Pullman: Quantum Biochemistry, Interscience, New York, 1963
[90] Kier, L. B.: Molecular Orbital Theory in Drug Research, Academic Press, New York, 1971
[91] Kier, L. B. (Ed.): Molecular Orbital Studies in Chemical Pharmacology, Springer-Verlag, New York, 1970
[92] Kier, L. B.: Adv. in Chemistry Series **114**, 278 (1972)
[93] Richards, W. G., and M. E. Black: Progr. Med. Chem. **11**, 68 (1975)
[94] Green, J. P., C. L. Johnson and S. Kang: Ann. Rev. Pharmacol. **14**, 319 (1974)
[94a] Weinstein, H., R. Osman and J. P. Green in E. C. Olson and R. E. Christoffersen (Eds.): Computer-Assisted Drug Design, ACS Symp. Ser. **112**, 161 (1979)

[95] Pullman, B., and E. Parr (Eds.): The New World of Quantum Chemistry, D. Reidl Publishing Company, Dordrecht, 1976
[96] Christoffersen, R. E., in E. C. Olson and R. E. Christoffersen (Eds.): Computer-Assisted Drug Design, ACS Symp. Ser. **112**, 3 (1979)
[97] Kaufmann, J. J., H. E. Popkie and P. C. Hariharan in E. C. Olson and R. E. Christoffersen (Eds.): Computer-Assisted Drug Design, ACS Symp. Ser. **112**, 415 (1979)
[98] Bergmann, E., and B. Pullman (Eds.): Molecular and Quantum Pharmacology, D. Reidl Publishing Company, Dordrecht, 1974
[99] Neely, W. B., in R. M. Featherstone (Ed.): Guide to Molecular Pharmacology-Toxicology, Marcel Dekker, New York, 1973, Part II
[100] Sklenar, H., and J. Jäger: Struktur-Wirkungs-Beziehungen auf quantenmechanischer Grundlage, Beiträge zur Wirkstofforschung, Heft 10, Akademie-Industrie-Komplex Arzneimittelforschung, Berlin, 1980
[101] Barnett, G., M. Trsic, and R. E. Willette (Eds.): Quantitative Structure-Activity Relationships of Analgesics, Narcotic Antagonists, and Hallucinogens, NIDA Res. Monograph 22, Rockville, 1978
[102] Pullmann, B.: Quantum Mechanics of Molecular Conformations, Wiley, New York, 1976
[103] Pople, J. A., and D. L. Beveridge: Approximate Molecular Orbital Theory, McGraw-Hill, New York, 1971
[104] Pullmann, B.: Adv. Quant. Chem. **10**, 251 (1977)
[105] Christoffersen, R.: Adv. Quant. Chem. **6**, 333 (1972)
[106] Fernandez-Alonso, E., in B. Pullman (Ed.): Quantum Mechanics of Molecular Conformations, Wiley, New York, 1976
[107] Lohr, L. L., and W. N. Lipscomb: J. Chem. Phys. **38**, 1607 (1963)
[108] Rein, R., N. Fukuda, H. Win and G. Clarke: J. Chem. Phys. **45**, 4743 (1966)
[109] Pople, J. A., and G. A. Segal: J. Chem. Phys. **44**, 3289 (1966)
[110] Pople, J. A., D. L. Beveridge and P. A. Dobosh: J. Chem. Phys. **44**, 3289 (1966)
[111] Halgren, T., and W. Lipscomb: J. Chem. Phys. **58**, 1569 (1973)
[112] Dewar, M., and E. Hasselbach: J. Chem. Phys. **58**, 1569 (1973)
[113] Diner, S., J. P. Malrieu, F. Jordan and M. Gilbert: Theor. Chim. Acta **15**, 100 (1969)
[114] Froimowitz, M., in G. Barnett, M. Trsic and R. E. Willette (Eds.): Quantitative Structure-Activity Relationships of Analgesics, Narcotic Antagonists, and Hallucinogens, NIDA Res. Monograph 22, Rockville, 1978, p. 359
[115] Froimowitz, M., and P. J. Gans: J. Am. Chem. Soc. **94**, 8020 (1972)
[116] Genson, D. W., and R. E. Christoffersen: J. Am. Chem. Soc. **95**, 362 (1973)
[117] Pullman, A., and G. N. J. Port: Theor. Chim. Acta **32**, 77 (1973)
[118] Gregory, A. R., and M. N. Paddon-Row: J. Am. Chem. Soc. **98**, 7521 (1976)
[119] Dyott, T. M., A. J. Stuper and G. S. Zander: J. Chem. Inf. Comput. Sci. **20**, 28 (1980)
[120] Scharfenberg, P., and H. Sklenar in R. Franke and P. Oehme (Eds.): Quantitative Structure-Activity Analysis, Akademie-Verlag, Berlin, 1978
[121] Scharfenberg, P.: Theor. Chim. Acta, **58**, 73 (1980)
[122] Scharfenberg, P., and J. Sauer: Int. J. Quant. Chem. **18**, 1309 (1980)
[123] Scheraga, H.: Adv. Phys. Org. Chem. **6**, 103 (1968)
[124] Balasubramanian, R., R. Chidambaran and G. Ramachandran: Biochim. Biophys. Acta **221**, 196 (1970)
[125] Engler, E., J. Andose and P. Schlever: J. Am. Chem. Soc. **98**, 8005 (1973)
[126] Hopfinger, A. J.: Conformational Properties of Macromolecules, Academic Press, New York, 1974
[127] Wilson, E. B.: Chem. Soc. Rev. **1**, 293 (1972)
[127a] Golebiewski, A., and A. Parczewski: Chem. Rev. **74**, 519 (1974)
[128] McGuire, R. F., F. A. Momany and H. A. Scheraga: J. Phys. Chem. **76**, 375 (1972)

[129] Altona, C., and D. H. Faberi: Top. Curr. Chem. **45**, 1 (1974)
[130] Lorongiu, G., and E. Clementi: Gazz. Chim. Ital. **108**, 273 (1978)
[131] Bogis, Y., and E. Clementi: J. Am. Chem. Soc. **99**, 5550 (1977)
[132] Clementi, E., F. Cavallone and R. Scordamaglia: J. Am. Chem. Soc. **99**, 5531 (1977)
[133] Gund, P.: Tables Rondes Roussel Uclaf **38**, 9 (1980)
[133a] Gund, P., and H. B. Schlegel in H. Weinstein and J. P. Green (Eds.): Quantum Chemistry in Biomedical Sciences, Ann. N. Y. Acad. Sci. **367**, 510 (1981)
[134] Gund, P., J. D. Andose and J. B. Rhodes: Proc. III Int. Conf. on Computers in Chem. Res. Educ. Technol., Plenum Press, 1977, p. 226
[135] Weintraub, H. J. R., and A. J. Hopfinger: Int. J. Quant. Chem. QBS **2**, 203 (1975)
[136] Potenzone, R., E. Cavicchi and H. J. R. Weintraub: Comput. Chem. **1**, 187 (1977)
[137] Weintraub, H. J. R., in E. C. Olson and R. E. Christoffersen (Eds.): Computer-Assisted Drug Design, ACS Symp. Ser. **112**, 353 (1979)
[138] Wilson, S. R., and J. C. Hofman: J. Org. Chem. **45**, 560 (1980)
[139] Marshall, G. R., C. D. Barry, H. F. Bosshard, R. A. Dammkoehler and D. A. Dunn in E. C. Olson and R. E. Christoffersen (Eds.): Computer-Assisted Drug Design, ACS Symp. Ser. **112**, 205 (1979)
[140] Cohen, C., P. Colin and G. Lemoine: Tables Rondes Roussel Uclaf **38**, 14 (1980)
[141] Hodges, D., and D. H. Nordby: Abstr. COMP 169th Am. Chem. Soc. Nat. Meeting, Philadelphia, USA
[142] Stuper, A. J., T. M. Dyott and G. S. Zander in E. C. Olson and R. E. Christoffersen (Eds.): Computer-Assisted Drug Design, ACS Symp. Ser. **112**, 383 (1979)
[143] Eaton, D. F., and D. A. Pensak: J. Am. Chem. Soc. **100**, 7428 (1978)
[143a] White, D. N. J., and C. Morrow: Tet. Letters **38**, 3385 (1977)
[143b] Tute, M. S., in S. H. Yalkowsky, A. A. Sinkula and S. C. Valvani (Eds.): Physical Chemical Properties of Drugs, Marcel Dekker, New York, 1980, p. 141
[143c] Warshel, A., and M. Levitt: QCPE No. 247
[143d] Browman, M., A. Burgess, L. Dunfield, S. Rumsey and H. A. Scheraga: QCPE No. 361.
[143e] Allinger, N. L., J. T. Sprague and T. Liljefors: J. Am. Chem. Soc. **96**, 5100 (1974)
[143f] Weiner, P. K., and P. A. Kollman: J. Comput. Chem. **2**, 287 (1981)
[143g] Humblet, C., and G. R. Marshall: Drug Devel. Res. **1**, 409 (1981)
[144] Dammkoehler, R. A.: Tables Rondes Roussel Uclaf **38**, 18 (1980)
[145] Grunewald, G. L., in E. C. Olson and R. E. Christoffersen (Eds.): Computer-Assisted Drug Design, ACS Symp. Ser. **112**, 439 (1979)
[146] Horn, A. S., and J. R. Rogers: Tables Rondes Roussel Uclaf 38, 1 (1980)
[147] Goldberg, L. I., P. H. Volkman, J. D. Kohli and A. N. Kotake: Adv. Biochem. Psychopharmac. **16**, 251 (1977)
[147a] Randall, W. C., P. S. Anderson, E. L. Cresson, C. A. Hunt, T. F. Lyon, K. E. Rittle, D. C. Remy, J. P. Springer, J. M. Hirshfield, K. Hoogsteen, M. Williams, E. A. Risley and J. A. Totaro: J. Med. Chem. **22**, 1222 (1979)
[147b] Olson, G. L., H.-C. Cheung, K. D. Morgan, J. F. Blount, L. Torado, L. Berger, A. B. Davidson and E. Boff: J. Med. Chem. **24**, 1026 (1981)
[148] Humber, L. G., A. H. Philipp, F. T. Bruderlein, M. Götz and K. Voith in E. C. Olson and R. E. Christoffersen (Eds.): Computer-Assisted Drug Design, ACS Symp. Ser. **112**, 227 (1979)
[149] Nichols, D. E., H. J. R. Weintraub, W. R. Pfister and G. K. W. Gim in G. Barnett, M. Trsic and R. E. Willette (Eds.): Quantitative Structure-Activity Relationships of Analgesics, Narcotic Antagonists, and Hallucinogens, NIDA Res. Monograph 22, Rockville, 1978, p. 70
[150] Veber, D. F., F. W. Holly, W. J. Paleveda, R. F. Nutt, S. J. Bergstrand, M. Torchiana,

M. S. Glitzer, R. Saperstein and R. Hirschmann: Proc. Natl. Acad. Sci. (USA) **75**, 2636 (1979)
[151] Veber, D. F., F. W. Holly, R. F. Nutt, S. J. Bergstrand, S. F. Brady, R. Hirschmann, M. S. Glitzer and R. Saperstein: Nature **280**, 512 (1979)
[152] Arison, B. H., R. Hirschmann and D. F. Veber: Bioorg. Chem. **7**, 447 (1978)
[153] Veber, D. F., and R. Saperstein: Ann. Rep. Med. Chem. **14**, 209 (1979)
[154] Veber, D. F., in E. Gross and J. Meienhofer (Eds.): Peptides: Proceedings of the 6th American Peptide Symposium, Pierce Chemical Company, Rockford, 1979, p. 409
[155] Veber, D. F.: Tables Rondes Roussel Uclaf **38**, 41 (1980)
[156] Seprodi, J., D. H. Coy, J. A. Vilchez-Martinez, E. Pedroza, W. Y. Huang and A. V. Schally: J. Med. Chem. **21**, 993 (1978)
[157] Go, N., and H. A. Scheraga: Macromolecules **3**, 178 (1970)
[158] Marshall, G. R., and H. E. Bosshard: Circulation Res. **31**, II-143 (1972)
[159] Pullman, A., and B. Pullman: Quart. Rev. Biophys. **7**, 505 (1974)
[160] Pullman, B. (Ed.): Environmental Effects on Molecular Structure and Properties, D. Reidl Publishing Company, Dordrecht, 1976
[161] Pullman, A., in B. Pullman and R. Parr (Eds.): The New World of Quantum Chemistry, D. Reidl Publishing Company, Dordrecht, 1976
[162] McCreery, J., R. E. Christoffersen and G. Hall: J. Am. Chem. Soc. **98**, 7191 (1976)
[163] Christoffersen, R. E., in B. Pullman (Ed.): Quantum Mechanics of Molecular Conformation, Wiley, New York, 1976
[164] Weintraub, H. J. R., and A. J. Hopfinger: J. theor. Biol. **41**, 53 (1973)
[165] Weintraub, H. J. R., and A. J. Hopfinger in E. Bergmann and B. Pullman (Eds.): Molecular and Quantum Pharmacology, D. Reidl Publishing Company, Dordrecht, 1974, p. 131
[166] Hopfinger, A. J.: Intermolecular Interactions and Biomolecular Organization, Wiley, New York, 1977
[167] Hopfinger, A. J., and R. D. Battershell: J. Med. Chem. **19**, 569 (1976)
[167a] Hodes, Z. I., G. Nemethy and H. A. Scheraga: Biopolymers **18**, 1565 (1979)
[167b] Hodes, Z. I., G. Nemethy and H. A. Scheraga: Biopolymers **18**, 1611 (1979)
[167c] Nemethy, G., Z. I. Hodes and H. A. Scheraga: Proc. Natl. Acad. Sci. (USA) **75**, 5760 (1978)
[167d] Paterson, Y., G. Nemethy and H. A. Scheraga in H. Weinstein and J. P. Green (Eds.): Quantum Chemistry in Biomedical Sciences, Ann. N.Y. Acad. Sci. **367**, 133 (1981)
[168] Kumbar, M.: J. Med. Chem. **19**, 1232 (1976)
[169] Kumbar, M., in G. Barnett, M. Trsic and R. E. Willette (Eds.): Quantitative Structure Activity Relationships of Analgesics, Narcotic Antagonists, and Hallucinogens, NIDA Res. Monograph 22, Rockville, 1978
[170] Marshall, G. R., H. E. Bosshard and R. A. Ellis in W. T. Wipke, S. R. Heller, R. J. Feldmann and E. Hyde (Eds.): Computer Representation and Manipulation of Chemical Information, Interscience, New York, 1974, p. 203
[171] Feldmann, R. J., in W. T. Wipke, S. R. Heller, R. J. Feldmann and E. Hyde (Eds.): Computer Representation and Manipulation of Chemical Information, Interscience, New York, 1974, p. 55
[172] Feldmann, R. J.: Ann. Rev. Biophys. Bioeng. **5**, 477 (1976)
[173] Katz, L., and C. Levinthal: Ann. Rev. Biophys. Bioeng. **1**, 465 (1972)
[174] Newman, W. M., and R. J. Sproull: Principles of Interactive Computer Graphics, McGraw-Hill, New York, 1979
[175] Sutton, L. E.: Tables of Interatomic Distances, Chemical Society, London, 1965
[176] Gordon, M. S., and J. A. Pople: QCPE 135 (1969)
[177] Kier, L. B.: Mol. Pharmacol. **3**, 487 (1967)
[178] Kier, L. B.: J. Med. Chem. **11**, 441 (1968)
[179] Kier, L. B.: Mol. Pharmacol. **4**, 70 (1968)

[180] Kier, L. B.: J. Pharmac. Exptl. Ther. **164**, 75 (1968)
[181] Kier, L. B.: J. Pharmac. Sci. **57**, 1188 (1968)
[182] Kier, L. B.: J. Med. Chem. **11**, 915 (1968)
[183] Kier, L. B.: J. Pharm. Pharmac. **21**, 93 (1969)
[184] Kier, L. B.: J. Pharm. Sci. **59**, 112 (1970)
[185] Kier, L. B., and E. B. Truitt: J. Pharmac. Exptl. Ther. **174**, 94 (1970)
[186] Kier, L. B., and E. B. Truitt: Experientia **26**, 988 (1970)
[187] Kier, L. B., in J. F. Canielli, J. F. Moran and D. J. Triggle (Eds.): Fundamental Concepts in Drug Receptor Interactions, Academic Press, New York, 1970, p. 15
[188] Kier, L. B., and J. M. George: J. Med. Chem. **14**, 80 (1971)
[189] George, J. M., L. B. Kier and J. R. Hoyland: Mol. Pharmacol. **7**, 328 (1971)
[190] Kier, L. B.: J. Pharm. Sci. **61**, 1394 (1972)
[191] Kier, L. B.: J. theor. Biol. **40**, 211 (1973)
[192] Kier, L. B., and J. M. George: Experientia **29**, 501 (1973)
[193] Kier, L. B., J. M. George and H.-D. Höltje: J. Pharm. Sci. **63**, 1435 (1974)
[194] Pullmann, B., in E. D. Bergmann and B. Pullman (Eds.): Molecular and Quantum Pharmacology, D. Reidl Publishing Company, Dordrecht, 1974
[195] Ham, S. H., A. F. Casy and R. R. Ison: J. Med. Chem. **16**, 470 (1973)
[196] Farnell, L., W. G. Richards and C. R. Ganellin: J. Med. Chem. **18**, 662 (1975)
[197] Beers, W. H., and E. Reich: Nature **228**, 917 (1970)
[198] Bustard, R. M., and Y. C. Martin: J. Med. Chem. **15**, 1101 (1972)
[199] Ganellin, C. R., E. S. Pepper, G. N. J. Port and W. G. Richards: J. Med. Chem. **16**, 610 (1973)
[200] Ganellin, C. R., G. N. J. Port and W. G. Richards: J. Med. Chem. **16**, 616 (1973)
[201] Ganellin, C. R.: J. Med. Chem. **16**, 620 (1973)
[202] Ganellin, C. R.: J. Appl. Biotechnol. **28**, 183 (1978)
[203] Ganellin, C. R.: Tables Rondes Roussel Uclaf **38**, 71 (1980)
[204] Farnell, L., W. G. Richards and C. R. Ganellin: J. theor. Biol. **43**, 389 (1974)
[205] Durant, G. J., C. R. Ganellin and M. E. Parsons: J. Med. Chem. **18**, 905 (1975)
[205a] Ganellin, C. R.: Ann. Rep. Med. Chem. **14**, 91 (1979)
[205b] Ganellin, C. R., in E. Bergman and B. Pullman (Eds.): Molecular and Quantum Pharmacology, D. Reidl Publishing Company, Dordrecht, 1974, p. 45
[205c] Durant, G. J., in A. Simkin (Ed.): Medicinal Chemistry VI, Cotswold Press, 1979, p. 189
[205d] Richards, W. G., and J. Wallis: Eur. J. Med. Chem. **14**, 9 (1979)
[206] Durant, G. J., J. C. Emmett, C. R. Ganellin, P. D. Miles, M. E. Parsons, H. P. Prain and G. R. White: J. Med. Chem. **20**, 901 (1977)
[207] Höltje, H.-D., and L. B. Kier: J. theor. Biol. **48**, 197 (1974)
[208] Kier, L. B., and H. S. Aldrich: J. theor. Biol. **46**, 529 (1974)
[209] Höltje, H.-D., and L. B. Kier: J. Med. Chem. **17**, 814 (1974)
[210] Höltje, H.-D., and L. B. Kier: J. Pharm. Sci. **63**, 1722 (1974)
[211] Höltje, H.-D., and L. B. Kier: J. Pharm. Sci. **64**, 418 (1975)
[212] Höltje, H.-D.: Archiv Pharmazie **308**, 438 (1975)
[213] Dipaolo, T., L. H. Hall and L. B. Kier: J. theor. Biol. **71**, 295 (1978)
[214] Kier, L. B., and R. A. Glennon in G. Barnett, M. Trsic and R. E. Willette (Eds.): Quantitative Structure-Activity Relationships of Analgesics, Narcotic Antagonists, and Hallucinogens, NIDA Res. Monograph 22, Rockville, 1978, p. 159
[215] Höltje, H.-D., and L. Vogelsang in J. Knoll and F. Darvas (Eds.): Chemical Structure — Biological Activity Relationships, Quantitative Approaches, Akedémiai Kiadó, Budapest, 1980
[216] Claverie, P., and R. Rein: Int. J. Quant. Chem. **3**, 535 (1969)
[217] Huron, M. J., and P. Claverie: Chem. Phys. Lett. **4**, 429 (1969)

[218] Bonaccorsi, R., E. Scrocco and J. Tomasi: J. Chem. Phys. **52**, 5270 (1970)
[219] Srebrenik, S., H. Weinstein and R. Pauncz: Chem. Phys. Lett. **20**, 419 (1973)
[220] Scrocco, E., and J. Tomasi: Top. Curr. Chem. **42**, 95 (1973)
[221] Scrocco, E., and J. Tomasi: Adv. Quant. Chem. **11**, 115 (1978)
[221a] Politzer, P., and D. G. Truhlar (Eds.): Chemical Applications of Atomic and Molecular Electrostatic Potentials, Plenum Publishing Corporation, New York, 1981
[222] Weinstein, H., S. Maayani, S. Srebrenik, S. Cohen and M. Sokolovsky: Mol. Pharmacol. **9**, 820 (1973)
[223] Weinstein, H., S. Srebrenik, R. Pauncz, S. Maayani, S. Cohen and M. Sokolovsky in E. Bergmann and B. Pullman (Eds.): Chemical and Biochemical Reactivity, D. Reidl Publishing Company, Dordrecht, 1974, p. 493
[224] Maayani, S., H. Weinstein, S. Cohen and M. Sokolovsky: Proc. Natl. Acad. Sci. (USA) **70**, 3103 (1973)
[225] Weinstein, H., S. Maayani, S. Srebrenik, S. Cohen and M. Sokolovsky: Mol. Pharmacol. **11**, 671 (1975)
[226] Weinstein, H.: Int. J. Quant. Chem. QBS **2**, 59 (1975)
[227] Loew, G. H., D. Berkowitz, H. Weinstein and S. Srebrenik in E. Bergmann and B. Pullman (Eds.): Molecular and Quantum Pharmacology, D. Reidl Publishing Company, Dordrecht, 1974, p. 355
[227a] Loew, G. H., D. S. Berkowitz and S. K. Burt in G. Barnett, M. Trsic and R. E. Willette (Eds.): Quantitative Structure Activity Relationships of Analgesics, Narcotic Antagonists, and Hallucinogens, NIDA Res. Monograph 22, Rockville, 1978, p. 278
[228] Weinstein, H., D. Chou, C. L. Johnson, S. Kang and J. P. Green: Mol. Pharmacol. **12**, 738 (1976)
[229] Weinstein, H., D. Chou, S. Kang, C. L. Johnson and J. P. Green: Int. J. Quantum Chem. QBS **3**, 135 (1976)
[230] Weinstein, H., and R. Osman: Int. J. Quant. Chem. **4**, 253 (1977)
[231] Weinstein, H., R. Osman, W. D. Edwards and J. P. Green: Int. J. Quant. Chem. QBS **5**, 449 (1978)
[232] Weinstein, H., J. P. Green, R. Osman and W. D. Edwards in G. Barnett, M. Trsic and R. W. Willette (Eds.): Quantitative Structure Activity Relationships of Analgesics, Narcotic Antagonists, and Hallucinogens, NIDA Res. Monograph 22, Rockville, 1978, p. 333
[232a] Weinstein, H., R. Osman, J. P. Green and S. Topiol in P. Politzer and D. G. Truhlar (Eds.): Chemical Applications of Atomic and Molecular Electrostatic Potentials, Plenum Publishing Corporation, New York, 1981, p. 309
[232b] Reggio, P. H., H. Weinstein, R. Osman and S. Topiol: Internat. J. Quant. Chem. QBS **8**, 373 (1981)
[232c] Weinstein, H., R. Osman, S. Topiol in H. Weinstein and J. P. Green (Eds.): Quantum Chemistry in Biomedical Sciences, Ann. N.Y. Acad. Sci. **367**, 434 (1981)
[233] Pullman, A., in E. Bergmann and B. Pullman (Eds.): Chemical and Biochemical Reactivity, D. Reidl Publishing Company, Dordrecht, 1974, p. 1
[234] Petrongolo, C., J. Tomasi, B. Macchia and F. Macchia: J. Med. Chem. **17**, 501 (1974)
[234a] Martin, M., R. Carbó, C. Petrongolo and J. Tomasi: J. Am. Chem. Soc. **97**, 1338 (1975)
[235] Petrongolo, C., B. Macchia, F. Macchia and A. Martinelli: J. Med. Chem. **20**, 1645 (1977)
[236] Petrongolo, C.: Gaz. Chim. Ital. **108**, 445 (1978)
[237] Martinelli, A., and C. Petrongolo: J. Phys. Chem. **80**, 105 (1980)
[238] Macchia, B., F. Macchia and A. Martinelli: Eur. J. Med. Chem. **15**, 515 (1980)
[239] Agresti, A., F. Buffoni, J. J. Kaufman and C. Petrongolo: Mol. Pharmacol. **18**, 461 (1980)
[240] Hadži, D., D. Kocjan and T. Šolmajer: Period. Biol. **83**, 13 (1981)
[241] Kaufmann, J. J.: Int. J. Quant. Chem. **16**, 221 (1978)

[241a] Kaufmann, J. J., P. C. Hariharan and H. E. Popkie in H. Weinstein and J. P. Green (Eds.): Quantum Chemistry in Biomedical Sciences, Ann. N.Y. Acad. Sci. **367**, 542 (1981)

[242] Kaufmann, J. J., in G. Barnett, M. Trsic and R. Willette (Eds.): Structure Activity Relationships of Analgesics, Narcotic Antagonists, and Hallucinogens, NIDA Res. Monograph 22, Rockville, 1978, p. 250

[243] Baldwin, S., L. B. Kier and D. Shilladay: Mol. Pharmacol. **18**, 455 (1980)

[244] Hayes, D. M., and P. Kollman: J. Am. Chem. Soc. **98**, 3335 (1976)

[245] Hayes, D. M., and P. Kollman: J. Am. Chem. Soc. **98**, 7811 (1976)

[245a] Hayes, D. M., and P. A. Kollman in B. Pullman (Ed.): Catalysis in Chemistry and Biochemistry. Theory and Experiment, D. Reidl Publishing Company, Dordrecht, 1979, p. 77

[246] Ranghino, G., and E. Clementi: Gazz. Chim. Ital. **108**, 157 (1978)

[247] Clementi, E., G. Ranghino and R. Scordamaglia: Chem. Phys. Lett. **49**, 218 (1979)

[248] Koppenol, W. H., C. A. J. Vroonland and R. Braams: Biochim. Biophys. Acta **503**, 499 (1979)

[249] Sheridan, R. P., and L. C. Allen: J. Amer. Chem. Soc. **103**, 1544 (1981)

[249a] Lavery, R., and B. Pullman: Internat. J. Quant. Chem. **20**, 259 (1981)

[249b] Jen, T., and C. Kaiser: J. Med. Chem. **20**, 693 (1977)

[249c] Gadret, M., J.-M. Légar and A. Capry: Eur. J. Med. Chem. **13**, 367 (1978)

[250] Cohen, N. C., in E. C. Olson and R. E. Christoffersen (Eds.): Computer-Assisted Drug Design, ACS Symp. Ser. **112**, 371 (1979)

[251] Radna, R. J., D. L. Beveridge and A. L. Bender: J. Am. Chem. Soc. **95**, 3831 (1973)

[252] Marshall, G. R., and H. E. Bosshard: Circulation Res. **31**, II-143 (1972)

[253] Cheney, B. V., D. J. Duchamp and R. E. Christoffersen in G. Barnett, M. Trsic and R. E. Willette (Eds.): Quantitative Structure Activity Relationships of Analgesics, Narcotic Antagonists, and Hallucinogens, NIDA Res. Monograph 22, Rockville, 1978, p. 218

[254] Andrews, P. R., in E. C. Olson and R. E. Christoffersen (Eds).: Computer-Assisted Drug Design, ACS Symp. Ser. **112**, 149 (1979)

[254a] Diamond, R.: Acta Cryst. **21**, 253 (1966)

[254b] McLachlan, A. D.: Acta Cryst. **A 28**, 656 (1972)

[254c] Urata, Y., Y. Mitsui and K. T. Nakamura: Chem. Pharm. Bull. **29**, 2738 (1981)

[255] Sundaram, K.: Int. J. Quant. Chem. **9**, 393 (1975)

[256] Cheney, B. V.: J. Med. Chem. **17**, 590 (1974)

[257] Nyburg, S. C.: Acta Crystallogr. Sect. **B 30**, 251 (1974)

[258] Wilson, S. R., and J. C. Hoffman: J. Org. Chem. **45**, 560 (1980)

[259] Fullerton, D. S., K. Yoshioka, D. C. Rohrer, A. H. L. From and K. Ahmed: Science **205**, 917 (1979)

[260] Hopfinger, A. J.: J. Am. Chem. Soc. **102**, 7196 (1980)

[260a] Hopfinger, A. J.: Arch. Biochem. Biophys. **206**, 153 (1981)

[260b] Battershell, C., D. Malhotra and A. J. Hopfinger: J. Med. Chem. **24**, 812 (1981)

[261] Hopfinger, A. J.: J. Med. Chem. **24**, 818 (1981)

[262] Gund, P., and T. Y. Shen: J. Med. Chem. **20**, 1146 (1977)

[263] Hahn, F. E., and P. Gund in J. Drews and F. E. Hahn (Eds.): Topics in Infectious Diseases, Vol. I, Drug Receptor Interactions in Antimicrobial Chemotherapy, Springer-Verlag, New York, 1975

[264] Green, J. P., C. L. Johnson and H. Weinstein in M. A. Lipton, A. DiMascio and K. F. Killam (Eds.): Psychopharmacology: A Generation of Progress, Raven Press, New York, 1978, p. 319

[265] Green, J. P., H. Weinstein and S. Maayani in G. Barnett, M. Trsic and R. E. Willette (Eds.): Quantitative Structure Activity Relationships of Analgesics, Narcotic Antagonists, and Hallucinogens, NIDA Res. Monograph 22, Rockville, 1978, p. 38

266] Rohrer, D. C., D. S. Fullerton, K. Yoshioka, A. H. L. From and K. Ahmed in E. C. Olson

and R. E. Christoffersen (Eds.): Computer-Assisted Drug Design, ACS Symp. Ser. **112**, 259 (1979)
[267] Gorin, F. A., and G. R. Marshall: Proc. Natl. Acad. Sci. (USA) **74**, 5179 (1977)
[267a] Gorin, F. A., and G. R. Marshall in M. Goodman and J. Meienhofer (Eds.): Peptides, Wiley, New York, 1977, p. 277
[267b] Gorin, F. A., T. M. Balasubramanian, C. D. Barry and G. R. Marshall: J. Supramol. Struc. **9**, 27 (1978)
[267c] Gorin, F. A., T. M. Balasubramanian, T. J. Cicero, J. Schwietzer and G. R. Marshall: J. Med. Chem. **23**, 1113 (1980)
[268] Burt, S. K., G. H. Loew and G. M. Hashimoto in H. Weinstein and J. P. Green (Eds.): Quantum Chemistry in Biomedical Sciences, Ann. N.Y. Acad. Sci. **367**, 219 (1981)
[268a] Humblet, C., and G. R. Marshall: Ann. Rep. Med. Chem. **15**, 267 (1980)
[269] Humblet, C., and G. R. Marshall: Tables Rondes Roussel Uclaf **38**, 38 (1980)
[270] Boyd, D. B.: J. Med. Chem. **22**, 533 (1979)
[271] Green, J. P., C. L. Johnson, H. Weinstein and S. Maayani: Proc. Natl. Acad. Sci. (USA) **74**, 5697 (1977)
[272] Soudijn, W., and I. van Wijngaarden in J. A. Keverling Buisman (Ed.): Biological Activity and Chemical Structure, Pharmacochemistry Library (Eds.: W. Th. Nauta and R. F. Rekker), Vol. 2, Elsevier, Amsterdam, 1977, p. 195
[273] Bradbury, A. F., D. G. Smyth and C. R. Snell: Nature **260**, 165 (1976)
[274] Horn, A. S., and J. R. Rogers: Nature **260**, 795 (1976)
[275] Smith, G. D., and J. F. Griffin: Science **199**, 1214 (1978)
[276] Loew, G. H., D. S. Berkowitz and S. K. Burt in G. Barnett, M. Trsic and R. E. Willette: Quantitative Structure Activity Relationships of Analgesics, Narcotic Antagonists, and Hallucinogens, NIDA Res. Monograph 22, Rockville, 1978, p. 278
[277] Loew, G. H., and S. K. Burt: Proc. Natl. Acad. Sci. (USA) **75**, 7 (1978)
[278] Andrews, P. R., and G. A. R. Johnston: J. theor. Biol. **79**, 263 (1979)
[279] Andrews, P. R., and G. A. R. Johnston: Biochem. Pharmacol. **28**, 2697 (1979)
[280] Johnston, G. A. R., R. D. Allan, P. R. Andrews, S. M. E. Kennedy and B. Twitchin: Adv. Pharmacol. Therap. **2**, 11 (1979)
[281] Marshall, G. R., F. A. Gorin and M. L. Moore: Ann. Rep. Med. Chem. **13**, 227 (1978)
[282] Marshall, G. R., in M. A. Simkin (Ed.): Medicinal Chemistry VI., Cotswold Press, Oxford, 1979, p. 225
[283] Weaver, D. C., C. D. Barry and P. E. Lacy: Diabetes **27**, 456 (1978)
[284] Weaver, D. C., M. L. McDaniel, S. P. Naber, C. D. Barry and P. E. Lacy: Diabetes **27**, 1205 (1978)
[285] Sufrin, J. R., and G. R. Marshall: Fed. Proc. **38**, 562 (1979)
[286] Humber, L. G.: Tables Rondes Roussel Uclaf **38**, 4 (1980)
[287] Cobb, M. H., G. R. Marshall, W. Heagy, J. Danner and H. M. Lenhoff: Fed. Proc. **37**, 1822 (1978)
[288] Balaban, A. T., A. Chiriac, I. Motoc and Z. Simon: Steric Fit in Quantitative Structure-Activity Relations, Springer-Verlag, Berlin, 1980
[289] Pauling, L.: Amer. Scientist **36**, 51 (1948)
[290] Jencks, W. P., in N. O. Kaplan and E. P. Kennedy (Eds.): Current Aspects of Biochemical Energetics, Academic Press, New York, 1966, p. 273
[291] Lumry, R., in P. D. Boyer, H. Lardy and K. Myrbacks (Eds.): The Enzymes, 2nd ed., Vol. 1, Academic Press, New York, 1959, p. 157
[292] Wolfenden, R.: Acc. Chem. Res. **5**, 10 (1972)
[293] Lienhardt, G. E.: Science **180**, 149 (1973)
[294] Lienhardt, G. E.: Ann. Rep. Med. Chem. **7**, 249 (1972)
[295] Wolfenden, R.: Ann. Rev. Biophys. Bioeng. **5**, 271 (1976)

[296] Lindquist, R. N., in E. J. Ariens (Ed.): Drug Design, Vol. V, Adademic Press, New York, 1975, p. 24
[297] Andrews, P. R., in E. C. Olson and R. E. Christoffersen (Eds.): Computer-Assisted Drug Design, ACS Symp. Ser. **112**, 259 (1979)
[298] Andrews, P. R.: Tables Rondes Roussel Uclaf **38**, 67 (1980)
[299] Brodbeck, U.: Chimia **34**, 415 (1980)
[300] Ngo, T. T., and G. Tunnicliff: Gen. Pharmacol. **12**, 129 (1981)
[301] Bingham, R. C., M. J. S. Dewar and D. H. Lo: J. Am. Chem. Soc. **97**, 1285 (1975)
[302] Dewar, M. J. S.: Science **187**, 1037 (1975)
[303] Jencks, W. P.: Catalysis in Chemistry and Enzymology, McGraw-Hill, New York, 1969
[304] Collins, K. D., and G. R. Stark: J. Biol. Chem. **246**, 6599 (1971)
[304a] Barth, A.: Wiss. Z. Univ. Halle **28**, 23 (1979)
[305] Ondetti, M. A., B. Rubin and D. W. Cushman: Science **196**, 441 (1977)
[306] Cushman, D. W., H. S. Cheung, E. F. Sabo and M. A. Ondetti: Prog. Cardiovasc. Dis. **21**, 176 (1978)
[307] Tipper, D. J., and J. L. Strominger: Proc. Natl. Acad. Sci. (USA) **54**, 1133 (1965)
[308] Lee, B.: J. Mol. Biol. **61**, 463 (1971)
[309] Boyd, D.B.: Proc. Natl. Acad. Sci. (USA), **74**, 5239 (1977)
[310] Boyd, D. B.: J. Med. Chem. **22**, 533 (1979)
[311] Boyd, D. B., in H. Weinstein and J. P. Green (Eds.): Quantum Chemistry in Biomedical Sciences, Ann. N.Y. Acad. Sci. **367**, 531 (1981)
[312] Boyd, D. B., and W. H. W. Lunn: J. Med. Chem. **22**, 778 (1979)
[314] Boyd, D. B., D. K. Herron, W. H. W. Lunn and W. A. Spitzer: J. Am. Chem. Soc. **102**, 1812 (1980)
[315] Gibson, F., and J. Pittard: Bacteriol. Rev. **32**, 465 (1968)
[316] Andrews, P. R., G. D. Smith and I. G. Young: Biochemistry **12**, 3492 (1973)
[317] Andrews, P. R., E. N. Cain, E. Rizzardo and G. D. Smith: Biochemistry **16**, 4848 (1977)
[318] Andrews, P. R., and R. C. Haddon: Aust. J. Chem. **32**, 1921 (1979)

13. Response Profiles

Drugs are usually investigated in not only one but in a battery of biological tests, the main reasons and objectives being:

1. Elimination of undesired effects and optimization of drug selectivity.
2. Several different biological tests exist to characterize the same biological effect which, however, may lead to different results. Since it is sometimes difficult if not impossible to select the most representative test on the grounds of biological knowledge alone, it has become common practice in such cases to use several pharmacological models in parallel.
3. A special situation of this type arises in the search for agents acting against parasites and abnormal cells. Since it is not possible to include all relevant species (e.g., bacteria, fungi, viruses, plants, etc.) in a screening program a selection has to be made which is felt to be representative.
4. A multipotent drug with a defined response profile is searched for.
5. Although classical random screening in a multitude of biological tests tends to be gradually replaced by more rational approaches aiming at selected pharmacological properties, it is still worthwhile routinely to investigate newly synthesized compounds in a standard set of basic pharmacological tests in order not to miss possibly important effects not anticipated at the time when the compounds were made.

Multiple biological data may have quite a complex internal structure and be interrelated in various ways. An analysis of such data can be approached via different routes with different objectives:

1. Evaluation of multivariate QSARs for series of compounds with the primary objective of a multidimensional optimization of drug structures. This problem has already been dealt with in chapter 9. and is, therefore, not a topic of this chapter. Only the special case of quantitative structure-selectivity relationships which are of great importance will be discussed here (13.1.) since they have not been considered in detail yet.
2. Investigation of the relatedness of tests and of multiple data structures independently of variations of drug structures. The resulting information can substantially aid the pharmacologist in the design of optimal systems of biological tests, in the interpretation of results and in a better understanding of what the biological answers from his tests really mean.

As compared to the huge number of QSARs published, investigations of this type are surprisingly scarce (for a recent review, see [27]). Since they are of great value a somewhat detailed discussion is appropriate (cf. 13.2.).

In the last section, finally, some possible screening strategies in systems of parallel or hierachically organized tests will be briefly outlined.

13.1. Structure-Selectivity Relationships

Safety is as important for a useful new drug as its potency with respect to the desired pharmacological effects. In other words, such a drug should not induce undesired side effects at therapeutic dose levels. The ability of a drug to elicit the desired response while being devoid of undesired side effects is called *selectivity*, which may be defined as [1]:

$$S = \log A_d/A_u = \log A_d - \log A_u \qquad (13/1)$$

S = selectivity
A_d = desired activity
A_u = undesired activity

Relationships between structure and selectivity can be determined using any of the procedures so far referred to for quantitative structure-activity analysis, the only difference being that instead of one biological activity two or more are studied at a time. This can be achieved along various lines. In the simplest case, the QSARs for the activities of interest are compared with the result that more or less qualitative or semi-quantitative conclusions can be drawn with respect to the nature of the structural variations that enhance selectivity. An advantage of this method is that the relationships to be compared must not necessarily be evaluated with the aid of the same training series. What is important is to understand exactly the molecular properties of relevance for the various biological effects and in particular their differences. This is especially true when drugs inhibiting a specific enzyme of a pathogen without inhibiting the corresponding enzyme in the host are to be designed. An example of this type has already been discussed concerning the selective inhibition of succinate dehydrogenase from liver fluke (cf., eqns. (4/84)–(4/86)). Another interesting case is the selective inhibition of bacterial dihydrofolate reductase (DHFR) which has extensively been investigated by Hansch and colleagues [2–10] and recently by Hyde and Roth [11] using QSAR methods. For a series of benzylpyrimidines of structure XLVI the following QSARs were obtained for the inhibitory potency against DHFR from bovine liver [8] and from *E. coli* [9]:

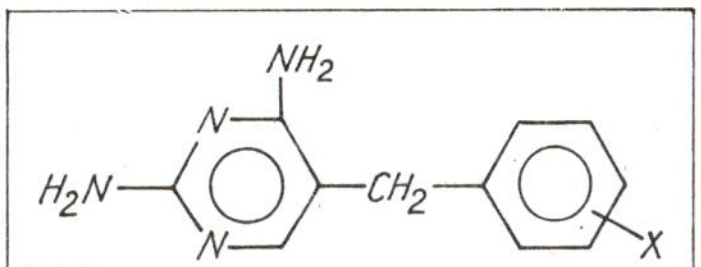

XLVI

Bovine liver enzyme

$$\log A = 0.62\pi_3 + 0.33 \sum \sigma + 4.99 \qquad (13/2)$$

$n = 23 \qquad r = 0.931 \qquad s = 0.146$

E. coli enzyme

$$\log A = 1.38\ \mathrm{MR}'_{3,5} + 0.82\ \mathrm{MR}_4' + 5.77 \qquad (13/3)$$

$n = 23 \qquad r = 0.918 \qquad s = 0.250$

with

$$MR' = \begin{cases} MR & \text{for} \quad MR \leqq 0.79 \\ 0{,}79 & \text{for} \quad MR > 0.79 \end{cases} \tag{13/4}$$

The electronic term in eqn. (13/2) accounts for not more than about 10% of the data variance and is thus only of marginal importance. HANSCH et al. [8] therefore concluded that the inhibition of the mammalian enzyme is primarily related to the hydrophobicity of 3-substituents, and the same conclusion was also reached by HYDE and ROTH [11]. The situation with the bacterial enzyme is quite different in that hydrophobic effects are absent and the inhibitory potency depends on substituent bulk. This dependence, however, is not a simple one since substitution of MR for MR′ leads only to a very poor correlation [9]. The idea of using MR′ instead of MR was based on the assumption that only a certain fraction of larger substituents in the 3 and 4 positions contacts the enzyme so that inhibitory potency does not change with substituent bulk above a certain size defined by MR = 0.79. The results of this study allow one to conclude that a selective and potent inhibitor for the bacterial enzyme should have hydrophilic groups in the meta position(s) (decreases inhibition of the mammalian enzyme) while taking care that the substituents in positions 3, 4 and 5 have optimal steric properties for inhibiting bacterial DHFR. These conclusions have been confirmed and refined by the work of HYDE and ROTH [11] who investigated in more detail the steric substituent effects operating in the inhibition of *E. coli* DHFR by XLVI type compounds. They suggested that these effects do not simply depend on substituent bulk (which is expressed by MR) but also on shape and introduced a new steric distance parameter, λ, on the basis of the following assumptions:

1. The effect of a substituent on *E. coli* DHFR inhibition is associated with its ability to fill space in the direction perpendicular to the axis of attachment.
2. A relevant parameter to characterize this ability is the distance λ which is a measure of substituent width in this direction.
3. For a substituent X which is free to rotate (no adjacent substituent present), λ is equal to the smallest STERIMOL B parameter (B_1) (see chapter 6.).
4. Inhibition of free rotation by an adjacent substituent increases the capacity of X to fill space in the desired direction. Hence a larger λ value is required, and the largest B value (B_4) is used in this case.
5. The adjacent substituent effect is only allowed for until the second atom. For example, the value required for λ for a higher alkoxy group would be the same as for methoxy.

The important aspect of this approach is that the steric substituent effect on *E. coli* DHFR inhibiting potency depends on both the environment and the nature of a substituent which leads to the following excellent relationship for 5-substituted compounds:

$$\log A = 0.826\lambda + 1.150I - 3.099 \tag{13/5}$$

$$n = 22 \qquad r = 0.966 \qquad F = 132.37$$

with

$$I = \begin{cases} 1, & \text{if methoxy groups are present in positions 3 and 4} \\ 0, & \text{if not} \end{cases} \tag{13/6}$$

The requirements for high selective toxicity against the bacterial enzyme can now be refined:

— hydrophilic substituents in meta-positions (see eqn. (13/2))
— high λ values of substituents which implies 3,4,5-trisubstitution

With this in mind it is easy to understand why trimethoprim (the 3,4,5-$(OCH_3)_3$ derivative of XLVI), a widely used antibacterial compound, is such a safe and at the same time potent drug (see also [9]). The presence of the hydrophilic meta methoxy groups and their conformational constrain due to the presence of the para substituent represent an extraordinarily effective fulfilment of the criteria of selective potency [11].

Another area where comparing QSARs seems to be a promising approach to selectivity is cancer chemotherapy (for a short review, see [12]). Here the objective is to establish molecular properties that will minimize toxicity to normal cells while maintaining (and possibly maximizing) toxicity to cancer cells. One means of achieving this, pointed out by Hansch et al. as early as 1972 [13], would be through appropriate adjustment of passive transport properties assumed to be different for tumour and normal cells [13, 14] by modelling hydrophobicity. A comparative QSAR analysis of antitumour activity and toxicity of nitrosoureas, for example, indicated that neutral and more hydrophilic compounds may have a higher selectivity than those currently in use [13, 15]. Other examples where the selectivity of potential anticancer drugs primarily depends on hydrophobicity concern the localization rate of boronic acids in normal and cancerous brain tissue (cf., eqns. (4/112)—(4/114)), the selectivity of antileukemic bisquaternary ammonium heterocycles [16] (cf., eqn. (13/12)) and the selective inhibition of tumour cell respiration in comparison with liver cell respiration by copper chelates [17—19]. In the last case, selectivity could be directly correlated with molecular parameters of substituents in an aromatic ring so affording eqn. (13/7):

$$S = -0.26\pi - 0.10\pi^2 - 0.650\sigma^+ + 2.27 \qquad (13/7)$$

$$n = 14 \qquad r = 0.81 \qquad s = 0.37$$

Thus, the concept of adjusting hydrophobicity as a key to selectivity may be regarded a worthwhile approach although one cannot always expect such clear-cut differences as in the above cases to emerge. An identical dependence of antitumour activity and toxicity on hydrophobicity was found, for example, for colchicines [20] and anthracyclines [21] so that other principles must be used here in order to increase selectivity. Generally speaking, hydrophobicity is always a useful quantity to look at but it is clearly not the only key to selectivity (cf., eqns. (13/5), (13/7), (4/112)—(4/114) and (13/8)).

An alternative to comparing QSARs for desired and undesired effects is directly to evaluate *quantitative structure-selectivity relationships* with selectivity defined as in eqn. (13/1) (cf., eqns. (4/84)—(4/86) and (13/7)). Some additional examples are:

1. *Herbicidal activity of phenylthioureas against cucumber versus wheat* [22]:

$$S = -0.38\,\mathrm{MR} - 0.69I - 3.28 \qquad (13/8)$$

$$n = 7 \qquad r = 0.999 \qquad s = 0.043$$

with

$$I = \begin{cases} 1, & \text{for oxygen-containing substituents} \\ 0, & \text{otherwise} \end{cases} \quad (13/9)$$

It follows from eqn. (13/8) that compounds acting selectively against cucumber should contain large and oxygen-free substituents.

2. *β-adrenergic versus α-adrenergic activity of dopamine derivatives* [1]:

$$S = -0.58\pi^2 + 2.91\pi - 0.46 \quad (13/10)$$

$$n = 6 \qquad r = 0.939 \qquad s = 0.570$$

3. *Antibacterial activity of* N,N-*dimethylbenzylammonium analogues against Cl. welchii versus S. typhosa* [1]:

$$S = -0.04\,(\log P)^2 + 0.35\log P - 0.220 \quad (13/11)$$

$$n = 10 \qquad r = 0.960 \qquad s = 0.132$$

4. *Antileukemic activity versus toxicity of bisquaternary ammonium heterocycles* [16]:

$$S = -0.56R_M{}^2 - 0.42R_M + 0.62\log(\mathrm{C}[_{50}(\mathrm{G{-}C})]/[\mathrm{C}_{50}(\mathrm{A{-}T})]) + 0.39 \quad (13/12)$$

$$n = 169 \qquad r = 0.62 \qquad s = 0.31$$

C_{50}(G—C) concentration necessary to displace 50% of bound ethidium from poly[D(G—C)]

C_{50}(A—T) concentration necessary to displace 50% of bound ethidium from poly[D(A—T)]

Although statistically highly significant, eqn. (13/12) explains only a small part of the data variance. This may be related to the fact that significant QSARs can only be obtained for antitumour activity but not for toxicity, indicating that toxicity may be brought about by more than one mechanism of action. An important aspect of eqn. (13/12) is that it suggests that, in addition to hydrophobicity, selectivity is related to the ability of the drugs to distinguish particular DNA sequences (the same is true of antitumour potency).

Applying QSAR methods including, in addition to Hansch analysis also Free-Wilson analysis (e.g., [23]) or, in particular, the classification methods discussed in chapters 9. and 11. (e.g., [24]) directly to selectivity data has the possible advantage of providing the investigator with a sharper picture of molecular features relevant to selectivity and of facilitating predictions. The disadvantage is that the same set of compounds must be studied in all relevant tests, and it should also be kept in mind that an analysis of such a complex quantity as selectivity is not without pitfalls. When the biological effects to be compared are entirely different in the way they depend on molecular properties, the structure dependence of the selectivity index may increase in complexity so much that it renders impossible the evaluation of meaningful relationships; this will be especially true of large and diverse data sets where for toxicity, for example, a constant mechanism of action cannot necessarily be anticipated. It is also conceivable that the two effects to be compared are directly correlated with each other, thus precluding selectivity. However, statistically significant structure-selectivity relationships may still sometimes be obtained in such cases which are, of course, of no predictive value.

The most important approaches to selectivity at the level of drug-receptor interactions undoubtedly are the methods outlined in chapter 12. since differences in such interactions may depend on subtle steric and electronic changes (cf., also eqn. (13/5)). Although some work in this direction has already been done (see 12.), systematic applications of such methods to the design of drugs with a pre-defined response profile are still rare. An interesting example which demonstrates what can be achieved by detailed steric considerations is provided by the work of UNGER et al. on the design of a new highly selective and non-depressive β-blocker [25, 26] based on tazolol (substituents varied at the heterocyclic ring). Using simple DREIDING models and an entirely static approach, steric parameters could be derived which yielded excellent correlations with both β_1- as well as β_2-blocking aktivity for about 40 different side-chains and offered a straightforward explanation for the extremely high cardioselectivity (high blockade of heart β_1-receptors and no blockade of lung β_2-receptors) imposed by the endobicyclo[3.1.0.]-hexylethyl group.

13.2. Multiple Response Data and Activity-Activity Relationships

Many drugs are multipotent and capable of interacting with more than a single receptor (see e.g. [26a, 26b]). As a consequence the observable global response will be a composite of contributions from different receptors, and even for identical responses these contributions may be different. With such data, the evaluation of structure-activity relationships is a hopeless task, and it is impossible to draw any conclusions on the pharmacological mechanism of action. This problem can be overcome if results from a battery of tests each differing in the single receptor contributions to the observable global response are analysed. The objectives of such an analysis may be:

1. separation of the single receptor contributions,
2. classification of compounds with respect to the receptor(s) they preferentially interact with,
3. classification of compounds with respect to a response profile or a particular therapeutic effect (e.g., classification of antidepressants using a general screen which does not contain any direct measure of antidepressant action [26]),
4. classification of tests with respect to similarities or dissimilarities.

Several methods may be used for that purpose. If the single receptor contributions to the global response can be assumed to be additive a simple linear model can be formulated:

$$\log A_{ij} = \sum_k a_{ik} x_{kj} \qquad (13/13)$$

with

A_{ij} global response of the j-th compound in the i-th test

x_{kj} contribution from the k-th receptor in a (hypothetical) test where only this receptor is present

a_{ik} weighting factor expressing the extent to which x_{kj} is realized in the i-th test

Such a situation clearly lends itself to factor or principal component analysis (cf., chapters 8. and 9.). As far as the model according to eqn. (13/13) is correct, the components extracted will represent the individual receptor contributions so that "pure" individual receptor responses can, in principle, be obtained from global response data of multipotent drugs in an appropriate set of pharmacological tests.[1]) This interesting possibility has not yet been explicitly explored although both factor and principal component analysis have been frequently applied to multiple response data (for reviews, see [27, 27a]). Even though these investigations were not aimed at and, consequently, did not result in the evaluation of individual receptor contributions, they provided interesting information about the tests considered. A first example of this type was presented in 9.1.2.2. concerning the antibacterial activity of rifamycine B amides against *M. aureus*, *S. faecalis*, *S. hemolyticus* and *B. subtilis*. Principal component analysis showed that these tests are highly interrelated and are, in fact, redundant. A similar result was also obtained by LUKOVITS and LOPATA [28] considering the same data set in an attempt to derive activity-activity relationships.

Table 13.1. Factor pattern (after Varimax rotation) obtained from multiple biological response data of a series of 27 piperidinoacetanilides (structure XXV) investigated in eight biological tests. Significant non-zero loadings are indicated by a cross [29, 30]

No.	Biological test	1st Factor	2nd Factor	3rd Factor
1	Growth inhibition in *S. alba* seedlings	+		
2	Amylase activity in *Triticum aleurone* cells		+	
3	Growth inhibition in *S. alba* hypocotyl	+		
4	Dry weight of seedlings		+	
5	Antihelmintic activity			+
6	Fungistatic activity			+
7	Bacteriostatic activity			
8	Inhibition of ribosomal protein synthesis	+		

Table 13.1. shows the factor pattern obtained for eight different biological activities measured in a series of substituted piperidinoacetanilides (structure XXV). Again, the system of tests is obviuosly redundant since only three factors are needed for data reproduction. Bearing in mind that variables (in our case: the tests) which are loaded in the same factor are interrelated while those which are loaded only in different factors are independent (cf., 8.4.1.), Table 13.1 leads to the following conclusions:

1. The first factor may be labelled "plant growth inhibition" also indicating that this effect may be related to the inhibition of protein synthesis (at least for the piperidinoacetanilides).
2. The second factor reveals that tests 2 and 4 are related which is biologically meaningful.
3. Somewhat surprising is the relationship between tests 5 and 6 shown by the third factor. This relationship indicates that, for the piperidinoacetanilides, similar

[1]) Possible influences of transport processes must, of course, adequately be accounted for if present.

molecular interactions operate in both biological effects (that does not mean, however, that the point of attack is similar).
4. Test 7 shows a completely unique behaviour and is not related to any other test.

This and some other examples summarized in Table 13.2 show that multiple biological response data are usually interrelated so that many batteries of biological tests are redundant. The results of factor or principal component analysis not only allow one to judge the information content of tests but also provide a means of showing which tests or compounds are grouped together and exhibit similarities. This can also be illustrated graphically by plotting either the tests or the compounds in a coordinate system spanned by the corresponding factors or components. Provided that the first two factors or components account for a sufficiently large part of the data variance, two-dimensional maps are obtained in which similar points are clustered together (for a detailed discussion of such mapping techniques and many examples, see [27, 27a]). A mapping of objects (compounds) has already been presented in Fig. 8.1. In this case the similarity of substituents with respect to a set of substituent constants was considered, but a completely analogous map can also be obtained with principal components extracted from multiple biological response data. Mapping techniques with the aim of classifying compounds with respect to the type of biological response can also be performed with principal components extracted from a data matrix of molecular parameters [e.g. 35, 36]. Provided that the parameters selected are connected with the type of response, compounds with different biological profiles will then be siutated in different regions of the resulting map. This is a classification problem in the classical QSAR sense as already discussed (cf., 9. and 11.) and will, therefore, not be considered again in this section.

Other useful methods to investigate the structure of multiple biological response data are cluster analysis (cf., 8.1.) and the classification methods discussed in chapters 9. and 11. with biological response data as descriptors. Unger [26] applied cluster analysis to the metabolic profile of amphetamine in five mammals (rat, rabbit, man, dog, horse). The results showed that the profiles of rabbit and horse are closest while the profile of man most closely resembles that of the dog; the rat is seen as an outlier. Examples of the application of classification methods will be presented below.

Obviously, a definite pattern frequently exists in multiple response data which manifests itself in *activity-activity relationships* allowing the prediction of potencies in one bioassay from the multiple results in other bioassays. The biological potency of benzodiazepines in the foot shock test, for example, can be calculated from principal components (PC) obtained from a data matrix containing the results from the other four bioassays listed in Table 13.2 [28]:

$$\log A = 0.39\ \mathrm{PC}_1 + 0.65\ \mathrm{PC}_3 + 0.42 \qquad (13/14)$$

$$n = 22 \qquad r = 0.995 \qquad s = 0.21$$

This equation shows better statistics than any two-term equation with molecular parameters as independent variables.

When such relationships which frequently also exist between pairs of tests (see e.g. [26]) are derived only from data of homologous series it cannot be concluded that they

Table 13.2. Interrelated biological tests investigated by factor or principal component analysis

Type of compounds	Biological test	Number of factors or components	References
Various neuroleptics	12 pharmacological test (see [31])	2	[27a]
Various hypnotic, anti-epileptic and muscle-relaxant drugs	6 tests for anticonvulsive activity	2	[27a]
Non-hormonal anti-inflammatories	Mouse phenylquinone writhing Rat carageenin paw Inhibition of human platelet cyclooxygenase Inhibition of bull seminal vesicle PGE_2 Inhibition of collagen-induced platelet aggregation	2	[26]
Benzodiazepines	Incl. screen Foot-shock Pentylene-tetrazole Electroshock max. Electroshock min.	2	[28]
8-Quinolinoles	*A. niger* *A. oryzae* *Trichoderma viride* *Trichophyton mentagrophytes* *M. verrucaria*	2	[28]
Ryfamycin B amides	*M. aureus* *S. faecalis* *S. hemolyticus* *S. subtilis*	2	[28, 32]
Various standard compounds	36 tests; mouse behaviour and symptomatology screen	11	[26]
Piperidinoacetanilides	see Table 13.1	3	[29, 30]
Cl-substituted biphenyles	Barbiturate sleeping time and effect on 5 liver enzymes in rats	3	[33]
Neuroleptics	Antimanic effect antiautistic effect antidelusional effect ataractic effect extrapyramidal effect adrenolytic effect	2	[27]
Various antianginal drugs	7 cardiovascular pharmacological tests	2	[34]

are of general validity and hold for any type of compound. More general conclusions require that structurally sufficiently diverse compounds are included in such an analysis.

Of great practical importance are attempts to predict clinical profiles or types of effects from animal pharmacology data. This problem has been dealt with in detail by

Lewi [27, 37—41]. Using discriminant functions obtained from biological response data for six screening tests in rats (descriptors), it was possible to predict whether a newly synthesized compound would be a neuroleptic or a morphinomimetic [27, 39]. None of the six tests alone would have allowed a complete discrimination between the two pharmacological classes.

Most of the methods mentioned thus far require continuous response data of sufficient precision. As already pointed out, however, many biological response data (especially from large screening programs) are discrete and not continuous, representing potency in terms of a classification (cf., 9.2.). A convenient method to investigate multiple data structures in such cases can be derived from *information theory* using Shannons *entropy* as a measure of information content [30, 42, 43]. The information $I(T_i, T(k))$, contained in a set of k tests, $T(k)$, about a given test T_i, can be calculated according to:

$$I(T_i, T(k)) = H(T_i) - H_{T(k)}(T_i) \qquad (13/15)$$

$H(T_i)$ Shannons entropy of test T_i
$H_{T(k)}(T_i)$ Shannons entropy of test T_i conditional to the set of tests $T(k)$

The entropies can easily be computed from the results of a sufficiently large set of compounds in the test T_i and the set $T(k)$. $H(T_i)$ characterizes the uncertainty in T_i, and $H_{T(k)}(T_i)$ the remaining uncertainty in T_i if the results from $T(k)$ are known. Hence, the quantity

$$I_q = [I(T_i, T(k))/H(T_i)] \cdot 100\% \qquad (13/16)$$

represents the gain in information (or decrease in uncertainty) of T_i if the results from $T(k)$ are known (as a percentage of the original uncertainty in T_i). A high value of I_q indicates that $T(k)$ yields much information about T_i and that T_i and the tests contained in $T(k)$ are closely interrelated. Instead of a single test T_i, a group of tests can also be considered in a completely analogous manner so that complete information about the grouping of tests can be obtained.

Such an analysis was performed, for example, with antifungal potencies (expressed as "active" or "inactive") of a series of thioureas against the fungi *Aspergillus niger* (AN), *Botrytis cinerea* (BC), *Sclerotinia fructigena* (SF), *Fusarium nivale* (FN) and *Alternaria solani* (AS) (for details, see [42]; experimental data from [44]). Table 13.3 presents the stepwise development of I_q for SF as test T_i and all possible combinations of the other four tests as $T(k)$. As can be seen BC shows the highest information about SF followed by AN and AS. The best combination of two tests is that of AN and BC, and the most information is obtained from the set AN, BC and AS (the small increase in I_q after adding FN to $T(k)$ is considered to be insignificant). The result shows that a multiple activity-activity relationship should exist for the potency against FS and the potencies against AN, BC and AS. The evaluation of this relationship amounts to the evaluation of a classificator with the results from AN, BC and AS as descriptors. Since the descriptors are discrete quantities the best method to apply here is the linear learning machine (cf., 11.2.5.). The classificator obtained for the activity against SF using the results from all the other fungi as descriptors reads

$$\boldsymbol{w}^T\boldsymbol{x} = 2.61 - 0.82[\mathrm{BC}] - 0.23\,[\mathrm{AN}] - 0.58[\mathrm{AS}] - 0.05[\mathrm{FN}] \qquad (13/17)$$

[ ] activity against the fungus indicated

Table 13.3. Stepwise development of I_q (eqn. (13/16) for *Sclerotinia fructigena* as test T_i and all possible combinations (indicated by a cross) of AN, BC, AS and FN as $T(k)$[1])

$T(k)$				I_q (in %)
AN	BC	AS	FN	
	+			23.4
+				14.5
		+		12.0
			+	0.1
+	+			40.8
	+	+		34.6
	+		+	26.9
+		+		24.6
+			+	16.8
		+	+	12.4
+	+	+		57.7[2])
+	+		+	43.6
	+	+	+	39.3
+		+	+	30.6
+	+	+	+	61.2

[1]) AN *Aspergillus niger*
BC *Botrytis cinerea*
AS *Alternaria solani*
FN *Fusarium nivale*

[2]) optimal combination of tests

Table 13.4. Optimal sets of tests $T(k)$ and the corresponding I_q values for all 5 fungi[1])

Test T_i	Set $T(k)$	I_q (in %)
AN	BC, SF	46.4
BC	AN, SF	53.5
SF	AN, BC, AS	57.7
AS	SF	11.9
FN	—	—

[1]) AN *Aspergillus niger*
BC *Botrytis cinerea*
SF *Sclerotinia fructigena*
AS *Alternaria solani*
FN *Fusarium nivale*

and correctly reclassifies 80% of the compounds. As was to be expected, FN makes only a marginal contribution to the separation of classes in agreement with the results presented in Table 13.3 and can, in fact, be neglected.

The results for all five tests are summarized in Table 13.4. Quite obviously the system of tests is redundant since much information about AN, BC and SF can be obtained from the other tests. Only AS and FN show a unique behaviour (high information content). This pattern should be reflected by the pattern of QSARs describing antifungal activity in terms of molecular parameters. When comparing Table 13.4 with results from non-elementary discriminant analysis (cf., 9.2.2.) performed with the same data set [45], it is seen that this is indeed the case. Since, for example, the set BC, SF provides much information about AN, the discriminant function describing antifungal activity against AN should be more or less a composite of the discriminant functions obtained for BC and SF. Table 13.5 shows that this is indeed the case.

Table 13.5. Molecular parameters appearing in the discriminant function describing the antifungal potency of thioureas (R_1—NH—CS—NH—R_2) against AN, in comparison to the occurrence of the same parameters in the discriminant functions obtained for BC and SF[1]). The sign of the corresponding weight coefficients is indicated by "+" or "—". Superimposition of the columns for BC and SF exactly yields the column for AN (compare with Table 13.4)

Part of the molecule	Molecular parameters[2])	Discriminant function for		
		BC	SF	AN
R_1	$\Sigma\ \sigma$	n.s.[3])	—	—
	E_S (para)	n.s.	+	+
	I_3	n.s.	—	—
R_2	$\Sigma\ \pi$	n.s.	—	—
	$\Sigma\ E_S$	—	—	—
	I_1	+	n.s.	+
	MW	n.s.	—	—

[1]) AN *Aspergillus niger*
BC *Botrytis cinerea*
SF *Sclerotinia fructigena*

[2]) $\Sigma\ \sigma$ = sum of HAMMETT σ for aromatic substituents in phenylthioureas (phenyl in R_1)
E_S (para) = steric substituent constant for para-substituents in phenylthioureas (phenyl in R_1)
I_3 = indicator variable (= 1 for 2.5-Cl_2 in phenyl at R_1)
$\Sigma\ \pi$ = sum of π values of aromatic substituents (phenyl in R_2)
$\Sigma\ E_S$ sum of E_S values of aromatic substituents (phenyl in R_2)
I_1 = indicator variable (= 1, if phenyl in R_2)
MW = molecular weight

[3]) corresponding term not significant

This indicates another important aspect of multiple response data analysis. Once a pattern has been obtained it can be used to check QSARs and QSAR predictions. If they fit the pattern their reliability can be regarded as fairly high, if they do not, care is in order.

To summarize, the investigation of data structure in batteries of bioassays is of great practical importance and can aid in:

- recognizing redundant and unique tests
- predicting potencies or types of effects directly from the biological data
- controlling predictions made from QSARs
- differentiating biological effects and/or separating global effects into intrinsic components

13.3. Possible Test Strategies in Screening

Resting on a better understanding of biological data structures, an algorithmic test strategy is an important target of drug research. However, more time will have to elapse before such an aim can really be achieved. Experience suggests a more heuristic approach, which will be discussed for the following two basic situations of biological screening [46]:

1. *hierarchic arrangement* of tests for the same biological effect,
2. *parallel arrangement* of biological tests for different biological effects, e.g., main activity and side effects.

In biological screening, tests for the same biological effect are often organized into a *hierarchy* in the sense of a system made up by a series of gradually finer sieves, the ability to predict active compounds (but also research expenditure) increasing as the tests move upward in the hierarchy. The procedure schematized in Fig. 13.1 may be

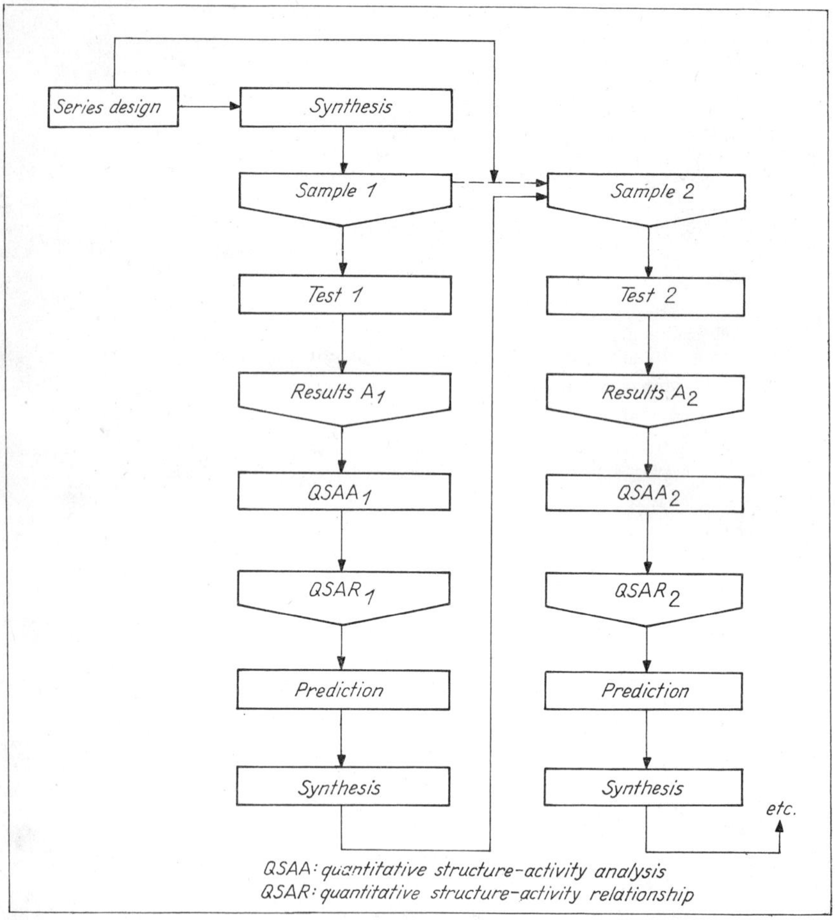

Fig. 13.1. Test procedure in hierarchically organized tests

helpful here. A sample composed according to the principles set forth in 8.1. (sample 1) is tested at the first test level (test 1). The outcome, A_1, is expressed in terms of a QSAR ($QSAR_1$), which serves for the prediction of more active compounds. These compounds are then synthesized and subjected to testing at the subsequent step (test 2). In addition, so many compounds from sample 1 are included that another training series according to the criteria indicated under 8.1. arises (sample 2) to which quantitative structure-activity analysis is again applied. The resulting QSAR ($QSAR_2$) serves as the basis of the synthesis of new compounds, which are tested in the next step, together with compounds selected from sample 2. This procedure is repeated at all levels of the hierarchy, and has the advantage that at each of them optimization takes place, the predictive capacity of the tests increasing as a higher level is attained.

Further advantages are as follows:

1. False results are detected immediately so that, in contrast to conventional screening, the risk of potentially very active compounds being erroneously eliminated is minimized.
2. Compounds that are extremely active at the lowest test level are not necessarily the most active ones at a higher test level or vice versa. This is allowed for by the stepwise alteration of the sample.

The strategy displayed in Fig. 13.1 should, of course, not taken to be a rigid scheme. Thus, tests at the top of the hierarchy may not be needed for a whole set. It is also possible that at a given stage of the test hierarchy the quantitative structure-activity analysis does not reveal a compound more active than the ones already available. In this case, one can proceed with the most active compounds and repeat quantitative structure-activity analyses (after testing again a corresponding number of compounds) at the highest stages only when these compounds suddenly show weak activity or change considerably in their biological activity sequence. In any case, the quantitative structure-activity analysis should be carried out as systematically as possible at an opportune moment. This is particularly true of tests arranged with reference to their biological integration stage, test 1 involving, for example, an isolated enzyme and the last test an intact organism. In such instances, the procedure outlined here enables pharmacodynamic and pharmacokinetic properties to be optimized simultaneously (see e.g. [47, 48]).

It will be obvious that in any search for new drugs side effects also need to be evaluated, thus requiring *parallel test arrangements* with respect to different biological activities. A simple example is that which only refers to two parallel tests: test 1 where the main activity and test 2 where an undesired effect is examined. Three strategical variants are possible here.

Variant 1 is schematized in Fig. 13.2, where the quantitative structure-activity analysis in cyclic stages (cf., Fig. 8.2) first serves to optimize only the desired activity, A_1. Only the most active compounds are then examined in test 2. The risk of this procedure is that precisely those compounds may also display a marked side effect and in extreme cases it is even possible that along with the main activity A_1 the side effect, A_2, has also been maximized so that all operations have been in vain. In the case that compounds with the highest activity A_1 only have a minimal side effect A_2 — which is, of course, not *a priori* known — unnecessary experimentation in test 2 can be avoided through the use of this variant.

When the second variant (*variant 2*; Fig. 13.3) is used, the sample in its entirety is examined in both tests and a quantitative structure-activity analysis is performed with both activity values. The quantitative structure-activity and structure-selectivity relations so determined provide an opportunity to predict whether better compounds of high selectivity can be made. If more selective compounds are possible, they are synthesized and tested, and another quantitative structure-activity analysis follows. Again, there is an optimization cycle (see Fig. 8.2) which is run through until the best compounds of the series in question are found with sufficient certainty. This variant is free from the risk that variant 1 entails, but quite unnecessary expenditure is involved if compounds showing the highest activity in test 1 appear to have little activity in test 2.

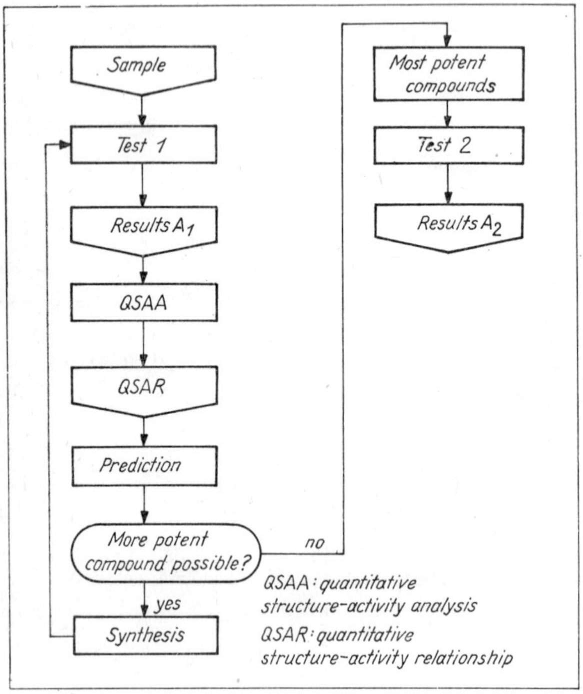

Fig. 13.2. Test procedure in parallelly organized tests, variant 1

None of these disadvantages pertains to the use of the third variant shown in Fig. 13.4 (*variant 3*), as it helps to decide on the use of variant 1 or variant 2 at an opportune time on the basis of available data. As regards the main activity (test 1), the usual cyclic optimization process is carried out, the most active compounds being examined at each cycle in test 2. If these compounds are also active in test 2, variant 2 can be used for further processing (while avoiding the risks of variant 1); if not, variant 1 can be used (while avoiding the risks of unnecessary testing).

In real screening systems, both of the two basic situations outlined here frequently occur simultaneously in that tests are ordered in a parallel as well as hierarchic fashion. Such systems tend to be extremely complex, requiring widely differing heuristics, but the

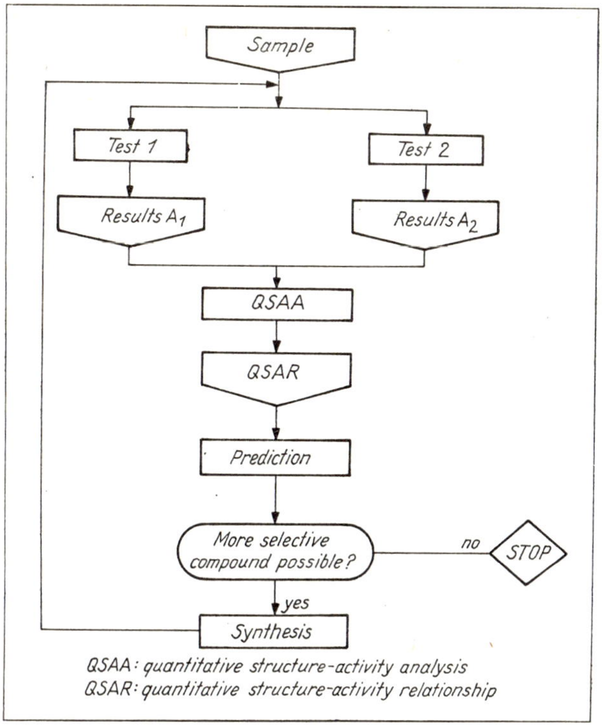

Fig. 13.3. Test procedure in parallelly organized tests, variant 2

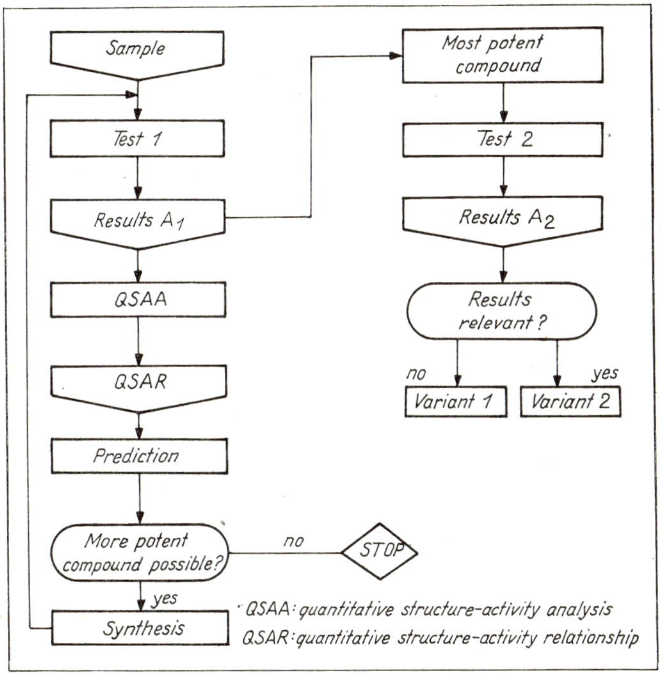

Fig. 13.4. Test procedure in parallelly organized tests, variant 3

basic elements mentioned above will invariably appear. A complex approach including the application of multivariate procedures for multiple data and quantitative structure-activity analyses in the sense of what has been said at the beginning of this chapter is of particular significance.

References

[1] Tichý, M., in R. Franke and P. Oehme (Eds.): Quantitative Structure-Activity Analysis, Akademie-Verlag, Berlin, 1978, p. 359
[2] Silipo, C., and C. Hansch: J. Am. Chem. Soc. **97**, 6849 (1975)
[3] Hansch, C., C. Silipo and E. E. Steller: J. Pharm. Sci. **64**, 1186 (1975)
[4] Fukunaga, J. Y., C. Hansch and E. E. Steller: J. Med. Chem. **19**, 605 (1976)
[5] Hansch, C., J. Y. Fukunaga, P. Y. C. Jow and J. B. Hynes: J. Med. Chem. **20**, 96 (1977)
[6] Dietrich, S. W., R. N. Smith, J. Y. Fukunaga, M. Olney and C. Hansch: Arch. Biochem. Biophys. **194**, 600 (1979)
[7] Dietrich, S. W., R. N. Smith, S. Brendler and C. Hansch: Arch. Biochem. Biophys. **194**, 612 (1979)
[8] Blaney, J. M., S. W. Dietrich, M. A. Reynolds and C. Hansch: J. Med. Chem. **22**, 614 (1979)
[9] Dietrich, S. W., J. M. Blaney, M. A. Reynolds, P. Y. C. Jow and C. Hansch: J. Med. Chem. **23**, 1205 (1980)
[10] Li, R.-L., S. W. Dietrich and C. Hansch. J. Med. Chem. **24**, 538 (1981)
[11] Hyde, R. M., and B. Roth in J. A. Keverling Buisman (Ed.): Strategy in Drug Research, Pharmacochemistry Library (Eds.: W. Th. Nauta and R. F. Rekker), Vol. 4, Elsevier, Amsterdam, 1981, p. 385
[12] Hansch, C.: Il Farmaco **33**, 89 (1979)
[13] Hansch, C., R. N. Smith, R. Engle and H. Wood: Cancer Chemother. Rep. **56**, 443 (1972)
[14] Lien, E. J., and G. C. Tong: Cancer Chemother. Rep. **57**, 251 (1973)
[15] Hansch, C., A. Leo, C. Schmidt and P. Y. C. Jow: J. Med. Chem. **23**, 1095 (1980)
[16] Denny, W. A., G. J. Atwell, B. C. Baguley and B. F. Cain: J. Med. Chem. **22**, 134 (1980)
[17] Coats, E. A., S. R. Milstein, G. Holbein, J. McDonald, R. Reed and H. G. Petering: J. Med. Chem. **19**, 131 (1976)
[18] Coats, E. A., S. R. Milstein, M. A. Pleiss and J. A. Roesner: J. Med. Chem. **21**, 804 (1978)
[19] Coats, E. A., in S. H. Yalkowsky, A. A. Sinkula and S. C. Valvani (Eds.): Physical Chemical Properties of Drugs, Marcel Dekker, New York, 1980, p. 111
[20] Quinn, F. R., Z. Neiman and J. A. Beisler: J. Med. Chem. **24**, 636 (1981)
[21] Funk, S. I., A. Leo, M. Yamakawa and C. Hansch: Il Farmaco **35**, 965 (1980)
[22] Franke, R., E. Karañov and J. Kaneti: C. R. Acad. Sci. Bulg. **31**, 1051 (1978)
[23] Grassy, G., A. Terol, Y. Robbe, J.-P. Chapat, R. Granger, M. Fatome and L. Andrieu: Eur. J. Med. Chem. **10**, 14 (1975)
[24] Bercher, H., W. Laass, E. Wendig, A. Grisk and R. Franke in J. Knoll and F. Darvas (Eds.): Chemical Structure — Biological Activity Relationships, Akadémiai Kiadó, Budapest, 1980, p. 365
[25] Unger, S. H., K. Untch, B. Lewis, B. Berkoz, J. Edwards, A. Strosberg, R. Weissberg and R. Alvarez in J. Knoll and F. Darvas (Eds.): Chemical Structure — Biological Activity Relationships, Akadémiai Kiadó, Budapest, 1980, p. 3
[26] Unger, S. H., in E. J. Ariens (Ed.): Drug Design, Vol. IX, Academic Press, New York, 1980, p. 48
[26a] Ariens, E. J., in E. J. Ariens (Ed.): Drug Design, Vol. I, Academic Press, New York, 1971, p. 1
[26b] Terenius, L., in J. A. Keverling Buisman (Ed.): Biological Activity and Chemical Struc-

ture, Pharmacochemistry Library, (Eds.: W. Th. Nauta and R. F. Rekker), Vol. 2, Elsevier, Amsterdam, 1977, p. 161
[27] Lewi, P. J., in E. J. Ariens (Ed.): Drug Design, Vol. X, Academic Press, New York, 1980, 307
[27a] Lewi, P. J., in E. J. Ariens (Ed.): Drug Design, Vol. VII, Academic Press, New York, 1976, p. 209
[28] Lukovits, I., and A. Lopata: J. Med. Chem. **23**, 449 (1980)
[29] Franke, R., A. Barth, S. Dove and W. Laass: Pharmazie **35**, 181 (1980)
[30] Franke, R., in J. A. Keverling Buisman (Ed.): Strategy in Drug Research, Pharmacochemistry Library (Eds.: W. Th. Nauta and R. F. Rekker), Vol. 4, Elsevier, Amsterdam, 1982, p. 355
[31] Janssen, P. A. J., C. J. E. Neimegeers and K. H. L. Schellekens: Drug Res. **15**, 104 (1965)
[32] Dove, S.: Thesis, Martin-Luther-Universität Halle—Wittenberg, 1978
[33] Franke, R., G. Schwarz, S. Dove, A. Dietrich and W. Klinger: Zentralblatt Pharmazie **122**, 459 (1983)
[34] Laass, W., D. Modersohn and E. Scheer in J. Knoll and F. Darvas (Eds.): Chemical Structure — Biological Activity Relationships, Akadémiai Kiadó, Budapest, 1980, p. 165
[35] Cammarata, A., and G. K. Menon: J. Med. Chem. **19**, 739 (1976)
[36] Menon, G. K., and A. Cammarata: J. Pharm. Sci. **66**, 304 (1977)
[37] Lewi, P. J.: Pharmacopsych. Neuro-Psychopharmacol. **8**, 375 (1975)
[38] Lewi, P. J.: Int. Pharmacopsychiatry **11**, 181 (1976)
[39] Lewi, P. J., W. F. M. Van Bever and P. A. J. Jansson: Eur. J. Pharmacol. **35**, 403 (1976)
[40] Lewi, P. J., and F. C. Colpaert: Psychopharmacologia **49**, 219 (1976)
[41] Lewi, P. J.: Pharm. Ther. **B 3**, 481 (1978)
[42] Krause, G., W. J. Streich and R. Franke: Pharmazie **35**, 488 (1980)
[43] Krause, G., W. J. Streich and R. Franke in J. Knoll and F. Darvas (Eds.): Chemical Structure — Biological Activity Relationships, Akadémiai Kiadó, Budapest, 1980, p. 145
[44] Vassilev, G. N., Z. Tomaleva and E. Karanov: C. R. Acad. Sci. agric. bulg. **2**, 259 (1969)
[45] Krause, G., R. Franke and G. N. Vassilev: Biochem. Physiol. Pflanzen **174**, 128 (1979)
[46] Franke, R.: Wiss. Beiträge der Martin-Luther-Universität Halle—Wittenberg **41**, 22 (1977)
[47] Seydel, J. K.: Int. J. Quant. Chem. **20**, 131 (1981)
[48] Seydel, J. K., in J. A. Keverling Buisman (Ed.): Strategy in Drug Research, Pharmacochemistry Library (Eds.: W. Th. Nauta and R. F. Rekker), Vol. 4, Elsevier, Amsterdam, 1982, p. 179

14. Concluding Remarks

Recent years have witnessed two clear-cut trends in the field of quantitative structure-activity analysis. On the one hand, there is an explosion of publications describing their application with the emphasis on Hansch and Free-Wilson analysis and, on the other hand, a systematic development of new methods tailored to particular problems and objectives such as those discussed in chapter 12. In view of this development it is obvious that these two methods, now widely used, were only the first steps in what is still running a stormy course, but it cannot be stressed enough that they constitute extremely important advances. It is, in fact, astonishing to see the services they have already rendered. They have been successfully employed at all possible levels of biological integration (molecular, subcellular, cellular, organic, organismic) as well as for a large variety of biological objects (microbes, plants, animals) and a huge spectrum of biological activities, encompassing an extremely wide range of chemical structures. The resulting QSARs, in general, show high descriptive power although it is not unusual for individual compounds to behave as outliers. Such compounds which show a peculiar behaviour compared with the other analogues and which can usually only be detected with the help of QSARs are of special interest since they may highlight possible mechanisms of action and serve as starting points for the development of novel drugs (see e.g. [1—7]).

The ultimate objective of QSARs is the prediction of either hypotheses on the mechanism of action or new analogues with high potency. Their predictive potential is limited to the feature space considered. As the application of quantitative structure-activity analysis to actual problems in drug research acquires greater prominence in relation to the retrospective analyses dominating in the sixties, an increasing number of experimentally verified examples of QSAR predictions are reported. Some of these are shown in Table 14.1, and many more may be hidden in the files of pharmaceutical companies (see also [89]). Some of the drugs found through the use of structure-activity analysis have already attained the stage of clinical trials (see e.g. [4, 22, 23, 61, 78—80, 90]). Nevertheless, there is as yet no unambiguous evidence of a drug introduced for therapeutic use as a direct consequence of predictions or conclusions based on quantitative structure-activity analysis. One of the reasons is, of course, that the systematic use of QSARs on an industrial scale was started only a few years ago. Much time must elapse, currently at least 8 years, before a new drug can be brought onto the market. Patent matters and strategic considerations are a also responsible for the fact that at the present time and in the near future the publication of such results is scarcely to be expected (e.g. [90—92]).

It would be essentially incorrect to evaluate the economic utility of quantitative structure-activity analysis preferentially in terms of the number of new compounds obtained directly through precalculations, for this criterion says nothing as to whether the likelihood of detecting new compounds of interest has been enhanced. For eco-

Table 14.1. Examples of correct predictions from QSARs

Type of compounds	Biological activity	References
Benzothiadiazines	Antihypertensive	[8—10]
Clonidine analogues	Antihypertensive	[11]
	α-adrenergic	[12]
Propynylamines	Inhibition of monoamino oxidase	[13]
N-(phenoxyethyl)-cyclopropylamines	Inhibition of monoamino oxidase	[14]
β-carbolines	Inhibition of monoamino oxidase	[15]
Fusaric acids	Inhibition of dopamine-β-hydroxylase	[16]
Sulfonamides	Inhibition of carboanhydrase	[17, 18]
Carbamoylpiperidines	Inhibition of cholinesterase	[19, 20]
Ketones	Inhibition of chymotrypsin	[21]
Thiazole-β-blockers	Inhibition of adenylate cyclase	[22, 23]
Benzylpyridinium ions	Inhibition of complement	[24]
Miscellaneous	Binding to BSA	[24]
Steroids	Binding to the progesterone receptor	[25]
Esters	Hydrolysis by papain	[2]
Dopamine amides	Hydrolysis by arylamidases	[16]
Peptidyl-p-nitroanilides	Hydrolysis by subtilisin	[26]
Polycyclic aromatic hydrocarbons	Hydroxylation by microsomal oxidase	[27]
	Carcinogenicity	[28]
Isatin-β-isothiosemicarbazones	Antiviral	[29]
Pyrazoles	Antiviral	[30]
Miscellaneous	Cytostatic	[31, 32]
ara-Cytidine derivatives	Cytostatic, Immunosuppressive	[33]
Nitrosoureas	Cytostatic	[34]
Mitomycins	Cytostatic	[35]
Hydantoin derivatives	Cytostatic	[36]
Rifamycin B amides	Antibacterial	[37]
Sulfonamides	Antibacterial, Pharmacokinetics	[38—41]
Erythromycins	Antibacterial	[16]
Quinoxaline 1,4-dioxides	Antibacterial	[42]
Phenanthrenes	Antimalaria	[1, 2]
Naphtoquinones	Antimalaria	[43]
Phenylamidinoureas	Antimalaria	[44, 45]
Tuberins	Antimycoplasma	[23]
Methoxychlors	Insecticidal	[46]
N-Hydroxypyridones	Antifungal	[47]
Pyridine derivatives	Antifungal	[48]
Trifluormethanesulfonamides	Herbicidal	[49, 50]
Aryl-alkyl-carbonylcompounds	Herbicidal	[51]
Arylethers	Herbicidal	[52]
Piperidinoacetanilides	Phytoactive	[53]
Pyrimidones	Inhibition of HILL reaction	[54]
Ureas	Herbicidal	[55]
Phenylacetamides	Hypnotic	[56]
Pyridylmethanes	Spasmolytic	[57]
Promazines	Neuroleptic	[58]
Miscellaneous	Cholinergic	[59, 60]

Tab. 14.1 (continued)

Type of compounds	Biological activity	References
Aromatic and aliphatic acids	Antiphlogistic	[61]
Benzothiepine derivatives	Neuroleptic	[62]
Carboxylate esters	Clot lysis	[2]
Thyroxine analogues	Thyroxin	[63]
Acrylates	Toxic	[64]
Miscellaneous	Toxic	[65]
Copper chelates	Cytotoxic	[66]
Pyranenamines	Immunosuppressive	[67]
Azapurine-6-ones	Immunosuppressive	[68]
Phenyloxazolidines	Radioprotective	[69]
Carbamoylethylamines	Cholinolytic	[70]
Miscellaneous	Affinity for the muscarinic receptor	[71]
Mescaline analogues	Hallucinogenic	[72]
Triazines	Inhibition of dihydrofolate reductase	[73]
Benzodiazepines	Antipentilene-tetrazol activity	[74]
Cyanocyclohexylamines	Antifungal	[74]
Cycloalkanolethers	Several	[74]
Piperidinoacetanilides	Antiserotonin	[75]
Miscellaneous	H_2-Antagonistic	[76]
Analogues of Somatostatin	Antidiabetic	[77]
Steroids	Progestational	[78–80]
Azacycloalkanes	Analgesic	[81]
Organosilicon amines	Antifungal	[32, 82]
Indandione-1,3	Toxic	[32]
derivatives	Anticonvulsive	
Sulfones	Antibacterial	[83]
1,3-Benzodioxoles	Synergism of carbaryl toxicity	[84]
Chlorinated hydrocarbons	Bioconcentration in fish	[85]
Alkoxybenzylalkylamines	Toxic	[86]
Spirobarbituric acids	Sedative	[87]
Cannabiniod analogues	Ataxia, Analgesis, Irritability	[88]
Adenosine analogues	Antihypertensive	[88]
Trimetoprim analogues	Antibacterial	[88]

nomic utility it is equally important to reduce synthesis operations and testing, and this is where methods of quantitative structure-activity analysis have their greatest potential. They make it possible to take the paths which offer the greatest promise and to avoid unpromising directions so that the search for new drugs can be performed with greater speed, less cost and a substantially increased chance of success. Even if in a given search area no new drug can be found, the utility of QSARs may be substantial. The reason is that QSARs can tell one when to stop thus avoiding large sums possibly spent on unsuccessful syntheses and biological testing.

A decisive factor in any efficient use of the methods of quantitative structure-activity analysis in drug research is an exact understanding of what can be obtained with each single technique and within what limits. A few selected aspects are summarized once more in Table 14.2.

As already stated, the relations between structure and biological activity are coded in the chemical structure of the drug in an extremely complex manner. Comparison of the various methods of quantitative structure-activity analysis from the viewpoint of molecular description presents the following picture where decoding is concerned. Methods based on structural parameters cannot decode but do provide data on the chief code elements and their contribution to biological activity. This allows a new encoding (new combinations of substructures) and thus the formulation of proposals for synthesis without the previous code being explicitly known. Similarly, the code is not "broken" at the level of the extrathermodynamic approach, i.e., of molecular description using external molecular parameters. Some partial decoding takes place at this level, providing the chemist with understandable information which, within certain limits, admits of manipulations. Full understanding and application of the code are only possible at the level of pharmacophoric pattern searching and interaction calculations, and this is what makes the development of these techniques so important, even though it calls for much further investment.

On inspection of Table 14.2 it will be seen that the majority of the methods of quantitative structure-activity analysis now routinely used are more or less restricted to congeneric series of compounds. The domain of QSAR work in the current practice of drug research therefore still is the optimization of a given lead, approaches to theoretical lead generation being in their infancy. This situation will probably gradually change as the methods outlined in chapters 11. and especially 12. are developed further and are applied systematically.

It must always be remembered that predictions derived from QSARs have a statistical character and, thus, always a certain probability of being in error. Predictions should, therefore, never be taken as a dogma and always considered and used critically in a close interaction with experimental work.

The development of structure-activity analysis has not yet advanced to the point where it always yields correct results or can be applied to problems of any nature. In its present stage it cannot be used as the sole basis of overall drug research, and enough room for intuitive manoeuvre must remain. In an effectively organized search, intuition or experience and the evaluation as well as interpretation of QSARs actually are only two sides of the same coin.

A basic limitation of structure-activity analysis lies in the fact that only such information can be extracted as is present in the biological data. Thus, structure-activity analysis by itself cannot lead to new concepts in therapy, although the manipulation of the information contained in biological data and chemical structures through the use of large computers and appropriate programs may also aid in developing new concepts. In summary, it may be said that methods of quantitative structure-activity analysis in their current stage of development have already been found to be extremely helpful instruments without which no effective search for new drugs is possible and which will undoubtedly offer further possibilities in both drug research and the elucidation of biological mechanisms.

An important trend resulting from the further development of QSAR methods and their systematic practical application is the implementation of what may be called "theoretical drug design systems" in many pharmaceutical companies and research

Table 14.2. Review of important QSAR methods

Molecular description	Mathematical procedure	Basic conditions for application	Results make possible		
			Directed synthesis	Hypothesis on molecular mechanisms	Generation of new lead compounds
1. *External molecular parameters*	1.1. Multiple regression analysis (Hansch analysis)	— Congeneric series — Biological activity is a continuous quantity with sufficient precision and variance	++	+	—
— Must be available or calculable		Systematic variation of all important molecular properties by a proper selection of substituents (many substituents present in only a few positions (compare with 2.1.))			
— Must account adequately for all molecular properties relevant for biological activity	1.2. Rank correlation analysis	As for 1.1., but activity data may be less precise and must not be more accurate as to allow a ranking of compounds	+	(+)	—
	1.3. Discriminant analysis	As for 1.1.; biological activity is not a continuous but a discrete quantity (classification) according to an activity score	+	(+)	—
	1.4. SIMCA analysis	As for 1.3. (within-class structure of objects can be described)	+	(+)	—
	1.5. Pattern recognition methods	As for 1.3., but less strict mathematical requirements	+	(+)	—
	1.6. Principal component analysis with target rotation	As for 1.1.; the method allows for a simultaneous (multivariate) analysis of several interrelated biological activities	+	+	—
	1.7. Multivariate regression analysis	As for 1.6.	+	+	—

2. *Sub-structural molecular descriptors*	2.1. Multiple regression analysis (FREE-WILSON analysis)	— Congeneric series with constant basic structure	+	—	—
		— Substituent contributions to biological activity must be constant and additive			
Can be directly derived from molecular topology or topography		— Especially suitable if only a few substituents are present at many positions (compare with 1.1.)			
		— Elimination of linear dependencies between columns ot the structure matrix			
	2.2. Pattern recognition methods	— Congeneric series and limitation with respect to structural variations not required	+	—	(+)
		— Biological activity is a discrete quantity (classification) according to an activity score			
	2.3. Logical and/or information theoretical methods	As for 2.2.	(+)	(+)	+
3. Molecular matching, various potentials, interaction calculations etc. (chapter 12.)	Various	— No limitation with respect to structural variation	+	++	++
		— Biological activity data relevant for drug-receptor interactions			
		— Effective methods for three-dimensional molecular manipulation and for describing intra- and intermolecular interactions			

centres (see p. 327). The basic features of such systems are (see also [89]):

1. graphic and tabular input and output,
2. data bases:
   - chemical substances and related physicochemical, biological and geometrical properties
   - substituent constants
   - QSARs
   - libraries of substructures
   - standard bond lengths and angles,
3. programs to calculate molecular properties and descriptors
   - log *P* from hydrophobic fragmental constants
   - molar volumes
   - cavity surface areas
   - connectivities
   - conformations
   - substructural descriptors,
4. programs for molecular manipulation (translation, rotation and superposition of molecules),
5. mathematical QSAR programs.

After entering molecules, those parts of the system can be activated which are needed to solve the problem concerned. This can be done in a stepwise manner, and several different programs can be applied to the same set of compounds if required. The advantage of such systems is that they allow a very effective use of the whole spectrum of QSAR and related methods in one package. They usually also include programs for computer-assisted chemical synthesis (for reviews, see e.g. [93—97]) which may greatly facilitate the derivation of synthetic routes to new compounds (e.g. [98, 99]).

References

[1] Hansch, C., and J. Y. Fukunaga: Chem. Technol. **7**, 120 (1977)

[2] Hansch, C., in J. A. Keverling Buisman (Ed.): Biological Activity and Chemical Structure, Pharmacochemistry Library (Eds.: W. Th. Nauta and R. F. Rekker), Vol. 2, Elsevier, Amsterdam, 1977, p. 47

[3] Kuchař, M., in R. Franke and P. Oehme (Eds.): Quantitative Structure-Activity Analysis, Akademie-Verlag, Berlin, 1978, Contribution to general discussion, p. 449

[4] Zeelen, F. J., in R. Franke and P. Oehme (Eds.): Quantitative Structure-Activity Analysis, Akademie-Verlag, Berlin, 1978, Contribution to general discussion, p. 450

[5] Seydel, J. K., in R. Franke and P. Oehme (Eds.): Quantitative Structure-Activity Analysis, Akademie-Verlag, Berlin, 1978, Contribution to general discussion, p. 449

[6] Seydel, J. K., and K.-J. Schaper in J. A. Keverling Buisman (Ed.): Strategy in Drug Research, Pharmacochemistry Library (Eds.: W. Th. Nauta and R. F. Rekker), Vol. 4, Elsevier, Amsterdam, 1982, p. 337

[7] Franke, R., in J. A. Keverling Buisman (Ed.): Strategy in Drug Research, Pharmacochemistry Library (Eds.: W. Th. Nauta and R. F. Rekker), Vol. 4, Elsevier, Amsterdam, 1982, p. 355

[8] Wohl, J. A., in L. B. Kier (Ed.): Molecular Orbital Studies in Chemical Pharmacology, Springer, New York, 1970, p. 262
[9] Aranda, A.: C. R. Acad. sci. **276**, 1301 (1973)
[10] Topliss, J. G., and M. D. Yudis: J. Med. Chem. **15**, 394 (1972)
[11] Rouot, B., G. Leclerc, C. G. Wermuth and F. Miesch: J. Pharmac. **8**, 95 (1977)
[12] Rouot, B., G. Leclerc, C. G. Wermuth, F. Miesch and J. Schwartz: J. Med. Chem. **19**, 1049 (1976)
[13] Martin, Y. C., W. B. Martin and J. D. Taylor: J. Med. Chem. **18**, 883 (1975)
[14] Fuller, R. W., M. M. Marsh and J. J. Mills: J. Med. Chem. **11**, 397 (1968)
[15] Martin, Y. C., and J. H. Biel in E. Usdin (Ed.): Neuropsychopharmacology of Monoamines and their Regulatory Enzymes, Raven Press, New York, 1974, p. 37
[16] Martin, Y. C.: Quantitative Drug Design, Marcel Dekker, New York, 1978
[17] Kakeya, N., M. Aoki, A. Kamada and N. Yata: Chem. Pharm. Bull. **17**, 1010 (1969)
[18] Kakey, N., N. Yata, A. Kamada and M. Aoki: Chem. Pharm. Bull. **17**, 2558 (1969)
[19] Purcell, W. P.: Biochim. Biophys. Acta **105**, 201 (1965)
[20] Beasley, J. C., and W. P. Purcell: Biochim. Biophys. Acta **178**, 175 (1969)
[21] Grieco, G., C. Silipo, A. Vittorio and C. Hansch: J. Med. Chem. **20**, 586 (1977)
[22] Unger, S. H., L. Untch, B. Lewis, B. Bertoz, J. Edwards, A. Strosberg, R. Weissberg and R. Alvarez in J. Knoll and F. Darvas (Eds.): Chemical Structure — Biological Activity Relationships, Akadémiai Kiadó, Budapest, 1980, p. 3
[23] Unger, S. H., in E. J. Ariens (Ed.): Drug Design, Vol. IX, Academic Press, New York, 1980, p. 48
[24] Hansch, C., M. Yoshimoto and M. H. Doll: J. Med. Chem. **19**, 1068 (1976)
[25] Lee, D. L., P. A. Kollman, F. J. Marsh and M. E. Wolff: J. Med. Chem. **20**, 1139 (1977)
[26] Pozsgay, M., R. Gaspar, J. Beejusz, and P. Elodi: Eur. J. Biochem. **95**, 115 (1979)
[27] Franke, R.: Chem. Biol. Interactions **6**, 1 (1973)
[28] Rösner, R., K. Türschman, R. Franke, D. Schönfelder and S. Unger: Paper presented at the 17th congress of the Pharmacological Society of the GDR, Berlin, 1975
[29] Franke, R., D. Labes, M. Tonew, W. Zschiesche and L. Heinisch: Acta biol. med. germ. **34**, 491 (1975)
[30] Michel, H.-J., R. Franke and H. Willitzer in R. Franke and P. Oehme (Eds.): Quantitative Structure-Activity Analysis, Akademie-Verlag, Berlin, 1978, p. 89
[31] Chu, K. C., R. J. Feldmann, M. B. Shapiro, G. F. Hazard and R. I. Geran: J. Med. Chem. **18**, 539 (1975)
[32] Golender, V. F., and A. B. Rozenblit in E. J. Ariens (Ed.): Drug Design, Vol. IX, Academic Press, New York, 1980, p. 300
[33] Wechter, W. J., M. A. Johnson, C. M. Hall, D. T. Warner, A. E. Berger, H. A. Wenzel, D. T. Gish and G. L. Neil: J. Med. Chem. **18**, 339 (1975)
[34] Montero, J. L., and J. L. Imbach: C. R. Acad. Sci. Ser. C **279**, 809 (1974)
[35] Remers, W. A., and C. S. Schepman: J. Med. Chem. **17**, 729 (1974)
[36] Peng, G. W., V. E. Marquez and J. S. Driscoll: J. Med. Chem. **18**, 846 (1975)
[37] Quinn, F. R., J. S. Driscoll and C. Hansch: J. Med. Chem. **18**, 332 (1975)
[38] Seydel, J. K., and E. Wempe: Arzneimittel-Forsch. **21**, 187 (1971)
[39] Seydel, J. K., and K.-J. Schaper: Chemische Struktur und biologische Aktivität von Wirkstoffen, Verlag Chemie, Weinheim, 1979
[40] Seydel, J. K.: Int. J. Quant. Chem. **20**, 131 (1981)
[41] Seydel, J. K., in J. A. Keverling Buisman (Ed.): Strategy in Drug Research, Pharmacochemistry Library (Eds.: W. Th. Nauta and R. F. Rekker), Vol. 4, Elsevier, Amsterdam, 1982, p. 179
[42] Dirmla, J. P., L. J. Czuba, B. W. Domminy, R. B. James, R. M. Pezzullo, J. E. Presslitz and R. M. Windisch: J. Med. Chem. **22**, 1118 (1979)

[43] Martin, Y. C., T. M. Bustard and K. R. Lynn: J. Med. Chem. **16**, 1089 (1973)

[44] Goodford, P. J., and F. E. Norrington in M. Tichý (Ed.): Quantitative Structur-Activity Relationships, Akadémiai Kiadó, Budapest, 1976, p. 79

[45] Goodford, P. J., F. E. Norrington, W. Richards and L. P. Walls: Br. J. Pharmac. **48**, 650 (1973)

[46] Goodford, P. J., A. T. Hudson, G. Sheppey, R. Wootton, M. Black, G. J. Sutherland and J. C. Wickham: J. Med. Chem. **19**, 1239 (1976)

[47] Dittmar, W., E. Druckrey and H. Urbach: J. Med. Chem. **17**, 753 (1974)

[48] Druckrey, E., and W. Dittmar in M. Tichý (Ed.): Quantitative Structure-Activity Relationships, Akadémiai Kiadó, Budapest, 1976, p. 59

[49] Yapel, A. F.: Adv. in Chemistry Series **114**, 183 (1972)

[50] Yapel, A. F.: Adv. in Chemistry Series **114**, 252 (1972)

[51] Franke, R., and E. Gäbler: unpublished results

[52] Schönfelder, D., and R. Franke: unpublished results

[53] Scholz, S., H. Sprinz, R. Hagemann, R. Franke, G. Hübner and A. Barth: Pharmazie **31**, 162 (1976)

[54] Gibbons, L. K., E. F. Koldenboven, A. A. Nethery, R. E. Montgomery and W. P. Purcell: J. Agr. Food Chem. **24**, 203 (1976)

[55] Magee, P. S.: ACS Symp. Ser. **112**, 319 (1979)

[56] Druckrey, E., H. Schwarz and H. Leditschke: Chim. Ther. **7**, 188 (1972)

[57] Cousse, H., C. Mouzin and L. D. D'Hinterland: Chim. Ther. **4**, 466 (1973)

[58] Kaufman, J. J., and W. S. Koski: Int. J. Quant. Chem. QBS **2**, 35 (1975)

[59] Weinstein, H., S. Maayani, S. Srebrenik, S. Cohen and M. Sokolovsky: Mol. Pharmacol. **9**, 820 (1973)

[60] Weinstein, H.: Int. J. Quant. Chem. QBS **2**, 59 (1975)

[61] Kuchař, M., in J. Knoll and F. Darvas (Eds.): Chemical Structure — Biological Activity Relationships, Akadémiai Kiadó, Budapest, 1980, p. 15

[62] Tollenaere, J. P., H. Moereels and M. Protiva: Eur. J. Med. Chem. **11**, 298 (1976)

[63] Jorgensen, E. C., and J. A. Reid: J. Med. Chem. **8**, 533 (1965)

[64] Bass, G. E., W. H. Lawrence, W. P. Purcell and U. Autrian: J. Dent. Res. **53**, 756 (1974)

[65] Enslein, K.: Genesee Statistic Newsletter **6**, 714 (1978)

[66] Coats, E. A., S. R. Milstein, G. Holbein, J. McDonald, R. Reed and H. G. Petering: J. Med. Chem. **19**, 131 (1976)

[67] Cramer, R. D., K. M. Snader, C. R. Willis, L. W. Chakrin, J. Thomas and B. M. Sutton: J. Med. Chem. **22**, 714 (1979)

[68] Broughton, B. J., P. Chaplen, P. Knowles, E. Lunt, S. M. Marshall, D. L. Pain and K. R. H. Woolridge: J. Med. Chem. **18**, 1117 (1975)

[69] Fernandez, J., G. Grassy, A. Terol, Y. Robbe, P. Chapar, R. Granger and H. Sentanay-Roumanou: Eur. J. Med. Chem. **13**, 245 (1978)

[70] Bowden, K., and R. C. Young: J. Med. Chem. **13**, 225 (1970)

[71] Kier, L. B., and L. H. Hall: J. Pharm. Sci. **67**, 1408 (1978)

[72] Glennon, R. A., L. B. Kier and A. T. Shulgin: J. Pharm. Sci. **68**, 906 (1979)

[73] Hopfinger, A. J.: J. Am. Chem. Soc. **102**, 7196 (1980)

[74] Darvas, F., in J. Knoll and F. Darvas (Eds.): Chemical Structure — Biological Activity Relationships, Akadémiai Kiadó, Budapest, 1980, p. 25

[75] Henkel, H. J., V. Hagen, A. Hagen, I. Schimke and A. Barth in J. Knoll and F. Darvas (Eds.): Chemical Structure — Biological Activity Relationships, Akadémiai Kiadó, Budapest, 1980, p. 39

[76] Green, J. P., H. Weinstein and S. Maayani: NIDA Res. Monograph **25**, 38 (1979)

[77] Gund, P.: Science **208**, 1425 (1980)

[78] Broek v. d., A. J., A. I. A. Broess, M. J. v. d. Heuvel, H. P. de Jongh, J. Leemhuis, K. H. Schönemann, J. Smits, J. de Visser, N. P. van Vliet and F. J. Zeelen: Steroids **30**, 481 (1977)

[79] Zeelen, F. J., in J. A. Keverling Buisman (Ed.): Biological Activity and Chemical Structure, Pharmacochemistry Library (Eds.: W. Th. Nauta and R. F. Rekker), Vol. 2., Elsevier, Amsterdam, 1977, p. 147

[80] Zeelen, F. J., in J. Knoll and F. Darvas (Eds.): Chemical Structure — Biological Activity Relationships, Akadémiai Kiadó, Budapest, 1980, p. 43

[81] Humblet, C., and G. Marshall: Tables Rondes Roussel Uclaf **38**, 38 (1980)

[82] Hiller, A. S., V. E. Golender, A. B. Rozenblit, E. S. Sturkovich and E. Ya. Lukevic: Khim.-Farm. Zh. **10**, 29 (1976)

[83] Tute, M. S., in S. H. Yalkowsky, A. A. Sinkula and S. C. Valvani (Eds.): Physical Chemical Properties of Drugs, Marcel Dekker, New York, 1980, p. 141

[84] Desmarchelier, J., R. I. Krieger, P. W. Lee and T. R. Fukuto: J. Econ. Entomol. **66**, 631 (1973)

[85] Neely, W. B., D. R. Branson and G. E. Blau: Environm. Sci. Technol. **8**, 1113 (1974)

[86] Buznikov, G. A., A. S. Kabankin, V. M. Kolbanov, M. A. Landau, A. A. Aroyan, T. R. Ovespyan and N. A. Teplits: Khim.-Farm. Zh. **10**, 23 (1976)

[87] Voronin, V. G., O. Y. Polevaya, V. G. Mukhanova, M. A. Landau, V. M. Kolbanov, T. P. Privolneva, V. V. Chugnov and E. F. Lavretskaya: Khim.-Farm. Zh. **10**, 43 (1976)

[88] Martin, Y. C., in J. A. Keverling Buisman (Ed.): Strategy in Drug Research, Pharmacochemistry Library (Eds.: W. Th. Nauta and R. F. Rekker), Vol. 4, Elsevier, Amsterdam, 1982, p. 269

[89] Martin, Y. C.: J. Med. Chem. **24**, 229 (1981)

[90] Purcell, W. P., in E. Bergmann and B. Pullman (Eds.): Molecular and Quantum Pharmacology, D. Reidl Publishing Company, Dordrecht, 1974, p. 37

[91] Humber, L. G., A. Albert, E. Campaigne, J. F. Cavalla, N. Arnand, M. Protiva, A. I. Rachlin and P. Sensi: IUPAC Information Bulletin **49**, 12 (1975)

[92] Nauta, W. Th., in J. A. Keverling Buisman (Ed.): Biological Activity and Chemical Structure, Pharmacochemistry Library (Eds.: W. Th. Nauta and R. F. Rekker), Vol. 2, Elsevier, Amsterdam, 1977, Contribution to the second round table discussion

[93] Wipke, W. T., and W. J. Howe (Eds.): Computer-Assisted Organic Synthesis, ACS Symp. Ser. **61**, (1977)

[94] Wipke, W. T., in W. T. Wipke, S. R. Heller, R. J. Feldmann and E. Hyde (Eds.): Computer Representation and Manipulation of Chemical Information, Interscience, New York, 1974, p. 147

[95] Gund, P.: Ann. Repts. Med. Chem. **12**, 288 (1977)

[96] Bersohn, M., and E. Esacks: Chem. Rev. **76**, 269 (1976)

[97] Bersohn, M., in E. C. Olson and R. E. Christoffersen (Eds.): Computer-Assisted Drug Design ACS Symp. Ser. **112**, 341 (1979)

[98] Gund, P., E. J. J. Grabowski, G. M. Smith, J. D. Andose, J. B. Rhodes and W. T. Wipke in E. C. Olson and R. E. Christoffersen (Eds.): Computer-Assisted Drug Design, ACS Symp. Ser. **112**, 527 (1979)

[99] Gund, P., E. J. J. Grabowski, D. R. Hoff, G. M. Smith, J. D. Andose, J. B. Rhodes and W. T. Wipke: J. Chem. Inf. Comput. Sci. **20**, 88 (1980)

15. Appendix: Some Principles of Linear Regression Analysis

At present the most widely employed mathematical method in quantitative structure-activity analysis is linear regression analysis (extrathermodynamic approach, FREE-WILSON analysis) and it is, therefore, certainly worth considering a few of its basics in greater detail.

What matters is not so much the compilation of a set of guidelines for the practical performance of regression analyses as the ability to interpret their outcome in a meaningful manner, and it may thus be sufficient to refer to the literature [1—3] with respect to mathematical details. A number of aspects of the theory underlying linear equations in quantitative structure-activity analysis have been treated elsewhere [4]. To make the present considerations more accessible to those who have no particular training in the discipline concerned, some concepts such as *estimate* and *statistical test* and the meaning of *random variables* will be dealt with first.

15.1. Series of Measurements and Random Variables

Quantitative structure-activity analyses are invariably based on data sets (e.g., biological activities). Such a set arises when one particular feature is measured on a number of n objects (e.g., drugs). The result is n numbers z_i ($i = 1, \ldots, n$), z_i indicating the extent to which the i-th object possesses the selected property (feature). Depending on the nature of that property, z_i values represent continuous (ED_x, etc.) or discrete (classification) variables, both of which serve to quantify pertinent features.

In mathematical statistics the features are abstracted as so-called *random variables* which may take certain values (the possible values of the quantity measured); each value can be regarded as the realization of a random variable. The designation random variable is meaningful in that measurements performed on a number of objects randomly selected from a population (the total of all objects sharing a given feature; in the present case, all compounds in a subsystem) will result in a set of randomly varying values. The series of measurements allows one to predict how probable it is that the feature under consideration will appear in all objects of the population, and to what extent.

Random variables will assume given values with a certain probability which means that they follow a *probability distribution*. This can be described by a *distribution function*, $F(a)$, representing the probability that the random variable will take a value smaller than or at most equal to a. For continuous variables the so-called *normal distribution* is the most important. Continuous random variables are usually normally distributed when they are influenced by several mutually independent factors.

Normal distribution of a variable x can be analytically expressed as

$$f(x) = \frac{1}{\sigma\sqrt{2\pi}} \exp\left[-\frac{(x-\mu)^2}{2\sigma^2}\right] \qquad (15/1)$$

which results in a bell-shaped curve. Its course is symmetric to a maximum at $x = \mu$, having inflection points at $x = \mu \pm \sigma$ (see below).

Important characteristics of a random variable, x, and of its distribution are its *expected value*, $E(x)$, and *variance*, D^2x. In the case of discrete variables the expected value is the mean of the possible values, x_i, of the random variable x weighted by their corresponding probabilities of occurrence, p_i[1]:

$$E(x) = p_1x_1 + p_2x_2 + p_3x_3 + \cdots \tag{15/2}$$

If, for example, the random variable x takes the values 1 and 4 with the probabilities 1/4 and 3/4, the expected value is:

$$E(x) = \frac{1}{4} \cdot 1 + \frac{3}{4} \cdot 4 = 3.25 \tag{15/3}$$

The variance provides a measure of the dispersion of the random variable around the expected value and in the discrete case is defined as:

$$D^2x = p_1[x_1 - E(x)]^2 + p_2[x_2 - E(x)]^2 + p_3[x_3 - E(x)]^2 + \cdots \tag{15/4}$$

As a measure of dispersion the *standard deviation*, σ, is usually applied which is to be defined as:

$$\sigma = \sqrt{D^2x} \tag{15/5}$$

In the case of a normal distribution, the expectated value $E(x)$ is equal to parameter μ and the standard deviation is equal to parameter σ in eqn. (15/1).

It is important that functions of random variables are also random variables. If the distribution of a random variable is known, the distribution of its functions can also be calculated. Functions of random variables emerge when regression analysis is carried out as indicated below. They also emerge when a set of measured values is transformed in a uniform manner. Such transformed values may then be considered as values of a uniformly transformed random variable.

Different random variables are either dependent on or independent of each other. When, for example, the π values of n compounds are measured in the two partition systems I and II the following n pairs of values will present themselves

$$(\pi_{I,1}, \pi_{II,1}), \ldots, (\pi_{I,i}, \pi_{II,i}), \ldots, (\pi_{I,n}, \pi_{II,n})$$

where the measured values $\pi_{I,i}$ and $\pi_{II,i}$ may be considered as the realization of two random variables. Within the validity range of eqn. (4/12), there appears to be a close connection between the two variables. Random variables of this type are said to be *correlated*. The degree of linear dependence between two random variables x and y can be characterized by the so-called *correlation coefficient*, $\varrho(x, y)$ which lies between -1 and $+1$. Its absolute value will be the higher the stronger is the linear dependence. If the correlation coefficient is 0, the random variables are not correlated. This con-

[1]) Integral-formulae result for the continuous case.

clusion is, however, only valid when the two random variables possess a normal distribution.

In many instances, the statistical independence of random variables is essential for the application of statistical procedures.

15.2. Statistical Estimation of Parameters

Statistics are fundamentally concerned with parameter estimation for a given population on the basis of samples randomly selected from this population. There are two types of such estimations, namely *point estimations* and *confidence estimations.*

In the case of *point estimation*, the parameters sought are determined by the use of an appropriate estimating function from the measured data sampe[1]). As estimate of the expected value $E(x)$ of a random variable x, it is customary to make use of the empirical mean, $\overline{x}$, of the data set:

$$\hat{E}(x) = \overline{x} = \frac{1}{n} \sum_{i=1}^{n} x_i \tag{15/6}$$

A suitable estimate of the variance D^2x is the sample variance, s^2:

$$\hat{D}^2x = s^2 = \frac{1}{n-1} \sum_{i=1}^{n} (x_i - \overline{x})^2 \tag{15/7}$$

Quantity

$$\hat{\sigma} = s = \sqrt{s^2} \tag{15/8}$$

provides an estimate of the standard deviation. The correlation coefficient between two random variables x and y can be estimated according to (15/9):

$$\hat{\varrho}(x, y) = r = \frac{\sum_{i=1}^{n} (x_i - \overline{x})(y_i - \overline{y})}{\sqrt{\sum_{i=1}^{n} (x_i - \overline{x})^2} \sqrt{\sum_{i=1}^{n} (y_i - \overline{y})^2}} \tag{15/9}$$

With respect to the *confidence estimation* only a lower and upper limit are given for the parameter to be estimated, the range between the two estimates being called the *confidence interval.* Any confidence interval is accompanied by a preassigned *confidence level,* which may, for example, be set at 0.95 (or 95%), indicating that the true value of the parameter is covered by the confidence interval with a probability of not less than 95%. The magnitude of the confidence interval, therefore, does not depend only on the data set but also on the confidence level selected increasing with the latter. A few relations for this kind of confidence estimation are referred to below.

---

[1]) In general, various estimating functions for a certain parameter are available; it depends on the type of problem which one to choose. In order to distinguish true parameters from their estimates the latter will be indicated by a hat (^).

15.3. Statistical Tests

In order to garner extensive information from data sets, it is necessary to test the estimated parameters for certain properties. This is based on formulating a so-called *null hypothesis*, representing a given assumption about the parameter of interest. Such a hypothesis may, for example, imply that the actual value of the parameter is equal to a given number or lies in a given interval, that two (unknown) parameters are equal or unequal, etc. The first step in testing a null hypothesis usually comprises the calculation of the value of what is called a *test variable*, the definition of which depends on the null hypothesis concerned. Next, this test variable is compared with a corresponding tabulated value. The null hypothesis will be rejected if the test variable exceeds this value and not rejected in the opposite case. Some examples of such tests will be provided below. The magnitude of the tabulated comparison value and thus the outcome of the test are dependent on the predetermined *confidence probability*, P, or the *error probability*, p, ($P + p = 1$ or $P \cdot 100\% + p \cdot 100\% = 100\%$). These probabilities refer to the so-called *error of the first type* which means that, although correct, a hypothesis is rejected; the probability of such an error occurring is smaller than or at most equal to p. On the other hand, it is possible that, although false, a hypothesis is accepted, in which case the term *error of the second type* is used. The probability of the latter error may be considerably greater than p, in general increasing as p decreases. It thus follows that a clear decision can only be made when the null hypothesis is rejected. This decision will be correct with a statistical probability of $P \cdot 100\%$. In the event of the null hypothesis not being rejected, the only — and less informative conclusion — to be drawn is that the data are not with certainty in conflict with the null hypothesis no decision that the null hypothesis can be accepted being justified.

15.4. Linear Regression Model

The objective of regression analysis is to find an equation on the basis of data samples for the relation between an dependent and a set of independent variables (features). The *simple linear regression*, which deals with the relation between only two variables (such as that between $\log A$ and π), will be considered first. The values for n objects of a sample are indicated by y_i and x_i for, respectively, dependent and independent variables ($i = 1, \ldots, n$). The y_i values are to be regarded as realizations of random variables η_i. The model of simple regression then assumes the existence of n equations of the form (15/10):

$$\eta_i = ax_i + b + \varepsilon_i \tag{15/10}$$

The coefficients a and b are independent of i, and the ε_i are random variables with the expected value of 0, which represent interferences with the systematic, linear relation between y and x (due, for example, to measuring errors). It is assumed that the ε_i are independent of each other, share the same variance and have an n-dimensional normal distribution, by which is meant that all ε_i possess a normal distribution. Coefficients a and b are the true parameters of the correlation (15/10), valid for the whole population which are now to be estimated as accurately as possible from the data of a sample taken from that population. It is implied here that the estimated values, $\hat{a}$ and $\hat{b}$, which are called *regression coefficients*, permit the regression equation

$$y = \hat{a}x + \hat{b} \tag{15/11}$$

closely to approximate the relation between y and x. By means of certain test variables one can establish the probability of the assumption being correct.

Geometrically, (15/11) denotes that straight line that provides the best possible fit of n points $(x_1, \ldots, y_1), (x_n, y_n)$ in a Cartesian coordinate system with the coordinates x (abscissa) and y (ordinate). If the relation between y and two independent variables has to be described, linear regression implies a fitting of a plane to a collection of points in three-dimensional space, and if there are k independent variables one has to deal with a so-called hyperplane in $k + 1$-dimensional space. In such cases, the designation *multiple regression* is used, as distinct from simple regression, and the regression equation for k independent variables reads[1]):

$$y = \sum_{j=1}^{k} \hat{a}_j x_j + \hat{a}_{k+1} = \hat{a}_1 x_1 + \cdots + \hat{a}_k x_k + \hat{a}_{k+1} \tag{15/12}$$

$\hat{a}_{k+1}$ = ordinate (absolute term).

The manner in which regression coefficients are estimated can be illustrated by the example of the simple regression equation (15/11). As already pointed out, they will be so estimated that a straight line is obtained having the best possible fit for the data point collection. Intuitively, one realizes that such a fit leads to the smallest possible total of the distances of the points from the straight regression line. Based on this concept, the *method of least squares* is employed to evaluate the coefficients $\hat{a}$ and $\hat{b}$ in (15/11) so that the sum of the squares of the deviations between measured y_i and values estimated from (15/11) is minimized according to:

$$\sum_{i=1}^{n} (y_i - \hat{y}_i)^2 = \sum_{i=1}^{n} (y_i - \hat{a}x_i - \hat{b})^2 = \text{Min!} \tag{15/13}$$

Partial differentiation with respect to $\hat{a}$ and $\hat{b}$ and equating the two derivatives with 0 affords the following equations for the determination of the coefficients:

$$\hat{a} = \frac{\sum_{i=1}^{n} (x_i - \overline{x})(y_i - \overline{y})}{\sum_{i=1}^{n} (x_i - \overline{x})^2} = \frac{\sum_{i=1}^{n} x_i \sum_{i=1}^{n} y_i - n \sum_{i=1}^{n} x_i y_i}{\left(\sum_{i=1}^{n} x_i\right)^2 n - \sum_{i=1}^{n} x_i^2} \tag{15/14}$$

$$\hat{b} = \overline{y} - \hat{a}\overline{x} \tag{15/15}$$

An entirely analogous procedure is used in multiple regression although here, of course, a larger number of equations (as many as there are coefficients) ensues for the determination of coefficients.

The multiple correlation coefficients, r, serves as a measure of goodness of fit of the regression equation to the data point collection. For its calculation, the measured values y_i and the values $\hat{y}_i$ estimated from regression equation (15/12) (see footnote) are

---

[1]) Equation (15/12) of course includes the simple regression according to (15/11) as a special case.

regarded as two data sets, the use of eqn. (15/9) resulting in:

$$r = \frac{\sum_{i=1}^{n} (y_i - \bar{y})(\hat{y}_i - \bar{\hat{y}})}{\sqrt{\sum_{i=1}^{n} (y_i - \bar{y})^2} \sqrt{\sum_{i=1}^{n} (\hat{y}_i - \bar{\hat{y}}_i)^2}} = \frac{\sum_{i=1}^{n} (y_i - \bar{y})(\hat{y}_i - \bar{y})}{\sqrt{\sum_{i=1}^{n} (y_i - \bar{y})^2} \sqrt{\sum_{i=1}^{n} (\hat{y}_i - \bar{y})^2}} \tag{15/16}$$

with

$$\bar{\hat{y}} = \bar{y} \tag{15/17}$$

and

$$\hat{y}_i = \sum_{j=1}^{k} \hat{a}_j x_{ij} + \hat{a}_{k+1} \tag{15/18}$$

The value of r is exactly 1 if all points are located in the hyperplane described by the regression equation, 0 if the dependent variable is not related with the features considered.

The multiple correlation coefficient r can also be represented in another way, the starting point being

$$\sum_{i=1}^{n} y_i^2 = \sum_{i=1}^{n} \hat{y}_i^2 + \sum_{i=1}^{n} (y_i - \hat{y}_i)^2 \tag{15/19}$$

which will not be explained further. It follows from (15/19):

$$\sum_{i=1}^{n} (y_i - \bar{y})^2 = \sum_{i=1}^{n} (\hat{y}_i - \bar{y})^2 + \sum_{i=1}^{n} (y_i - \hat{y}_i)^2 \tag{15/20}$$

with (see eqn. (15/7)

$$s_y^2 = \frac{1}{n-1} \sum_{i=1}^{n} (y_i - \bar{y})^2 \tag{15/21}$$

$$s_{\hat{y}}^2 = \frac{1}{n-1} \sum_{i=1}^{n} (\hat{y}_i - \bar{y})^2 \tag{15/22}$$

$$u_i = y_i - \hat{y}_i$$

$$s_{\hat{u}}^2 = \frac{1}{n-1} \sum_{i=1}^{n} (y_i - \hat{y}_i)^2 \tag{15/23}$$

an expression for the dispersion distribution results from eqn. (15/2)):

$$s_y^2 = s_{\hat{y}}^2 + s_{\hat{u}}^2 \tag{15/24}$$

Equation (15/24) can be so interpreted that the total variance of data set y_i is a composite of the variance of the estimated $\hat{y}_i$ and a residual variance, $s_{\hat{u}}^2$. The smaller the residual variance relative to the total variance, the better is the description of the sample by the corresponding regression equation; hence, the residual variance, and the standard deviation, s, respectively

$$s = \sqrt{s_{\hat{a}}^2} \tag{15/25}$$

also provide a measure of the goodness of fit of the regression equation. An additional criterion of this type is furnished by the coefficient of determination, R^2, which is expressed as

$$R^2 = \frac{s_{\hat{y}}^2 - s_{\hat{a}}^2}{s_{\hat{y}}^2} \tag{15/26}$$

and lies between 0 and 1. It denotes the percentage of the total variance of y "explained" by the regression equation. It is easy to demonstrate that:

$$R^2 = r^2 \tag{15/27}$$

As a result, the multiple correlation coefficient can be interpreted in two different manners, according to either eqn. (15/16) or (15/26).

Regression models based on (15/12) are called inhomogeneous, and differ from homogeneous models which do not include an absolute term, as shown in:

$$y = \sum_{j=1}^{k} \hat{a}_j x_j \tag{15/28}$$

This implies the *a priori* definition that the regression hyperplane passes through the origin of the coordinate system. In general, however, there is no *a priori* reason to impose this limitation. Another important point is that relations (15/17), (15/19), (15/24) and (15/27) are always applicable only in the event of regression being inhomogeneous.

15.5. Statistical Tests after Regression Analysis and the Calculation of Confidence Intervals

Once regression coefficients have been estimated, it is necessary to judge their accuracy and reliability. For the sake of convenience, the procedure will be exemplified for the case of simple linear regression (eqn. (15/11)), the various operations for multiple regression being analogous.

1. Tests of coefficient a

The null hypothesis to be tested is that a is equal to a preset value a_0. To this end the test quantity, $\tilde{F}$, is calculated from:

$$\tilde{F} = \frac{(\hat{a} - a_0)^2 \sum_{i=1}^{n} (x_i - \bar{x})^2}{\frac{1}{(n-2)} \sum_{i=1}^{n} (y_i - \hat{y}_i)^2} \tag{15/29}$$

After the level of significance (usually $p = 0.01$ or $p = 0.05$) has been chosen, $\tilde{F}$ will be compared with a tabulated F value, $F_{(p;1,n-2)}$[1]) (*F-test*). The null hypothesis is rejected if:

$$\tilde{F} \geqq F_{(p;1,n-2)} \tag{15/30}$$

[1]) Value of the central F-distribution at significance level p; the numbers 1 and $n-2$ are the degrees of freedom of the F-distribution in the case of simple regression.

Rejection of the null hypothesis implies that the true regression coefficient is different from a_0. Of particular importance is the case $a_0 = 0$, where with eqn. (15/14) the calculation of $\tilde{F}$ simplifies to:

$$\tilde{F} = \frac{\sum_{i=1}^{n} (\hat{y}_i - \bar{y})^2}{\frac{1}{(n-2)} \sum_{i=1}^{n} (y_i - \hat{y}_i)^2} \tag{15/31}$$

Where the null hypothesis $a = 0$ is not rejected, the regression coefficient a is not significantly different from 0 and the regression line cannot be distinguished significantly from a line parallel to the abscissa. This means that feature x has no influence on the dependent variable y. On this basis, no regression equation can be accepted as being significant unless the hypothesis $a = 0$ is rejected. Another possibility of testing the hypothesis $a = a_0$ is based on what is called the t-distribution (*t-test*). For this purpose

$$\tilde{t} = \frac{(\hat{a} - a_0) \sqrt{\sum_{i=1}^{n} (x_i - \bar{x})^2}}{\frac{1}{(n-2)} \sqrt{\sum_{i=1}^{n} (y_i - \hat{y}_i)^2}} \tag{15/32}$$

is calculated and compared with the tabulated value, t, at a level of significance, p, and $n = 2$ degrees of freedom. The null hypothesis is then rejected if:

$$|\tilde{t}| \geqq t_{p/2,n-2} \tag{15/33}$$

2. Tests of coefficient b

The hypothesis $b = b_0$ can also be checked by the use of the F-test or the t-test. The test quantities concerned are:

$$\tilde{F} = \frac{(\hat{b} - b_0) \sum_{i=1}^{n} (x_i - \bar{x})^2}{\frac{1}{(n-2)} \sum_{i=1}^{n} (y_i - \hat{y}_i)^2 \frac{1}{n} \sum_{i=1}^{n} x_i^2} \tag{15/34}$$

$$\tilde{t} = \frac{(\hat{b} - b_0)}{\sqrt{\frac{\sum_{i=1}^{n} (y_i - \hat{y}_i)^2}{n-2}}} \cdot \frac{\sum_{i=1}^{n} (x_i - \bar{x})^2}{\sqrt{\frac{1}{n} \sum_{i=1}^{n} x_i^2}} \tag{15/35}$$

If

$$\tilde{F} \geqq F_{p;1,n-2} \tag{15/36}$$

or

$$|\tilde{t}| \geqq t_{p/2,n-2} \tag{15/37}$$

the hypothesis is rejected. Again, the case $b_0 = 0$ is of special importance; if the null hypothesis is not rejected, the intercept does not differ significantly from 0 and the presumption is that the straight regression line passes through the origin of the coordinate system. Where this happens, a homogeneous regression model according to eqn. (15/28) should be applied.

3. Simultaneous test of a and b

The null hypothesis $a = a_0$ and $b = b_0$ is tested using the test quantity:

$$\tilde{F} = \frac{n(\hat{b} - b_0)^2 + 2(\hat{a} - a_0)(\hat{b} - b_0)\sum_{i=1}^{n} x_i + (\hat{a} - a_0)\sum_{i=1}^{n} x_i^2}{2\sum_{i=1}^{n}(y_i - \hat{y}_i)^2} \tag{15/38}$$

The hypothesis is rejected with the probability of error, p, when:

$$\tilde{F} > F_{p;2,n-2} \tag{15/39}$$

4. Confidence estimates for a and b

The standard deviations of coefficients a and b are as follows:

$$s_a = \sqrt{\frac{\sum_{i=1}^{n}(y - \hat{y}_i)^2}{(n-2)\sum_{i=1}^{n}(x_i - \bar{x})^2}} \tag{15/40}$$

$$s_b = \sqrt{\frac{\sum_{i=1}^{n}(y_i - \hat{y}_i)^2}{(n-2)\,n\sum_{i=1}^{n}(x_i - \bar{x})^2}} \tag{15/41}$$

With s_a and s_b the confidence intervals for a and b can be calculated at a preset probability of error, p, according to

$$\hat{a} - t_{p/2,n-2} \cdot s_a \leqq a \leqq \hat{a} + t_{p/2,n-2} \cdot s_a \tag{15/42}$$

and

$$\hat{b} - t_{p/2,n-2} \cdot s_b \leqq b \leqq \hat{b} + t_{p/2,n-2} \cdot s_b \tag{15/43}$$

Thus calculated, the intervals overlap the true values of a and b at statistical probability $P \cdot 100\%$ $\left(= (1 - p)\,100\%\right)$.

5. Confidence interval for a single y value at a given x value

The introduction of a given value, say x_0, for parameter x into the regression equation (15/11) yields a corresponding y_0 value. The confidence interval for this value at the probability of error, p, is:

$$\hat{y}_0 - t_{p/2,n-2}\sqrt{\frac{\sum_{i=1}^{n}(y_i - \hat{y}_i)^2}{n-2}}\sqrt{1 + \frac{1}{n} + \frac{(x_0 - \bar{x})^2}{\sum_{i=1}^{n}(x_i - \bar{x})^2}} \leqq y_0$$

$$\leqq \hat{y}_0 + t_{p/2,n-2}\sqrt{\frac{\sum_{i=1}^{n}(y_i - \hat{y}_i)^2}{n-2}}\sqrt{1 + \frac{1}{n} + \frac{(x_0 - \bar{x})^2}{\sum_{i=1}^{n}(x_i - \bar{x}_i)^2}} \tag{15/44}$$

If for each potential value of x confidence intervals according to eqn. (15/44) are introduced into the graphical representation of the straight regression line, the so-called confidence region around that line is obtained (see Fig. 15.1). The confidence region is formed by hyperbolas, having its narrowest shape at $x_0 = \bar{x}$. The value calculated for the independent variable becomes less accurate as x_0 is removed from $\bar{x}$. This also follows from the last summation in the second root of eqn. (15/44). As a consequence, uncertainty increases rapidly on extrapolation outside the feature x space covered by the sample, precluding a meaningful prediction of y outside this space.

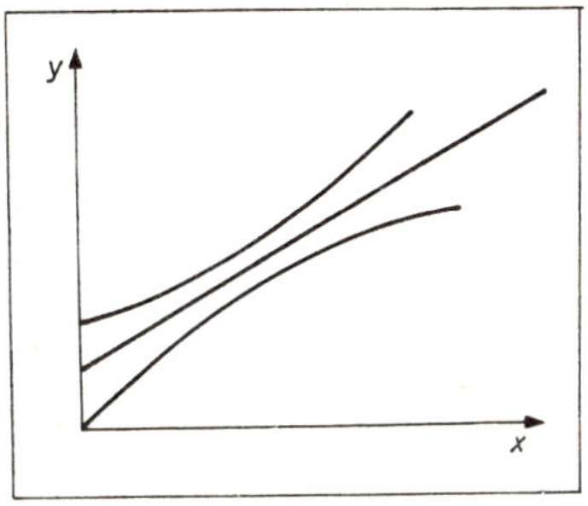

Fig. 15.1. Confidence region around a regression line

15.6. Generalization of the Linear Regression Model

Frequently, the relation between y and x is not simply linear but of a different type, as for example, eqns. (15/45) and (15/46):

$$y = a \ln x + b \tag{15/45}$$

$$y = ax^2 + b \tag{15/46}$$

In such cases, the features are so transformed that a linear relation appears. Regression is then calculated using the transformed features. In the two instances described above, the respective transformations would be as

$$x' = \ln x$$

and

$$x' = x^2$$

with the regression model:

$$y = \hat{a}x' + \hat{b} \tag{15/48}$$

A similar procedure is followed for multiple regression. If the coefficients $\hat{a}_j$ ($j = 1, \ldots k + 1$) of a regression equation of the form

$$y = \sum_{j=1}^{k} \hat{a}_i f_j(x_j) + \hat{a}_{k+1} \tag{15/49}$$

are to be determined, new variables of the form

$$x_j' = f_j(x_j) \tag{15/50}$$

are introduced so that again a linear regression is obtained according to the notation:

$$y = \sum_{j=1}^{k} \hat{a}_j x_j' + \hat{a}_{k+1} \tag{15/51}$$

Where such a transformation is not possible, methods of the so-called non-linear regression analysis, which will not be discussed here, are to be applied.

15.7. Some Remarks about Regression Calculations and Judgement on Regression Equations

Certain dangers and sources of errors may occur in the process of the regression calculation and have been referred to in preceding sections. A special problem arises in the case of multiple regression. An assumption made when carrying out the usual regression procedure is that the columns of the feature matrix

$$\boldsymbol{X} = (x_{ij})_{i=1,\ldots,n;j=1,\ldots,k} \tag{15/52}$$

(where x_{ij} = the value of the jth feature for the i-th object), are neither simply nor multiply correlated. This condition is not satisfied in the case that the determinant of matrix $\boldsymbol{X}^T\boldsymbol{X}$ ($\boldsymbol{X}^T$ is the transposed matrix of $\boldsymbol{X}$) has a value close to 0. In such an instance the customary regression procedure needs modification, a subject not within the scope of this treatise.

As discussed in preceding chapters, it is frequently necessary to study the relations of many features x_i with y. In principle, it is, of course, possible to perform a regression calculation for any conceivable combination of features and to compare the results. Such a procedure may be named regression analysis with fixed basis. In practice, the number of equations to be calculated can be decreased by stepwise strategies based on hypotheses along the lines already discussed in detail in 8.2. This is advisable since if k features are available, $2^k - 1$ different equations are possible, and such a number could be rather difficult to digest under practical circumstances.

When comparing regression equations, any correlation is rejected where one or more regression coefficients are not significantly different from 0 at $p \leq 0.05$. Of the remaining equations the best in statistical terms is the one that shows the highest goodness of fit at the smallest number of features. Among the criteria to be applied in this context are the multiple correlation coefficient, the standard deviation, the F value and the confidence intervals of the regression coefficients. Once again it must be emphasized that these statistical criteria for selecting the "best" equations must be supplemented by chemical and biological reasoning and common sense.

An alternative is presented by a feature reduction prior to regression analysis. This step is intended to eliminate non-relevant features and to permit the selection of features which do not correlate with each other while providing the largest possible amount of information on y. A suitable procedure is factor analysis (cf., 8.4.).

Feature reduction and regression can also be combined into one procedure, as is the case in stepwise regression, by which individual features are included in or excluded from a regression equation in a stepwise manner according to certain criteria (for example, the F test) until an optimum is reached. To a certain extent, the outcome depends on the method used and on the properties and collinearities of the features and, herefore, does not necessarily represent the best solution. Thus, instead of a variable, x_j, which is, in fact, causally coupled to y, another variable highly correlated with x_j may occur in the regression equations; hence, it is to be recommended that the outcome of stepwise regression analysis be checked — and extended — by calculating some selected equations on a fixed basis.

Finally, a short discussion of *statistical degrees of freedom* seems appropriate. A straight line is unambiguously determined by two points. Therefore, there is only one way of describing a relation between an independent variable, y, and a feature, x, namely precisely the straight line determined by the two points (y_1, x_1) and (y_2, x_2). The number of degrees of freedom is 0, and neither considerations based on probability theory nor statistical tests are feasible. By including a third point, there is more than one possibility to connect the points, and the number of degrees of freedom is 1. For a multiple relationship with k features derived from a sample with n objects, the number of degrees of freedom, f, is:

$$f = n - (k + 1) \tag{15/53}$$

As the number of degrees of freedom increases, the results of the statistical tests become more definite and therefore it is always necessary to aim at sufficient degrees of freedom.

References

[1] Draper, N. R., and H. Smith: Applied Regression Analysis, Wiley, New York, 1966
[2] Daniel, C., and F. S. Wood (with the assistence of J. W. Gorman): Fitting Equations to Data, 2nd Ed., Wiley, New York, 1980
[3] Snedecor, G. W., and W. C. Cochran: Statistical Methods, 6th Ed., The Iowa State University Press, Ames, 1967
[4] Schaad, L. J., and B. A. Hess, Jr.: J. Med. Chem. **20**, 619 (1977)

16. Index